Clinical Nursing Calculations

D0507362

The Pedagogy

Clinical Nursing Calculations drives comprehension through various strategies that meet the learning needs of students while also generating enthusiasm about the topic. This interactive approach addresses different learning styles, making this the ideal text to ensure mastery of key concepts. The pedagogical aids that appear include the following:

Case Consideration

As you begin each chapter, read and analyze real-life situations in clinical calculations. Then use your critical thinking skills to answer questions.

The CASE Approach

This step-by-step method of performing dosage calculations is applied to every dosage calculation. CASE is an acronym for: Convert, Approximate, Solve, Evaluate.

Case Consideration … Calculation Choices

After learning about each medication, the nursing student was ready to prepare the medications for administration. The patient needed an intravenous (IV) antibiotic, a liquid cough medicine, and several other medications that were dispensed as tablets and capsules. The student reviewed the medication administration record (MAR) and realized dosage calculations were indicated.

1. How is dosage calculation performed?
2. Is there one approach that can be used for all dosage calculations?

■ INTRODUCTION

When administering medications, each *case* should be considered separately. Because medications may be supplied in varying dosage strengths, varying amounts may be required to administer the same dosage of medication. For example, Paxil® CR is supplied as 12.5 mg tablets and 25 mg tablets. Administration of a 25 mg dose would require two 12.5 mg tablets or only one 25 mg tablet. Even though the dose is the same, the amount to administer is different.

The patient's needs may change; a patient who was able to take an oral dose of medication may be ordered to take nothing by mouth (NPO), and will then require a different form and route of medication. Medications should be ordered on a case-by-case basis; safe dosages vary depending on the patient's age, weight, kidney function, liver function, and individual response. The authorized prescriber will order the dosage and route, but the nurse will have to consider the individual patient and supplied medication prior to administration.

To ensure safety and accuracy with dosage calculations, use the **CASE approach**. *CASE* is an acronym for four steps of safe dosage calculation, which are:

- **C**: *Convert*—convert to like units of measurement
- **A**: *Approximate*—estimate the amount to administer
- **S**: *Solve*—perform dosage calculation
- **E**: *Evaluate*—check the dosage calculation and compare to approximated amount

The word *CASE* also reminds the nurse to consider the appropriateness of the medication and dose ordered in each individual case.

7-1   Comparing the Supply to the Ordered Dose

The first two steps of the *CASE* approach, *C*: *Convert* and *A*: *Approximate*, require the comparison of the dosage strength (referred to as "supply") to the ordered dose. For example, the ordered dose may be in grams (g), while the supply is in milligrams (mg). Step *C*: *Convert*, requires comparing the supply to the ordered dose and converting to the same unit of measurement, if they are different. If the supplied dosage strength and the ordered dose are in the same unit of measurement, the conversion step is not applicable (N/A).

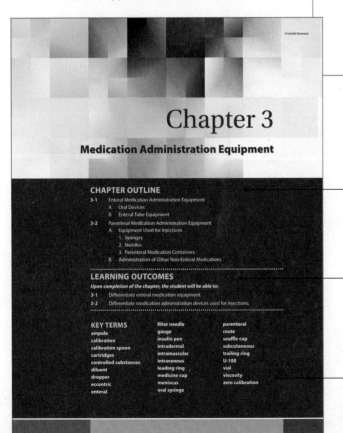

Chapter 3

Medication Administration Equipment

CHAPTER OUTLINE

3-1   Enteral Medication Administration Equipment
   A.   Oral Devices
   B.   Enteral Tube Equipment
3-2   Parenteral Medication Administration Equipment
   A.   Equipment Used for Injections
     1.   Syringes
     2.   Needles
     3.   Parenteral Medication Containers
   B.   Administration of Other Non-Enteral Medications

LEARNING OUTCOMES

Upon completion of the chapter, the student will be able to:
3-1   Differentiate enteral medication equipment.
3-2   Differentiate medication administration devices used for injections.

KEY TERMS

ampule	filter needle	parenteral
calibration	gauge	route
calibration spoon	insulin pen	souffle cup
cartridges	intradermal	subcutaneous
controlled substances	intramuscular	trailing ring
diluent	intravenous	U-100
dropper	leading ring	vial
eccentric	medicine cup	viscosity
enteral	meniscus	zero calibration
	oral syringe	

Chapter Outline

Each chapter begins with a brief but clear outline to give students and instructors a preview of the content that will be covered.

Learning Outcomes

Learning Outcomes provide instructors and students with a snapshot of the key information they will encounter in each chapter, and serve as a checklist to help guide and focus study.

Key Terms

Found in a list at the beginning of each chapter, these terms will create an expanded vocabulary.

Three Methods of Calculation

Ratio-Proportion, Formula Method, and Dimensional Analysis are all introduced, demonstrating the distinct advantage of each approach. The three methods are presented side-by-side in a tabled format for every dosage calculation.

Learning Activities

Practice what you learn as you read through the text.

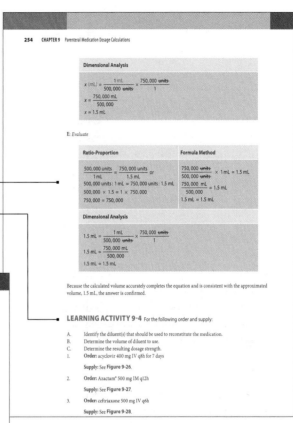

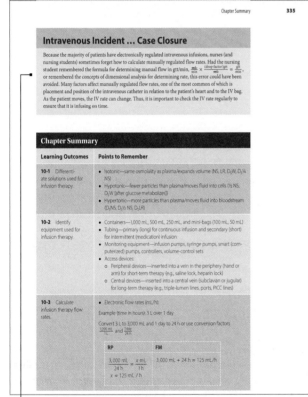

Case Closure

As you finish the chapter, the Case Closure uses information learned in the chapter to wrap up the case from the beginning of the chapter.

Clinical Clues

These notes reinforce correct methods and techniques and provide information on matters in day-to-day practice.

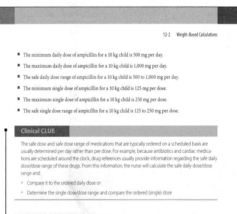

Warning!

These notes caution the student about common pitfalls and errors to be aware of in nursing practice.

NCLEX®-Style Review Questions

NCLEX-style questions that test your comprehension of the material.

Answer Key

Answers to the Learning Activities, Homework, and NCLEX®-Style Review Questions, available at the end of the chapter.

Homework

Test your comprehension of the material at the end of the chapter.

---

242   CHAPTER 9   Parenteral Medication Dosage Calculations

WARNING!
Device Devised for Full Doses!

Reconstitution devices are to be used only when the full dose of medication in the vial is ordered.

The medication package insert, and often the label, will provide directions for reconstitution. Reconstitution directions are also found in many drug guides. Included in these directions are the acceptable diluent, the required volume of diluent, and the resulting dosage strength (**Figure 9-17**). The volume of the reconstituted medication may be larger than the volume of diluent added due to expansion of the powdered medication. Therefore, the nurse must refer to the package insert or label for the new dosage strength and not calculate strength based on the volume injected into the vial of medication.

The reconstituted medication should be labeled if the dose is not immediately withdrawn from the vial. The label should include the preparation date and time, dosage strength, storage information, discard date, and preparer's initials (**Figure 9-18**).

WARNING!
Manufacturer's Recommendations for Reconstitution Rule!

Some powdered medications may expand significantly after reconstituting with a diluent. For example, 1 gram of powdered medication may result in a dosage strength of 100 mg/mL, (1,000 mg/10 mL) after only

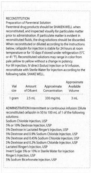

FIGURE 9-17   The package insert provides reconstitution information.

---

340   CHAPTER 10   Infusion Therapy and Calculations

NCLEX-Style Review Questions

For questions 1–4, select the best response.

1. To infuse 3 L over 24 hours using tubing with a drop factor of 15, the nurse should establish a flow rate of:
   a. 31 gtt/min
   b. 125 gtt/min
   c. 188 mL/h
   d. 1,875 mL/h

2. To infuse ampicillin 500 mg in 50 mL D₅W over 30 minutes, the nurse should:
   a. Set the infusion pump to 10 mL/h.
   b. Establish the flow rate of 17 gtt/min.
   c. Establish the flow rate of 25 gtt/min.
   d. Set the secondary IV infusion rate on the pump to 100 mL/h.
   e. Not enough data to answer the question.

3. The nurse initiates the order for continuous intravenous infusion, D₅½ NS @ 50 mL/h, with a 1-liter bag of solution at 0900 and anticipates that the next liter bag should be ready to hang at:
   a. 1500
   b. 1540
   c. 1600
   d. 1607

4. The home care nurse is preparing to visit a patient ordered to receive long-term intravenous antibiotic therapy. The nurse expects that the patient will have which access device?
   a. Saline lock
   b. Heparin lock
   c. PICC line
   d. Large-volume infusion pump

For questions 5–6, select all that apply.

5. To administer an intermittent infusion of Zosyn 3.375 g in 100 mL D₅W IVPB over 30 minutes via infusion pump, the nurse should:
   a. Flush the saline lock prior to injecting the medication.
   b. Prime the secondary tubing.
   c. Set the IV infusion pump to 100 mL/h.
   d. Swab the injection port closest to the IV bag with alcohol.
   e. Establish a flow rate of 200 gtt/min.
   f. Calculate the flow rate in mL/h.
   g. Verify compatibility of the medication with the secondary IV solution.

6. Nursing responsibilities regarding intravenous therapy include:
   a. Checking the IV site at regular intervals, according to institutional policy
   b. Calculating the IV flow rate in mL/h
   c. Hanging the primary solution above the secondary solution
   d. Counting the flow rate in gtt/min
   e. Ordering the correct IV solution
   f. Observing the patient for complications
   g. Programming the infusion pump

REFERENCES

Centers for Disease Control and Prevention. (2011). 2011 guidelines for the prevention of intravascular catheter-related infections. Retrieved from http://www.cdc.gov/hicpac/BSI/07-bsi-background-info-2011.html#s-2011.html

Crawford, A., & Harris, H. (2011, May). IV fluids: What nurses need to know. *Nursing 2011, 41*(5), 30–38.

David, K. (October 2007). IV fluids: Do you know what's hanging and why? *Modern Medicine.* Retrieved from http://www.modernmedicine.com/modernmedicine/article/articleDetail.jsp?id=463604

Grissinger, M. (2007). How fast is too fast for delivering IV push medications? *Pharmacy & Therapeutics, 32*(3). Retrieved from http://www.ptcommunity.com/system/files/PTJ3203124.pdf

Infusion Nurses Society. (2012). Recommendations for frequency of assessment of the short peripheral catheter site. Retrieved from http://www.insl.org/i4a/pages/index.cfm?pageid=3412

Institute of Safe Medication Practices. (2003, May 15). Medication safety alert: How fast is too fast for IV push medications? Retrieved from http://www.ismp.org/newsletters/acutecare/articles/20030515.asp

Kaufman, M. B. (2009, July 20). New IV smart pump technologies prevent medication errors, ADRs. *Formulary ENews.* Retrieved from http://formularyjournal.modernmedicine.com/formulary/Technology+News/New-IV-smart-pump-technologies-prevent-medication-/ArticleStandard/Article/detail/611706

---

90   CHAPTER 3   Medication Administration Equipment

REFERENCES

Khan, A. (2010, January 4). A spoonful of medicine may be too much or not enough. Retrieved from http://latimesblogs.latimes.com/booster_shots/2010/01/spoon-teaspoon-medicine-tylenol-study-annals-internal-medicine-cornell.html

Perry, A. G., & Potter, P. A. (2012). *Clinical nursing skills and techniques* (8th ed.). St. Louis: Elsevier.

Potter, P. A., Perry, A. G, Stockhart, P., & Hall, A. (2013). *Fundamentals of nursing* (8th ed.). St. Louis: Elsevier.

Chapter 3   ANSWER KEY

Learning Activity 3-1
1. d
2. a
3. b
4. a, b, c

Learning Activity 3-2
1. d
2. e
3. a
4. b

Learning Activity 3-3
1. The second syringe, with the leading ring at the 3.4 mL calibration, contains 3.4 mL of medication.
2. The first syringe, with the leading ring at the 1.5 mL calibration, contains 1.5 mL of medication. NOTE: The space between the leading ring and the trailing ring is dead space and contains no medication.
3. 2.7 mL
4. 7.2 mL

Homework
1. False: Enteral medication administration refers to medicine given directly into the gastrointestinal (GI) tract.
2. False: To ensure accurate measurement of medication in a medicine cup, the medication should be poured at eye level and measured at the bottom of the meniscus.
3. True

6. False: The oral syringe can measure volumes of liquid medication up to 10 mL. The medicine cup can measure volumes up to 1 ounce.
7. False: The eccentric or off-centered tip alerts the nurse that a needle should not be attached to this syringe.
8. False: The appropriate device for administration of 7 mL of liquid medication is an oral syringe.
9. True
10. True
11. False: The 1 mL syringe should be used to measure liquid volumes of less than 1 mL.
12. True
13. True
14. False: One teaspoon cannot be accurately measured in all calibrated oral medication administration equipment. Droppers may not be calibrated in teaspoons.
15. False: A medicine cup is calibrated to deliver volumes up to 1 ounce (2 tablespoons) of liquid.
16. False: A subcutaneous injection is delivered below all of the layers of the skin. An intramuscular injection is delivered directly into a muscle.
17. True
18. True
19. False: The more viscous the solution, the lower the needle gauge number should be, because the lower the gauge, the wider the needle diameter.
20. False: The primary purpose of safety syringes is to prevent needlestick injury (i.e., to promote safe medication administration).
21. False: Cartridges need to be loaded into a syringe holder for medication administration.
22. True
23. False: Insulin syringes are used to administer U-100 insulin only.
24. True
25. True
26. False: Medication volumes are determined by reading the calibration on the leading ring.
27. False: Medication is withdrawn from a vial by inserting a needle in to the rubber stopper on the top. Medication is withdrawn from an ampule by inserting a filter needle into the solution after the ampule neck is snapped open.
28. False: Each calibration on a 1 mL syringe is one-hundredth milliliter.

Clinical Nursing Calculations

Susan Sienkiewicz, MA, RN
Professor
Community College of Rhode Island
Warwick, Rhode Island

Jennifer Palmunen, MSN/Ed, RN
Case Manager
Assisted Daily Living, Inc.
Warwick, Rhode Island

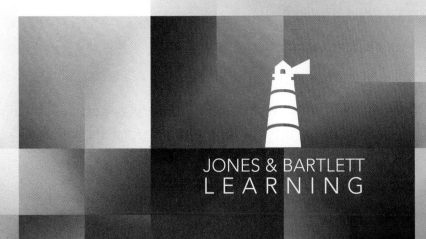

JONES & BARTLETT
LEARNING

World Headquarters
Jones & Bartlett Learning
5 Wall Street
Burlington, MA 01803
978-443-5000
info@jblearning.com
www.jblearning.com

Jones & Bartlett Learning books and products are available through most bookstores and online booksellers. To contact Jones & Bartlett Learning directly, call 800-832-0034, fax 978-443-8000, or visit our website, www.jblearning.com.

Substantial discounts on bulk quantities of Jones & Bartlett Learning publications are available to corporations, professional associations, and other qualified organizations. For details and specific discount information, contact the special sales department at Jones & Bartlett Learning via the above contact information or send an email to specialsales@jblearning.com.

Copyright © 2017 by Jones & Bartlett Learning, LLC, an Ascend Learning Company

All rights reserved. No part of the material protected by this copyright may be reproduced or utilized in any form, electronic or mechanical, including photocopying, recording, or by any information storage and retrieval system, without written permission from the copyright owner.

The content, statements, views, and opinions herein are the sole expression of the respective authors and not that of Jones & Bartlett Learning, LLC. Reference herein to any specific commercial product, process, or service by trade name, trademark, manufacturer, or otherwise does not constitute or imply its endorsement or recommendation by Jones & Bartlett Learning, LLC and such reference shall not be used for advertising or product endorsement purposes. All trademarks displayed are the trademarks of the parties noted herein. *Clinical Nursing Calculations* is an independent publication and has not been authorized, sponsored, or otherwise approved by the owners of the trademarks or service marks referenced in this product.

There may be images in this book that feature models; these models do not necessarily endorse, represent, or participate in the activities represented in the images. Any screenshots in this product are for educational and instructive purposes only. Any individuals and scenarios featured in the case studies throughout this product may be real or fictitious, but are used for instructional purposes only.

The authors, editor, and publisher have made every effort to provide accurate information. However, they are not responsible for errors, omissions, or for any outcomes related to the use of the contents of this book and take no responsibility for the use of the products and procedures described. Treatments and side effects described in this book may not be applicable to all people; likewise, some people may require a dose or experience a side effect that is not described herein. Drugs and medical devices are discussed that may have limited availability controlled by the Food and Drug Administration (FDA) for use only in a research study or clinical trial. Research, clinical practice, and government regulations often change the accepted standard in this field. When consideration is being given to use of any drug in the clinical setting, the health care provider or reader is responsible for determining FDA status of the drug, reading the package insert, and reviewing prescribing information for the most up-to-date recommendations on dose, precautions, and contraindications, and determining the appropriate usage for the product. This is especially important in the case of drugs that are new or seldom used.

08177-0

Production Credits
VP, Executive Publisher: David D. Cella
Executive Editor: Amanda Martin
Associate Acquisitions Editor: Rebecca Myrick
Editorial Assistant: Danielle Bessette
Senior Production Editor: Amanda Clerkin
Senior Marketing Manager: Jennifer Scherzay
VP, Manufacturing and Inventory Control: Therese Connell
Composition: Cenveo Publisher Services
Cover and Interior Design: Scott Moden
Rights & Media Manager: Joanna Lundeen
Rights & Media Research Assistant: Wes DeShano
Media Development Editor: Shannon Sheehan
Cover Image: © Forfunlife/Shutterstock
Printing and Binding: RR Donnelley
Cover Printing: RR Donnelley

Library of Congress Cataloging-in-Publication Data
Sienkiewicz, Susan, author.
  Clinical nursing calculations / Susan Sienkiewicz and Jennifer Plamunen.
    p. ; cm.
  Includes bibliographical references and index.
  ISBN 978-1-284-05752-2
  I. Plamunen, Jennifer, author. II. Title.
  [DNLM: 1. Drug Dosage Calculations--Nurses' Instruction. 2. Pharmaceutical Preparations--administration & dosage--Nurses' Instruction. QV 748]
  RS57
  615.1'4--dc23
                    2015010018

6048

Printed in the United States of America
19 18 17 16   10 9 8 7 6 5 4 3 2

© Forfunlife/Shutterstock

Contents

© Forfunlife/Shutterstock

Acknowledgments

To our husbands, Tom & Greig:
Thank you for your support and sacrifice.
Your encouragement kept us on track.

To Kenneth Kasee, II:
Thank you for believing in us.
Without you, this book would never have been written.
You have our deepest gratitude.

To the marvelous team at Jones & Bartlett Learning:
Thank you for your help in making this text a reality.
You are a hardworking, dynamic, and professional group of people.
It has been a pleasure collaborating with you on this project.

To future and practicing nurses, we hope this text makes safe practice a little easier.
We wish you success.

© Forfunlife/Shutterstock

Preface

While teaching nursing in both associate and baccalaureate nursing programs, we discovered that while some students are very comfortable and competent with math, others are not. Even when a dosage calculation course or math proficiency is a requirement for admission to a nursing program, testing at the start of each semester in a nursing program reveals that some students need continued support and remediation to perform dosage calculations.

Students weak in long division and basic math rely on calculators to problem solve. They appear to have lost the understanding of numerical values, thus are not able to discern whether or not a solution is realistic. An example of a common error: If the dose is 5 mg, and the patient is supplied 10 mg tablets, the student might suggest administering two tablets (20 mg) instead of half a tablet (5 mg). This answer is yielded when the problem is set up incorrectly and the student fails to estimate a reasonable amount to administer.

Students observe staff nurses' reliance on technology to establish infusion rates and determine amounts to administer without performing calculations. "Smart pumps" generate infusion rates after the nurse inputs the volume and time, and electronic medication administration records (eMAR) include (computer-generated) amounts to administer. While these devices assist the nurse and reduce medication error potential, they may provide a false sense of security, prompting the nurse to eliminate double-checking via calculation. Thus, we set out to write a text that would strengthen students' and nurses' comfort with performing calculations in the clinical setting.

This text offers a step-by-step approach to basic math and dosage calculation. We have included approximation as a critical thinking step to evaluate the calculated answer. Believing students have different learning styles, we have color-coded steps to appeal to visual learners, provided narrated PowerPoint slides to appeal to auditory learners, and have provided suggested activities for clinical instructors to support kinesthetic learners. Student engagement is supported through "clicker questions" provided in a PowerPoint. Adult learners may recognize the relevance of the material presented, as each chapter begins with a case study. In addition to demonstrating three different dosage calculation techniques side-by-side, we provide tips for performing dosage calculation efficiently in the clinical setting. Learning activities and practice problems are designed in response to actual clinical errors or common student errors, in addition to reinforcing the content presented. Faculty will appreciate this practical text, which students can use throughout the nursing program and into professional practice.

© Forfunlife/Shutterstock

Introduction

Clinical Nursing Calculations can be used as a primary text for a dosage calculations course or as a supplemental text for a nursing course/program or pharmacology course. It also can be used by practicing nurses. This text is intended to appeal to faculty who teach online or in the classroom, have a strong clinical background, and want to apply math concepts to clinical practice. Content can be integrated into a medical-surgical curriculum, and clinical instructors can use content for remediation or assigned clinical exercises. Students will enjoy and benefit from the features that distinguish *Clinical Nursing Calculations* from other dosage calculations texts, such as:

- The CASE approach, a step-by-step process of performing dosage calculations
- A tabled side-by-side comparison of three methods of dosage calculation (ratio-proportion, formula method, dimensional analysis) for each calculation
- A case study that opens and closes each chapter
- Color-coding of values and labels to appeal to visual learners
- Advantages of each approach presented:
  - Ratio-proportion promotes critical thinking.
  - Formula method is a shortcut tactic useful for individuals who easily grasp math.
  - Dimensional analysis is most useful when multiple conversions are required.

CASE is an acronym for a four-step calculation process, developed by the authors, that will prompt the student to methodically proceed with calculations:

- Convert
- Approximate
- Solve
- Evaluate

First, the student must determine if it is necessary to convert the ordered dose and the supplied dose to like units of measurement. After converting, the student can approximate the amount to administer. The approximation step promotes confidence in the answer if the approximated value is close to the solved value. To solve the dosage calculation, the student uses one of three methods of dosage calculations: ratio-proportion, formula method, or dimensional analysis. In the evaluate step, the student compares the solved value to the approximated value and checks the answer by repeating the calculation, replacing the unknown (x) with the solved value.

© Forfunlife/Shutterstock

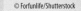

Numerous pedagogical features are included in every chapter. An outline, followed by Learning Outcomes and Key Terms, begins every chapter. When defined in the text, the key terms are in bold. Expanding on the CASE acronym, each chapter includes a case study: opening with a Case Consideration in which a clinical issue is presented that includes a dosage error or potential error (relevant to the chapter material), and then concluding with a Case Closure in which the clinical issue is explained and resolved.

Learning Activities are inserted after each new concept is taught. Many of these activities are designed to be used as "clicker questions" in the classroom. Because many students have difficulty remembering when and how far to round, Rounding Rules are emphasized as a key feature. Warnings and Clinical Clues provide helpful tips that apply to clinical practice. Chapter Summaries provide a quick reference to chapter material and are organized by learning outcomes. Each chapter concludes with 50 questions that can be assigned as homework or that students can use for practice. Homework is followed by NCLEX®-style Review Questions. All questions are referenced to learning outcomes, allowing students and faculty to select questions by outcome for practice or homework.

General features throughout the text include:

- Expanded clinical content, including nutrition and insulin pen calculations
- Legal implications of medication administration
- Exercises targeting safe practice with high-alert medications
- Examples given in eMAR and electronic health record format
- Information from The Joint Commission and the Institute for Safe Medication Practices regarding safe medication administration

Faculty and students will appreciate the use of current medications presented with large readable labels in this text. Realistic dosages, practical clinical application, and case studies should assist students and nurses to perform clinical calculations with competence.

© Forfunlife/Shutterstock

Chapter 1

Basic Math

LEARNING OUTCOMES

Upon completion of the chapter, the student will be able to:

1-1   Perform calculations with fractions.

1-2   Perform calculations with decimals.

1-3   Convert quantities.

1-4   Calculate percentages.

1-5   Calculate unknown quantities using ratio-proportion.

KEY TERMS

addend

complex fraction

cross-multiplication

decimal

denominator

dividend

divisor

fraction

improper fraction

leading zero

mixed number

numerator

proper fraction

quotient

subtrahend

trailing zero

Case Consideration ... Death by Decimal

On an exam, a nursing student correctly calculated a quantity to be 62.5 mg, but recorded the answer as 6.25 mg. The student exclaimed, "I can't believe the instructor marked the entire question wrong! I did all of the math right; I just put the decimal point in the wrong place. What's the big deal? It probably won't make a difference in medication administration; it's only a fraction off. I should have at least received partial credit!"

1. Where is the error in the student's reasoning?

2. How can this error be avoided?

■ INTRODUCTION

Nurses perform basic math without a calculator. Even when a calculator is used to perform dosage calculations, checking the accuracy of calculations requires the ability to perform basic math without a calculator. This is sometimes referred to as "mental math." As a nurse, mental math is performed on a daily basis. In this and other chapters, color is used to enhance mathematical operations by matching the color of the text font with the corresponding numbers in an equation.

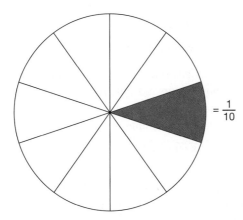

FIGURE 1-1   The shaded part of the circle, which is one (1) part, reflects the numerator and the total number of parts (10) is the denominator. Therefore $\frac{1}{10}$ means 1 of 10 equal parts.

| 1-1 | **Calculating with Fractions** |

Fractions are used when calculating dosages, converting metric to household measurement, and when critically evaluating the relationship of one quantity to another quantity. A **fraction** represents a portion of a whole (**Figure 1-1**). It is written as two quantities: a **numerator** (part[s] of a whole) and a **denominator** (the whole). The denominator represents the number of equal parts that make up a whole. Because a fraction is the division of a whole quantity, it is written using a division sign, with the numerator as the first number and the denominator as the second number.

$$\frac{\text{numerator}}{\text{denominator}} \quad \leftarrow \quad \text{division sign}$$

The horizontal line above the denominator is a division sign that indicates the numerator is divided by the denominator.

Types of Fractions

There are various types of fractions:

- **Proper fraction**—Numerator is less than the denominator, so the value is less than 1 (e.g., $\frac{3}{5}$).

- **Improper fraction**—Numerator is greater than the denominator, so the value is greater than 1 (e.g., $\frac{5}{3}$), or the numerator is the same as the denominator, so the value is equivalent to 1 (e.g., $\frac{5}{5}$).

- **Mixed number**—Whole number and fraction (e.g., $1\frac{3}{5}$).

- **Complex fraction**—A fraction in which the numerator and/or the denominator is a fraction (e.g., $\frac{\frac{1}{2}}{1\frac{1}{4}}, \frac{3}{5}{2}$, or $\frac{1}{\frac{2}{3}}$). Calculations with complex fractions are included in Appendix A.

LEARNING ACTIVITY 1-1   Refer to the following fractions and answer the questions that follow:

$$\frac{3}{5}, \quad \frac{9}{8}, \quad 2\frac{1}{2}$$

1.   Identify the improper fraction(s). _____
2.   Identify the fraction(s) that are greater than one (1). _____
3.   Identify the proper fraction(s). _____

Creating Equivalent Fractions

Performing calculations with fractions requires the ability to:

- *Convert fractions to equivalent fractions with common denominators.* Converting fractions to equivalent fractions with common denominators most often involves enlarging the fraction. This is done by multiplying both the numerator and denominator by the same number. Select a number that will produce the common denominator. For example, to convert $\frac{2}{3}$ to twelfths (12ths), multiply both the numerator and denominator by 4: $\frac{2(\times 4)}{3(\times 4)} = \frac{8}{12}$. This skill is necessary for addition and subtraction of fractions.

- *Convert mixed numbers to improper fractions.* To convert mixed numbers to improper fractions, multiply the denominator by the whole number and add the numerator and place that number over the existing denominator. For example, to convert $4\frac{4}{5}$ to an improper fraction, $\frac{(5\times 4)+4}{5} = \frac{24}{5}$.

- *Reduce fractions to lowest terms and convert improper fractions to mixed numbers.* To reduce fractions to lowest terms, find the largest number that will divide evenly into both the numerator and denominator. For example, to reduce $\frac{24}{18}$ to lowest terms, divide the largest number (6) that goes evenly into both the numerator and denominator: $\frac{24(\div 6)}{18(\div 6)} = \frac{4}{3} = 1\frac{1}{3}$.

Comparing Fractions by Size

Why it is important to know if the value of one fraction is equivalent to (=), less than (<), or greater than (>) the value of another fraction?

- Estimating the correct answer is an important step in dosage calculation.

- Estimating involves comparing values.

- Comparing reduces accidental over or under dosage.

When the numerator and the denominator are the same, the value equals one (1).

Example: Six (6) slices of a pizza cut into 6 equal parts is considered $\frac{6}{6}$ (or 1) pizza (**Figure 1-2**).

$$\frac{6}{6} = 1$$

When the denominators are both the same, the fraction with the smaller numerator has the lesser value.

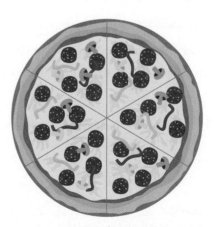

FIGURE 1-2 $\frac{6}{6}$ of a pizza equals 1 whole pizza.

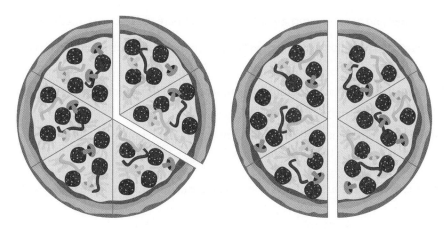

FIGURE 1-3   When the slices are the same size (i.e. the denominators are the same) 2 slices is less than 3 slices.

Example: Two slices, or $\frac{2}{6}$ of a pizza, are less than 3 slices, or $\frac{3}{6}$ of a pizza of the same size (**Figure 1-3**).

$\dfrac{2}{6}$ is less than $\dfrac{3}{6}$ because the denominators are the same and 2 is less than 3.

When the numerators are the same, the fraction with the smaller denominator has the greater value.

Example: If one pizza is sliced into 5 equal parts, and the other same-sized pizza is sliced into 10 equal parts, each of the 10 slices will be smaller than the slices from the pizza cut into 5 pieces. So, 4 slices from the pizza cut into 5 pieces, or $\frac{4}{5}$ of a pizza, is a larger quantity than slices from the pizza cut into 10 pieces, or $\frac{4}{10}$ of a pizza.

$\dfrac{4}{5}$ is greater than $\dfrac{4}{10}$ because the numerators are the same, and the denominator, 5, is less than 10 (**Figure 1-4**).

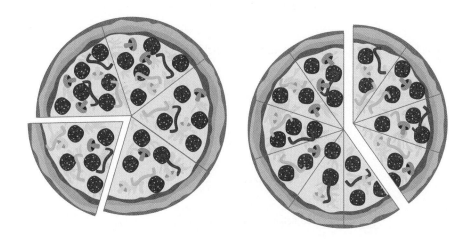

FIGURE 1-4   The fraction with the smaller denominator, $\frac{4}{5}$ (of a pizza), is a larger quantity than $\frac{4}{10}$ (of a pizza), a fraction with the same numerator, but larger denominator.

When the numerators and denominators are different, to compare the fractions, do the following:

- Convert the fractions to equivalent fractions with a common denominator, and then compare the numerators.

- To find a common denominator, multiply the numerator and denominator of the first fraction by the denominator of the other fraction.

- Next, multiply the numerator and denominator of the other fraction by the denominator of the first fraction as demonstrated in the following examples.

Example 1:   Determine if the first fraction is less than, greater than, or equal to the second fraction.

$$\frac{5}{6} \; ? \; \frac{3}{5}$$

Find a common denominator:

- Multiply the numerator and denominator of the first fraction by 5 (the denominator of the second fraction).

$$\frac{5(\times 5)}{6(\times 5)} = \frac{25}{30}$$

- Multiply the numerator and denominator of the second fraction by 6 (the denominator of the first fraction).

$$\frac{3(\times 6)}{5(\times 6)} = \frac{18}{30}$$

Compare the numerators of the resulting fractions, $\frac{25}{30}$? $\frac{18}{30}$. Because the numerator of the first fraction, $\frac{25}{30}$, is larger than the numerator of the second fraction, $\frac{18}{30}$, the first fraction has greater value:

$$\frac{25}{30} \text{ is larger than } \frac{18}{30}$$

$$\text{Therefore, } \frac{5}{6} \text{ is larger than } \frac{3}{5}.$$

Example 2:   The patient had $\frac{3}{5}$ of breakfast and $\frac{2}{3}$ of lunch. Did the patient eat more for breakfast or lunch?

$$\frac{3}{5} ? \frac{2}{3}$$

$$\frac{3(\times 3)}{5(\times 3)} \; ? \; \frac{2(\times 5)}{3(\times 5)}$$

$$\frac{9}{15} \text{ is less than } \frac{10}{15}$$

$$\text{Therefore, } \frac{3}{5} \text{ is less than } \frac{2}{3}.$$

So, the patient ate more for lunch.

Example 3: The patient walked $\frac{2}{3}$ of the hall in the morning, and then $\frac{3}{4}$ of the hall in the evening. Did the patient walk farther in the morning or evening?

$$\frac{2}{3} \; ? \; \frac{3}{4}$$

$$\frac{2(\times 4)}{3(\times 4)} \; ? \; \frac{3(\times 3)}{4(\times 3)}$$

$$\frac{8}{12} \text{ is less than } \frac{9}{12}$$

$$\text{Therefore, } \frac{2}{3} \text{ is less than } \frac{3}{4}.$$

So, the patient walked farther in the evening.

If the denominators are large, find the least common denominator (LCD) by dividing the numerator and denominator of each fraction by a number that will yield the smallest denominator that is the same in both fractions.

Example: Determine if the first fraction is less than or greater than the second fraction.

$$\frac{30}{80} \; ? \; \frac{29}{40}$$

$$\frac{30(\div 2)}{80(\div 2)} \; ? \; \frac{29}{40}$$

$$\frac{15}{40} \text{ is less than } \frac{29}{40}$$

$$\text{Therefore, } \frac{30}{80} \text{ is less than } \frac{29}{40}.$$

LEARNING ACTIVITY 1-2 Determine if the first fraction is less than, greater than, or equal to the second fraction.

1. $\frac{2}{3}$? $\frac{2}{5}$ _____

2. $\frac{5}{8}$? $\frac{7}{8}$ _____

3. $\frac{4}{7}$? $\frac{2}{3}$ _____

Calculations Using Fractions

Healthcare professionals must acquire proficiency with addition, subtraction, multiplication, and division of fractions. Addition and subtraction of fractions require common denominators, whereas common denominators are not needed for multiplication and division.

Addition of Fractions

Fractions are added by following these steps:

- Convert **addends** (numbers that are added together) to fractions with common denominators, if needed.

- Add the numerators, but maintain the common denominator.

- **Reduce, if necessary.**

Adding fractions *with* common denominators. When common denominators exist, skip step 1 and simply add the numerators and maintain the common denominator (e.g., $\frac{1}{5} + \frac{2}{5} = \frac{3}{5}$). Because $\frac{3}{5}$ is not reducible, step 3, reducing to lowest terms is also eliminated.

Adding fractions *without* common denominators. To add $\frac{1}{5} + \frac{4}{15}$, begin with step 1:

- Determine a common denominator (15) and convert $\frac{1}{5}$ to 15ths by multiplying both the numerator and denominator by 3:

$$\frac{1(\times 3)}{5(\times 3)} = \frac{3}{15}$$

- Add the numerators and maintain the common denominator, $\frac{3}{15} + \frac{4}{15} = \frac{7}{15}$, a fraction that is already in lowest terms.

Adding mixed numbers. Adding mixed numbers can be accomplished by converting the mixed numbers to improper fractions or by keeping the mixed numbers intact.

Adding Mixed Numbers Converted to Improper Fractions	Adding Intact Mixed Numbers
1. Reduce fractions, if desired. 2. Convert mixed number addends to improper fractions. 3. Convert fractions to equivalent fractions with common denominators. 4. Add the numerators, but maintain the common denominator. 5. **Reduce, if necessary.** Example: $2\frac{2}{8} + 3\frac{2}{3} = $ _____ $$2\frac{1}{4} + 3\frac{2}{3} =$$ $$\frac{9(\times 3)}{4(\times 3)} + \frac{11(\times 4)}{3(\times 4)} =$$ $$\frac{27}{12} + \frac{44}{12} =$$ $$\frac{71}{12} = 5\frac{11}{12}$$	1. Reduce fractions, if desired. 2. Convert addends to mixed numbers with common denominators. 3. Add the whole numbers; add the numerators; maintain the common denominator. 4. **Reduce, if necessary.** Example: $2\frac{2}{8} + 3\frac{2}{3} = $ _____ $$2\frac{1}{4} + 3\frac{2}{3} =$$ $$2\frac{1(\times 3)}{4(\times 3)} + 3\frac{2(\times 4)}{3(\times 4)} =$$ $$2\frac{3}{12} + 3\frac{8}{12} =$$ $$5\frac{11}{12} = 5\frac{11}{12}$$

LEARNING ACTIVITY 1-3 Add the fractions.

1. $\frac{2}{7} + \frac{1}{3} = $ _____

2. $\frac{5}{16} + \frac{1}{4} + \frac{1}{2} = $ _____

3. $2\frac{1}{3} + 3\frac{1}{2} = $ _____

Subtraction of Fractions

Subtracting proper fractions.   To subtract fractions, follow these steps:

1. Convert **subtrahends** (numbers involved in subtraction) to fractions with common denominators.

2. Subtract the numerators, but maintain the common denominator.

3. Reduce, if necessary.

Example: $\frac{1}{2} - \frac{1}{3} =$

$$\frac{1}{2} - \frac{1}{3} = \frac{1(\times 3)}{2(\times 3)} - \frac{1(\times 2)}{3(\times 2)} = \frac{3}{6} - \frac{2}{6} = \mathbf{\frac{1}{6}}$$

Subtracting mixed numbers.   As with addition, subtracting mixed numbers can be accomplished by converting the mixed numbers to improper fractions or by keeping the mixed number intact.

Keeping the mixed number intact may require borrowing from the whole number in order to enlarge the first fraction. To borrow from the whole number, reduce the whole number by 1, convert 1 to a fraction with the needed denominator, and then add this fraction to the existing fraction. For example, to solve $4\frac{1}{8} - 2\frac{3}{8}$, borrow 1 from 4 (making it 3), convert 1 to $\frac{8}{8}$, and then add $\frac{8}{8}$ to $\frac{1}{8}$ (making $\frac{9}{8}$), for a total of $3\frac{9}{8}$. Now the problem can be solved: $3\frac{9}{8} - 2\frac{3}{8} = 1\frac{6}{8}$, which reduces to $1\frac{3}{4}$.

Subtracting Mixed Numbers Converted to Improper Fractions	Subtracting Intact Mixed Numbers
1. Convert mixed numbers to improper fractions. 2. Convert subtrahends to fractions with common denominators. 3. Subtract the numerators, but maintain the common denominator. 4. **Reduce, if necessary.**	1. Convert subtrahends to fractions with common denominators. 2. Borrow from the whole number to make an improper fraction, if needed. 3. Subtract the whole number, subtract the numerators, but maintain the common denominator. 4. **Reduce, if necessary.**

Example: $3\frac{1}{4} - 1\frac{3}{8} =$

$$\frac{13}{4} - \frac{11}{8} =$$

$$\frac{26}{8} - \frac{11}{8} =$$

$$\frac{15}{8} =$$

$$1\frac{7}{8}$$

Example: $3\frac{1}{4} - 1\frac{3}{8}$

$$3\frac{1 \times 2}{4 \times 2} = 3\frac{2}{8}$$

$$-1\frac{3}{8}$$

Because $\frac{3}{8}$ cannot be subtracted from $\frac{2}{8}$, convert $3\frac{2}{8}$ to $2\frac{10}{8}$: Borrow $\frac{8}{8}$ (1) from 3 and reduce to 2; add $\frac{8}{8}$ to $\frac{2}{8}$, which results in $2\frac{10}{8}$.

$$2\frac{10}{8}$$

$$-1\frac{3}{8}$$

$$1\frac{7}{8}$$

LEARNING ACTIVITY 1-4 Subtract the fractions.

1. $\frac{5}{6} - \frac{1}{4} =$ _____

2. $2\frac{3}{5} - 1\frac{1}{4} =$ _____

3. $6\frac{1}{3} - 2\frac{3}{5} =$ _____

Multiplication of Fractions

Converting mixed numbers is required for multiplication and division of fractions, whereas it is optional for addition and subtraction. Steps for multiplying fractions include:

1. Convert the whole or mixed number(s) to improper fractions, if necessary.

2. Reduce to lowest terms (cancel terms). NOTE: This step is optional, but recommended.

3. Multiply the numerators.

4. Multiply the denominators.

5. **Reduce, if necessary.**

Example 1: $2\frac{3}{5} \times 1\frac{1}{4}$

$$2\frac{3}{5} \times 1\frac{1}{4} = \frac{13}{5} \times \frac{5}{4} = \frac{13}{5} \times \frac{\cancel{5}^{1}}{4} = \frac{13 \times 1}{1 \times 4} = \frac{13}{4} = 3\frac{1}{4}$$

Example 2: $\frac{100}{400} \times \frac{1}{5}$

$$\frac{100}{400} \times \frac{1}{5} = \frac{\cancel{100}^{1}}{\cancel{400}_{4}} \times \frac{1}{5} = \frac{1 \times 1}{4 \times 5} = \frac{1}{20}$$

Example 3: $5 \times \frac{2}{3}$

$$5 \times \frac{2}{3} = \frac{5}{1} \times \frac{2}{3} = \frac{5 \times 2}{1 \times 3} = \frac{10}{3} = 3\frac{1}{3}$$

LEARNING ACTIVITY 1-5 Multiply the fractions.

1. $\frac{1}{3} \times \frac{1}{4} =$ _____

2. $3 \times \frac{9}{10} =$ _____

3. $2\frac{3}{5} \times 1\frac{1}{4} =$ _____

Division of Fractions

The first fraction or number in the equation is referred to as the **dividend** (i.e., the fraction or number being divided). The second number or fraction in the equation—the number the dividend is being divided by—is called the **divisor**. The result of the division is the **quotient**. The steps in the division of fractions include:

1. Convert dividend and/or divisor to improper fractions, if necessary.

2. Invert the divisor by placing the denominator over the numerator.

3. Cancel terms (optional, if needed).

4. Multiply the inverted divisor by the dividend.

5. Reduce, if necessary.

Example 1: $\frac{3}{4} \div \frac{1}{2}$

$$\frac{3}{4} \div \frac{1}{2} = \frac{3}{\underset{2}{\cancel{4}}} \times \frac{\overset{1}{\cancel{2}}}{1} = \frac{3}{2} \times \frac{1}{1} = \frac{3}{2} = 1\frac{1}{2}$$

Example 2: $3\frac{1}{2} \div 1\frac{4}{5}$

$$3\frac{1}{2} \div 1\frac{4}{5} = \frac{7}{2} \div \frac{9}{5} = \frac{7}{2} \times \frac{5}{9} = \frac{35}{18} = 1\frac{17}{18}$$

LEARNING ACTIVITY 1-6 Determine the quotient.

1. $\frac{5}{9} \div \frac{3}{4} =$ _____

2. $\frac{8}{16} \div \frac{1}{3} =$ _____

3. $1\frac{1}{2} \div 2\frac{1}{4} =$ _____

Clinical CLUE

Most dosage calculations are performed using *fractions,* but most amounts to administer are *decimal* quantities.

1-2   Calculating with Decimals

Dosage quantities less than one (1) are written using decimals. The metric system, the system of measurement used in dosage calculations, is a decimal system. Patient deaths have occurred due to misplaced or poorly written decimal points:

> In 2002, a cancer patient received a 10-fold overdose of the blood thinner, warfarin, which resulted in an eventually fatal cerebral hemorrhage. A common term for this is "death by decimal," which involves a patient getting 10 times or one-tenth what the doctor prescribed. (*Quality Digest*, 2008)

Therefore, nurses must understand the value of each decimal place, and how to calculate accurately with decimals. **Decimals** are fractions with a denominator that is a multiple of 10. The most common decimal places used in health care are:

- $0.1 = \frac{1}{10}$ (one-ten*th*)

- $0.01 = \frac{1}{100}$ (one-hundred*th*)

- $0.001 = \frac{1}{1,000}$ (one-thousand*th*)

The decimal point separates a whole number from the fraction. The whole number is placed to the left of the decimal point, and the fraction (quantity ending in *th*) is placed to the right of the decimal point (**Figure 1-5**).

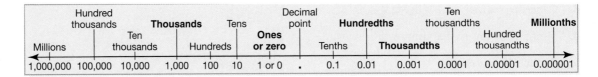

FIGURE 1-5   Number line with with whole numbers to the left of the decimal point and decimal fractions to the right of the decimal point.

WARNING!

Avoid "Death by Decimal" Medication Errors!

To prevent medication errors, The Institute for Safe Medication Practices (ISMP, 2012) recommends:

- Placing a **leading zero** (0) in front of a "naked" decimal point, one that has no whole number preceding it, for example:

  - Write 0.2 not .2

- Omitting a **trailing zero** after a decimal point, for example:

  - Write 3.5 not 3.50

  - Write 1 not 1.0

Including a leading zero emphasizes the decimal point and minimizes the potential for overdose due to an overlooked or missed decimal point. Omitting a trailing zero also decreases the potential for giving the patient 10 times the ordered dose or more.

Adding Decimals

1. Align the decimals.

2. Annex zeros to make the numbers the same length after the decimal.

3. **Add the numbers.**

Example: 0.24 + 3.46 + 12.345 =

$$\begin{array}{r} 0.240 \\ 3.460 \\ + \ 12.345 \\ \hline \mathbf{16.045} \end{array}$$

LEARNING ACTIVITY 1-7   Add the numbers.

1.   5 + 2.1 + 0.225 = _____

2.   2.5 + 3.49 + 4.01 = _____

3.   0.001 + 7.25 + 500 = _____

Subtracting Decimals

1. Align the decimals.

2. Annex zeros to make the number the same length after the decimal.

3. Subtract numbers.

Example: 5.67 − 1.422 =

$$
\begin{array}{r}
5.670 \\
- 1.422 \\
\hline
4.248
\end{array}
$$

LEARNING ACTIVITY 1-8 Subtract the numbers.

1.   2.67 − 0.125 = _____
2.   3.012 − 1.954 = _____
3.   14 − 1.025 = _____

Multiplying Decimals

1. Multiply the numbers together.

2. Count the number of decimal places.

3. Move the decimal point by that many spaces to the left.

Example: 12.5 × 0.45 =

$$
\begin{array}{r}
12.5 \quad \text{1 decimal place} \\
\times \ 0.45 \quad \text{2 decimal places} \\
\hline
6\,2\,5 \\
5\,0\,0 \\
0 \\
\hline
5.625
\end{array}
$$

Because 1 decimal place + 2 decimal places = 3 decimal places, move the decimal point 3 places to the left.

LEARNING ACTIVITY 1-9 Multiply the decimals.

1.   25 × 0.33 = _____
2.   6.2 × 1.04 = _____
3.   0.85 × 1.009 = _____

Multiplying Decimals by the Power of 10

When multiplying decimals by numbers that are powers (multiples) of 10, move the decimal as many places to the right as there are zeros in the multiplier.

Examples:

$$0.5 \times 10 = 5 \qquad 0.5 \times 100 = 50 \qquad 0.5 \times 1,000 = 500$$

LEARNING ACTIVITY 1-10 Determine the product by moving the decimal as many places to the right as there are zeros in the multiplier.

1. $0.003 \times 10 =$ _____
2. $2.5 \times 10 =$ _____
3. $0.75 \times 1,000 =$ _____

Dividing Decimals

1. Move the decimal point of the divisor as many places as necessary to make a whole number.

2. Move the decimal point of the dividend to the right by the same number of places.

3. Place the new decimal point above the dividend in the quotient.

Example: $54 \div 0.2 =$

$$0.2\overline{)54}$$
$$02.\overline{)540.}$$
$$\rightarrow \quad \rightarrow$$

$$\begin{array}{r} 270. \\ 2\overline{)540.} \\ \underline{4} \\ 14 \\ \underline{14} \\ 00 \end{array}$$

LEARNING ACTIVITY 1-11 Determine the quotient using long division.

1. $100 \div 2.5 =$ _____
2. $75 \div 0.05 =$ _____
3. $9.5 \div 5 =$ _____

Dividing Decimals by the Power of 10

When dividing decimals by numbers that are powers (multiples) of 10, move the decimal as many places to the left as there are zeros in the divisor.

Examples:

$$0.5 \div 10 = 0.05 \qquad 0.5 \div 100 = 0.005 \qquad 0.5 \div 1,000 = 0.0005 \qquad 1,500 \div 1,000 = 1.5$$

LEARNING ACTIVITY 1-12 Determine the quotient by moving the decimal as many places to the left as there are zeros in the divisor.

1. $0.003 \div 10 =$ _____
2. $2.5 \div 10 =$ _____
3. $0.75 \div 1{,}000 =$ _____

Rounding Decimals

Typically, for dosage calculation, the nurse will round decimals to the nearest tenth or hundredth. If rounding to tenths, the end value will be tenths; if rounding to hundredths, the end value will be hundredths. To round:

- Evaluate the digit one decimal place to the right of the desired end value (one decimal place to the right of tenths or one decimal place to the right of hundredths).

- Increase the digit in the end value by 1 if the digit to the right of the end value is 5 or higher, and delete all digits to the right of the end value. For example, 1.25 rounded to the nearest tenth becomes 1.3.

- Leave the digit in your end value unchanged if the digit to the right of the end value is 4 (four) or less, and delete all digits to the right of the end value. For example 1.24 rounded to the nearest tenth becomes 1.2.

Rounding RULE

To round, evaluate *only one* digit to the right of the level to be rounded to. For example, if rounding to the whole number, 6.45 is rounded to 6, not 7, because only the numeral 4 is evaluated. *Do not* perform successive rounding, i.e., round 6.45 to 7 by rounding 4 up to 5 and then 6 up to 7.

LEARNING ACTIVITY 1-13 Round the decimal number as indicated.

1.   2.68 to the nearest tenth   _____
2.   0.322 to the nearest hundredth   _____
3.   0.446 to the nearest hundredth   _____

1-3   Converting Quantities

Fractions and decimals are expressions of relationships of quantities. For example, the fraction $\frac{1}{2}$ expresses 1 of 2 equal parts. Because a decimal is a fraction with a denominator that is a multiple of 10, a decimal also expresses a relationship between quantities. Other expressions of quantity relationships include percent and ratio. Ratios are fractions with the numerator written to the left of the denominator and separated by a colon (:). Percent means "per hundred," referring to a quantity expressed in hundredths. Healthcare professionals must be able to interpret and convert quantities expressed as fractions, decimals, percentages, and ratios.

Converting Fractions

- Fraction to decimal: Divide the numerator by the denominator:

$$\frac{1}{2} = 1 \div 2 = \mathbf{0.5}$$

- Fraction to ratio: Write the fraction side by side using a colon as the division sign:

$$\frac{1}{2} = 1:2$$

- Fraction to percentage:

  - Convert the fraction to a decimal (by dividing the numerator by the denominator).

  - Convert the decimal to a percentage by moving the decimal point to the right two places, and then add a percent sign:

$$\frac{1}{2} = 1 \div 2 = 0.5 = 50\%$$

Converting Decimals

- Decimal to fraction:

  1. The denominator is written as the decimal place value.

  2. The numerator is the decimal number without the decimal point.

  3. **Reduce, if necessary.**

$$0.02 = \frac{2}{100} = \frac{1}{50}$$

- Decimal to ratio: Convert the decimal to a fraction, then convert to a ratio:

$$0.02 = \frac{2}{100} = \frac{1}{50} = 1:50$$

- Decimal to percentage: Move the decimal point to the right two places; add a percent sign:

$$0.02 = 2\%$$

Converting Ratios

- Ratio to fraction: Write first quantity, numerator, over the second quantity, denominator:

$$3:4 = \frac{3}{4}$$

- Ratio to decimal: First quantity, numerator, divided by second quantity, denominator:

$$3:4 = 3 \div 4 = 0.75$$

- Ratio to percentage:

  - Convert the ratio to a decimal (by dividing the numerator by the denominator).

  - Convert the decimal to a percentage by moving the decimal point to the right by two places, and then add a percent sign:

$$3:4 = 3 \div 4 = \mathbf{0.75} = 75\%$$

Converting Percentages

- Percentage to fraction: Eliminate the percent sign; convert the quantity to a numerator and place it over a denominator of 100; reduce the fraction:

$$95\% = \frac{95}{100} = \mathbf{\frac{19}{20}}$$

- Percentage to decimal: Eliminate the percent sign; move the decimal point to the *left* two places:

$$95\% = 0.95$$

- Percentage to ratio: Convert the percent to a fraction; **reduce**; write the fraction as a ratio:

$$95\% = \frac{95}{100} = \mathbf{\frac{19}{20}} = 19:20$$

LEARNING ACTIVITY 1-14 Convert the quantity to its equivalent as indicated.

1. 1.5 = _____ (percentage) _____ (ratio)
2. ½ = _____ (decimal) _____ (percentage)
3. 1:5 = _____ (percentage) _____ (fraction)

| 1-4 | **Calculating Percentages** |

Calculating the Percentage of a Whole Quantity

Nurses may need to calculate percentages of quantities. To answer the question, "What is 6% of 120?":

- First translate the words to math:

  - *What* means x (the unknown)

  - *Is* means = (equals)

  - *Of* means × (multiplied by)

  - $x = 6\% \times 120$

- Next, convert the percentage to decimal, write the equation, and solve:

  - $6\% = \frac{6}{100} = 0.06$

  - $x = 0.06 \times 120$

  - $x = 7.2$

Calculating the Percentage of a Partial Quantity

Nurses will also be required to calculate percentages of partial quantities. For example, the nurse may answer the question, "If the patient ate 300 calories at breakfast, what percentage of a 2,000-calorie diet was consumed?" For the nurse to determine that 300 *is what* percentage *of* 2,000:

- First, translate the words to math:

  - *What* means x (the unknown)

  - *Is* means = (equals)

  - *Of* means × (multiplied by)

- Next, write the equation and solve:

  - $300 = x \times 2,000$

  - $300 = 2,000\,x$

    To solve for x, divide both sides of the equation by the quantity in front of x.

  - $\frac{300}{2,000} = \frac{2,000\,x}{2,000}$

  - $0.15 = x$

  - $x = 15\%$ (by converting the decimal to percent)

- Simple method:

  - Create a fraction.

  - Convert to a decimal.

  - **Convert to a percent.**

Example: 300 *is what* percentage [or portion] *of* 2,000?

$$\frac{300}{2,000}$$

$$300 \div 2,000 = 0.15$$

$$\mathbf{0.15 = 15\%}$$

1-5   Calculating Unknown Quantities Using Ratio-Proportion

Unknown quantities can be determined by equating equivalent fractions or ratios. This process is used to calculate the amount of medication to administer. Nurses should become proficient in using ratio-proportion to determine an unknown quantity.

Cross-Multiplication to Determine if Fractions Are Equivalent

Equivalent fractions will have equivalent products when cross-multiplied. **Cross-multiplication** is the product of the numerator of the first fraction and the denominator of the second fraction equal to the product of the numerator of the second fraction and the denominator of the first fraction. Equivalent cross products mean that the fractions are equivalent.

Example:

$$\text{Cross-multiply } \tfrac{3}{5} = \tfrac{6}{10}$$

$$\text{Cross-multiply } 3 \times 10 = 5 \times 6$$

$$\text{producing } 30 = 30$$

Multiplying Extremes and Means to Determine if Ratios Are Equivalent

Fractions can be written as linear ratios, in which case the numerator of the first fraction and the denominator of the second fraction are called the *extremes* (outer quantities), while the denominator of the first fraction and the numerator of the second fraction are called the *means* (inner quantities). The ratios are equivalent if the product of extremes equals the product of the means. Multiplication of extremes and means to determine if ratios are equivalent is similar to cross-multiplication of fractions.

Clinical CLUE

The colon (:) in a linear ratio is read as "to," and the double colon (::)—used to compare two ratios to determine if they are proportionate (equivalent)—is read as "as." The ratio-proportion, 1:2 :: 4:8, is interpreted, "1 is to 2 as 4 is to 8." An equal sign (=) can take the place of a double colon (::).

Example: Determine if the following ratios are equivalent:

$$3:5 = 6:10$$

The product of the extremes *(the outer numbers)* **equals the product of the** means *(the inner numbers)*.

$$3 \times 10 = 5 \times 6$$
$$30 = 30$$

Finding the Value of *x* in a Proportion

To find the value of x in a proportion, set up the equation and perform the calculation until x stands alone.

Example: Solve for x to create two proportionately equivalent fractions: $\frac{3}{5} = \frac{x}{10}$

$$\frac{3}{5} = \frac{x}{10}$$

- Cross-multiply:

$$5 \times x = 3 \times 10$$
$$5x = 30$$

- Divide each side of the equation by 5:

$$\frac{\cancel{5} \, x}{\cancel{5}} = \frac{30}{5}$$

- Solve for x:

$$x = 6$$

Finding *x* When a Fraction Is Multiplied By a Whole Number

- Convert the whole number to an improper fraction using 1 as the denominator.

- **Perform the calculation.**

Example: $\frac{4}{9} \times 2 = x$

$$\frac{4}{9} \times 2 = x$$

$$\frac{4}{9} \times \frac{2}{1} = x$$

$$\frac{8}{9} = x$$

LEARNING ACTIVITY 1-15 Determine the value of *x*.

1. $\frac{250}{500} = \frac{x}{2}$ _____

2. $250:750 = x:3$ _____

3. $\frac{5}{20} = \frac{1}{x}$ _____

Death by Decimal … Case Closure

If the decimal point is in the wrong place, the dose is incorrect by a power of 10. How well the mathematical steps are followed does not matter to the patient if the dose administered is wrong. If the nurse correctly calculates a dose of 62.5 mg, but administers 6.25 mg, a serious under-dosing of medication will occur. In the event that the medication is ordered to treat a life-threatening situation, under-dosing will lead to ineffective (or no) treatment. This type of error has resulted in the death of patients. A nurse can prevent decimal point errors by:

- Memorizing the steps for performing decimal calculations outlined in this chapter.

- Following the ISMP guidelines to use leading zeros before naked decimal points and avoid trailing zeros when recording quantities.

- Practicing calculations (practice promotes fluency and every nurse should strive to become fluent in math).

- When in doubt, double-checking calculations with another nurse.

Chapter Summary

Learning Outcomes	Points to Remember
1-1 Perform calculations with fractions: a. Types of Fractions b. Creating Equivalent Fractions c. Comparing Fractions	*Proper fraction*: Numerator is less than denominator $\frac{3}{5}$ *Mixed*: Whole number and fraction $1\frac{3}{5}$ *Improper*: Numerator is greater than denominator $\frac{5}{3}$ or numerator is the same as the denominator $\frac{5}{5}$ *Enlarging fractions*: Multiply the numerator and denominator by the same number: $\frac{2(\times 4)}{3(\times 4)} = \frac{8}{12}$ *Comparing fractions*: If denominators are the same, the smaller the numerator, the lesser the value: $\frac{2}{4}$ is less than $\frac{3}{4}$ If the numerators are the same, the smaller the denominator, the greater the value: $\frac{4}{5}$ is greater than $\frac{4}{10}$
d. Calculating with Fractions 1. Addition	*Adding proper fractions*: $$\frac{1}{3} + \frac{2}{6} = \frac{2}{6} + \frac{2}{6} = \frac{4}{6} = \mathbf{\frac{2}{3}}$$ *Adding mixed numbers by*: • Converting addends to improper fractions: $$2\frac{2}{8} + 3\frac{2}{3} = 2\frac{1}{4} + 3\frac{2}{3} = \frac{9}{4} + \frac{11}{3} = \frac{27}{12} + \frac{44}{12} = \frac{71}{12} = \mathbf{5\frac{11}{12}}$$ • Keeping the mixed number(s) intact: $$2\frac{2}{8} + 3\frac{2}{3} = 2\frac{1}{4} + 3\frac{2}{3} = 2\frac{3}{12} + 3\frac{8}{12} = \mathbf{5\frac{11}{12}}$$
2. Subtraction	*Subtracting proper fractions*: $$\frac{5}{8} - \frac{1}{4} = \frac{5}{8} - \frac{2}{8} = \mathbf{\frac{3}{8}}$$ *Subtracting mixed numbers by*: • Converting subtrahends to improper fractions: $$3\frac{1}{4} - 1\frac{3}{8} = \frac{13}{4} - \frac{11}{8} = \frac{26}{8} - \frac{11}{8} = \frac{15}{8} = \mathbf{1\frac{7}{8}}$$ • Keeping the mixed number intact and borrowing from the whole number: $$3\frac{1}{4} - 1\frac{3}{8} = 3\frac{2}{8} - 1\frac{3}{8} = 2\frac{10}{8} - 1\frac{3}{8} = \mathbf{1\frac{7}{8}}$$

3. Multiplication	$\dfrac{100}{400} \times \dfrac{1}{5} = \dfrac{\cancel{100}^{1}}{\cancel{400}_{4}} \times \dfrac{1}{5} = \dfrac{1 \times 1}{4 \times 5} = \dfrac{1}{20}$
	Multiplying a whole number by a fraction:
	$5 \times \dfrac{2}{3} = \dfrac{5}{1} \times \dfrac{2}{3} = \dfrac{10}{3} = 3\dfrac{1}{3}$
	Multiplying mixed numbers:
	$2\dfrac{3}{5} \times 1\dfrac{1}{4} = \dfrac{13}{5} \times \dfrac{5}{4} = \dfrac{13}{\cancel{5}_{1}} \times \dfrac{\cancel{5}^{1}}{4} = \dfrac{13}{4} = 3\dfrac{1}{4}$
4. Division	*Dividend*—the fraction being divided
	Divisor—the fraction the dividend is being *divided by*
	Quotient—the result of the division
	Dividing proper fractions:
	$\dfrac{3}{4} \div \dfrac{1}{2} = \dfrac{3}{\cancel{4}_{2}} \times \dfrac{\cancel{2}^{1}}{1} = \dfrac{3}{2} \times \dfrac{1}{1} = \dfrac{3}{2} = 1\dfrac{1}{2}$
	Dividing mixed numbers:
	$3\dfrac{1}{2} \div \dfrac{4}{5} = \dfrac{7}{2} \div \dfrac{4}{5} = \dfrac{7}{2} \times \dfrac{5}{4} = \dfrac{35}{8} = 4\dfrac{3}{8}$
1-2 Perform calculations with decimals: a. Addition	$0.24 + 3.46 + 12.345 =$ $\begin{array}{r} 0.240 \\ 3.460 \\ +12.345 \\ \hline 16.045 \end{array}$
b. Subtraction	$5.67 - 1.422 =$ $\begin{array}{r} 5.670 \\ -1.422 \\ \hline 4.248 \end{array}$

c. Multiplication	$12.5 \times 0.45 =$

12.5 1 decimal place
$\times\, 0.45$ 2 decimal places
——————
625
500
$\ \ 0$
——————
$5.625.$

← Because 1 decimal place + 2 decimal places = 3 decimal places, move the decimal point 3 places to the left.

Multiplying decimals by the power of 10:
Move the decimal as many places to the right as there are zeros in the multiplier.

$$0.5 \times 10 = 5, \quad 0.5 \times 100 = 50, \quad 0.5 \times 1,000 = 5,000$$

d. Division	

$0.2)\overline{54}$

$02.)\overline{540.}$

$\underset{2)\overline{540.}}{\overset{\mathbf{270.}}{}}$

$\ \ 4$
——
14
14
——
000

e. Rounding	Round 0.569411

- Tenths: 0.6
- Hundredths: 0.57

1-3 Convert quantities: a. Fractions	

- Fraction to ratio: $\frac{1}{2} = 1:2$
- Fraction to decimal: $\frac{1}{2} = 1 \div 2 = 0.5$
- Fraction to percent: $\frac{1}{2} = 1 \div 2 = 0.5 = 50\%$

b. Decimals	

- Decimal to fraction: $0.02 = \frac{2}{100} = \frac{1}{50}$
- Decimal to ratio: $0.02 = \frac{2}{100} = \frac{1}{50} = 1:50$
- Decimal to percent: $0.02 = 2\%$

c. Ratios	• Ratio to fraction: $75:100 = \frac{75}{100} = \frac{3}{4}$ • Ratio to decimal: $75:100 = 75 \div 100 = 0.75$ • Ratio to percent: $75:100 = 75 \div 100 = 0.75 = 75\%$
d. Percentages	• Percent to fraction: $25\% = \frac{25}{100} = \frac{1}{4}$ • Percent to ratio: $25\% = \frac{25}{100} = \frac{1}{4} = 1:4$ • Percent to decimal: $25\% = 0.25$
1-4 Calculate percentages	What is 6% of 120? • $6\% = \frac{6}{100} = 0.06$ • $x = 0.06 \times 120$ • $x = 7.2$ 300 is what percentage of 2,000? • $300 = x \times 2{,}000$ • $\frac{300}{2{,}000} = \frac{x \times 2{,}000}{2{,}000}$ • $0.15 = x$ • $x = 15\%$ (by converting the decimal to percent)
1-5 Calculate quantities using ratio-proportion	$\dfrac{3}{5} = \dfrac{6}{10}$ **cross-multiply** $3 \times 10 = 5 \times 6$ producing $30 = 30$ As a ratio equation: $3:5 = 6:10$ Multiply the extremes: $3 \times 10 = 30$ Multiply the means: $5 \times 6 = 30$ producing $30 = 30$ Finding the value of x in a proportion: $\dfrac{3}{5} = \dfrac{x}{10}$ Cross-multiply $3 \times 10 = 5 \times x$ $30 = 5x$ $\dfrac{30}{5} = \dfrac{5x}{5}$ $6 = x$

Homework

For exercises 1–3, circle the correct answer. (LO 1-1)

1. Identify the fraction(s) greater than 1
$$\frac{3}{16}, \frac{5}{4}, \frac{3}{3}$$

2. Identify the fraction(s) equal to 1 $\frac{27}{25}, \frac{3}{4}, \frac{9}{9}$

3. Identify the fraction(s) less than 1 $\frac{24}{25}, \frac{4}{4}, \frac{12}{9}$

For exercises 4–7, match the fractions with the corresponding type. (LO 1-1)

4. $\frac{7}{5}$ _____

5. $2\frac{9}{16}$ _____

6. $\frac{4}{4}$ _____

7. $\frac{6}{7}$ _____

A. Improper fraction

B. Proper fraction

C. Mixed number

For exercises 8–25, perform the calculations with fractions and reduce to lowest terms. (LO 1-1)

8. $\frac{3}{4} + \frac{5}{16} =$ _____

9. $\frac{3}{7} + \frac{2}{3} =$ _____

10. $2\frac{5}{6} + \frac{1}{8} =$ _____

11. $7\frac{2}{3} + 2\frac{11}{12} + \frac{3}{4} =$ _____

12. $\frac{5}{9} - \frac{3}{6} =$ _____

13. $\frac{2}{3} - \frac{5}{24} =$ _____

14. $15\frac{12}{14} - 3\frac{1}{7} =$ _____

15. $32\frac{1}{3} - 4\frac{3}{4} =$ _____

16. $\frac{2}{5} \times \frac{7}{8} =$ _____

17. $6\frac{1}{2} \times 2\frac{1}{3} =$ _____

18. $25 \times \frac{2}{5} =$ _____

19. $\frac{4}{7} \div \frac{2}{9} =$ _____

20. $5 \div \frac{3}{8} =$ _____

21. $\frac{1}{4} \div 9 =$ _____

22. $5\frac{1}{2} \div 3\frac{1}{3} =$ _____

23. $2\frac{5}{9} \div \frac{1}{4} =$ _____

24. $\frac{3}{4} \div 1\frac{1}{2} =$ _____

25. $\frac{100}{1} \times \frac{25}{1} \times 1\frac{1}{2} =$ _____

For exercises 26–35, solve the decimal equations and round to the hundredth, when necessary. (LO 1-2)

26. $3.84 + 0.1 + 10.25 =$ _____

27. $7 + 9.1 + 0.003 =$ _____

28. $10 - 6.3 =$ _____

29. $7.5 - 0.205 =$ _____

30. $3.5 \times 2 =$ _____

31. $1.5 \times 8.95 =$ _____

32. $4.75 \times 100 =$ _____

33. $0.5 \times 1000 =$ _____

34. $125 \div 2.5 =$ _____

35. $5.75 \div 0.25 =$ _____

For exercises 36–41, convert the quantity as indicated. Convert fractions and ratios to lowest terms. Round decimals to the hundredths, if necessary. Round percentages to the whole number. (LO 1-3)

36. $\frac{3}{25} =$ _____ (decimal)
    $=$ _____ (ratio)

37. $0.45 =$ _____ (fraction)
    $=$ _____ (percent)

38. $\frac{8}{12} =$ _____ (ratio)
    $=$ _____ (decimal)

39. $4:5 =$ _____ (decimal)
    $=$ _____ (percent)

40. $1:5 =$ _____ (percent)
    $=$ _____ (fraction)

41. $\frac{21}{50} =$ _____ (percent)
    $=$ _____ (decimal)

For exercises 42–45, solve the word problems, rounding percentages to the whole number. (LO 1-4)

42. What is 8% of 50? _____

43. What is 10.5% of 1,200? _____

44. 40 is what percent of 90? _____

45. 500 is what percent of 1,700? _____

For exercises 46–50, solve for x using ratio-proportion. (LO 1-5)

46. $\frac{5}{15} = \frac{x}{21}$ _____

47. $2:3 = x:12$ _____

48. $\frac{1,000}{250} = \frac{25}{x}$ _____

49. $\frac{100}{5} = \frac{250}{x}$ _____

50. $\frac{80}{20} = \frac{65}{x}$ _____

NCLEX®-Style Review Questions

For questions 1–6, select the best response.

1. A newborn weighs 3,751 grams at birth and 3,352 grams just prior to discharge from the hospital 2 days later. Knowing that newborns may lose 5–10% of their body weight in the first few days of life, the nurse correctly calculates that this newborn's weight loss is:

   a. less than 5%.

   b. within the 5–10% range.

   c. more than 10%.

   d. not able to be determined from the information given.

® NCLEX and NCLEX-RN are registered trademarks of the National Council of State Boards of Nursing, Inc.

2. A patient is ordered to maintain a fluid restriction of 1,500 milliliters per day. If the patient has an intravenous solution running continuously at 30 milliliters per hour, how much fluid can the patient have by mouth per day?
   a. 120 milliliters
   b. 720 milliliters
   c. 780 milliliters
   d. 1,470 milliliters

3. A patient is ordered to take one tablet of "baby aspirin" per day. Each tablet contains 81 milligrams of aspirin. If a regular adult tablet contains 325 milligrams of aspirin, what portion of an adult aspirin tablet does this "baby aspirin" tablet represent?
   a. $\frac{1}{4}$
   b. $\frac{1}{3}$
   c. $\frac{3}{8}$
   d. $\frac{1}{2}$

4. A patient's total caloric intake should consist of 15% protein. If the patient consumes 1,800 calories a day, how many calories should be from protein?
   a. 120
   b. 240
   c. 270
   d. 360

5. A patient consumes 2,000 calories; 1,100 calories were from carbohydrates. What percent of calories were from carbohydrates?
   a. 45%
   b. 55%
   c. 60%
   d. 65%

6. The nurse receives an order to prepare a ¼-strength feeding solution. Which other quantities also represent ¼? Select all that apply.
   a. 25%
   b. 0.75
   c. 4:1
   d. 1:4
   e. $\frac{100}{25}$
   f. 75%
   g. 0.25

REFERENCES

Quality Digest. (2008, January 8). *Will new Medicare rules lead to better health care quality?* Retrieved from http://www.qualitydigest.com/inside/health-care-article/will-new-medicare-rules-lead-better-health-care-quality

Institute for Safe Medication Practices (ISMP). (2015). *Guidelines for standard order sets.* Retrieved from http://www.ismp.org/tools/guidelines/StandardOrderSets.asp

Chapter 1 ANSWER KEY

Learning Activity 1-1

1. $\frac{9}{8}$
2. $\frac{9}{8}, 2\frac{1}{2}$
3. $\frac{3}{5}$

Learning Activity 1-2

1. Greater than
2. Less than
3. Less than

Learning Activity 1-3

1. $\frac{13}{21}$
2. $\frac{17}{16} = 1\frac{1}{16}$
3. $5\frac{5}{6}$

Learning Activity 1-4

1. $\frac{7}{12}$
2. $1\frac{7}{20}$
3. $3\frac{11}{15}$

Learning Activity 1-5

1. $\frac{1}{12}$
2. $2\frac{7}{10}$
3. $3\frac{1}{4}$

Learning Activity 1-6

1. $\frac{20}{27}$
2. $1\frac{1}{2}$
3. $\frac{2}{3}$

Learning Activity 1-7
1. 7.325
2. 10
3. 507.251

Learning Activity 1-8
1. 2.545
2. 1.058
3. 12.975

Learning Activity 1-9
1. 8.25
2. 6.448
3. 0.85765

Learning Activity 1-10
1. 0.03
2. 25
3. 750

Learning Activity 1-11
1. 40
2. 1,500
3. 1.9

Learning Activity 1-12
1. 0.0003
2. 0.25
3. 0.00075

Learning Activity 1-13
1. 2.7
2. 0.32
3. 0.45

Learning Activity 1-14
1. 150%, 3:2
2. 0.5, 50%
3. 20%, $\frac{1}{5}$

Learning Activity 1-15
1. 1
2. 1
3. 4

Homework

1. $\frac{5}{4}$
2. $\frac{9}{9}$
3. $\frac{24}{25}$
4. A
5. C

6. A
7. B
8. $1\frac{1}{16}$
9. $1\frac{2}{21}$
10. $2\frac{23}{24}$
11. $11\frac{1}{3}$
12. $\frac{1}{18}$
13. $\frac{11}{24}$
14. $12\frac{5}{7}$
15. $27\frac{7}{12}$
16. $\frac{7}{20}$
17. $15\frac{1}{6}$
18. 10
19. $2\frac{4}{7}$
20. $13\frac{1}{3}$
21. $\frac{1}{36}$
22. $1\frac{13}{20}$
23. $10\frac{2}{9}$
24. $\frac{1}{2}$
25. 3,750
26. 14.19
27. 16.103
28. 3.7
29. 7.295
30. 7
31. 13.425
32. 475
33. 500
34. 50
35. 23
36. 0.12, 3:25
37. $\frac{9}{20}$, 45%
38. 2:3, 67%
39. 0.8, 80%
40. 20%, $\frac{1}{5}$
41. 42%, 0.42
42. 4
43. 126
44. 44%
45. 29%
46. 7
47. 8
48. 6.25
49. 12.5
50. 16.25

NCLEX-Style Review Questions

1. c

   Rationale: The weight loss is 399 grams (3,751 grams − 3,352 grams). The percent weight loss is $\frac{399}{3,751} = 0.106 = 10.6\%$ weight loss

2. b

   Rationale: 30 milliliters per hour × 24 hours per day = 720 milliliters of IV fluid per day; 1,500 milliliters total intake − 720 milliliters IV fluid = 780 milliliters remaining for oral intake.

3. a

   Rationale: Each baby aspirin tablet is $\frac{81}{325}$ of an adult tablet. $\frac{81}{325} = 0.249 = 24.9\% = 25\% = \frac{1}{4}$

4. c

   Rationale: 15% of 1,800 calories = 0.15 × 1,800 = 270 calories

5. b

   Rationale: 1,100 carbohydrate calories out of 2,000 total calories $= \frac{1,100}{2,000} = 0.55 = 55\%$

6. a, d, g

   Rationale: $\frac{1}{4} = 1:4 = 1 \div 4 = 0.25 = 25\%$

© Forfunlife/Shutterstock

Chapter 2

Systems of Measurement

CHAPTER OUTLINE

LEARNING OUTCOMES

Upon completion of the chapter, the student will be able to:

2-1 Calculate using metric and household measurements.

2-2 Convert between systems of measurement.

2-3   Convert between centigrade and Fahrenheit temperature scales.

2-4   Express international and traditional time.

KEY TERMS

apothecary system

Celsius scale

centigrade

conversion factor method

dimensional analysis

Fahrenheit scale

gram

household system

International System of Units (SI)

international time

international unit

liter

meter

metric system

military time

milliequivalent (mEq)

traditional time

United States Pharmacopeia

United States Pharmacopeia units (USP units)

World Health Organization

Case Consideration ... What Time Is It?

At midnight, the night nurse administered vancomycin 1 g intravenously (scheduled for 12:00 p.m. daily) to an elderly patient with renal insufficiency. The next day, lab work, drawn before and after the scheduled dose, indicated that the patient had a toxic serum level of vancomycin. This result suggests that the dose was too high or the dosage intervals were too close together.

1. What went wrong?
2. How could this error be avoided?

■ INTRODUCTION

Depending on the setting, the nurse will use different systems for measuring time, temperature, and amount. It is important to be able to convert from one system of measurement to another in order to "translate" measurements used by a healthcare agency to measurements used by patients. Understanding time, temperature, and quantity conversions will directly affect the nurse's ability to care for and teach patients. Skilled nurses can think in multiple systems of measurement.

2-1   Systems of Measurement Used to Calculate Dosages

Metric System

The **metric system** is the preferred system of measurement used in health care. A significant advantage of the metric system is that water weight can easily be converted to volume. In the metric system 1 milliliter (volume) of pure water weighs 1 gram (weight), and occupies 1 cubic centimeter (volume) of space. Because of this, by weighing their patients, physicians and nurses are able to calculate how much body fluid needs to be removed during dialysis, for example, or how much body fluid a person with heart failure needs to diurese. Weighing a patient to determine fluid volume status is done routinely in health care. The house-hold system of measurement cannot easily determine volume by weight. However, weights measured in either system should be rounded to the tenth.

The metric system uses powers of 10. Amounts are written as whole numbers or as decimals, not fractions, e.g. 0.1 instead of 1/10 as noted in Figure 2-1. It was first adopted by France as the official system of measurement in the late 1700s. In 1960 the metric system was the system of measurement used by the scientific community and most nations. At that time, it was renamed the Système International d'Unité, **International System of Units (SI)** (Metricconverson.us, 2014). The SI is still commonly referred to as the metric system. The metric system includes three base units of measurement: liter, gram, and meter. Metric measures are determined by their prefixes. Common metric prefixes include:

- Kilo—one thousand (1,000) times larger than the base

- Deci—one-tenth (0.1) of the base

- Centi—one-hundredth (0.01) of the base

- Milli—one-thousandth (0.001) of the base

- Micro—one-millionth (0.000001) of the base

Metric prefixes can be remembered by their location on the metric prefix scale as related to the base unit. **Figure 2-1** shows the base unit (gram, liter, or meter) in relation to the prefixes. Prefixes to the left of the base unit are factors of the base unit. Prefixes to the right of the base unit are fractions, expressed as decimal numbers.

To memorize prefix placement and value, some use the mnemonic "*King Henry Died* from *a Disease Called Mumps*," to recall kilo-, hecto-, deca-, base, deci-, centi-, milli-.

Base Units

The **liter** (L) is the base unit of volume. The **gram** (g) is the base unit of weight and the **meter** (m) is the base unit of length.

Volume.   The liter (L) is a common measure of intravenous (IV) fluid (**Figure 2-2**), and is slightly larger than one household quart:

- Milliliter (mL), a small volume, is one-thousandth of a liter and is commonly used in dosage calculations. Milliliters are used to measure intake and output (I&O), and are also used in IV flow rate calculations.

- Deciliter (dL) is one-tenth of a liter and is used in some laboratory measurements.

The most common metric volume equivalency used in health care is 1 L = 1,000 mL.

Clinical CLUE

To prevent errors, in healthcare, metric amounts less than one are written as a decimal with a leading zero (0.25 mg not .25 mg). Although a leading zero should always be used, a trailing zero should never be used (1.5 L not 1.50 L)

kilo-	hect-	deca-	base	deci-	centi-	milli-	decimilli-	centimilli-	micro-
1000	100	10	0	0.1	0.01	0.001	0.0001	0.00001	0.000001

FIGURE 2-1   Metric prefix scale. Notice there is no prefix for the ones (base) column. The colored prefixes are common values used in health care. Because there are 3 decimal places between the red prefixes, conversion between these units occurs by moving the decimal point 3 places to the left or right. Because the green prefix, centi, is 1 decimal place from milli, conversions between these units occur by moving the decimal point 1 place to the left or right.

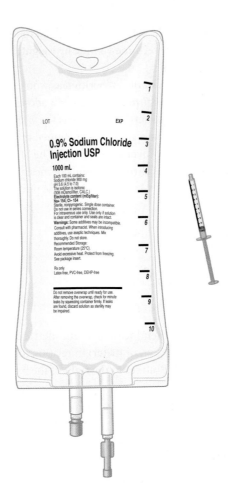

FIGURE 2-2   One liter is a large quantity as shown by the 1 L bag of intravenous fluid. One milliliter is a small quantity as shown by the syringe containing 1 mL.

WARNING!

Watch Out for Error-Prone Abbreviations!

A cubic centimeter (cc) is the amount of space occupied by 1 mL of pure water, therefore, 1 cc has been used interchangeably for 1 mL. According to the Institute for Safe Medication Practices (ISMP), cc is an error-prone abbreviation and should not be used. Another error-prone abbreviation, U (a former abbreviation for "units"), has been misinterpreted for cc when written with insulin orders. For example, when handwritten, "4 U insulin" would be misinterpreted as 4 cc, and a patient would be given 4 milliliters of insulin (the volume equivalent of 400 units), instead of 0.04 milliliters; this is 100 times the prescribed dose of insulin and a very dangerous dosage error! (NSW Therapeutic Advisory Group, 2007)

Weight.   The gram (g) is often used to measure IV medications:

- Kilogram (kg) is 1,000 times the weight of 1 gram and is heavy. People are weighed in kg (**Figure 2-3**). A kilogram is approximately twice as heavy as a pound.

- Milligram (mg) is one-thousandth of a gram and is the common unit used to measure a specific dose of medication.

- Microgram (mcg) is one-millionth of a gram and is used to measure very potent medications.

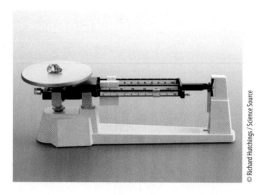
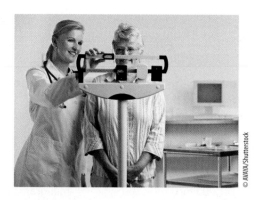

FIGURE 2-3   This small stone is measured in g, just as powdered medications are measured in g, as well as mg, and mcg. The larger weight of a person is measured in kg.

The most common metric weight equivalencies used in dosage calculations are:

- 1 kilogram (kg) = 1,000 grams (g)

- 1 gram (g) = 1,000 milligrams (mg)

- 1 milligram (mg) = 1,000 micrograms (mcg)

- 1 microgram (mcg) = 0.000001 gram (g) = 0.001 milligram (mg)

Length.   The meter (m) is used to measure length or height:

- A meter is approximately 3 inches longer than 1 yard.

- Centimeter (cm) is one-hundredth of a meter. It is used to measure body surface area, length of babies, wound size, and so forth.

- Millimeter (mm) is one-thousandth of a meter (**Figure 2-4**). A millimeter is very short and is used to measure pupil size, skin lesions, skin swelling, and so forth.

LEARNING ACTIVITY 2-1 Fill in the blank.

1.   The base SI unit of measurement for weight is _____.
2.   The base SI unit of measurement for length is _____.
3.   The base SI unit of measurement for volume is _____.

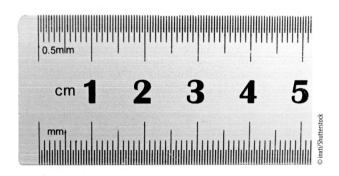

FIGURE 2-4   Each cm is made up of 10 mm.

TABLE 2-1   Common Metric Equivalencies Used in Dosage Calculations with Corresponding Conversion Factors

Equivalency (for Ratio-Proportion)	Conversion	Conversion Factor (for Dimensional Analysis)
1 kg = 1,000 g	grams to kilograms kilograms to grams	1 kg/1,000 g 1,000 g/1 kg
1 g = 1,000 mg	milligrams to grams grams to milligrams	1 g/1,000 mg 1,000 mg/1 g
1 mg = 1,000 mcg	micrograms to milligrams milligrams to micrograms	1 mg/1,000 mcg 1,000 mcg/1mg
1 L = 1,000 mL	milliliters to liters liters to milliliters	1 L/1,000 mL 1,000 mL/1L
1 cm = 10 mm	millimeters to centimeters centimeters to millimeters	1 cm/10 mm 10 mm/1 cm

Metric Conversions

Sometimes medication is supplied in a different unit of measurement than is ordered for the patient. When this occurs, the nurse must convert either the order or the supply, so that the units of measurement are the same. To convert, the nurse must know the equivalency for the amount to convert. Equivalencies (**TABLE 2-1**) should be memorized so that conversions are accurate.

Metric conversion using ratio-proportion.   To convert quantities within the metric system using ratio-proportion, select the appropriate equivalency from Table 2-1 and write it as a ratio or fraction (e.g., 1 kg = 1,000 g is written as $\frac{1\ kg}{1,000\ g}$), then follow these steps:

1. Set up the proportion with the known equivalency on the left and the unknown quantity on the right.

2. Keep the unit of measure in the numerators the same.

3. Keep the unit of measure in the denominators the same.

4. Cross-multiply and divide to solve for x and express the final answer in decimal form, if fractional.

5. Label the answer with the unit of measure next to x.

Example 1:   Convert 750 mg to g; use equivalency 1 g = 1,000 mg, or $\frac{1\ g}{1,000\ mg}$.

$$\frac{1\ g}{1,000\ mg} = \frac{x\ g}{750\ mg}$$

The numerators of each fraction have the same unit of measurement.

$$1,000 \times x = 1 \times 750$$

$$\frac{\cancel{1,000}x}{\cancel{1000}} = \frac{750}{1,000}$$

$$x = 0.75 \ g$$

Example 2:   Convert 0.5 g to mg; use equivalency 1 g = 1,000 mg, or $\frac{1 \ g}{1,000 \ mg}$.

$$\frac{1 \ g}{1,000 \ mg} = \frac{0.5 \ g}{x \ mg}$$

$$1 \times x = 1,000 \times 0.5$$

$$x = 500 \ mg$$

Example 3:   Convert 0.8 L to mL; use equivalency 1 L = 1,000 mL, or $\frac{1 \ L}{1,000 \ mL}$.

$$\frac{1 \ L}{1,000 \ mL} = \frac{0.8 \ L}{x \ mL}$$

$$1 \times x = 1,000 \times 0.8$$

$$x = 800 \ mL$$

Example 4:   Convert 450 mL to L; use equivalency 1 L = 1,000 mL, or $\frac{1 \ L}{1,000 \ mL}$.

$$\frac{1 \ L}{1,000 \ mL} = \frac{x \ L}{450 \ mL}$$

$$1,000 \times x = 1 \times 450$$

$$1,000x = 450$$

$$x = 0.45 \ L$$

Example 5:   Convert 2 mm to cm; use equivalency 1 cm = 10 mm, or $\frac{1 \ cm}{10 \ mm}$.

$$\frac{1 \ cm}{10 \ mm} = \frac{x \ cm}{2 \ mm}$$

$$10 \times x = 1 \times 2$$

$$10x = 2$$

$$x = 0.2 \ cm$$

Example 6:   Convert 0.8 cm to mm; use equivalency 1 cm = 10 mm, or $\frac{1 \ cm}{10 \ mm}$.

$$\frac{1 \ cm}{10 \ mm} = \frac{0.8 \ cm}{x \ mm}$$

$$1 \times x = 10 \times 0.8$$

$$x = 8 \ mm$$

LEARNING ACTIVITY 2-2 Convert the following using the appropriate equivalency in a ratio-proportion equation.

1. Convert 1.5 g to mg.   _____
2. Convert 1,400 mL to L.   _____
3. Convert 12 mm to cm.   _____

Metric conversion using dimensional analysis (conversion factor method).   Another way to convert within the metric system is to use **dimensional analysis**, also known as the **conversion factor method**. In this method, the quantity to be converted is multiplied by the appropriate conversion factor in Table 2-1. This method has the following steps:

1. Place the unknown, x, on the left side of the equal sign. As a prompt, place the desired unit of measurement in parentheses next to x.

2. Choose the conversion factor with the desired unit as the numerator, and the original unit as the denominator. (This allows the original unit of measurement to be canceled out, leaving only the desired unit.)

3. Multiply by the quantity to be converted/1.

4. Convert the answer to decimal form, if the product is fractional.

Example 1:   Convert 500 mg to g.

To convert mg to g, choose the conversion factor with g in the numerator $\frac{1\ g}{1,000\ mg}$.

$$x\ (g) = \frac{1\ g}{1,000\ mg} \times \frac{500\ mg}{1}$$

$$x = \frac{1\ g}{1,000\ \cancel{mg}} \times \frac{500\ \cancel{mg}}{1}$$

$$x = \frac{500\ g}{1,000}$$

$$x = 0.5\ g$$

Example 2:   Convert 1,600 mcg to mg.

To convert mcg to mg, choose the conversion factor with mg in the numerator $\frac{1\ mg}{1,000\ mcg}$.

$$x\ (mg) = \frac{1\ mg}{1,000\ mcg} \times \frac{1,600\ mcg}{1}$$

$$x = \frac{1\ mg}{1,000\ \cancel{mcg}} \times \frac{1,600\ \cancel{mcg}}{1}$$

$$x = \frac{1,600\ mg}{1,000}$$

$$x = 1.6\ mg$$

Example 3:   Convert 1.8 L to mL.

To convert L to mL, choose the conversion factor with mL in the numerator $\frac{1,000 \text{ mL}}{1 \text{ L}}$.

$$x \text{ (mL)} = \frac{1,000 \text{ mL}}{1 \text{ L}} \times \frac{1.8 \text{ L}}{1}$$

$$x = \frac{1,000 \text{ mL}}{1 \text{ L}} \times \frac{1.8 \text{ L}}{1}$$

$$x = \frac{1,800 \text{ mL}}{1}$$

$$x = 1,800 \text{ mL}$$

Example 4:   Convert 0.3 g to mg.

To convert g to mg, choose the conversion factor $\frac{1,000 \text{ mg}}{1 \text{ g}}$.

$$x \text{ (mg)} = \frac{1,000 \text{ mg}}{1 \text{ g}} \times \frac{0.3 \text{ g}}{1}$$

$$x = \frac{1,000 \text{ mg}}{1 \text{ g}} \times \frac{0.3 \text{ g}}{1}$$

$$x = \frac{300 \text{ mg}}{1}$$

$$x = 300 \text{ mg}$$

LEARNING ACTIVITY 2-3 Perform the metric conversion by using the dimensional analysis.

1.   Convert 1.7 g to mg.   _____
2.   Convert 1,600 mL to L. _____
3.   Convert 15 mm to cm. _____

Metric conversion by moving the decimal point.   Because metric system equivalencies are powers of 10, conversion within the system is easily accomplished by moving the decimal point. Recall from Chapter 1:

- When multiplying by a power of 10, *move the decimal as many places to the right as there are zeros in the multiplier.*

- When dividing by a power of 10, *move the decimal as many places to the left as there are zeros in the divisor.*

Think of a number line with the larger amounts to the left and the smaller amounts to the right; move the decimal point as many places to the left or right as the equivalency has zeros. Remember, move the decimal point toward the position of the desired unit. For example, when converting from mg *to* g, move the decimal place to the left, because grams are to the left of milligrams on the number line (**Figure 2-5**). Move the decimal place to the right if you are converting from g *to* mg (**Figure 2-6**).

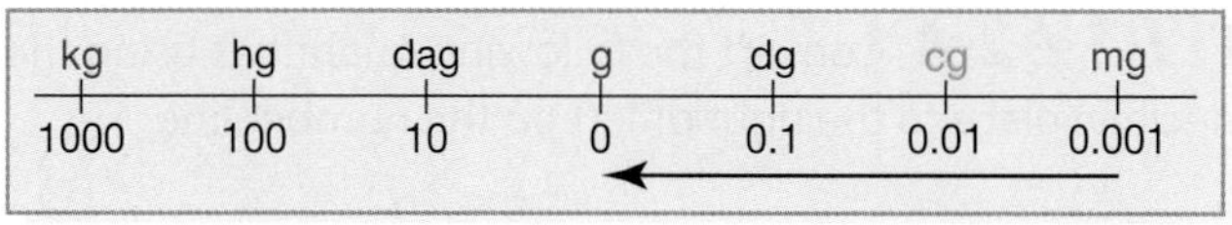

kg	hg	dag	g	dg	cg	mg
1000	100	10	0	0.1	0.01	0.001

FIGURE 2-5   Grams (g) are to the left of milligrams (mg), so the decimal place will be moved to the left when converting from mg to g.

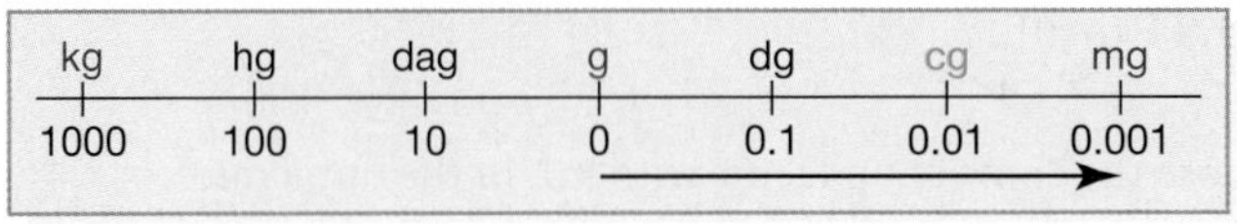

kg	hg	dag	g	dg	cg	mg
1000	100	10	0	0.1	0.01	0.001

FIGURE 2-6   Milligrams (mg) are to the right of grams (g), so the decimal place will be moved to right when converting from g to mg.

Example 1:   Convert 5 mm to cm.

Move the decimal toward the unit of conversion as many places as there are zeros in the equivalency.

Equivalency: 1 cm = 10 mm

Centimeter is to the left of mm on the number line, and there is one zero in the equivalency, so *move the decimal one place to the left* (**Figure 2-7**).

5 mm = 0.5 cm

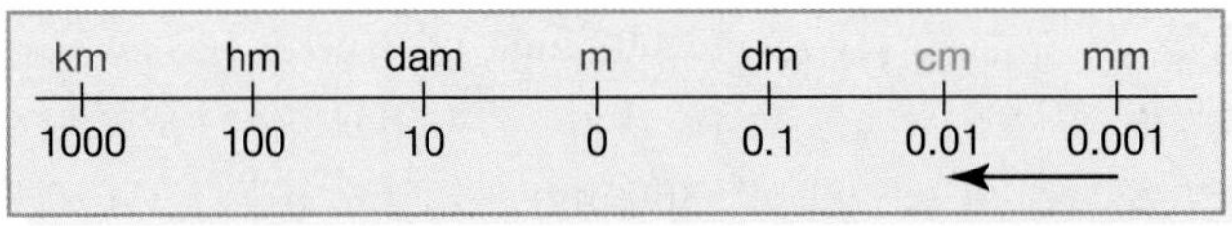

km	hm	dam	m	dm	cm	mm
1000	100	10	0	0.1	0.01	0.001

FIGURE 2-7   Move the decimal point one place to the left when converting millimeters (mm) to centimeters (cm).

Example 2:   Convert 1.5 g to mg.

Move the decimal toward the unit of conversion as many places as there are zeros in the equivalency.

Equivalency: 1 g = 1,000 mg

Milligram is to the right of gram on the number line, and there three zeros in the equivalency, so *move the decimal three places to the right* (**Figure 2-8**).

1.5 g = 1,500 mg

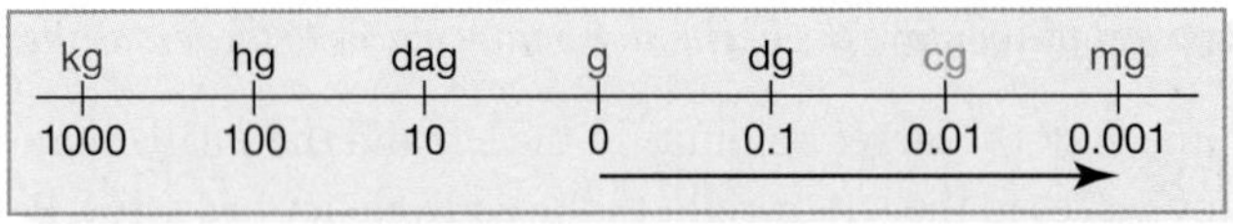

kg	hg	dag	g	dg	cg	mg
1000	100	10	0	0.1	0.01	0.001

FIGURE 2-8   Move the decimal point three places to the right on the metric number line when converting grams (g) to milligrams (mg).

LEARNING ACTIVITY 2-4 Convert the following quantities using the appropriate equivalency and moving the decimal place to the right or left on the number line.

1.   Convert 568.1 g to kg.   _____
2.   Convert 750 mL to L.   _____
3.   Convert 11 mm to cm.   _____

Clinical CLUE

Look at the red quantities on the metric number line (Figure 2-1) and notice that "kilo" is 1,000 times bigger than the base unit (e.g., kilogram is 1,000 times larger than gram); the base unit is 1,000 times bigger than "milli" (e.g., gram is 1,000 times larger than milligram); "milli" is one 1,000 times bigger than "micro" (e.g., milligram is 1,000 times larger than microgram).

To perform "red conversions" (i.e., convert kilo to base to milli to micro), move the decimal point to the right three places for each conversion (e.g., 3.2 kg = 3,200 g = 3,200,000 mg). When converting micro to milli to base to kilo, move the decimal point to the left three places for each conversion (e.g., 5,400 mcg = 5.4 mg = 0.0054 g = 0.0000054 kg).

Because the green quantity, "centi," is 10 times bigger than "milli," to convert centi to milli (e.g., centimeters to millimeters) move the decimal one place to the right (e.g., 66 cm = 660 mm); to convert millimeters to centimeters, move the decimal point one place to the left (e.g., 17 mm = 1.7 cm).

Apothecary System

The **apothecary system** is an antiquated system of measurement based on the weight of one grain of wheat; therefore, the base unit of weight is one grain. The smallest measure of volume is one minim, which is a drop of water that weighs the same amount as one grain of wheat. Use of the apothecary system has resulted in numerous medication errors, so it is currently out of favor. For this reason, conversions using the apothecary system are not covered in this chapter, but they are included in Appendix B.

Household System

The **household system** of measurement is the system of measurement currently used in the United States. It requires the measuring tools used for cooking (measuring cups and measuring spoons). The household system of measurement is derived from the apothecary system. The household system is the least accurate system of measurement and is not recommended for medication administration. In 2009, the ISMP called upon "prescribers, pharmacists, and other healthcare professionals, as well as pharmacy computer system and e-prescribing system vendors, to remove or prevent the use of 'teaspoonful' and other non-metric measurements in prescription directions in order to better protect patients" (ISMP, 2009, para 1). In 2011 the ISMP issued the "Statement on the Use of Metric Units of Measurements to Prevent Errors with Oral Liquids." This statement recommends the exclusive use of metric measurements for dosing and measuring oral liquids (ISMP, 2011).

Despite this recommendation from the ISMP, medications are sometimes ordered in household measurements. A nurse may use the household system to determine how much liquid the patient has had to drink, or when instructing the patient regarding fluid requirements. In addition, household measurements of weight and height might be used in an outpatient setting.

The household system is not based on powers of 10 and does not use decimals. Instead partial units are written as proper fractions. It is important to memorize the equivalencies within the household system.

Volume Equivalencies

Household volume measurements include: teaspoon (t), tablespoon (T), fluid ounce (fl oz, commonly referred to as ounce [oz]), cup (c), pint (pt), quart (qt), and gallon (gal) (**Figure 2-9** and **Figure 2-10**). Equivalencies that may be used in health care include those listed in **TABLE 2-2**.

TABLE 2-2   Household Volume Equivalencies and Conversion Factors

Volume Equivalency (for Ratio-Proportion)	Conversion	Conversion Factors (for Dimensional Analysis)
1 T = 3 t	teaspoons to tablespoons tablespoons to teaspoons	1T/3t 3t/1T
1 fl oz = 2 T	tablespoons to fluid ounces fluid ounces to tablespoons	1 fl oz/2 T 2 T/1 fl oz
1 c = 8 fl oz	fluid ounces to cups cups to fluid ounces	1 c/8 fl oz 8 fl oz/1 c
1 pt = 2 c	cups to pints pints to cups	1 pt/2 c 2 c/1 pt
1 qt = 2 pt	pints to quarts quarts to pints	1 qt/2 pt 2 pt/1 qt
1 qt = 4 c	cups to quarts quarts to cups	1 qt/4 c 4 c/1 qt
1 qt = 32 fl oz	fluid ounces to quarts quarts to fluid ounces	1 qt/ 32 fl oz 32 fl oz/1 qt

			1 quart
		1 pint	2 pints
	1 cup	2 cups	4 cups
	8 fl oz	16 fl oz	32 fl oz

FIGURE 2-9   Volume measurements with equivalencies.

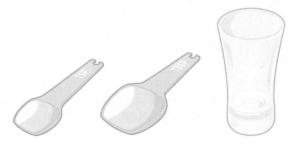

FIGURE 2-10   Teaspoon, tablespoon, and a 1-fluid-ounce (fl oz) shot glass. There are 3 teaspoons in 1 tablespoon, and 2 tablespoons in 1 fl oz.

TABLE 2-3 Household Weight Equivalency and Conversion Factors		
Weight Equivalency (for Ratio-Proportion)	**Conversion**	**Conversion Factors (for Dimensional Analysis)**
1 lb = 16 oz	pounds to ounces ounces to pounds	16 oz/1 lb 1 lb/16 oz

Weight Equivalency

Household weight measurements include: ounce (oz), pound (lb), and ton. Healthcare professionals must know the equivalency: 1 lb = 16 oz (**TABLE 2-3**).

Length Equivalencies

Household length measurements include: inch (in), foot (ft), yard (yd), and mile (mi) (**Figure 2-11**). Household length equivalencies that are helpful for the healthcare professional to know include: 1 ft = 12 in and 1 yd = 3 ft (**TABLE 2-4.**)

Household Conversions

Converting quantities within the household system can be done using ratio-proportion or dimensional analysis.

Household conversions using ratio-proportion.   To convert within the household system using ratio-proportion, choose the appropriate equivalency, then:

- Set up the proportion with the known equivalency on the left and the unknown quantity on the right.

- Keep the unit of measure in the numerators the same.

- Keep the unit of measure in the denominators the same.

- Convert any fractions in the numerator or denominator to decimal form.

- Cross-multiply and divide to solve for x, then label answer with unit of measure next to x.

TABLE 2-4 Household Length Equivalencies and Conversion Factors		
Length Equivalencies (for Ratio-Proportion)	**Conversion**	**Conversion Factors (for Dimensional Analysis)**
1 ft = 12 in	inches to feet feet to inches	1 ft/12 in 12 in/1 ft
1 yd = 3 ft	feet to yards yards to feet	1 yd/3 ft 3 ft/1 yd

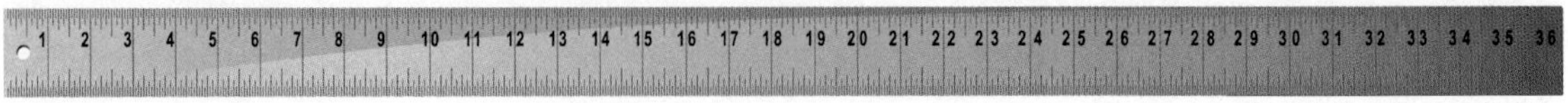

© John Takai / Hemera/Getty Images Plus / Getty

FIGURE 2-11 This yardstick shows inches, feet, and 1-yard measurements.

Household Conversion Using Dimensional Analysis. To convert within the household system using dimensional analysis:

- Place the unknown, x, with the desired unit of measure in parentheses on the left side of the equal sign.
- Choose the conversion factor with desired unit as the numerator.
- Multiply the conversion factor by the quantity to be converted/1.

Example 1: Convert 2 cups to quarts.

For ratio-proportion, use equivalency, 1 qt = 4 c; for dimensional analysis, use conversion factor $\frac{1\ qt}{4\ c}$.

Ratio-Proportion	Dimensional Analysis
$\dfrac{1\ qt}{4\ c} = \dfrac{x\ qt}{2\ c}$ $4 \times x = 1 \times 2$ $\dfrac{4x}{4} = \dfrac{2}{4}$ $x = \dfrac{1}{2}\ qt$	$x\ (qt) = \dfrac{1\ qt}{4\ c} \times \dfrac{2\ c}{1}$ $x = \dfrac{1\ qt}{4\ \cancel{c}} \times \dfrac{2\ \cancel{c}}{1}$ $x = \dfrac{2}{4}\ qt$ $x = \dfrac{1}{2}\ qt$

Example 2: Convert 1 ½ pints to cups.

For ratio-proportion, use equivalency, 1 pt = 2 c; for dimensional analysis, use conversion factor $\frac{2\ c}{1\ pt}$.

Ratio-Proportion	Dimensional Analysis
$\dfrac{1\ pt}{2\ c} = \dfrac{1.5\ pt}{x\ c}$ $1 \times x = 2 \times 1.5$ $x = 3\ c$	$x\ (c) = \dfrac{2\ c}{1\ pt} \times \dfrac{1.5\ pt}{1}$ $x = \dfrac{2\ c}{1\ \cancel{pt}} \times \dfrac{1.5\ \cancel{pt}}{1}$ $x = \dfrac{3\ c}{1}$ $x = 3\ c$

Example 3:   Convert 12 ounces (oz) to pounds (lb).

For ratio-proportion, use equivalency, 1 lb = 16 oz; for dimensional analysis, use conversion factor $\frac{1\ lb}{16\ oz}$.

Ratio-Proportion	Dimensional Analysis
$\dfrac{1\ lb}{16\ oz} = \dfrac{x\ lb}{12\ oz}$	$x\ (lb) = \dfrac{1\ lb}{16\ oz} \times \dfrac{12\ oz}{1}$
$16 \times x = 1 \times 12$	$x = \dfrac{1\ lb}{16\ \cancel{oz}} \times \dfrac{12\ \cancel{oz}}{1}$
$16x = 12$	
$\dfrac{16\ x}{16} = \dfrac{12}{16}$	$x = \dfrac{1\ lb}{4} \times \dfrac{3}{1}$
$x = \dfrac{3}{4}\ lb$	$x = \dfrac{3}{4}\ lb$

Example 4:   Convert 5 feet 6 inches to inches.

For ratio-proportion, use equivalency 1 ft = 12 in; for dimensional analysis, use conversion factor $\frac{12\ in}{1\ ft}$.

Convert feet to inches then add 6 inches to give you the total amount of inches in 5 ft 6 in.

Ratio-Proportion	Dimensional Analysis
First, convert 5 ft to inches:	$x\ (in) = \left(\dfrac{12\ in}{1\ ft} \times \dfrac{5\ ft}{1} \right) + 6\ in$
$\dfrac{1\ ft}{12\ in} = \dfrac{5\ ft}{x\ in}$	$x = \left(\dfrac{12\ in}{1\ \cancel{ft}} \times \dfrac{5\ \cancel{ft}}{1} \right) + 6\ in$
$1 \times x = 12 \times 5$	
$x = 60\ in$	$x = (60\ in) + 6\ in$
Then add to 6 remaining inches:	$x = 66\ in$
$60\ in + 6\ in = 66\ in$	

LEARNING ACTIVITY 2-5 Convert the following using the appropriate equivalency.

1.   Convert 9 lb 8 oz to pounds.   _____
2.   Convert 6 ft 2 in to inches.   _____
3.   Convert 4 teaspoons to tablespoons. _____

| 2-2 | **Converting Between Systems** |

Nurses convert household weight (pounds, ounces) to metric weight (kilograms, grams) to determine the appropriate dose of medication or to perform advanced clinical calculations. Some drug doses are based on both weight and height (length), requiring the ability to convert household length to metric centimeters. Nurses also convert household volume measurements to metric liters and milliliters. For the purpose of patient teaching, the nurse may be required to convert metric measurements to household measurements.

Household-to-Metric Approximate Equivalencies

It is important to recognize that when converting between systems, the measurements are approximately equal, not actually equal. **TABLE 2-5** reveals approximate equivalencies between the metric and household systems that are commonly used in health care. Rough equivalencies, not routinely used for dosage calculation, are sometimes used for estimation:

- 1 quart is approximately equal to 1 liter (1,000 mL).

- 1 pint (½ qt) is approximately equal to 500 mL (one-half of a liter).

- 1 cup (½ pt or ¼ qt) is approximately equal to 250 mL (one-fourth of a liter).

TABLE 2-5 Household and Metric Approximate Equivalencies and Conversion Factors

Household–Metric Approximate Equivalency (for Ratio Proportion)	Conversion	Conversion Factor (for Dimensional Analysis)
1 in = 2.5 cm*	centimeters to inches inches to centimeters	1 in/2.5 cm 2.5 cm/1 in
1 t = 5 mL	milliliters to teaspoons teaspoons to milliliters	1 t/5 mL 5 mL/1 t
1 T = 15 mL	milliliters to tablespoons tablespoons to milliliters	1 T/ 15 mL 15 mL/1 T
1 fl oz = 30 mL	milliliters to fluid ounces fluid ounces to milliliters	1 fl oz = 30 mL 30 mL/1 fl oz
1 kg = 2.2 lb	pounds to kilograms kilograms to pounds	1 kg/2.2 lb 2.2 lb/1 kg

*2.5 cm/1 in is a common equivalency used in health care, although 2.54 cm/1 in is more precise.

Dosage and clinical calculations are generally calculated using the more precise equivalencies listed in Table 2-5.

Rounding RULE

- Round weights to the tenth.
- Scales used in health care are calibrated to tenths, however, when converting between systems, weights may result with decimal fractions beyond the tenth. Always round the final weight to the tenth, unless otherwise specified.

To convert between the household and metric systems using ratio-proportion:

- Choose the appropriate equivalency from Table 2-5 and convert any household fraction to a decimal.
- Set up a ratio-proportion, cross-multiply, and divide to solve for x; label answer with the unit of measure next to x.
- When converting household to metric, the final answer should be in decimal form; when converting metric to household, the final answer should be in fractional form.

To convert between the household and metric systems using dimensional analysis:

- Convert household fractions to decimals.
- Place the unknown, x, with the desired unit of measure in parentheses on the left side of the equal sign.
- Choose the conversion factor with the desired unit as the numerator.
- Multiply the conversion factor by the quantity to be converted/1.
- When converting household to metric, the final answer should be in decimal form; when converting metric to household, the final answer should be in fractional form.

Example 1:   Convert 20 in to cm.

For ratio-proportion, use equivalency 1 in = 2.5 cm; for dimensional analysis, choose conversion factor $\frac{2.5\ cm}{1\ in}$.

Ratio-Proportion	Dimensional Analysis
$\dfrac{1\ in}{2.5\ cm} = \dfrac{20\ in}{x\ cm}$ $1 \times x = 2.5 \times 20$ $x = 50\ cm$	$x\ (cm) = \dfrac{2.5\ cm}{1\ in} \times \dfrac{20\ in}{1}$ $x = \dfrac{2.5\ cm}{1\ \cancel{in}} \times \dfrac{20\ \cancel{in}}{1}$ $x = \dfrac{50\ cm}{1}$ $x = 50\ cm$

Example 2:   Convert 165 lb to kg.

For ratio-proportion, use equivalency 1 kg = 2.2 lb; for dimensional analysis, choose conversion factor $\frac{1\ kg}{2.2\ lb}$.

Ratio-Proportion	Dimensional Analysis
$\dfrac{1\ kg}{2.2\ lb} = \dfrac{x\ kg}{165\ lb}$ $2.2 \times x = 1 \times 165$ $\dfrac{2.2\ x}{2.2} = \dfrac{165}{2.2}$ $x = 75\ kg$	$x\ (kg) = \dfrac{1\ kg}{2.2\ lb} \times \dfrac{165\ lb}{1}$ $x = \dfrac{1\ kg}{2.2\ \cancel{lb}} \times \dfrac{165\ \cancel{lb}}{1}$ $x = \dfrac{165\ kg}{2.2}$ $x = 75\ kg$

Example 3:   Convert 1 ½ fl oz to mL.

For ratio-proportion, use equivalency 1 oz = 30 mL; for dimensional analysis, use conversion factor $\frac{30\ mL}{1\ oz}$.

Ratio-Proportion	Dimensional Analysis
$\dfrac{1\ fl\ oz}{30\ mL} = \dfrac{1.5\ fl\ oz}{x\ mL}$ $1 \times x = 30 \times 1.5$ $x = 45\ mL$	$x\ (mL) = \dfrac{30\ mL}{1\ fl\ oz} \times \dfrac{1.5\ fl\ oz}{1}$ $x = \dfrac{30\ mL}{1\ \cancel{fl\ oz}} \times \dfrac{1.5\ \cancel{fl\ oz}}{1}$ $x = \dfrac{45\ mL}{1}$ $x = 45\ mL$

It is important to reinforce that when converting between systems, approximate equivalences are used because exact equivalencies are impractical to use. For example, using a more precise equivalency for fluid ounces and milliliters, 1 oz = 29.625 mL, would be time-consuming and would require the use of a calculator, whereas using the conversion 1 oz = 30 mL can readily yield conversions without the aid of a calculator. Also note that using approximate equivalencies sometimes yields slight discrepancies. For example, if 1 L is approximately equivalent to 1 qt, then it should follow that 1,000 mL = 1 qt. However, to convert a quart to milliliters, you might first convert 1 qt to 32 oz and then multiply 32 oz by the conversion factor of 30 mL/1 oz to determine that there are 960 mL in 1 qt. So, how many milliliters are there in 1 qt, 960 mL or 1,000 mL? Although both answers are acceptable, it is preferable to use the conversion, 30 mL/1 oz, yielding 960 mL in 1 qt, when converting milliliters to ounces and vice versa.

LEARNING ACTIVITY 2-6 Convert the following using ratio-proportion or dimensional analysis.

1.   Convert 12 lb 8 oz to kg. _____
2.   Convert 5 ft 6 in to cm. _____
3.   Convert 45 mL to fl oz. _____

Other Units of Measurement

Some medications are measured by other units of measurement, such as:

- International units

- United States Pharmacopeia units (USP units)

- Milliunits (mU)

- Milliequivalents (mEq)

Nurses are not required to convert these units of measurement. However, because some medication dosages are ordered in these units of measurement, it is helpful to understand these terms.

International Units

The **international unit** is a standardized measurement determined by the **World Health Organization (WHO)**, a United Nations institute that is concerned with public health. The international unit is a measure of medication potency for the same medication, between nations and manufacturers. These units are substance specific. That is to say, the international unit for vitamin D is different from the international unit for vitamin E. However, an international unit for vitamin D made by one manufacturer will provide the same effect as an international unit of vitamin D made by another manufacturer, regardless of where in the world it was manufactured. The **United States Pharmacopeia unit (USP unit)** is a measurement standardized between manufacturers, determined by the **United States Pharmacopeia (USP)**, a U.S. government agency that sets standards for medicines. A USP unit is a measure of medication potency for the same medication (**Figure 2-12**). Like international units, these units are also substance specific. That is to say, the USP unit of heparin (a medication used to inhibit blood clotting) is different from the USP unit of insulin (a medication used to lower blood sugar). Most USP units are equivalent to the international units of the same substance, but determining their equivalency is not done by the nurse. Nurses do not convert units into any other system of measurement.

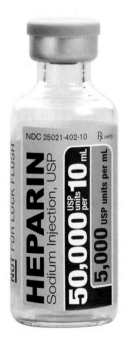

FIGURE 2-12   Heparin measured in units determined by the United States Pharmacopeia (USP).

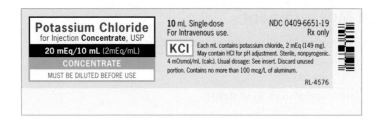

FIGURE 2-13   Potassium is measured in millequivalents (mEq).

Milliequivalents

A **milliequivalent (mEq)** is a measurement of chemical activity, not molecular weight. It is used to measure the combining power of ions. Electrolytes such as potassium are measured in milliequivalents (**Figure 2-13**).

WARNING!

U and IU Are Not Used!

International Unit was formerly abbreviated "IU," and unit was formerly abbreviated as "U." When handwritten, IU can be mistaken for 10 or IV, and U can be mistaken for 0. Such errors can lead to very dangerous medication errors. Use only approved abbreviations as indicated in Chapter 4.

Percentages and Ratios

Other medications may be labeled by the percentage of medication per volume, or as a ratio of medication to volume. Nurses need to know how to convert these medication quantities to metric equivalents. Percent is the concentration of medication in a mixture. The percent of liquid medication is the number of grams of powdered medication or the number of milliliters of liquid medication dissolved in 100 mL of solution. For example, 1% lidocaine contains 1 g of lidocaine per 100 mL of solution. The percent of solid medication is determined by the number of grams of powdered medication or the number of milliliters of liquid medication present within 100 grams of solid mixture. For example, 2.5% hydrocortisone contains 2.5 g of hydrocortisone per 100 g (or 25 mg/g) of solid mixture.

Concentrations expressed in ratio refer to number of grams per number of milliliters (grams : milliliter). For example, epinephrine 1:1,000 (**Figure 2-14**) means that there is 1 g in 1,000 mL (or 1 mg/mL). Dosage calculation of medication dosage strength expressed as ratio or percent is covered in Chapters 9 and 11.

LEARNING ACTIVITY 2-7   Fill in the blanks to make the sentence correct.

1.   Liquid concentrations expressed in percent represent the number of _____ of powdered medication or number of _____ of liquid medication dissolved in 100 _____ of solution.

2.   A unit of heparin _____ the same as a unit of insulin.

3.   International units are determined by _____ .

4.   Concentrations expressed as a ratio represent the number of _____ per the number of _____ .

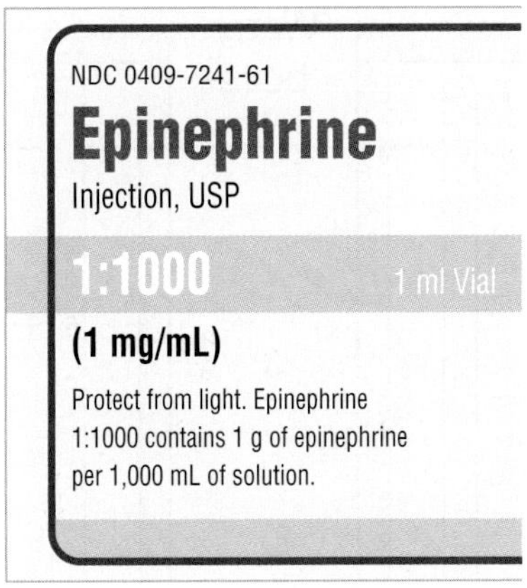

FIGURE 2-14   Epinephrine 1:1,000 contains 1 g of epinephrine per 1,000 mL of solution.

2-3   Centigrade and Fahrenheit Temperature Scales

WARNING!

Know Your Patient's Temperature!

A nurse, familiar with measuring body temperature using a Fahrenheit thermometer, moved to an agency that required the use of centigrade thermometers. Recalling from nursing school that 37°C is the equivalent of 98.6°F, the nurse thought that a patient temperature of 39°C was a low-grade fever, not high enough to require treatment. However, during change-of-shift report, the oncoming nurse, upon realizing that nothing was done to treat the patient's increased temperature exclaimed, "Don't you realize that 39°C is 102.2°F!" The provider was contacted, blood cultures were drawn, and antibiotics were started. Treatment would not have been delayed had the temperature been converted properly when obtained.

A patient's temperature is an indication of the presence or absence of infection and other abnormalities. Nurses measure temperature with thermometers that use the **Fahrenheit (F) scale** and the **Celsius (C) scale**. The Fahrenheit thermometer is calibrated with 212 degrees (°), and has a freezing point of 32°F and boiling point of 212°F. This means there are 180° between freezing and boiling in the Fahrenheit scale. The Celsius thermometer, also call **centigrade** (100 grades or calibrations) is calibrated with 100 degrees. Water freezes at 0°C and boils at 100°C. This means that the ratio between Fahrenheit and Celsius is 180:100 or the proportion $\frac{180}{100}$ which can be converted to 1.8; therefore, 1.8 is the conversion factor used to convert between the Fahrenheit and Celsius scales. To convert Fahrenheit to Celsius, divide by 1.8, after subtracting the baseline of 32. To convert Celsius to Fahrenheit, multiply by 1.8 and then add the baseline of 32. The formulas for converting Fahrenheit to Celsius and Celsius to Fahrenheit are:

$$\frac{°F - 32}{1.8} = °C \qquad (°C \times 1.8) + 32 = °F$$

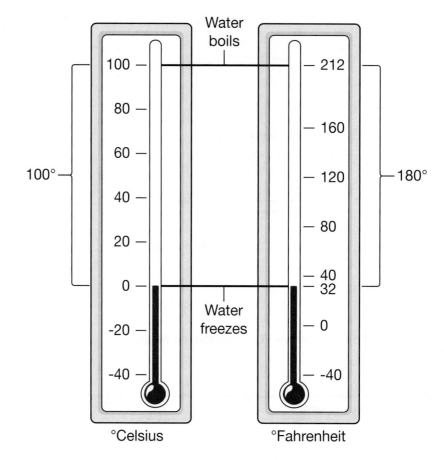

FIGURE 2-15 The Fahrenheit thermometer shows 180° between freezing and boiling and the Celsius thermometer shows 100° between freezing and boiling.

Example 1: Convert 98.6°F to °C.

$$\frac{98.6°\text{F} - 32}{1.8} = °\text{C} \qquad \frac{66.6}{1.8} = °\text{C} \qquad 37 = °\text{C}$$

Example 2: Convert 39°F to °C.

$$(°\text{C} \times 1.8) + 32 = °\text{F} \qquad (39°\text{C} \times 1.8) + 32 = °\text{F} \qquad 70.2 + 32 = °\text{F} \qquad 102.2 = °\text{F}$$

Rounding RULE

Because thermometers are calibrated to tenths, converted temperatures should be rounded to tenths. For example, when 102.5°F is converted to °C, the calculated answer includes a repeating decimal: $\frac{(102.5 - 32)}{1.8} = \frac{70.5}{1.8} = 39.1666$. This temperature should be recorded as 39.2°C.

LEARNING ACTIVITY 2-8 Convert the following temperatures.

1.   Convert 102°F to °C.   _____
2.   Convert 38.6°C to °F.   _____
3.   Convert 97.2°F to °C.   _____

| TABLE 2-6   Centigrade–Fahrenheit Equivalents of Body Temperatures ||
Fahrenheit	**Centigrade**
96.8	36
97.7	36.5
98.6 (normal body temperature)	**37 (normal body temperature)**
99.5	37.5
100.4	38
101.3	38.5
102.2	39
103.1	39.5

The temperature scales side by side reveal every 1°C equals 1.8°F therefore every 0.5°C equals 0.9°F. Normal body temperature is 98.6°F which is the equivalent of 37°C as determined in Example 1. **TABLE 2-6** compares body temperatures in both the centigrade and Fahrenheit scales.

2-4   International and Traditional Time

Traditionally, time has been measured using a 12-hour clock that repeats, at the meridian (midday or noon time), to account for 24 hours of the day. The day begins at midnight (12:00 a.m. or *ante meridian*), and the second 12 hours of the day begin at noon (12:00 p.m. or *post meridian*). This is known as **traditional time**. In traditional time, hours are represented by Arabic numerals to the left of a colon, and minutes are to the right of the colon. Medication administration errors have been made using traditional time, because 12:00 a.m. is at night, and 12:00 p.m. is during the day. Additionally, errors can arise if the prescriber does not mark a.m. or p.m.

To prevent errors, many healthcare agencies use **international time**, also known as **military time**. International time is based on 24 hours, not 12 hours. Because of this, each hour has a unique numerical representation. The day begins after 0000; the first minute of the day is 0001 and the day ends at 2400. Both 0000 and 2400 represent midnight. When documenting international time, no colon or a.m. or p.m. is used, but all four digits are always included. The first two numbers represent hours and the remaining two numbers represent minutes (**Figure 2-16**).

The first 12 hours of the day are noted very similarly in traditional and international time. For example, 1:00 a.m. is 0100, and 1:15 a.m. is 0115. This similarity holds true through 12:59 p.m.

At 1:00 pm international time is written as 1300 and the remaining post meridian hours, 2:00 p.m. through midnight, are written as 1400 through 2400.

Clinical CLUE

When converting traditional time after midnight, it is important to remember that the day ends at 2400. A common time conversion error made by students is to convert time between 12:01 a.m. and 12:59 a.m. to 2401 to 2459. Because 2400 ends one day and 0000 begins the next, time written between 12:01 a.m. and 12:59 p.m. is written as 0001 to 0059. For example, 12:15 a.m., documented as international time, is 0015.

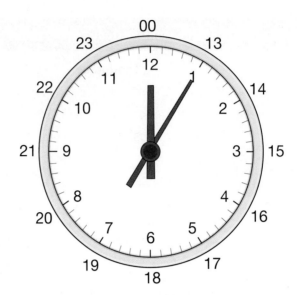

FIGURE 2-16 Clock depicting 0005 (12:05 a.m.) and 1205 (12:05 p.m.).

Converting Traditional Time to International Time

To convert traditional time to international time:

- From 12 a.m. to 12:59 a.m., replace 12 with 00 and delete the colon and term a.m.

- Up to 9:59 a.m., place a 0 in front of the time and delete the colon and the term *a.m.*

- From 10:00 a.m. to 12:59 p.m., remove the colon and the term *a.m.* or *p.m.*

- After 12:59 p.m., remove the colon and term *p.m.*, then add 12 hours to the traditional time.

Example 1: Convert 2:00 a.m. to international time.

Remove the colon and write 02 for 2 hours, and 00 for zero minutes.

$$2:00 \rightarrow 0200$$

Example 2: Convert 12:25 p.m. to international time.

Remove the colon and write 12 for 12 hours, and 25 for 25 minutes.

$$12:25 \rightarrow 1225$$

Converting International Time to Traditional Time

To convert international time to traditional time:

- Before 1000, remove the leading zero, insert a colon, and label a.m.

- Between 1000 and 1159, insert a colon and label a.m.

- After 1259, subtract 1200, insert a colon, and label p.m.

Example 1:   Convert 1400 to traditional time.

$$
\begin{array}{r}
1400 \\
- 1200 \\
\hline
200
\end{array}
$$ Rewrite as 2:00 p.m.

Example 2:   Convert 1620 to traditional time.

$$
\begin{array}{r}
1620 \\
- 1200 \\
\hline
420
\end{array}
$$ Rewrite as 4:20 p.m.

LEARNING ACTIVITY 2-9   Convert the following times.

1.   12:54 a.m.   _____
2.   1721   _____
3.   9:05 p.m.   _____

What Time Is It? ... Case Closure

Knowing time notation is a critical part of medication administration. The night nurse accidentally gave a dose of medication at midnight that was due at noon. This resulted in the patient receiving two doses after only 12 hours, the dose given 12 hours early at midnight, and the dose given at noon the next day. Overdosing a patient can be lethal, and, at the very least, it can increase the patient's risk for serious side effects. If the authorized prescriber was unaware of the additional dose, the laboratory data would guide an inappropriate change in dosage frequency. It is the nurse's duty to administer medications at the correct time. If the patient was harmed as a result of this error, the nurse is liable. The nurse could have avoided this error by knowing traditional time. The agency could have avoided this error by using international time, because it is clear that 1200 is not 2400.

Chapter Summary

Learning Outcomes	Points to Remember

2-1 Calculate using metric and household measurements.	*Metric system—decimal system based on powers of 10:*
	• Base units/conversion factors
	  o Weight—gram (g)
	    ▪ 1,000 g/1 kg; 1 kg/1,000 g
	    ▪ 1,000 mg/1g; 1 g/1,000 mg
	    ▪ 1,000 mcg/1 mg; 1 mg/1,000 mcg
	  o Volume—liter (L)
	    ▪ 1,000 mL/1 L; 1 L/1,000 mL
	  o Length—meter (m)
	    ▪ 10 cm/1 mm; 1 mm/10 cm

- Prefixes
  - o Deci—one-tenth of base
  - o Centi—one-hundredth of base
  - o Milli—one-thousandth of base
  - o Micro—one-millionth of base
  - o Kilo—one thousand times the base unit

Metric conversion using ratio-proportion:
- Known equivalency on left, unknown quantity on right.
- Keep unit of measure in the numerators the same.
- Keep unit of measure in the denominators the same.
- Express final answer in decimal form, if fractional.

Example :   Convert 750 mg to g.

$$\frac{1\,g}{1{,}000\ mg} = \frac{x\ g}{750\ mg}$$

$$1{,}000x = 1 \times 750$$

$$x = \frac{750}{1{,}000}$$

$$x = 0.75\ g$$

Metric conversion using dimensional analysis:
- Place the unknown, *x*, with the desired unit of measurement in parentheses on the left side of the equal sign.
- Use conversion factor with desired unit as numerator and original unit as denominator.
- Multiply by quantity/1; cancel terms; convert answer to decimal, if product is fractional.

Example :   Convert 500 mg to g.

$$x\,(g) = \frac{1\,g}{1{,}000\ \cancel{mg}} \times \frac{500\ \cancel{mg}}{1}$$

$$x = \frac{1\,g}{1{,}000\ \cancel{mg}} \times \frac{500\ mg}{1}$$

$$x = \frac{500\ g}{1{,}000}$$

$$x = 0.5\ g$$

Conversion by moving the decimal point:
- Multiplying by a power of 10—move decimal to right as many places as there are zeros in the multiplier.
- Dividing by a power of 10—move decimal to left as many places as there are zeros in the divisor.

Example 1:   Convert 5 mm to cm.
Equivalency: 1 cm = 10 mm; because cm is left of mm on number line and there is 1 zero in the equivalency, move the decimal 1 place to the left; 5 mm = 0.5 cm.

Example 2: Convert 1.5 g to mg.

Equivalency: 1 g = 1,000 mg; because mg is right of g on number line, and there are 3 zeros in the equivalency, move the decimal 3 places to the right; 1.5 g = 1,500 mg.

Household system—system used in the United States; not based on powers of 10; amounts less than 1 written as fractions.

Volume equivalencies:

- 1 T = 3 t; 1 fl oz = 2 T; 1 cup = 8 fl oz
- 1 pt = 2 cup; 1 qt = 2 pt

Weight equivalency: 1 lb = 16 oz

Length equivalencies: 1 ft = 12 in; 1 yd = 3 ft

2-2 Convert between systems of measurement.	*Household to metric approximate equivalencies*:

Household to metric approximate equivalencies:

- 1 in = 2.5 cm
- 1 t = 5 mL
- 1 t = 15 mL
- 1 fl oz = 30 mL
- 1 kg = 2.2 lb

Converting between systems:

1. Using ratio-proportion:
- Convert household fractions to decimals.
- Set up ratio-proportion with equivalency on left and unknown quantity on right.
- Keep same unit of measure for numerators and same unit of measure for denominators.

2. Using dimensional analysis:
- Convert household fractions to decimals.
- Use conversion factor with desired unit in numerator.
- Multiply conversion factor by given quantity/1.
- Convert final answer to decimal, if fractional.

Rounding rule—round weights to tenths, unless otherwise specified.

Other units of measurement:

Units—medication-specific quantity needed to achieve a specific response over a specified time; no conversions

- International units determined by WHO
- USP units determined by U.S. Pharmacopeia

Milliequivalent (mEq)—measurement of chemical activity; used for electrolytes; no conversions to other systems

Percent—concentration of medication in a mixture

- Liquids—number of grams or milliliters of medication in 100 mL of solution
- Solids—number of grams or milliliters of medication in 100 g of mixture

Ratio—number of grams per the number of milliliters, for example, epinephrine 1:1,000 is 1 g epinephrine per 1,000 mL

2-3 Convert between centigrade and Fahrenheit temperature scales.	*Fahrenheit*: • Freezing is 32°F; boiling is 212°F • $(°C \times 1.8) + 32 = °F$ *Celsius* (centigrade): • Freezing is 0°C; boiling is 100°C • $\dfrac{°F - 32}{1.8} = °C$

2-4 Express international and traditional time.	*International time (military time)*:
	• 24-hour measure
	• Four digits: first two are hours, last two are minutes
	• No colon; no a.m. or p.m.
	Traditional time:
	• 12-hour measure
	• Colon between hours and minutes
	• Before noon is a.m., after noon is p.m.
	Converting between systems:
	• Traditional to international:
	  o Remove colon and a.m./p.m. label.
	  o From 12 a.m. to 12:59 a.m., replace 12 with 00.
	  o Place zero (0) in front of hours prior to 10:00 a.m.
	  o Add 12 hours to time from 1:00 p.m. to 12:00 a.m.
	• International to traditional:
	  o Before 1000, remove the leading zero, insert colon, label a.m.
	  o Between 1000 and 1159, insert colon, label a.m.
	  o After 1259, subtract 1200, insert colon, label p.m.

Homework

For exercises 1–10, determine if the unit of measurement refers to weight, volume, or length. (LO 2-1)

1. Kilogram _____
2. Millimeter _____
3. Microgram _____
4. Fluid ounce _____
5. Milliliter _____
6. Meter _____
7. Pound _____
8. Gram _____
9. Centimeter _____
10. Pint _____

For exercises 11–20, determine the dimensional analysis conversion factors. (LO 2-1, 2-2)

11. Grams to milligrams _____
12. Inches to feet _____
13. Centimeters to inches _____
14. Centimeters to millimeters _____
15. Milliliters to liters _____
16. Milliliters to teaspoons _____
17. Tablespoons to ounces _____
18. Milliliters to ounces _____
19. Cups to quarts _____
20. Fluid ounce to cup _____

For exercises 21–30, convert each quantity as indicated. (LO 2-2)

21. 2 t = _____ mL
22. 740 mg = _____ g
23. 0.5 mg = _____ mcg
24. 0.25 L = _____ mL
25. 2½ c = _____ mL
26. 6 in = _____ cm
27. 5 lb 12 oz = _____ kg
28. 86 kg = _____ lb
29. 75 mL = _____ oz
30. 8.5 cm = _____ mm

For exercises 31–35, determine if the statement is true or false. If the statement is false, correct it to make a true statement. (LO 2-2)

31. _____ A unit of heparin is the same quantity as a unit of insulin.
32. _____ Electrolytes are measured in milliequivalents (mEq).
33. _____ The size of a USP unit is always the same as an international unit.
34. _____ 2% lidocaine contains 2 g of lidocaine per 100 mL of solution.
35. _____ Epinephrine 1:10,000 contains 10,000 mg of epinephrine per 1 L of solution.

For exercises 36–41, convert the temperatures as indicated. Round to the nearest tenth. (LO 2-3)

36. 97.4°F = _____ °C
37. 37.4°C = _____ °F
38. 95°F = _____ °C
39. 38.2°C = _____ °F
40. 101.6°F = _____ °C
41. 36°C = _____ °F

For exercises 42–50, convert the time as indicated. (LO 2-4)

42. 6:05 a.m. to international time _____
43. 9:30 a.m. to international time _____
44. 3:35 p.m. to international time _____
45. 8:00 p.m. to international time _____
46. 12:08 a.m. to international time _____
47. 1004 to traditional time _____
48. 1735 to traditional time _____
49. 0415 to traditional time _____
50. 0010 to traditional time _____

NCLEX-Style Review Questions

For questions 1–4, select the best response.

1. The patient drank ½ pint of Postum®, had ½ cup of milk with cereal, and 6 oz of juice. How many mL were consumed?
   a. 320 mL
   b. 480 mL
   c. 540 mL
   d. 1,320 mL

2. The incision is $7\frac{1}{5}$ inches long. What is the length in cm?
   a. 3 cm
   b. 3.4 cm
   c. 16.5 cm
   d. 18 cm

3. The patient is scheduled for a 10:45 a.m. surgery, which is expected to last 3½–4 hours. During what hours, in international time, is the surgery expected to finish?
   a. 1345–1415
   b. 1415–1445
   c. 1530–1600
   d. 1530–1645

4. The baby weighs 12 lb 5 oz. How much does the baby weigh in kg?
   a. 5.6 kg
   b. 5.7 kg
   c. 27.1 kg
   d. 27.5 kg

For question 5–6, select all that apply.

5. Lipitor should be stored between 20°C and 25°C. Identify all of the following temperatures that are appropriate for storing Lipitor.
   a. 47°F
   b. 50°F
   c. 68°F
   d. 75°F

6. The nurse instructs the new mother to drink 2 L of fluid per day to support lactation. Which quantities are equivalent or roughly equivalent to 2 L?
   a. 2 qt
   b. 10 c
   c. 4 pt
   d. 2,000 mL
   e. 8 qt
   f. 32 fl oz

REFERENCES

Institute for Safe Medication Practices (ISMP). (2009). *ISMP calls for elimination of "teaspoonful" and other non-metric measurements to prevent errors.* Retrieved from https://www.ismp.org/pressroom/PR20090603.pdf

Institute for Safe Medication Practices (ISMP). (2011). *Statement on the use of metric measurements to prevent errors with oral liquids.* Retrieved from http://www.ismp.org/pressroom/PR20110808.pdf

MetricConversion.us. (2014). *Metric system history.* Retrieved from http://www.metricconversion.us/system.htm

NSW Therapeutic Advisory Group, Inc. (2007). *Percentage of medication orders that include error-prone abbreviations.* Retrieved from http://www.safetyandquality.gov.au/wp-content/uploads/2012/02/SAQ127_National_QUM_Indicators_V14_indicator3.3.pdf

Chapter 2   ANSWER KEY

Learning Activity 2-1
1. Gram
2. Meter
3. Liter

Learning Activity 2-2
1. 1,500 mg
2. 1.4 L
3. 1.2 cm

Learning Activity 2-3
1. 1,700 mg
2. 1.6 L
3. 1.5 cm

Learning Activity 2-4
1. 0.5681 kg
2. 0.75 L
3. 1.1 cm

Learning Activity 2-5
1. 9½ lb
2. 74 in
3. $1\frac{1}{3}$ T

Learning Activity 2-6
1. 5.7 kg
2. 165 cm
3. 1½ fl oz

Learning Activity 2-7
1. grams, milliliters, mL
2. is not
3. the World Health Organization (WHO)
4. grams, milliliters

Learning Activity 2-8
1. 38.9°C
2. 101.5°F
3. 36.2°C

Learning Activity 2-9
1. 0054
2. 5:21 p.m.
3. 2105

Homework

1. Weight
2. Length
3. Weight
4. Volume
5. Volume
6. Length
7. Weight
8. Weight
9. Length
10. Volume
11. 1,000 mg/1 g
12. 1 ft/12 in
13. 1 in/2.5 cm
14. 10 mm/1 cm
15. 1 L/1,000 mL
16. 1 t/5 mL
17. 1 fl oz/2 T
18. 1 fl oz/30 mL
19. 1 qt/4 c
20. 1 c/8 fl oz
21. 10 mL
22. 0.74 g
23. 500 mcg
24. 250 mL
25. 625 mL or 600 mL
26. 15 cm
27. 2.6 kg
28. 189.2 lb
29. 2½ oz
30. 85 mm
31. False. A unit of heparin is not the same quantity as a unit of insulin; units are medication specific.
32. True.
33. False. Many USP units are the same quantity as international units, but some USP units are not the same as international units.
34. True.
35. False. Epinephrine 1:10,000 has 1 g epinephrine : 10,000 mL solution.
36. 36.3°C
37. 99.3°F
38. 35°C
39. 100.8°F
40. 38.7°C
41. 96.8°F
42. 0605

43. 0930
44. 1535
45. 2000
46. 0008
47. 10:04 a.m.
48. 5:35 p.m.
49. 4:15 a.m.
50. 12:10 a.m.

NCLEX-Style Review Questions

1. c
   Rationale: Because ½ pt = 240 mL and ½ c = 120 mL and 6 oz = 180, mL, the total intake is 540 mL.
2. d
   Rationale: Because $7\frac{1}{5}$ inches converts to 7.2 inches and there are 2.5 cm/inch, the length is recorded as 18 cm.
3. b
   Rationale: 3½–4 hours after 10:45 a.m. is 2:15 p.m.–2:45 p.m., which converts to 1415–1445.
4. a
   Rationale: 5 oz is $\frac{5}{16}$ lb or 0.3 lb, therefore 12 lb 5 oz is 12.3 lb. 12.3 lb ÷ 2.2. lb/kg = 5.6 kg.
5. c, d
   Rationale: Because 20°C converts to 68°F and 25°C converts to 77°F, 68°F and 75°F are appropriate temperatures for storing Lipitor. The other temperatures, 47°F and 50°F, are too low.
6. a, c, d
   Rationale: 2 L = 2,000 mL; because 1 L is approximately 1 qt and there are 2 pt in 1 qt, the household equivalents of 2 L are 2 qt and 4 pt.

© Forfunlife/Shutterstock

Chapter 3

Medication Administration Equipment

CHAPTER OUTLINE

3-1   Enteral Medication Administration Equipment
    A.   Oral Devices
    B.   Enteral Tube Equipment

3-2   Parenteral Medication Administration Equipment
    A.   Equipment Used for Injections
        1. Syringes
        2. Needles
        3. Parenteral Medication Containers
    B.   Administration of Other Non-Enteral Medications

LEARNING OUTCOMES

Upon completion of the chapter, the student will be able to:

3-1   Differentiate enteral medication equipment.

3-2   Differentiate medication administration devices used for injections.

KEY TERMS

ampule

calibration

calibration spoon

cartridges

controlled substances

diluent

dropper

eccentric

enteral

filter needle

gauge

insulin pen

intradermal

intramuscular

intravenous

leading ring

medicine cup

meniscus

oral syringe

parenteral

route

souffle cup

subcutaneous

trailing ring

U-100

vial

viscosity

zero calibration

Case Consideration ... Calibration Conundrum

A nursing student, preparing to administer a volume of 2.2 mL, selected a 3 mL syringe on clinical day 1 and drew up the medication to two calibrations past the 2 mL mark. To administer the same medication on clinical day 2, the student selected a 5 mL syringe and drew up the medication to two calibrations past the 2 mL mark.

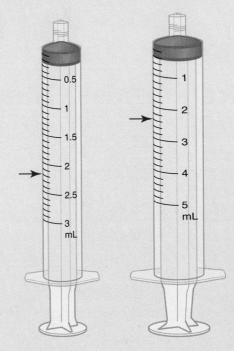

1. Where is the error in the nursing student's judgment on clinical day 2?

2. How can this error be avoided?

■ INTRODUCTION

Various types of equipment are available for medication administration. Selecting the proper device is based upon the medication type, amount, and **route** of administration. The route, named by the entry point, is the path by which the medication enters the body. The nurse must select appropriate equipment and accurately measure medications using each device.

3-1   Enteral Medication Administration Equipment

Enteral medication administration refers to medicine given through the gastrointestinal (GI) tract, which includes drugs given orally or through a tube into the stomach or intestines. Most enteral medications are supplied in the form of tablets, capsules, and liquids. Liquid medications are given with devices that are marked with **calibrations** or lines on equipment that represent a specific unit of measurement.

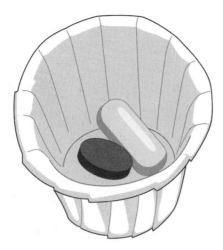

FIGURE 3-1   Solid oral medications, such as tablets and capsules, can be administered with a soufflé cup.

Oral Devices

- **Soufflé cup**—A small paper or plastic cup used to administer solid oral medications (**Figure 3-1**).

- **Medicine cup**—A plastic measuring cup used to administer liquid oral medications; medicine cups are open containers marked with household and metric calibrations (**Figure 3-2**). Liquids poured into an open container may form a **meniscus**, or concave curve in the upper surface of the liquid (**Figure 3-3**). Medicine cups should be placed on a flat surface and liquids should be poured at eye level, measured at the bottom of the meniscus (**Figure 3-4**). Medicine cups are calibrated in 2.5 mL increments up to 10 mL and in 5 mL increments up to 30 mL.

- **Dropper**—A device used to deliver small quantities of liquid medication; droppers have different sized openings that produce different quantities of medication with each drop. Because drop size varies, medications, such as children's vitamins, that are administered via dropper are often packaged with the device to ensure accurate dosing. Some droppers are calibrated with milliliter markings

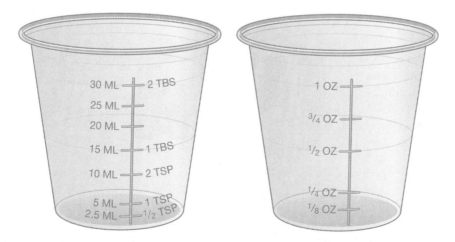

FIGURE 3-2   A medicine cup shows milliliter and teaspoon calibrations on one side and ounce calibrations on the other side.

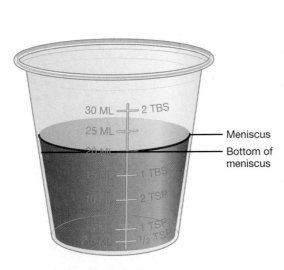

FIGURE 3-3 This liquid medication, in the amount of 20 mL, is measured at the bottom of the meniscus.

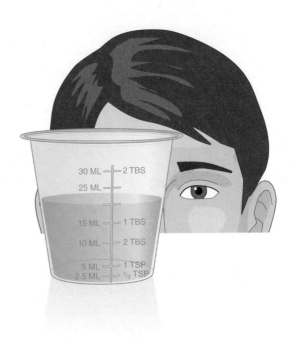

FIGURE 3-4 To accurately measure liquid medication, the nurse places the medicine cup on a flat surface and pours the prescribed amount at eye level.

(**Figure 3-5**). To avoid dosage errors, droppers should not be interchanged, but should be used only with the medication with which they are packaged.

■ **Calibrated spoon**—A device calibrated in 2.5 mL increments and fractional teaspoons that has a capacity of 10 mL (2 teaspoons [t]); designed for pediatric medication administration, some calibrated spoons are shaped like animals and have "legs" that allow the device to sit sideways without spilling (**Figure 3-6**).

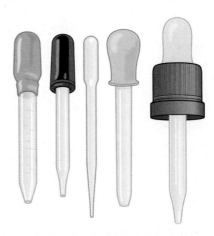

FIGURE 3-5 Because there is no standard drop size, droppers have varying calibrations and therefore should be used to measure only the medication with which they have been packaged.

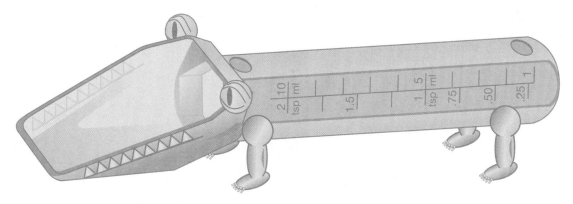

FIGURE 3-6   This "Kyle the Crocodile" medicine spoon appeals to children.

WARNING!

Use Calibrated Equipment for Household Medication Administration!

Researchers, testing the reliability of the average household spoons, asked student patients at a university health clinic to pour out 5 milliliters of cold medicine into different-sized kitchen spoons. The research revealed that participants underdosed by 8.4% when using the medium-sized spoon and overdosed by 11.6% when using the larger spoon (Khan, 2010). Repeating this dosing error for a drug that is ordered several times per day for a multiple-day regimen can be problematic. Overdosing can lead to troublesome side effects, while underdosing may undertreat or not treat the problem. Underdosing an antibiotic can lead to development of drug-resistant bacteria, ultimately rendering the medication ineffective. This study reveals the importance of using a calibrated device— a medicine cup, oral syringe, or dosing spoon— to administer oral liquid medication.

- **Oral syringe**—Used to deliver 5 to 10 mL of liquid and available in two sizes, 5 mL and 10 mL; calibrated in tenths of a milliliter and fractional teaspoon measurements, oral syringes are designed with specific features to differentiate them from syringes used for injections.

  - An **eccentric** or off-center tip alerts the nurse that a needle should not be attached to this syringe (**Figure 3-7**).

  - Some oral syringes are clear and labeled "for oral use only" to distinguish them from syringes used for injection (**Figure 3-8**).

Clinical CLUE

To determine the appropriate device for administration of medication:

- First compare the volume of the medication ordered to the device volume.

- Then determine if the device calibration is appropriate.

For example, to administer 9 mL of oral medicine, the nurse knows that an oral syringe, calibrated spoon, and medicine cup all have the capacity to hold 9 mL. However, because a medicine cup and some calibrated spoons do not have a 9-mL calibration, the nurse should select an oral syringe for administration of this medication.

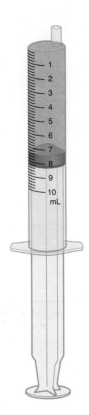

FIGURE 3-7   An oral syringe with an eccentric (off-center) tip differentiates it from a syringe to be used for injections.

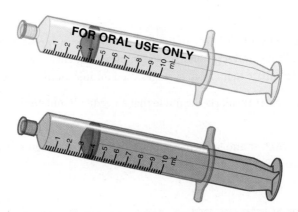

FIGURE 3-8   Oral syringes are distinguished from syringes used for injection by tinted color or a label on the barrel stating, "for oral use only."

LEARNING ACTIVITY 3-1 Select the appropriate device to deliver the amount of medication indicated in questions 1–4. Select all that apply.

1.   2 tab   _____   a.   medicine cup
2.   1 oz   _____   b.   oral syringe
3.   4 mL   _____   c.   calibrated spoon
4.   2 t   _____   d.   soufflé cup
                               e.   dropper

Enteral Tube Equipment

When medications intended for absorption in the stomach or intestines cannot be delivered by mouth, they can be administered through a tube (**Figure 3-9**). Types of enteral tubes used to deliver nutrients and medications are reviewed in Chapter 8. Equipment used to administer medications through enteral tubes varies according to the type and amount of medication to be administered. To administer solid medication through an enteral tube, the following equipment is needed:

- A pill crusher to crush solid medications (**Figure 3-10**)

- Liquid (usually water) to liquefy crushed medications (**Figure 3-11**)

- Catheter-tip syringe or bulb syringe to inject medication into feeding tube (**Figure 3-12**) or a Luer lock syringe and adapter inserted into feeding tube (**Figure 3-13**). By removing the barrel or bulb from these syringes (**Figure 3-14**), the nurse creates a funnel through which medications can be poured into an enteral tube.

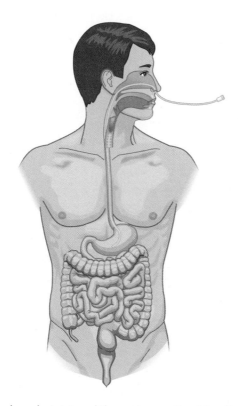

FIGURE 3-9   Medications can be administered through an enteral feeding tube when a patient is unable to take medications orally.

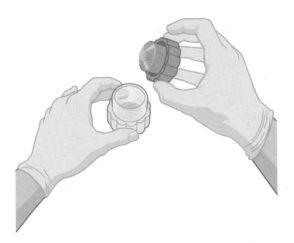

FIGURE 3-10   Pill crushers can make a powder from a solid medication.

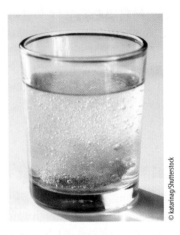

FIGURE 3-11   In order to administer solid medication through an enteral tube, the nurse must crush and liquefy the pill.

To administer liquid medication through an enteral tube, the following equipment is needed:

- A medicine cup or oral syringe to measure liquid medication

- A catheter-tip syringe, bulb syringe, or Luer lock syringe with which to inject the medication into the enteral tube (**Figures 3-15** and **3-16**)

The procedure for administration of medication through an enteral tube is provided in Chapter 8.

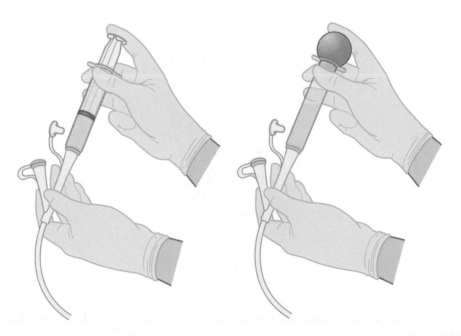

FIGURE 3-12   Catheter-tip and bulb syringes can be used to administer medications through an enteral tube.

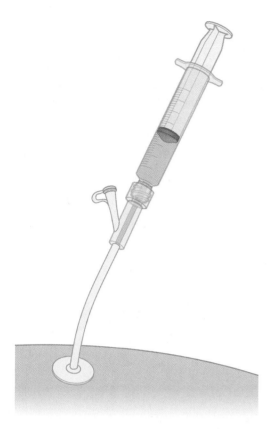

FIGURE 3-13   Some enteral tubes have an adapter at the end into which a medication can be delivered through a Luer lock syringe.

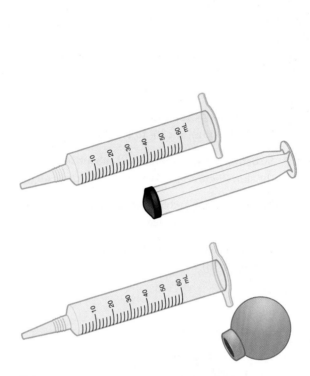

FIGURE 3-14   By removing the bulb or barrel from a large syringe, the nurse creates a funnel through which medications can be poured into an enteral tube.

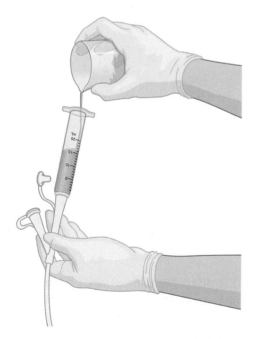

FIGURE 3-15   The nurse removes the bulb from a bulb syringe before attaching it to the feeding tube, then pours the medication into the open device and allows the medication to flow by gravity.

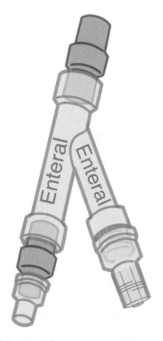

FIGURE 3-16   The nurse may inject medication into an enteral tube through a Luer lock adapter.

3-2   Parenteral Medication Administration Equipment

The word **parenteral** means outside the digestive tract. Parenteral medications, when administered, enter the bloodstream without first entering the intestines. Although parenteral literally refers to any non-enteral route, this text will generally refer to parenteral drug forms as injectable medications. A discussion of equipment used for administration of non-injectable, non-enteral medications is included in this section, but it is referred to as "other non-enteral medications."

The most common parenteral (injection) routes of medication administration include:

- **Intradermal**—Abbreviated ID, an intradermal injection is inserted into the dermis (connective tissue within the skin), at a 10- to 15-degree angle (**Figure 3-17**).

- **Subcutaneous**—Abbreviated subcut, a subcutaneous injection is delivered below all of the layers of the skin (Figure 3-17) at a 45- to 90-degree angle.

- **Intramuscular**—Abbreviated IM, an intramuscular injection is injected directly into a muscle (Figure 3-17) at a 90-degree angle.

- **Intravenous**—Abbreviated IV, an intravenous injection is administered directly into a vein (**Figure 3-18**).

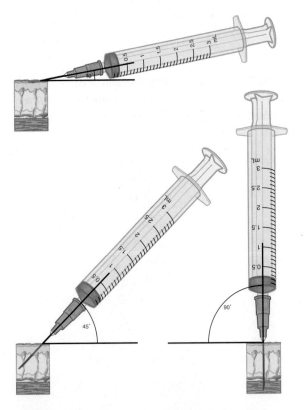

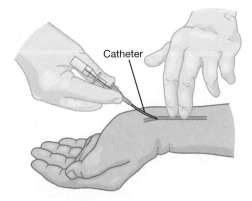

FIGURE 3-17   An intradermal injection is administered into the dermal layer; a subcutaneous injection is administered into the fat and connective tissue that lies below the skin; an intramuscular injection enters the deep vascular muscle bed.

FIGURE 3-18   Intravenous medications are administered directly into the bloodstream through a flexible catheter tip that is inserted into a vein.

Equipment Used for Injections

The nurse is responsible for selecting the proper medication administration equipment. Syringes and needles necessary for parenteral medication administration vary in size. Equipment selection depends upon multiple factors including:

- Route—Small-volume syringes are used for the subcut, IM, and IV routes, while large-volume syringes are typically used for IV medication administration. The length of the needle used to administer an injection is determined by route. The depth of a subcut injection is less than 1 inch, while the depth of an IM injection for the average adult is 1 inch or more. Therefore, the needle length for a subcut injection ranges from $\frac{3}{8}$ to $\frac{5}{8}$ inches and the needle length for the average adult IM injection ranges from 1 to 1½ inches.

- Volume—The maximum injectable amount into an adult subcutaneous site is 1 mL, therefore, small-volume syringes are often used for subcutaneous injections. The maximum volume that can be administered into an adult muscle is 3 mL, making the 3 mL syringe the most common device used to deliver IM injections.

- Viscosity—The **viscosity** or thickness of the solution to be administered will determine the needle **gauge** (diameter) required to administer a medication. Needles with lower gauge numbers have larger diameters and are needed to administer viscous medications. Needle gauges are differentiated in **TABLE 3-1**.

- Medication to be administered—Insulin may require the use of an insulin syringe. Medications packaged in cartridges may require special devices to deliver the medication (**Figure 3-19**).

Syringes

Syringes are available in a variety of sizes, including 0.5 mL, 1 mL, 3 mL, 5 or 6mL, 10 or 12 mL, 20 mL, 30 mL, 40 mL, and 60 mL. Syringes are calibrated in milliliters and the calibrations vary with size. Small-volume syringes deliver amounts of 1 mL or less and are calibrated to hundredths of a milliliter, while larger syringes have larger calibration increments.

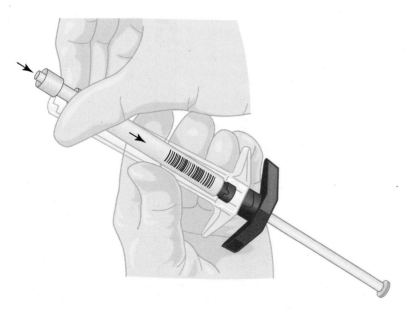

FIGURE 3-19   The nurse inserts a medication cartridge into the appropriate device in preparation for medication administration.

Tuberculin syringe.   Because the 1 mL syringe is typically used for tuberculin (TB) testing, it has been given the name "tuberculin (or TB) syringe." It is used for the administration of:

- Allergen extracts for allergy testing

- Heparin

- Hormones

- Vaccines

- Small volumes of medication given to children or critical care patients

Figure 3-20 shows each large calibration on the tuberculin syringe is 0.1 milliliter and each small calibration is 0.01 milliliters. Tuberculin syringes are available in two sizes: 1 mL and 0.5 mL (**Figure 3-21**). The smaller the volume to be administered, the greater the accuracy in measurement may be needed. Because the scale on the 0.5 mL syringe is expanded, it provides increased measurement accuracy and is, therefore, meant to be used to administer volumes less than 0.5 milliliters.

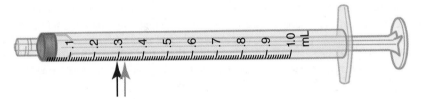

FIGURE 3-20   The 0.3 mL calibration (red arrow) is one of ten 0.1 mL increments on this syringe; the 0.33 mL calibration (blue arrow) is one of one hundred 0.01-mL increments on this syringe that is used to deliver small volumes of medication.

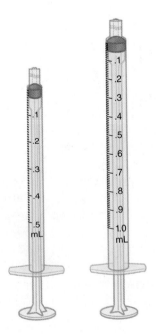

FIGURE 3-21   Although the 0.5 mL syringe holds half the volume of a 1 mL syringe, it is more than half the length of a 1 mL syringe, allowing for an expanded scale.

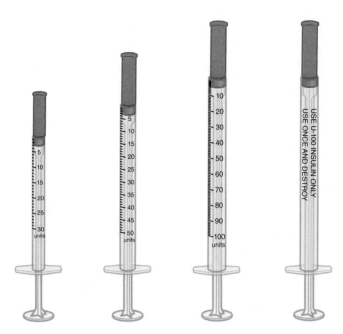

FIGURE 3-22   While the low-dose (30-unit and 50-unit) syringes have a lower volume capacity with their more narrow diameters, they are almost as long as a standard 1 mL insulin syringe, allowing for an expanded scale.

Insulin syringes.   *Insulin syringes are used only to deliver units of insulin.* To decrease dosage error, insulin syringes are calibrated in units and not milliliters. Insulin syringes are available in three sizes: 100 unit (1 mL), 50 unit (0.5 mL), and 30 unit (0.3 mL) (**Figure 3-22**). The 100-unit (1 mL) syringe is sometimes referred to as a "standard" insulin syringe. The 50-unit (0.5 mL) and 30-unit (0.3 mL) insulin syringes are called low-dose insulin syringes because, with their expanded scale, they are designed to deliver low doses of insulin with greater accuracy than the standard insulin syringe. If available, a 50-unit (0.5 mL) insulin syringe should be used to administer doses of 50 units or less and a 30-unit (0.3 mL) insulin syringe should be used to administer doses of 30 units or less. Insulin syringes are used for administration of **U-100** insulin only, which is insulin in the dosage strength of 100 units per milliliter.

Standard 3 mL syringes.   Because 3 mL is the maximum amount that should be injected into an adult muscle, the 3 mL syringe is the most common syringe used to deliver intramuscular injections. **Figure 3-23** displays a 3 mL syringe with a preattached needle and shows the parts of a syringe. The barrel or body of the syringe is marked with calibrations indicating volume amount. The beginning of the barrel is known as **zero calibration**. Each calibration after zero calibration on a 3 mL syringe is 0.1 mL or one-tenth milliliter. The plunger is used to pull fluid into the syringe or to eject fluid out of the syringe. The plunger has a black rubber tip with a leading ring and a trailing ring. The **leading ring** is closest to the needle, while the **trailing ring** is the ring farthest from the needle. Medication volumes are determined by the reading the calibration on the syringe barrel at the location of the leading ring.

Many syringes have safety devices that, when activated, will prevent needlestick injury. **Figures 3-23** and **3-24** show a needlestick prevention safety device. After administration of an injection, the nurse should activate the safety device (Figure 3-24 and **Figure 3-25**). Safety syringes are available in multiple sizes and styles.

Large-volume syringes.   Large-volume syringes include syringes with the capacity of 5 or 6 mL, 10 or 12 mL, 20 mL, 30 mL, 40 mL, and 60 mL. These syringes are used to deliver larger volumes of medications that are often ordered to be given via the intravenous route. Medications may be added to a primary

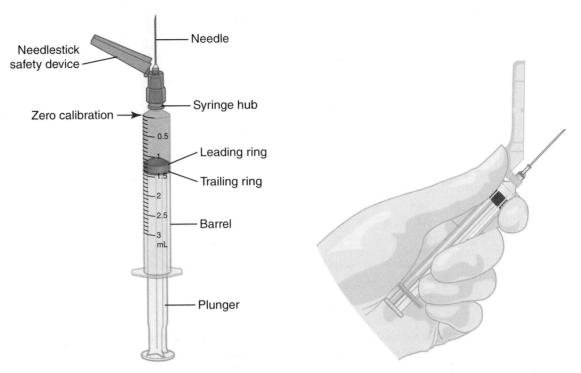

FIGURE 3-23 This syringe contains 1.2 mL of medication as revealed by the location of the leading ring which is two calibrations past the 1 mL mark.

FIGURE 3-24 The nurse activates the needlestick safety device by pushing up on it with the thumb or index finger.

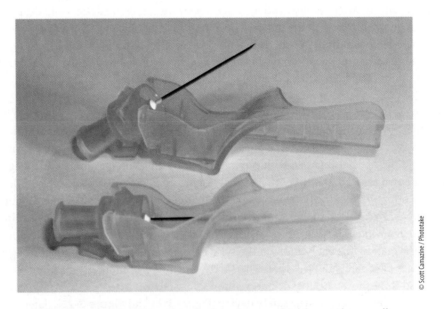

FIGURE 3-25 Activating a needlestick safety device places a shield over the needle.

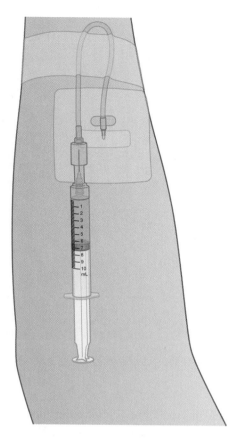

FIGURE 3-26   This 10 mL syringe, calibrated at 0.2 mL increments, contains 6.4 mL of an intravenous medication to be injected directly into an existing IV line.

IV infusion or may be administered intermittently through a secondary IV or by directly injecting a medication into an IV line (**Figure 3-26**). A needleless, large-volume syringe may also be used to administer medications via enteral tube as shown in Figure 3-13.

Rounding RULE

When medication volumes must be rounded, rounding is done according to syringe selection:

- Volumes less than 1 mL should be rounded to hundredths, because that is the calibration of a 1 mL syringe.
- Volumes of 1 to 12 mL should be rounded to tenths, because that is the calibration of the 3 mL, 5 to 6 mL, and 10 to 12 mL syringes.
- Volumes greater than 10 mL (or 12 mL, depending on manufacturer) should be rounded to the whole number, because that is the typical calibration of these large-volume syringes (see **Figure 3-27**).

Needles

Needles are used to draw up and administer medication. Needle sizes vary in length and gauge (G). For example, a 25 G needle has an outer diameter of 0.02 inches, whereas an 18 G needle has an outer diameter of 0.05 inches. For injections, depending on the size of the patient and the medication route (ID, IM, or subcut), the nurse will use a needle that is $\frac{3}{8}$ to 1.5 inches in length and 20 to 30 gauge. To

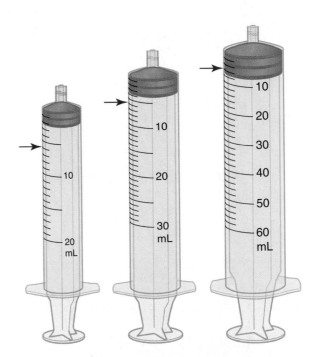

FIGURE 3-27 The 6 mL marking on each of these syringes is an example of the 1 mL or 2 mL calibration on large-volume syringes.

mix and draw up powdered and or viscous medications, the nurse may use a wider gauge (e.g., 18 G) needle, but should change the needle to a smaller gauge (e.g., 21 G) if the medication is to be administered intramuscularly. As revealed in Table 3-1, which differentiates needle sizes used for various injection types, the larger the gauge, the smaller the needle diameter and, conversely, the smaller the gauge, the larger the diameter.

TABLE 3-1	Needle Sizes for Injection Types				
Injection Type	Needle Diameter	Needle Length	Maximum Injection Volume	Injection Location	Needle Angle
ID	25–27 G	⅜–⅝ inch	0.1 mL	Inner aspect of forearm	5–15°
Subcut for infant/child	25–30 G	⅜ inch	0.5 mL	Anterior lateral thigh	45–90°
Subcut for adult	25–30 G	½–⅝ inch	1 mL	Thigh, upper arm, abdomen	45–90°
IM for infant/child	22–25 G	⅝–1 inch	0.5–1 mL	Vastus lateralis	90°
IM for adult	20–23 G	1–1½ inches	1 mL	Deltoid	90°
			3 mL	Ventrogluteal, vastus lateralis	

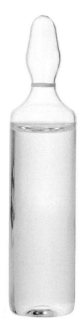

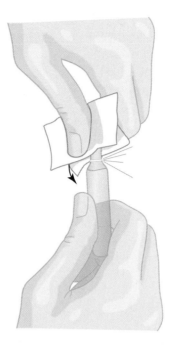

FIGURE 3-28   The ampule is scored at the neck to facilitate opening the device.

FIGURE 3-29   The thumb is placed against the scored neck and the neck is snapped away from (not toward) the nurse.

Parenteral Medication Containers

Parenteral medication is packaged in a variety of devices. An **ampule** (**Figure 3-28**) is a small glass container that contains a typical single dose of medication. Some narcotics are packaged in ampules to provide enhanced management of **controlled substances**—drugs that are regulated because of their potential for abuse. An ampule is opened by snapping the neck of the container as shown in **Figure 3-29**. To prevent injury, a plastic protective sleeve, 2 × 2 gauze, or alcohol wipes are placed around the neck, and the ampule is snapped away from the nurse to open it. Medication is withdrawn from an ampule with a **filter needle**, a needle that contains a filter inside to separate from the medication any glass fragments that occur as a result of breaking open the ampule.

A **vial** is a multiple-dose or single-dose container (**Figure 3-30**) of powdered or liquid medication with a rubber stopper (also called a diaphragm) on top. A powdered and viscous (thick) liquid medication

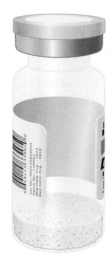

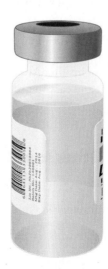

FIGURE 3-30   Medication vials contain single or multiple doses of liquid or powdered medication.

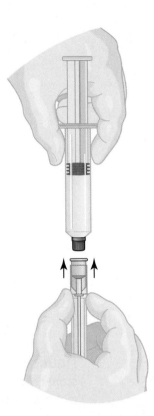

FIGURE 3-31   After calculating the amount of medication needed, the nurse discards what is not needed and then will attach a needle to this prefilled syringe to administer this medication.

must be mixed with an appropriate **diluent** (diluting agent), such as sterile water or sodium chloride, by injecting it through the rubber stopper.

A **cartridge** is a device that is prefilled with a typical single dose of medication. Drugs that are packaged in cartridges are administered with reusable devices into which the cartridge is loaded. Prefilled syringes (**Figure 3-31**) also provide a single typical dose of medication, but are distinguished from cartridges in that they come packaged with a plunger, therefore they do not need to be loaded into a syringe holder for medication administration. Many medications are available in prefilled syringes, including vaccines and emergency medications, such as atropine. Some advantages of using cartridges and prefilled syringes include ease of use, reduced risk of dosage error with a single-dose system, and reduced medication waste.

An **insulin pen** (**Figure 3-32**), an example of a prefilled syringe, is a device used to administer insulin. After the pen is loaded with an insulin cartridge and primed (air expelled), the dial on the pen is adjusted to the ordered dose of insulin. After a disposable needle is attached to the device, the insulin can be administered. Convenient and easy to use, this device is widely used for home insulin administration. The "dial-the-dose" feature on the pen reduces the incidence of dosage errors. More detail regarding insulin pens is included in Chapter 14.

Administration of Other Non-Enteral Medications

Other non-enteral medications that are commonly administered include:

- Medications absorbed through the skin:

    - Topical ointments and creams (**Figure 3-33**)

    - Transdermal patches containing medication (**Figure 3-34**)

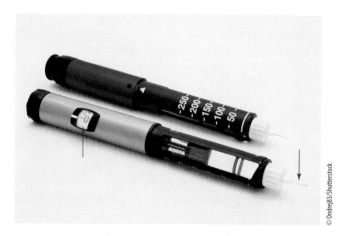

FIGURE 3-32   After dialing the correct dose (red arrow) and adding a 31 G, $\frac{5}{16}$-inch needle (blue arrow), specially made for this device, the patient can self-administer insulin.

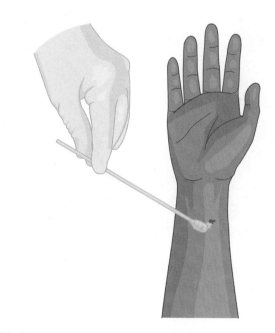

FIGURE 3-33   A tongue blade or cotton-tipped applicator may be used to administer topical medications.

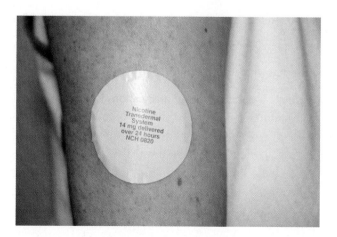

FIGURE 3-34   The transdermal patch, a medicated adhesive patch applied to the skin to deliver a specific dose of medication, must be applied whole; that is, it may not be cut or altered.

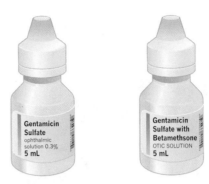

FIGURE 3-35 Medications given via dropper, such as eye (ophthalmic) drops and ear (otic) drops, are ordered by the number of drops.

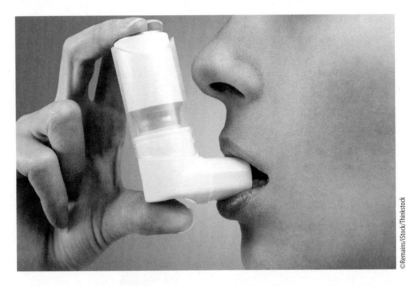

FIGURE 3-36 A meter-dosed inhaler (MDI) is used to deliver inhalant medications; a measure dose of medication is provided with each inhalation.

- Medicines given via dropper into the eye and ear (**Figure 3-35**)

- Inhaled medications administered through a variety of devices (**Figures 3-36** and **3-37**)

- Rectal suppositories inserted by gloved hand using lubricant (**Figure 3-38**)

- Vaginal suppositories inserted with an applicator (**Figure 3-39**)

Equipment used to administer other non-enteral medications is sometimes packaged with the medication. Calculations are rarely required to administer these non-enteral medications. However, in order to administer the proper dose of non-enteral medications, the nurse should follow the instructions supplied with the medication order and with the equipment used to deliver the medication.

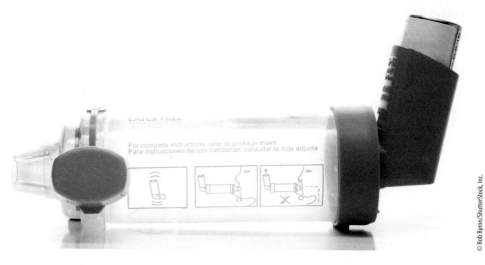

FIGURE 3-37   A spacer may be attached to an MDI to facilitate delivery of inhaled medications.

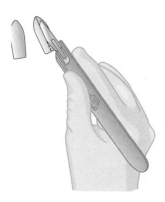

FIGURE 3-38   If a partial (half) dose of a rectal suppository is needed per provider order, it must be cut lengthwise to promote proper absorption.

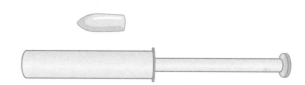

FIGURE 3-39   An applicator is used by the nurse or patient to insert a vaginal suppository.

LEARNING ACTIVITY 3-2   Select the appropriate device to deliver the volume of medication indicated in questions 1–4.

1.   30 units of U-100 insulin   _____   a.   5-mL syringe
2.   0.75 mL of medication   _____   b.   Standard 1 mL insulin syringe
3.   3.8 mL of medication   _____   c.   3 mL syringe
4.   85 units of insulin   _____   d.   Low-dose insulin syringe
                            e.   Tuberculin syringe

LEARNING ACTIVITY 3-3 Answer the questions regarding the volume of medication contained in each syringe.

1.   Which syringe contains 3.4 mL of medication?

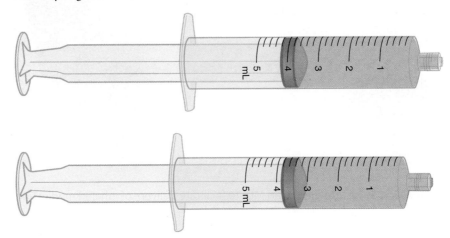

2.   Which syringe contains 1.5 mL of medication?

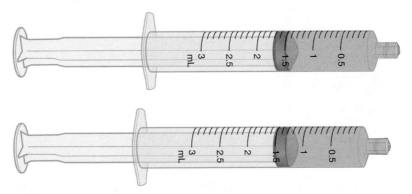

3.   What volume of medication is contained in this syringe?

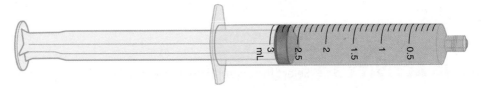

4.   What volume of medication is contained in this syringe?

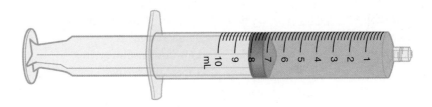

Calibration Conundrum ... Case Closure

It is important to differentiate syringe calibrations. The 3 mL syringe calibrations are 0.1 mL and the 5 mL syringe calibrations are 0.2 mL. To draw up 2.2 mL in a 3 mL syringe, the student correctly draws up the medication to the second calibration past the 2 mL marking. However, to draw up 2.2 mL in a 5 mL syringe, the student should draw up to the first calibration past the 2 mL marking. Drawing up the medication two calibrations past the 2 mL marking will deliver 2.4 mL of medication and will administer a 0.2 mL overdose. This situation can be avoided by learning to differentiate syringe calibrations and by careful syringe selection during the medication administration process.

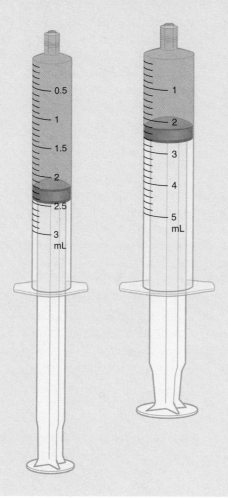

Chapter Summary

Learning Outcomes	Points to Remember
3-1 Differentiate enteral medication equipment.	*Enteral*— refers to medication given through the GI tract *Oral devices:* • Soufflé cup— paper or plastic cup for pills • Medicine cup— plastic cup with metric and household calibrations (lines that represent a unit of measurement); volume is read at the meniscus (concave curve in the upper surface of the liquid) • Dropper— device that delivers drops of medication; because drop size varies, should be used *only* with medication with which it is packaged • Calibrated spoon— device calibrated in milliliters and teaspoons used to deliver up to 10 mL (2 t) • Oral syringe— device calibrated in tenths of a milliliter and fractional teaspoons used to deliver up to 10 mL (2 t); may be differentiated from injection syringes with: an eccentric (off-center) tip, a tinted color, or "for oral use only" printed on barrel

3-2 Differentiate medication administration devices used for injections.	*Parenteral*— refers to medications given outside the GI tract; most common indicates the injection route
	Most common routes:
	• Intradermal (ID)— into the dermis
	• Subcutaneous (subcut)— below the skin, into the fat
	• Intramuscular (IM)— into the muscle
	• Intravenous (IV)— into the vein
	Equipment selection for parenteral medication administration depends upon: route (ID, subcut, IM, or IV), volume of medication, viscosity (thickness) of medication, medication to be administered, size of patient.
	Small-volume syringes:
	• 1 mL syringe (tuberculin syringe)
	  o Each calibration is 0.01 mL
	  o Also available in 0.5 mL size to deliver volumes of 0.5 mL or less
	• Insulin syringes
	  o Available in standard 100-unit and low-dose 50-unit and 30-unit sizes
	  o Used to administer U-100 (100 units/mL) insulin only
	  o Calibrated in units
	• 3 mL syringe
	  o Each calibration is 0.1 mL
	  o Most common syringe for IM injections because maximum injectable amount into adult muscle is 3 mL
	Large-volume syringes:
	• 5 mL to 12 mL syringes— each calibration is 0.2 mL
	• 20 mL, 30 mL, 40 mL, and 60 mL syringes
	  o Each calibration is 1 or 2 mL
	  o May be used to administer medications via enteral feeding tube

Needles—vary in length and gauge (outer diameter); the higher the gauge, the smaller the outer diameter

- Intradermal
  - $\frac{3}{8}$–$\frac{5}{8}$-inch, 25–27 G, 0.1 mL at 5–15°
- Subcutaneous
  - $\frac{5}{8}$-inch, 25 G, 1 mL for adult injection at 45–90°
  - $\frac{3}{8}$-inch, 27–30 G, 0.5 mL for infant/child injection at 45–90°
- Intramuscular
  - 1 to 1½ inch, 20–23 G, 3 mL for adult injection at 90°
  - $\frac{5}{8}$–1 inch, 22–25 G for infant/child injection at 90°

Ampule— glass container holding a typical single dose of medication; after opening the device by snapping the neck, medication is withdrawn with a filter needle (needle that filters glass fragments from medication)

Vial— container with a rubber stopper on top; medication is withdrawn by inserting a needle into the rubber stopper

Cartridges and pre-filled syringes— contain a typical single dose of medication; advantages include reducing medication waste and minimizing the chance of dosage error

Homework

For exercises 1–15, determine if the statement is true or false. If the statement is false, correct it to make a true statement. (LO 3-1)

1. _____ Enteral medication administration refers to medicine given directly into the bloodstream.

2. _____ To ensure accurate measurement of medication in a medicine cup, the medication should be poured at eye level and measured at the top of the meniscus.

3. _____ Droppers should be used only with the medication with which they are packaged.

4. _____ Tablets and capsules are administered in a soufflé cup.

5. _____ It is the responsibility of the nurse to select the appropriate equipment and accurately measure medications.

6. _____ The oral syringe can measure volumes of liquid medication up to 1 ounce.

7. _____ A Luer lock syringe tip alerts the nurse that a needle should not be attached to this syringe.

8. _____ The appropriate device for administration of 7 mL of liquid medication is the medicine cup.

9. _____ An oral syringe is calibrated in tenths of a milliliter and fractional teaspoon measurements.

10. _____ Calibrations are markings or lines on equipment that represent a specific unit of measurement.

11. _____ The medicine cup may be used to measure liquid volumes of less than 1 milliliter.

12. _____ The medicine cup is marked with both household and metric calibrations.

13. _____ Enteral tubes can be used for medication administration when medicine cannot be given by mouth.

14. _____ One teaspoon of liquid medication can be accurately measured in all calibrated oral medication administration equipment.

15. _____ A soufflé cup is calibrated to deliver volumes up to 1 tablespoon of liquid.

For exercises 16–30, determine if the statement is true or false. If the statement is false, correct it to make a true statement. (LO 3-2)

16. _____ A subcutaneous injection is delivered below the layer of muscle.

17. _____ Parenteral drug forms are typically injectable medications.

18. _____ The 3 mL syringe is the most common device used to administer IM injections.

19. _____ The more viscous the solution to be injected, the higher the needle gauge number will be needed to administer the medication.

20. _____ The primary purpose of safety syringes is to promote accurate medication administration.

21. _____ Prefilled syringes need to be loaded into a syringe holder for medication administration.

22. _____ A controlled substance is a drug that is regulated because of its potential for abuse.

23. _____ Because the 1 mL tuberculin syringe and the 1 mL insulin syringe are identical in size, they can be used interchangeably.

24. _____ Low-dose insulin syringes are used to administer U-100 insulin doses of 50 units or less.

25. _____ Each calibration on a 3 mL syringe is one-tenth milliliter.

26. _____ Medication volumes are determined by reading the calibration on the trailing ring.

27. _____ Medication is withdrawn from an ampule by inserting a needle into the rubber stopper on top.

28. _____ Each calibration on a 1 mL syringe is one-tenth milliliter.

29. _____ Insulin syringes are calibrated in units.

30. _____ Cartridges and prefilled syringes are designed to reduce medication waste and the risk of dosage error.

For exercises 31–40, mark the equipment where you would measure the required volume. (LO 3-1, 3-2)

31. 15 mL

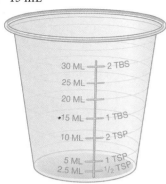

32. 15 mL

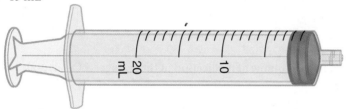

33. 1.6 mL

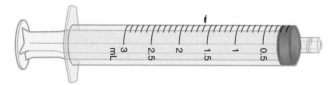

34. 1.6 mL

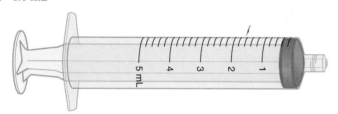

35. 0.7 mL

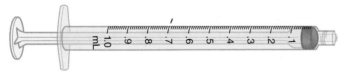

36. 0.7 mL

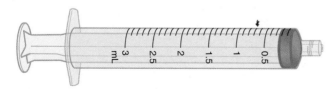

37. 1½ tsp

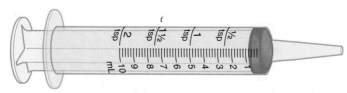

38. 1½ tsp

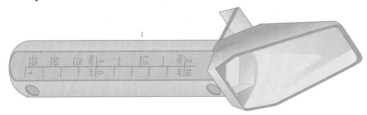

39. 0.65 mL

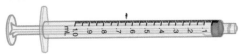

40. 65 units of U-100 insulin

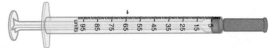

For exercises 41–50, identify the syringe type and the volume of medication in the syringe. (LO 3-1, 3-2)

41.

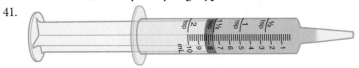

Syringe type: _____ Volume: _____

42.

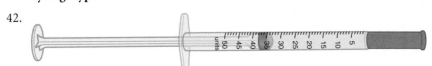

Syringe type: _____ Volume: _____

43.

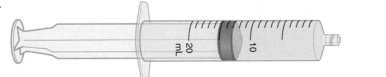

Syringe type: _____ Volume: _____

44.

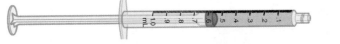

Syringe type: _____ Volume: _____

45.

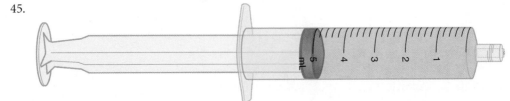

Syringe type: _____ Volume: _____

46.

Syringe type: _____ Volume: _____

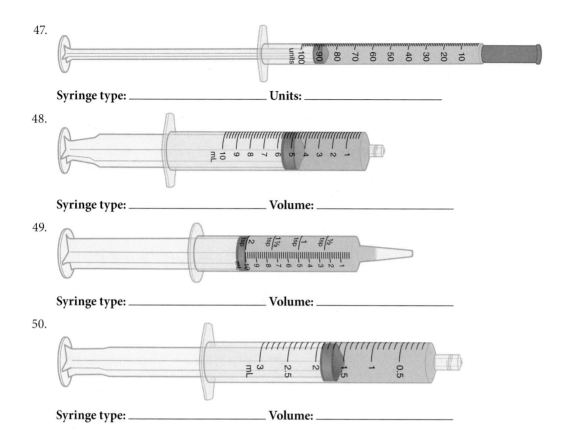

47.

Syringe type: _____ Units: _____

48.

Syringe type: _____ Volume: _____

49.

Syringe type: _____ Volume: _____

50.

Syringe type: _____ Volume: _____

NCLEX-Style Review Questions

For questions 1–4, select the best response.

1. The nurse preparing to administer an intramuscular injection to an adult patient should select which needle:
   a. 16 gauge
   b. 18 gauge
   c. 23 gauge
   d. 27 gauge

2. To administer 2 mL of medication intramuscularly to an adult, the nurse will select a:
   a. Small-volume syringe and a ⅞-inch needle
   b. 3 mL syringe and 1½-inch needle
   c. Tuberculin syringe and 1-inch needle
   d. Large-volume syringe and a ⅝-inch needle

3. To administer 15 mL of oral medication, the nurse will use a:
   a. Medicine cup
   b. Oral syringe
   c. Calibrated spoon
   d. All of the above

4. When drawing up a parenteral medication, the nurse will measure the medication:
   a. From the leading ring to the trailing ring
   b. From the zero calibration to the leading ring
   c. From the zero calibration to the trailing ring
   d. At the meniscus

For question 5–6, select all that apply.

5. Which factors will the nurse consider when determining the equipment needed to administer a parenteral injection?
   a. Route
   b. Volume of medication
   c. Viscosity of medication
   d. Type of medication
   e. Size of the patient

6. The physician orders 2 teaspoons of oral antibiotic. The nurse selects which device(s) to administer this medication?
   a. Oral syringe
   b. Calibrated spoon
   c. Medicine cup
   d. Dropper
   e. 10 mL syringe

REFERENCES

Khan, A. (2010, January 4). A spoonful of medicine may be too much or not enough. Retrieved from http://latimesblogs.latimes.com/booster_shots/2010/01/spoon-teaspoon-medicine-tylenol-study-annals-internal-medicine-cornell.html

Perry, A. G., & Potter, P. A. (2012). *Clinical nursing skills and techniques* (8th ed.). St. Louis: Elsevier.

Potter, P. A., Perry, A. G, Stockhart, P., & Hall, A. (2013). *Fundamentals of nursing* (8th ed.). St. Louis: Elsevier.

Chapter 3 ANSWER KEY

Learning Activity 3-1
1. d
2. a
3. b
4. a, b, c

Learning Activity 3-2
1. d
2. e
3. a
4. b

Learning Activity 3-3
1. The second syringe, with the leading ring at the 3.4 mL calibration, contains 3.4 mL of medication.
2. The first syringe, with the leading ring at the 1.5 mL calibration, contains 1.5 mL of medication. NOTE: The space between the leading ring and the trailing ring is dead space and contains no medication.
3. 2.7 mL
4. 7.2 mL

Homework

1. False: Enteral medication administration refers to medicine given directly into the gastrointestinal (GI) tract.
2. False: To ensure accurate measurement of medication in a medicine cup, the medication should be poured at eye level and measured at the bottom of the meniscus.
3. True
4. True
5. True
6. False: The oral syringe can measure volumes of liquid medication up to 10 mL. The medicine cup can measure volumes up to 1 ounce.
7. False: The eccentric or off-centered tip alerts the nurse that a needle should not be attached to this syringe.
8. False: The appropriate device for administration of 7 mL of liquid medication is an oral syringe.
9. True
10. True
11. False: The 1 mL syringe should be used to measure liquid volumes of less than 1 mL.
12. True
13. True
14. False: One teaspoon cannot be accurately measured in all calibrated oral medication administration equipment. Droppers may not be calibrated in teaspoons.
15. False: A medicine cup is calibrated to deliver volumes up to 1 ounce (2 tablespoons) of liquid.
16. False: A subcutaneous injection is delivered below all of the layers of the skin. An intramuscular injection is delivered directly into a muscle.
17. True
18. True
19. False: The more viscous the solution, the lower the needle gauge number should be, because the lower the gauge, the wider the needle diameter.
20. False: The primary purpose of safety syringes is to prevent needlestick injury (i.e., to promote safe medication administration).
21. False: Cartridges need to be loaded into a syringe holder for medication administration.
22. True
23. False: Insulin syringes are used to administer U-100 insulin only.
24. True
25. True
26. False: Medication volumes are determined by reading the calibration on the leading ring.
27. False: Medication is withdrawn from a vial by inserting a needle in to the rubber stopper on the top. Medication is withdrawn from an ampule by inserting a filter needle into the solution after the ampule neck is snapped open.
28. False: Each calibration on a 1 mL syringe is one-hundredth milliliter.
29. True
30. True

31.

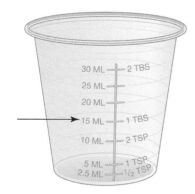

32.

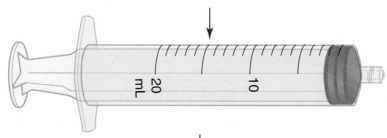

33.

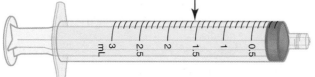

34.

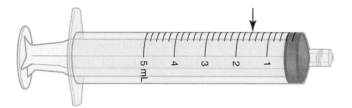

35.

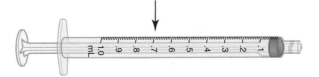

36.

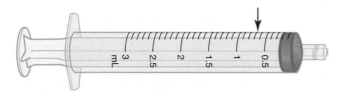

37.

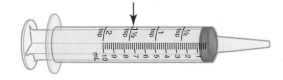

38.

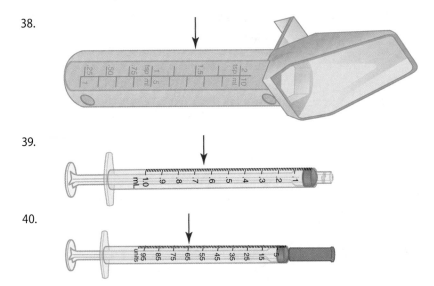

39.

40.

41. Oral syringe; 7.5 mL or 1½ t
42. Low-dose insulin syringe; 35 units (0.35 mL)
43. Large-volume, 20 mL syringe; 13 mL
44. Small-volume, 1 mL (tuberculin) syringe; 0.57 mL
45. Large-volume, 5 mL syringe; 4.8 mL
46. Small-volume, 1 mL (tuberculin) syringe; 0.08 mL
47. Standard 100 unit (1 mL) insulin syringe; 88 units
48. Large-volume, 10 mL syringe; 4.8 mL
49. Oral syringe; 10 mL or 2 t
50. Small-volume, 3 mL syringe; 1.7 mL

NCLEX-Style Review Questions

1. c
   Rationale: The typical needle gauge used for adult IM injections is 20–23.
2. b
   Rationale: The 3 mL syringe is most commonly used for adult IM injections, because the maximum injectable amount into an adult large muscle is 3 mL. The typical needle length used for adult IM injections is 1–1½ inches.
3. a
   Rationale: A medicine cup is used to measure medication volumes of 2.5, 5, 7.5, 10, 15, 20, 25, and 30 mL. Oral syringes and calibrated spoons can measure volumes up to 10 mL (or 2 tsp).
4. b
   Rationale: Using the plunger, the nurse will draw the medication through the needle into the syringe and measure the medication from the zero calibration (the starting point on the syringe barrel) to the leading ring, the ring on the plunger that is closest to the needle.
5. a, b, c, d, e
   Rationale: To determine the equipment needed for an injection, the nurse must consider:
   - Route/volume of medication/size of patient— small- or large-volume syringes are used for IV medication administration; small-volume syringes are used for subcut and IM injections
     o Adult IM injections require 1–1½-inch, 20–23 gauge needles; infant and child IM injections require ⅝-inch, 22–25 gauge needles
     o Adult subcut injections require ⅝-inch, 25–30 gauge needles; infant and child subcut injections require ⅜-inch, 25–30 gauge needles
   - Viscosity of the medication— the more viscous the medication, the lower the needle gauge used
   - Medication to be administered— for example, a U-100 insulin syringe is used to administer U-100 insulin
6. a, b, c
   Rationale: The oral syringe, calibrated spoon, and medicine cup are calibrated to deliver milliliters and teaspoons. A dropper should be used to administer only the medication with which it is packaged. A soufflé cup is not calibrated and is used for solid oral medications.

© Forfunlife/Shutterstock

Chapter 4

Medication Orders

CHAPTER OUTLINE

4-1 Medical Abbreviations
  - A. Frequency Abbreviations
  - B. Route Abbreviations
  - C. Form Abbreviations
  - D. General Abbreviations

4-2 Error-Prone Documentation
  - A. Error-Prone Abbreviations
    1. Error-Prone Frequency Abbreviations
    2. Error-Prone Route Abbreviations
    3. Error-Prone General Abbreviations
    4. Error-Prone Symbols
  - B. Error-Prone Drug Name Abbreviations

4-3 Components of a Medication Order

4-4 Verbal Orders

4-5 Medication Administration Records

LEARNING OUTCOMES

Upon completion of the chapter, the student will be able to:

4-1 Interpret common medical abbreviations.

4-2 Identify error-prone medical abbreviations.

4-3 Identify required elements of a medication order.

4-4 Apply the procedural guidelines for receiving verbal orders.

4-5 Recognize the components of a medication order on the medication administration record (MAR).

KEY TERMS

electronic medication
administration record (eMAR)
form
frequency

Institute for Safe Medication
Practices (ISMP)
The Joint Commission (TJC)
licensed independent
practitioner (LIP)

medication administration
record (MAR)
prescriptive authority
transcription
verbal order/telephone order

Case Consideration ... Order Error!

The nurse contacted the physician to report a child's fever. Over the telephone, the physician gave an order for Tylenol® 325 mg by mouth. Because the child's temperature remained elevated throughout the nurse's 12-hour shift, the medication was administered three times (i.e., every 4 hours), as is the usual time interval for acetaminophen (Tylenol). The physician, disturbed to find out that the child's temperature remained elevated for 12 hours, exclaimed, "Why was I not notified regarding this child's persistent fever?" The nurse replied, "You were notified when the child's temperature first spiked and your order to administer Tylenol every 4 hours was implemented." The physician responded, "The Tylenol order was for a single dose; it should not have been repeated without a new order. This child should have had orders to draw blood cultures and start on broad-spectrum antibiotics 8 hours ago!"

1. What went wrong?

2. How can this error be avoided?

■ INTRODUCTION

Preparation for medication administration begins with the medication order. Nurses must be able to interpret medication orders. Accurate interpretation of medication orders requires the ability to interpret common medical abbreviations and recognize the required components of a drug order. Committing these abbreviations to memory will increase efficiency and accuracy in interpreting medication orders.

4-1   Medical Abbreviations

Licensed independent practitioners (LIPs), also called prescribers, are licensed healthcare professionals that have **prescriptive authority**, the legal right to prescribe medication, granted by the state in which they are licensed. Examples of disciplines often authorized to prescribe include physicians, nurse practitioners, dentists, and physician assistants. The disciplines that have prescriptive authority vary from state to state. Authorized prescribers use many abbreviations when writing medication orders. There are several types of abbreviations used in drug orders, including frequency, route, form, and general abbreviations.

Frequency Abbreviations

Frequency refers to how often a medication is to be administered. Common frequency abbreviations are included in **TABLE 4-1**.

Some frequency abbreviations seem similar in meaning; however, they should be distinguished:

- **prn and ad lib**—*prn,* a Latin acronym for *pro re nata* that means as the need arises, is usually ordered with a time interval and a reason, such as q4h prn pain. This phrase means a medication may be given every 4 hours as needed for relief of pain. The phrase *ad lib* is short for ad libitum, the Latin phrase for "at one's pleasure." Medications ordered on an *ad lib* basis can be given as often as desired, generally without an assigned time interval, for example, artificial tears are often ordered to be administered on an *ad lib* basis. Few medications are ordered with the *ad lib* frequency designation.

- **bid and tid**—The Latin phrases *bis in die* and *ter in die*, abbreviated bid and tid, mean twice a day and three times a day. Some individuals confuse the meaning of these two abbreviations by thinking that the "t" in tid refers to twice, instead of three times daily. To help avoid this confusion, think of "b" in

TABLE 4-1 Frequency Abbreviations	
Frequency	**Meaning**
ac	before meals
ad lib	as desired
bid	twice a day
min	minute
pc	after meals
prn	as needed
qid	four times a day
q2h	every 2 hours
q3h	every 3 hours
q4h	every 4 hours
q6h	every 6 hours
q8h	every 8 hours
q12h	every 12 hours
stat	immediately
tid	three times a day

bid as "bi," the prefix meaning two as in bicycle; thus, bid means twice daily. Likewise, think of "t" in tid as "tri," a prefix meaning three, as in tricycle; thus, tid means three times daily.

- **q6h and qid**—Although medications ordered q6h and qid (Latin for *quater in die*) will be administered four times per day, medications ordered q6h must be separated by 6 hours, whereas drugs ordered qid are not required to be given around the clock. For example, a "qid" medication schedule might be 0900, 1300, 1700, 2100, while a q6h schedule would be 0600, 1200, 1800, 2400.

- **q8h and tid**—Both abbreviations indicate that a medication is ordered three times per day, but a q8h schedule is an around-the-clock order, such as 0600, 1400, 2200, while a tid schedule might be 1000, 1400, 1800.

- **q12h and bid**—Both abbreviations indicate a medication is ordered twice per day, but a q12h schedule is an around-the-clock order, such as 0800, 2000, while a "bid" schedule might be 1000, 1800.

Scheduled administration times may vary between healthcare facilities. It is the responsibility of nurses to learn the routine medication administration schedules at their healthcare institution.

Route Abbreviations

Route, as defined in Chapter 3, refers to the path by which a medication enters the body. Some enteral (PO, NG, GT) and parenteral (IM, IV, subcut) routes were reviewed in Chapter 3. Because of medication errors associated with the abbreviations SC and SQ, the subcutaneous route is now abbreviated as "subcut." Common route abbreviations are included in **TABLE 4-2**.

TABLE 4-2 Route Abbreviations	
Route	**Meaning**
GT	gastrostomy tube
ID	intradermal
IM	intramuscular
IV	intravenous
IVPB	intravenous piggyback
NG, NGT	nasogastric, NG tube
NJ	nasojejunal
PO	by mouth (*per os*, Latin)
PR	per rectum/rectally
subcut	subcutaneously
SL	sublingual

Form Abbreviations

The **form** of a drug refers to its composition, which may be solid or liquid. Time-release medications, formulated so that the active ingredient is released slowly and steadily over time, are identified (and abbreviated) as controlled-release (CR), delayed-release (DR), sustained-release (SR), extended-release (ER or XR), or long-acting (LA, XL) formulations. Common drug form abbreviations are included in **TABLE 4-3**.

Clinical CLUE

Medication given via GT, NG, or NJ tube must be in liquid form, such as a syrup or suspension. Some, but not all, solids (pills) can be crushed and mixed with liquid, for administration through an enteral tube (see Chapter 3, Figure 3-11). Examples of medications that cannot be crushed and mixed with liquid for enteral tube administration include enteric-coated and time-release drugs.

TABLE 4-3   Drug Form Abbreviations

Drug Form	Meaning
cap	capsule
EC	enteric-coated
elix	elixir
gt, gtt	drop, drops
LA, XL	long-acting
liq	liquid
CR, DR, SR, ER or XR	controlled-release, delayed-release, sustained-release, extended-release
supp	suppository
susp	suspension
syr	syrup
tab	tablet
tinc	tincture
ung, oint	ointment

TABLE 4-4	General Abbreviations
General	**Meaning**
ā,	before
p̄	after
aq	water
BP	blood pressure
c̄, s̄	with, without
et	and
NKA	no known allergies
NKDA	no known drug allergies
NPO	nothing by mouth
q	every
qs	quantity sufficient
×	times (× 1, × 2, × 3, etc., meaning once, twice, three times)

General Abbreviations

General abbreviations are those that do not refer to route, frequency, or form. These abbreviations may be used with drug orders or may pertain to medication administration. Common general abbreviations are included in **TABLE 4-4**.

LEARNING ACTIVITY 4-1 Interpret and identify the type of medical abbreviation (frequency, route, form, or general).

1. bid   _____ _____
2. q2h   _____ _____
3. PO   _____ _____
4. prn   _____ _____
5. IM   _____ _____

4-2   **Error-Prone Documentation**

A medication order must be clearly understood in order for the medication to be properly administered. Sometimes, abbreviations and documentation styles are misinterpreted, leading to potentially harmful medication errors.

As a result of an increasing number of medication errors made due to misinterpretation of medical abbreviations, various organizations have identified the abbreviations, symbols, and documentation that are prone to misinterpretation and, therefore, likely to lead to a medication error. **The Joint Commission (TJC)**, an organization whose mission is to improve health care by evaluating healthcare organizations for their compliance with federal regulations, has produced a list of abbreviations that should no longer be used because of their propensity for misinterpretation (The Joint Commission, 2009). This list, called the "Do Not Use" List (Appendix C), was issued in 2004. The **Institute for Safe Medication Practices (ISMP)**, an organization whose sole mission is to prevent medication errors and promote safe medication administration, also published a list of error-prone abbreviations, symbols, and dose designations, which includes TJC's "Do Not Use" List (Appendix D). According to ISMP recommendations, the abbreviations, symbols, and dose designations on this list should not be used in medication orders.

Error-Prone Abbreviations

Illegible handwriting is a contributing factor to medication errors related to error-prone abbreviations (see **Figures 4-1** and **4-2**). Computerized order-entry systems have decreased the number of medication order errors. According to a 2009 study, the reason for the decrease in medication order errors is that "computerized orders cannot be incomplete or illegible" (Walsh, 2009, para 19). Despite the fact that medication errors related to error-prone abbreviations are decreasing, the nurse should recognize error-prone abbreviations and learn their intended meaning and proper documentation. Nurses promote safe medication administration and avoid documentation errors by learning and not using error-prone abbreviations.

Error-Prone Frequency Abbreviations

One of the most common error-prone frequency abbreviations is q.d. or QD. This abbreviation was used to mean every day or daily, but has also been mistaken as q.i.d., especially if the period after the "q" or the tail of the "q" is misunderstood as an "i" (ISMP, 2013). This abbreviation, as well as q.o.d. (meaning every other day, but mistaken for q.d. or q.i.d. if the "o" is poorly written) appears on both TJC's Official "Do Not Use" List and the ISMP's "List of Error-Prone Abbreviations, Symbols, and Dose Designations." Common error-prone frequency abbreviations are listed in **TABLE 4-5.**

TABLE 4-5 Common Error-Prone Frequency Abbreviations			
Abbreviation	**Intended Meaning**	**Misinterpretation**	**Instead, Use:**
HS	hour of sleep (bedtime)	half-strength	bedtime
o.d. or OD	once daily	right eye (oculus dexter), leading to oral medication administered in the eye	daily
q.d. or QD	every day	q.i.d.	daily
qhs	bedtime	qhr or every hour	nightly
q.o.d. or QOD	every other day	q.d. or qid	every other day

TABLE 4-6　Common Error-Prone Route Abbreviations

Abbreviation	Intended Meaning	Misinterpretation	Instead, Use:
AD, AS, AU	right ear, left ear, both ears	OD, OS, OU (right eye, left eye, both eyes)	right ear, left ear, both ears
OD, OS, OU	right eye, left eye, both eyes	AD, AS, AU (right ear, left ear, both ears)	right eye, left eye, both eyes

Error-Prone Route Abbreviations

Both ear (otic) drops and eye (optic or ophthalmic) drops are liquid preparations available in similar packaging. The similarity in the drug route names, otic and optic, as well as the similar abbreviations OU (former abbreviation for both eyes) and AU (former abbreviation for both ears) has caused confusion regarding route of administration. Ear drops have been administered into the eyes, causing blurriness, redness, and pain. For this reason eye and ear route abbreviations (**TABLE 4-6**) are no longer used.

Error-Prone General Abbreviations

A 2007 analysis by Rutgers University of approximately 30,000 medication errors revealed that improper dose/quantity is one of the most common abbreviation-related medication errors (Texas Medical Association, 2008). Some commonly misinterpreted abbreviations cited in this study included "U" (former abbreviation for units) and "cc" (abbreviation for cubic centimeter), both of which have been mistaken as zeros after an Arabic number leading to a (potential) drug overdose. Other misinterpreted general abbreviations are noted in **TABLE 4-7**.

TABLE 4-7　Common Error-Prone General Abbreviations

Abbreviation	Intended Meaning	Misinterpretation	Instead, Use:
μg	microgram	mg	mcg
cc	cubic centimeters	U (units)	mL
IU	international unit	IV or 10	international unit
ss	sliding scale or ½	55	sliding scale or ½
SSRI	sliding scale regular insulin	selective serotonin reuptake inhibitor	sliding scale
U or u	unit	0 or 4, for example 4U mistaken as 40 or 44; also mistaken as cc, so 4u mistaken for 4cc	unit

WARNING!

Error-Prone Documentation May Lead to Overdose!

Consider the overdoses that could occur due to the *misinterpretation* of the handwritten orders in Figures 4-1 and 4-2. In Figure 4-1, because there is no space between the drug name and the dose, the "l" in Tegretol can easily be misunderstood as a one, in which case the order might be read as 1,300 mg, instead of 300 mg.

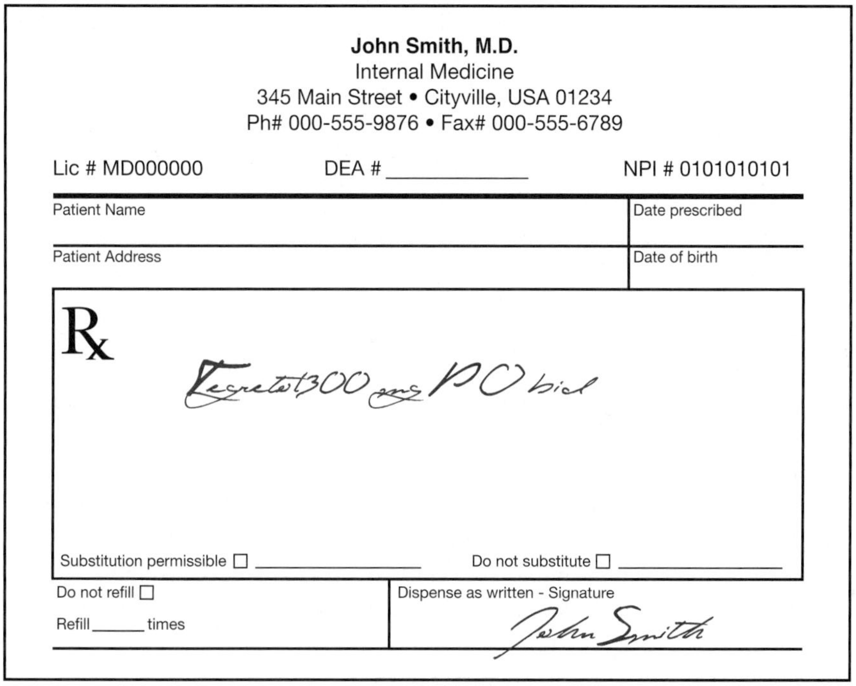

FIGURE 4-1   To avoid a medication error with handwritten medication orders, include a space between the drug name and dose.

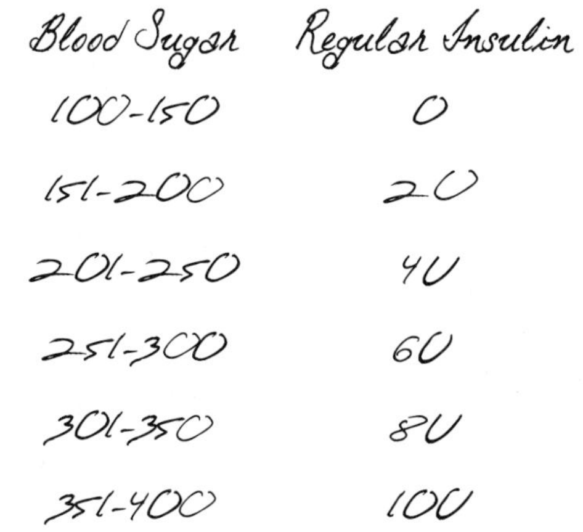

FIGURE 4-2   The error-prone abbreviation U, when handwritten, can easily be misinterpreted as a zero. To avoid this error, the authorized prescriber should write "units" and include a space between the quantity and the unit of measurement. (More information on sliding scales for insulin is included in Chapter 14.)

TABLE 4-8   Error-Prone Symbols

Abbreviation	Intended Meaning	Misinterpretation	Instead, Use:
> and <	greater than and less than	mistaken for each other	greater than and less than
@	at	2	at
&	and	2	and
+	plus or and	4	and
°	hour	zero (e.g., q2° mistaken for q 20)	h or hour

Error-Prone Symbols

The use of symbols can be a quick way of communicating information, but some symbols, such as < and > are confusing. An elderly patient was ordered to receive Vasotec® 1.25 mg IV for a systolic blood pressure (SBP) greater than 180 mm Hg. The order read, "hold Vasotec® for SBP < 180." The "<" symbol was misinterpreted and the patient received the medication when the systolic blood pressure was only 140 mm Hg, leading to a significant drop in the patient's blood pressure (Cohen, 2007). Another common symbol used when writing medication orders is "@" which has been misinterpreted as a 2. For example, an intravenous infusion with sodium bicarbonate that was ordered to run "@50 mL/h" was interpreted as 250 mL/h (Cohen, 2007). While a space between the "@" symbol and the numerical value (50) may have prevented this error, it is now recommended that use of symbols, such as those listed in **TABLE 4-8**, be avoided when writing medication orders.

Error-Prone Drug Name Abbreviations

The Joint Commission recommends that drug names not be abbreviated when writing medication orders. Despite TJC's recommendations regarding the avoidance of abbreviations, errors related to abbreviated drug names persist. A Pennsylvania physician wrote an intravenous order to "increase Mg to 1.5 grams per liter" for an elderly patient. The physician's order referred to magnesium sulfate, but the nurse that received the order misinterpreted the Mg for MS and prepared an intravenous solution with 1.5 grams of morphine sulfate, which led to respiratory arrest requiring resuscitation (Cohen, 2007). To avoid a potentially life-threatening medication error, prescribing practitioners should never abbreviate drug names when ordering medications and nurses should question medication orders with abbreviated drug names.

WARNING!

Be Aware of Drugs with Similar Names!

In June 2004, *The Pharmacy Times* issued a story about a child who had leukemia and missed 6 months of the chemotherapeutic drug Purethinol® because the pharmacy instead dispensed propylthiouracil, a medication used to treat hyperthyroidism. Conversely, the ISMP reported the tragic consequences in the case of a pregnant woman, ordered to receive PTU (the unapproved abbreviation for propylthiouracil), who was given Purethinol instead. Although the drug names are quite distinct, both start with P and end with L and both medications are available in a 50 mg tablet strength. The abbreviation, PTU, used for propylthiouracil, further increases the risk of an error as both drug names have in them a P, T, and U (Gaunt, 2009).

Clinical CLUE

The ISMP (2014) has published a list of look-alike, sound-alike (LASA) medications, called *ISMP's List of Confused Drug Names* (see Appendix E). "Tall man lettering" emphasizes the different medications. Some common LASA medications include:

- alprazOLam and lorazEPam
- buPROPion and busPIRone
- cycloSPORINE and cycloSERINE
- DOBUTamine and DOPamine
- glipiZIDE and glyBURIDE
- hydrOXYzine and hydrALAZINE
- oxyCODONE and HYDROcodone

Nurses should become familiar with the common LASA medications ordered for their patient population and double-check these orders. Determining the rationale for each medication to be administered, an important step in the medication administration process, will assist the nurse in avoiding errors related to LASA medications.

LEARNING ACTIVITY 4-2 Match the error-prone abbreviation with the correct documentation.

1.	OS	_____	a.	daily
2.	AU	_____	b.	left eye
3.	QD	_____	c.	international units
4.	U	_____	d.	both ears
			e.	units

4-3   Components of a Medication Order

Before carrying out a medication order, the nurse must ensure that the order is complete. The components of a complete medication order include:

1. Name of patient and date of birth (DOB)

2. Name of medication

3. Dose of medication

4. Route of administration

5. Frequency and/or time of administration

6. Date and time the order was written

7. Signature of the prescriber

The patient's name should be a full name, including a middle name or initial. The patient's DOB, though not required by all agencies, is typically used as a second identifier to differentiate patients with similar names. As previously mentioned, to avoid potential errors, the complete name of the drug should be used when ordering a medication. The drug dose is the specific amount of medication to be given at one time. The route or path by which the medication enters the body should be included with the medication order. The frequency indicates how often a medication should be given.

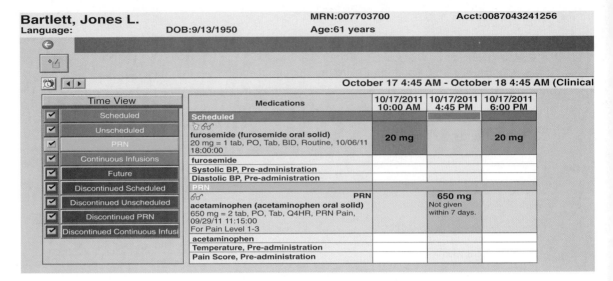

FIGURE 4-3   Medication orders generated through an electronic medical record.

Most healthcare facilities have a standard schedule for the frequencies listed in Table 4-1. Examples of standard frequency schedules include:

- q6h: 0600, 1200, 1800, 2400

- q8h: 0800, 1600, 2400 or 0600, 1400, 2200

- q12h: 0800, 2000

Some medications must be scheduled with meals or apart from meals. Nurses are responsible for ensuring that medications are properly scheduled. The final required component of a medication order is the signature of the prescriber, which may be a handwritten or electronic signature. **Figure 4-3** depicts five of the seven required components of a medication order on an electronic medical record—patient name and DOB, drug names, doses, routes, and frequencies. The electronic signature and date/time the order is generated, though accessible, is not readily visible on this screen shot.

Although most healthcare facilities utilize electronic medical records and generate medication orders electronically, sometimes medication orders are handwritten on paper forms. For agencies that do not have a computerized order-entry system in place or during unexpected computer downtimes, it is necessary for prescribing practitioners to generate medication orders via a paper documentation form as shown in **Figure 4-4**.

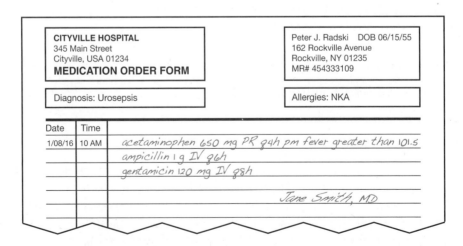

FIGURE 4-4   Handwritten orders on a medication order form.

Clinical CLUE

National Patient Safety Goals, published annually by The Joint Commission, are identified to improve the safety of patients. The first of the recent goals published is correct patient identification. Double identification of the patient, that is, using both the patient name and DOB on the medication order, will ensure that each patient gets the correct medication.

LEARNING ACTIVITY 4-3 Answer questions 1 and 2 as they relate to the order: "Give Mr. Smith (DOB 8/8/1959) ampicillin 500 mg q6h, Lucille Waterman, MD." Answer questions 3–5 as they relate to Figure 4-3.

1.   Identify each complete component included in this medication order.
2.   Cite the missing components of this medication order.
3.   Identify the patient's name and DOB in Figure 4-3.
4.   Identify the scheduled medication name, dose, route, and frequency.
5.   Identify the PRN medication name, dose, route, and frequency.

4-4   Verbal Orders

Typically, medication orders are written and signed by the prescribing practitioner. However, when the prescriber is unavailable to write an order such as in the event of an emergency, a verbal order, delivered in person or as a "telephone order," may be given to a registered nurse, pharmacist, or other personnel authorized to receive verbal orders. A **verbal/telephone order** is given orally instead of via documentation. Because of the potential for error with verbal orders, The Joint Commission recommends the following guidelines for the person accepting a verbal order:

1. *Document the order* carefully and legibly as the order is being delivered. While writing the order, ensure that all components of a medication order are included.

2. *Recite the order* back to the prescriber.

3. Ask the prescriber to *verify* that *the order* is correct.

Example: Dr. Lucille Waterman delivers a telephone order to the nurse caring for the patient, Lewis A. Clarke. The patient is confirmed by stating the full name and DOB. TJC's guidelines for accepting a verbal order are applied as follows:

1. The prescriber states the order, "Dilaudid 2 mg by mouth as needed for severe pain." The nurse *documents the order* as stated, leaving a space for frequency because it is recognized that that the frequency is missing. The nurse asks the prescriber, "How often can the medication be given?" The prescriber indicates, "every 4 hours," and the nurse writes the complete order.

2. The nurse *recites the* complete order back to the prescriber: "Dilaudid 2 mg PO q4h prn for severe pain."

3. The nurse asks the prescriber to *verify the order*, "Is the order I've stated for Lewis A. Clark correct?" The nurse documents the date and time that the order is received and labels the order as a verbal/telephone order with a V.O. or T.O. or per agency policy. The nurse signs the order and the prescriber must cosign the order when available to do so, usually within 24 to 48 hours, per agency policy.

LEARNING ACTIVITY 4-4 Answer the questions regarding the verbal order, "Give Paul M. Smythe diphenhydramine IV stat."

1. Cite three guidelines for accepting verbal orders.
2. What additional information should the nurse request from the prescribing practitioner?

4-5 Medication Administration Records

Medication administration records (MARs) are legal records that contain the same information as the medication order with the addition of the specified times for administration. After an order is generated electronically, it is (typically automatically) uploaded to a special form within the patient's electronic medical record that is used for documentation of drugs given to the patient and is called the **electronic medication administration record (eMAR)**. Handwritten medication orders are manually entered onto the eMAR or transcribed onto a paper MAR according to agency protocol for **transcription** of medication orders. Transcription is the process of copying or entering orders onto the MAR or eMAR and includes the assignment of times for administration. The person responsible for transcription depends upon agency policy and may be a nurse, pharmacist, secretary, or pharmacy technician. **Figure 4-5** reveals the transcription of the medication orders from the form in Figure 4-4 onto a MAR, while **Figure 4-6** shows orders on an eMAR.

As shown in Figures 4-5 and 4-6, the MAR/eMAR provides a place for documentation of medications given.

Cityville Hospital
345 Main Street • Cityville, USA 01234

Medication Administration Record

Patient Name: Peter J. Radski DOB: 06/15/55 MR#: 454333109			Allergies: NKA Diagnosis: Urosepsis			Week Ending: 1/12/16			
Order Date	Scheduled Medications	Times	1/06/16	1/07/16	1/08/16	1/09/16	1/10/16	1/11/16	1/12/16
1/08	Ampicillin 1 g IV q6h	0600			SS				
		1200							
		1800							
		2400							
1/08	Gentamicin 120 mg IV q8h	0800			SS				
		1600							
		2400							

PRN Medications

Order Date	Medication	Date	Time	Route	Reason	Result	Initials
1/08	Acetaminophen 650 mg PR q4h prn fever greater than 101.5	1/08	1000	PR	Temp 102.4	101.3 at 1030	SS

Initials	Signature/Title	Initials	Signature/Title	Initials	Signature/Title
SS	Sharon Schultz, RN				

FIGURE 4-5 This MAR indicates that gentamicin was administered at 0800, acetaminophen was given at 1000, and ampicillin was given at 0600 by Sharon Schultz, RN, on January 8.

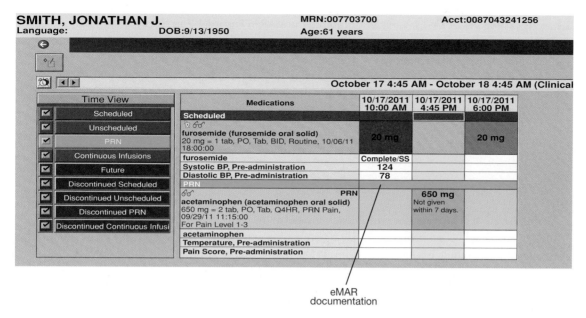

FIGURE 4-6   To access details regarding the administration of furosemide on the eMAR, such as the name of the individual that administered the medication or the blood pressure at the time of administration, the user hovers the mouse over the identified site on the eMAR.

Cityville Hospital
345 Main Street • Cityville, USA 01234

Medication Administration Record

Patient Name: Kevin L. Dunbar		Allergies: NKA					
DOB: 10/22/55					Week Ending: 5/11/16		
MR#: 54556120		Diagnosis: Congestive Heart Failure					

Order Date	Scheduled Medications	Times	5/05/16	5/06/16	5/07/16	5/08/16	5/09/16	5/10/16	5/11/16

PRN Medications

Order Date	Medication	Date	Time	Route	Reason	Result	Initials

Initials	Signature/Title	Initials	Signature/Title	Initials	Signature/Title

FIGURE 4-7   Medication administration record (MAR) to be completed for Kevin Dunbar.

LEARNING ACTIVITY 4-5 Complete the MAR in **Figure 4-7** as follows:

1. Enter this medication ordered on 5/5: Heparin 5,000 units subcut q12h (0800, 2000)
2. Enter this medication ordered on 5/6: Maalox® 30 mL via GT q6h (0600, 1200, 1800, 2400)
3. Sign the medication sheet with your initials as if you had given the medications on the day shift (0700–1500) on 5/8.

Order Error ... Case Closure

Administration of multiple doses of Tylenol® instead of the single dose that was intended resulted in delays in evaluation and treatment. Delaying evaluation of the cause of this child's fever and resulting treatment delays could have adverse effects. When taking telephone orders, the nurse should:

- Ensure that all of the components of medication orders are included.

- Follow the process for taking a verbal order: document the order, recite the order back, verify that the order is correct.

The nurse should have questioned the medical doctor (MD) regarding frequency. Had the nurse asked, "Did you want the Tylenol® given q4h prn fever greater than 101?" as was presumed, the physician would then have clarified that it was to be a single-dose order. Then the nurse should have recited back the order back for verification, saying something like, "Oh, so you want Tylenol® 325 mg PO now one time only and notify MD for persistent fever ... is that right?" After which the MD would reply, "Yes, that's correct!" This exchange reveals that the nurse correctly interpreted the order.

Chapter Summary

Learning Outcomes	Points to Remember

4-1 Interpret common medical abbreviations. See Tables 4-1, 4-2, 4-3, 4-4.	• *Frequency abbreviations*:
	  o ac/pc—before meals/after meals
	  o bid/tid/qid—two/three/four times per day
	  o prn—as needed
	  o q4h—every 4 hours
	  o stat—immediately
	 • *Route abbreviations:*
	  o PO—by mouth
	  o GT/NGT—gastrostomy/nasogastric tube
	  o IM—intramuscular
	  o IV—intravenous
	  o subcut—subcutaneously
	  o PR—rectally

- *Form abbreviations:*
  - o EC—enteric-coated
  - o LA/XL—long-acting
  - o gtt—drops
  - o CR/SR/XR—controlled/sustained/extended release
- *General abbreviations:*
  - o ā/p̄—before/after
  - o c̄/s̄—with/without
  - o NPO—nothing by mouth

4-2 Identify error-prone medical abbreviations. See Tables 4-5, 4-6, 4-7, 4-8.	**Per ISMP and TJC** *do not use* these abbreviations: • QD/qod—use daily/every other day • HS/qhs—use bedtime/nightly • OD/OS/OU—use right eye/left eye/both eyes • AD/AS/AU—use right ear/left ear/both ears • U/IU—use unit/international unit • µg—use mcg • cc—use mL • Symbols such as <, >, @, &, +, °—write the intended meaning instead
4-3 Identify required elements of a medication order.	Name of patient (& DOB), name of medication, dose, route, time/frequency of administration, date/time order is written, prescriber signature

4-4 Apply the procedural guidelines for receiving verbal orders.	• Personnel such as registered nurse or pharmacist must be authorized to accept verbal orders or telephone orders.
	• Order should be labeled with T.O. or V.O., signed by nurse upon verification, and cosigned by prescriber as soon as possible.
	• Guidelines:
	  1. Document the order
	  2. Recite the order
	  3. Verify the order

4-5 Recognize the components of a medication order on the MAR.	• The MAR/eMAR is a legal document. • The medication order is transcribed and specified times for medication administration are added. • The MAR/eMAR provides a place for documentation of medications given.

Homework

For exercises 1–10, differentiate the pairs of abbreviations. (LO 4-1)

1. q8h, tid
2. prn, ad lib
3. NG, GT
4. PO, NPO
5. SL, XL
6. bid, q12h
7. IM, IV
8. q6h, qid
9. subcut, ID
10. c̄, s̄

For exercises 11–15, circle the correct documentation for each error-prone abbreviation/symbol. (LO 4-2)

11. QD   a. right eye   b. daily
         c. every other day
12. <   a. less than   b. more than
         c. mL
13. IU   a. unit   b. insulin unit
         c. international unit
14. HS   a. bedtime   b. hourly
         c. half-strength
15. cc   a. units   b. mL
         c. cubic centimeter

For exercises 16–20, fill in the blanks.

16. The Institute for Safe Medication Practices is an organization whose mission is to prevent _____.
17. Illegible _____ is a contributing factor to medication errors related to error-prone abbreviations.
18. _____ is an organization whose mission is to evaluate healthcare organizations for their compliance with federal regulations.
19. TJC published a list of error-prone abbreviations called the _____ List.

20. One of the most common error-prone abbreviations is _____, which was used to mean daily.

For exercises 21–30, interpret (write out the abbreviations in) the medication orders and label these order components: medication name, dose, route, and frequency. Also label medication form and special instructions when provided. (LO 4-3)

21. Docusate sodium elix 100 mg per GT bid
22. Furosemide 40 mg IV stat
23. Propantheline 15 mg ac PO tid et bedtime
24. Simethicone 80 mg PO pc
25. Acetaminophen supp 650 mg PR qid prn fever greater than 101.5
26. EC aspirin 325 mg PO daily
27. Nitroglycerin tab 0.4 mg SL stat; may repeat q5min × 2
28. Amoxicillin susp, 200 mg/5mL, ½ tsp q6h
29. Timoptic® ophthalmic solution 0.25% 2 gtt both eyes bid; hold/contact MD for systolic BP less than 90
30. Topricin® oint, apply topically to hands ad lib

For exercises 31–35, indicate whether the statement is true or false and correct the false statements. (LO 4-4)

31. The nursing assistant must follow TJC's procedural guidelines for accepting verbal orders.
32. When accepting a telephone order, the patient should be verified by full name and DOB.
33. After the prescriber states the order, the nurse documents the verbal order.
34. Once the nurse has written a complete order, the order should be recited back to the prescriber as a final step in the verbal order process.
35. A verbal order should be signed immediately by the nurse and as soon as possible by the prescribing practitioner.

For exercises 36–45, answer the questions regarding the MAR. (LO 4-5)

Cityville Hospital
345 Main Street • Cityville, USA 01234

Medication Administration Record

Patient Name: Simon D. Jones		Allergies: NKA					
DOB: 01/11/66				Week Ending: 2/14/16			
MR#: 61061432		Diagnosis: Congestive Heart Failure					

Order Date	Scheduled Medications	Times	2/10/16	2/11/16	2/12/16	2/13/16	2/14/16
2/10	Lanoxin 0.25 mg PO every other day (Odd dates at 1000) hold for apical rate less than 60	1000					
2/10	Furosemide 10 mg IV q12h (0800-2000)	0800					
		2000					
2/10	Ferrous sulfate 325 mg PO bid before breakfast and dinner (0800-1700)	0800					
		1700					

PRN Medications

Order Date	Medication	Date	Time	Route	Reason	Result	Initials
2/10	Morphine sulfate 4 mg IV q4h prn severe pain						
2/10	Ibuprofen 600 mg q8h PO prn mild to moderate pain						

Initials	Signature/Title	Initials	Signature/Title	Initials	Signature/Title

36. Which component(s) of the medication order are not visible on this MAR/eMAR?

37. By what route and how often is furosemide to be administered?

38. Prior to administration of Lanoxin, what action should the nurse perform?

39. After administration of Lanoxin on 2/11, when is the next dose due to be administered?

40. What medications are scheduled to be given on the day shift, 0700–1500?

41. What medications are scheduled to be given on the evening shift, 1500–2300?

42. What medications are scheduled to be given on the night shift, 2300–0700?

43. If morphine sulfate is administered at 2045 on 2/10, when can the next dose be administered?

44. Differentiate Mr. Jones's scheduled and prn medications.

45. What medications does Mr. Jones take orally?

For exercises 46–50, indicate whether the statement is true or false. Correct the false statements.

46. If Simon Jones's heart rate is 66 at 0800 on 2/11, the nurse should not give the scheduled Lanoxin and contact the authorized prescriber.

47. Mr. Jones reports pain on 2/12 upon arising at 0730. He rates his pain 3 on a scale of 1 (mild) to 10 (severe). The nurse should administer morphine sulfate 4 mg IV.

48. Mr. Jones experiences chronic pain for which he prefers to take ibuprofen twice daily with meals, therefore he can take his ferrous sulfate and ibuprofen at the same time.

49. Furosemide is ordered to be given two times per day.

50. At bedtime, Mr. Jones complains of pain and rates it 8 on a scale of 1–10. The nurse should administer morphine sulfate 2 mg IV.

NCLEX-Style Review Questions

For questions 1–4, select the best response.

1. Select the properly written medication order.
   a. Acetaminophen with codeine 4cc PO q4h prn pain
   b. Furosemide 40 mg PO QD
   c. Heparin 5,000 U SC q12h
   d. Levothyroxine 150 mcg PO daily ā breakfast

2. A medication is ordered to be given q8h. If the first dose is administered at 1630, the next dose should be given at:
   a. 0130
   b. 2430
   c. 0030
   d. 0430

3. When taking a verbal order, the nurse should:
   a. Document the order as it is dictated by the prescriber
   b. Recite the order to the pharmacist
   c. Verify the order with another nurse
   d. Get the order cosigned by the pharmacist

4. Lasix 40 mg IV stat should be given:
   a. By injection
   b. As needed
   c. Immediately
   d. As soon as possible

For question 5–6, select all that apply.

5. Identify components of a medication order.
   a. Route of administration
   b. Name of pharmacy
   c. Signature of authorized prescriber
   d. Type of medication
   e. Patient's date of birth
   f. Dose of medication

6. Select the common medical abbreviations that indicate frequency of medication administration.
   a. bid
   b. GT
   c. NKA
   d. ac
   e. q4h
   f. NPO
   g. subcut

REFERENCES

Cohen, M. R. (Ed.). (2007). *Medication errors* (2nd ed.). Washington, DC: American Pharmacists Association.

Gaunt, M. J. (2009, August 15). Medication safety: Avoid the error-prone abbreviation PTU. *Pharmacy Times*. Retrieved from http://www.pharmacy-times.com/publications/issue/2009/August2009/MedSafety-0809

Institute for Safe Medication Practices. (2013). *List of error-prone abbreviations, symbols, and dose designations*. Retrieved from http://www.ismp.org/tools/errorproneabbreviations.pdf

Institute for Safe Medication Practices. (2014). *ISMP's list of confused drug names*. Retrieved from http://www.ismp.org/tools/confuseddrugnames.pdf

The Joint Commission. (2009). *Official "do not use" list*. Retrieved from http://www.jointcommission.org/assets/1/18/dnu_list.pdf

Texas Medical Association. (2008, May 30). Medication errors: A preventable risk. Retrieved from http://www.texmed.org/Template.aspx?id=6673

Walsh, N. (2009, August 10). Computerized system limits PICU medication errors. *MedPage Today*. Retrieved from http://www.medpagetoday.com/HospitalBasedMedicine/RiskManagement/15456

Chapter 4   ANSWER KEY

Learning Activity 4-1
1. Twice a day; frequency
2. Every 2 hours; frequency
3. By mouth or orally; route
4. As needed; frequency
5. Intramuscularly; route

Learning Activity 4-2
1. b
2. d
3. a
4. e

Learning Activity 4-3
1. DOB, drug name, dose, frequency, prescriber signature
2. Complete patient name, date and time order was written, route
3. Jonathan J. Smith, 9/13/1950
4. furosemide 20 mg PO bid
5. acetaminophen 650 mg PO q4h prn pain

Learning Activity 4-4
1. Document the order, recite the order back to the prescriber, verify the order
2. Patient's DOB, dose of medication

Learning Activity 4-5

Cityville Hospital
345 Main Street • Cityville, USA 01234

Medication Administration Record

Patient Name: Kevin L. Dunbar
DOB: 10/22/55
MR#: 54556120

Allergies: NKA

Diagnosis: Congestive Heart Failure

Week Ending: 5/10/16

Order Date	Scheduled Medications	Times	5/05/16	5/06/16	5/07/16	5/08/16	5/09/16	5/10/16
5/05	Heparin 5,000 units subcut q12h	0800			JP			
		2000						
5/06	Maalox 30 mL via GT q6h	0600						
		1200			JP			
		1800						
		2400						

PRN Medications

Order Date	Medication	Date	Time	Route	Reason	Result	Initials

Initials	Signature/Title	Initials	Signature/Title	Initials	Signature/Title
JP	Jennifer Palmunen, RN				

Homework

1. tid means three times per day and does not have to be spaced out every 8 hours; q8h is scheduled around the clock

2. prn means as often as needed and is usually ordered with a time interval; ad lib means as desired and is usually not ordered with a time interval

3. NG means via nasogastric tube—a tube inserted into the stomach through the nose; GT means via gastrostomy and is inserted into the stomach through the skin

4. PO means by mouth or orally; NPO means nothing by mouth

5. SL means sublingual; XL is an abbreviation attached to a medication name and indicates that it is an extended-release form of the medication

6. bid means twice a day and does not have to be spaced out every 12 hours; q12h is scheduled around the clock

7. IM and IV are both parenteral injection routes, however IM refers to the intramuscular injection route and IV refers to the intravenous injection route

8. q6h is scheduled around the clock; qid means four times a day and does not have to be spaced out every 6 hours

9. subcut is the abbreviation for the subcutaneous (into the fat, under the skin) injection route; ID is the abbreviation for intradermal (between the layers of the skin)

10. $\bar{c}$ means with; $\bar{s}$ means without

11. b

12. a

13. c

14. a

15. b

16. Medication errors

17. Handwriting

18. The Joint Commission

19. "Do Not Use"

20. QD or qd

21. Give docusate sodium (drug name) elixir (form) 100 mg (dose) through the gastrostomy tube (route) twice a day (frequency).

22. Give furosemide (drug name) 40 mg (dose) intravenously (route) immediately (time/frequency).

23. Give propantheline (drug name) 15 mg (dose) orally (route) before meals three times a day and at bedtime (frequency).

24. Give simethicone (drug name) 80 mg (dose) orally (route) after meals (frequency).

25. Give acetaminophen (drug name) suppository (form) 650 mg (dose) rectally (route) four times a day as needed for fever (frequency).

26. Give enteric-coated (form) aspirin (drug name) 325 mg (dose) orally (route) every day (frequency).

27. Give nitroglycerin (drug name) tablet (form) 0.4 mg (dose) sublingually (route) immediately and may repeat every 5 minutes two times (frequency).

28. Give amoxicillin (drug name) suspension (form) 200 mg/5 mL, ½ teaspoon (dose) every 6 hours (frequency).

29. Give Timoptic® (drug name) ophthalmic solution (form) 0.25% two drops (dose) in both eyes (route) twice a day (frequency); hold the medication and contact the MD if the systolic blood pressure is less than 90 (special instructions).

30. Apply Topricin® (drug name) ointment (form) topically to the hands (route) as often as desired (frequency).

31. False: The *nurse or other authorized personnel* must follow TJC's procedural guidelines for accepting verbal orders.

32. True

33. False: *While the prescriber* is stating the order, the nurse *is documenting* the verbal order.

34. False: Once the nurse has written a complete order, the order should be recited back to the prescriber, *after which the order should be verified*.

35. True

36. Date and time the order was written, signature of the authorized prescriber

37. Intravenous route, every 12 hours

38. Check Mr. Jones's heart rate.

39. On 2/13 at 1000

40. Lanoxin (odd days only), furosemide, ferrous sulfate (ibuprofen and morphine sulfate are not scheduled, but may be given if needed)

41. Furosemide, ferrous sulfate (ibuprofen and morphine sulfate are not scheduled, but may be given if needed)

42. None (ibuprofen and morphine sulfate are not scheduled, but may be given if needed)

43. 0045 on 2/11

44. Scheduled medicines, Lanoxin, furosemide, and ferrous sulfate, are given on a scheduled basis. PRN medications, morphine sulfate and ibuprofen, are given on an as needed basis, spaced by the ordered interval.

45. Lanoxin, ferrous sulfate, ibuprofen

46. False. If Simon Jones's heart rate is 66 at 0800 on 2/11, the nurse should administer the scheduled Lanoxin.

47. False. The nurse should administer ibuprofen 600 mg PO.

48. False. Mr. Jones must take his ferrous sulfate before breakfast and dinner and can take his ibuprofen with or after breakfast and dinner.

49. True

50. False. The nurse should administer morphine sulfate 4 mg IV.

NCLEX-Style Review Questions

1. d
   Rationale: The other orders contain these error-prone abbreviations: cc, QD, U; there should be a space between the quantity and unit of measurement, 4 mL (not 4mL).

2. c
   Rationale: The next dose is due 8 hours after 1630 (4:30p.m.), which is 12: 30a.m., documented as 0030 using international time.

3. a
   Rationale: The nurse should document the order as it is being stated by the prescribing practitioner, recite the order back to the prescriber, then verify the order with the prescriber.

4. c
   Rationale: A stat medication should be given immediately. Although IV is an injection route, it is more clearly interpreted as the intravenous route.

5. a, c, e, f
   Rationale: The components of a medication order are: patient's name and DOB, name of medication, dose, route, frequency/time, date and time the order is written, signature of prescribing practitioner.

6. a, d, e
   Rationale: bid (twice a day), ac (before meals), and q4h (every 4 hours) refer to frequency of medication administration. GT (gastrostomy tube) and subcut (subcutaneously) are route abbreviations, while NKA (no known allergies) and NPO (nothing by mouth) are general abbreviations.

© Forfunlife/Shutterstock

Chapter 5

Interpretation of Medication Labels and Package Inserts

CHAPTER OUTLINE

LEARNING OUTCOMES

Upon completion of the chapter, the student will be able to:

5-1   Differentiate information on a medication label.

5-2   Identify information on a medication package insert.

KEY TERMS

bar code

combination medication

control number

controlled substance

controlled substance schedule

dosage strength

dosage unit	reconstitution	total volume
generic name	single dose	trade name
lot number	single use	unit dose
multiple dose	supply/supply dosage/supply dose	*United States Pharmacopeia—National Formulary (USP-NF)*
National Drug Code (NDC)		
net weight	total number	warning

Case Consideration … What's on a Label?

The patient has an order for ofloxacin: 2 drops right eye. The student nurse was supplied a bottle with the following label.

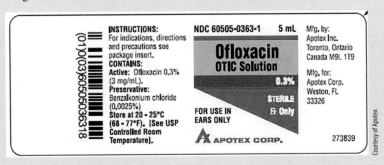

INSTRUCTIONS: For indications, directions and precautions see package insert.
CONTAINS: Active: Ofloxacin 0.3% (3 mg/mL). Preservative: Benzalkonium chloride (0,0025%). Store at 20 - 25°C (68 - 77°F). [See USP Controlled Room Temperature].

NDC 60505-0363-1   5 mL

Ofloxacin
OTIC Solution
0.3%
STERILE
Rx Only
FOR USE IN EARS ONLY

APOTEX CORP.

Mfg. by: Apotex Inc. Toronto, Ontario Canada M9L 1T9

Mfg. for: Apotex Corp. Weston, FL 33326

273839

Courtesy of Apotex

Should the student nurse administer this medication?

■ INTRODUCTION

To safely administer medications, the nurse must be able to identify essential information on the medication label and within the package insert. The label will reveal the drug name, form, dosage strength, total number or volume in container, route of administration, storage information, warnings, manufacturing information, and, if applicable, reconstitution information and control schedule. The package insert will provide more complete information about the drug, including chemical and physical description, clinical pharmacology, indications and usage, contraindications, warnings, precautions, adverse reactions, overdosage, dosage and administration, preparation for administration, and manufacturer supply information. Sometimes the label will make reference to the package insert for additional information not included on the label.

5-1   Information on a Medication Label

Generic Name

The **generic name** is the nonproprietary name assigned to the active substance of a medication. This name is registered with the United States Pharmacopeia for inclusion in the ***United States Pharmacopeia— National Formulary (USP-NF)***, a book that contains standards for medicines, dosage forms, drug substances, excipients (inactive substances), medical devices, and dietary supplements (*USP-NF*, 2014). This name is not specific to the manufacturer. Medications are usually ordered by generic name.

Trade Name

The **trade name**, also called a brand name, is the name that the manufacturer gives a medication to identify it as made by the manufacturer. This name is registered with the U.S. Department of Commerce, Patent and Trademark Office by the manufacturer, so that no other pharmaceutical company can use the same name. The trade name brands the medication and is used to market the medication. The symbol ® for registered trademark or ™ for trademark follow the trade name. It is customary for the trade name to be printed in larger font, above the generic name. Common practice is to capitalize a trade name, while the generic is in lower case letters. If there is only one name on the medication, it is the generic name.

Form

Medications are available in a variety of forms, including:

- Solids, such as capsules, tablets, gelcaps, or suppositories

- Liquids, such as oral liquids, injectable liquids, inhalants, drops, sprays, or mists

- Other forms, such as creams, ointments, or patches

Dosage Strength

The **dosage strength** (also referred to as **supply, supply dosage, or supply dose, or concentration**) is the amount of medication in each dosage unit (325 mg per tablet, 80 mg per mL, 200 mcg per metered spray). Dosage strength must include both the amount of medication (325 mg) and the unit of delivery (per tablet or per 5 mL). The dosage strength of the same medication may vary between age groups (**Figures 5-1** and **5-2**).

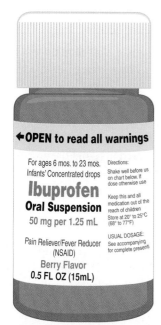

FIGURE 5-1   The dosage strength of this ibuprofen preparation is very concentrated, requiring smaller volumes to be administered. This facilitates the infant consuming the entire dose.

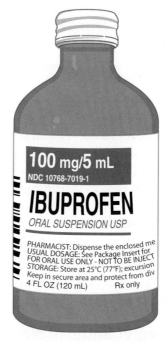

FIGURE 5-2   The dosage strength of this ibuprofen preparation is less concentrated than the infant preparation.

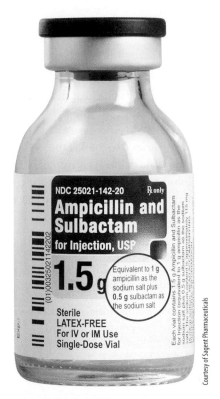

FIGURE 5-3   Ampicillin and sulbactam for injection, USP 1.5 g is a generic combination medication. The two generic names and dosage strengths are listed.

WARNING!
Follow Storage Information

Opening the multiple-dose container may shorten the expiration time—for example, a medication that has an expiration date 1 year away may need to be discarded 30 days after opening. Always read the storage information on the label.

Dosage unit refers to the quantity of solid or liquid in which the supplied dose is contained. When dosage strength is expressed as a percentage, the amount of medication is always measured in g, and the dosage unit is always 100 mL for liquid medications or 100 g for solid or semisolid medications, such as creams and ointments (Figure 5-6). Dosage strength does not refer to the amount of medication in the container.

Combination Medication

A **combination medication** is a combination of two or more medications in one form. For example, ampicillin and sulbactam 1.5 g is a combination of ampicillin 1 g and sulbactam 0.5 g per vial (**Figure 5-3**). The generic name and dosage strength of each medication are always listed on the label, under the trade name of a combination medication.

Total Number, Volume, or Net Weight

The **total number**, **total volume**, and **net weight** refer to the total amount of the medication form within the container, *not dosage strength*. That is to say, the total number refers to the number of tablets, suppositories, capsules, or other form/unit in the container (**Figure 5-4**), or the total number of milliliters in the bottle (**Figure 5-5**). The total number, total volume, and net weight does not refer to the number

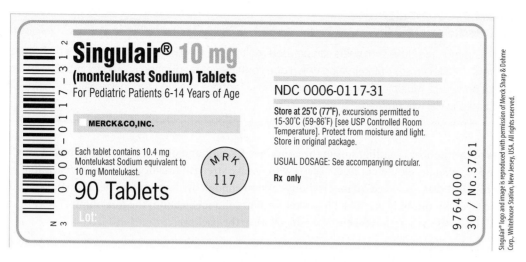

Singulair® logo and image is reproduced with permission of Merck Sharp & Dohme Corp., Whitehouse Station, New Jersey, USA. All rights reserved.

FIGURE 5-4   The total number of tablets in this bottle of Singulair® is 90 tablets, and the dosage strength is 10 mg per tablet.

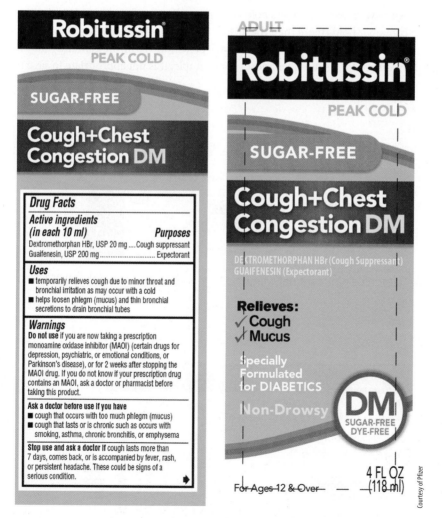

FIGURE 5-5   Robitussin® Cough Sugar-Free DM total volume 4 fl oz (118 mL) is a combination medication with two dosage strengths: Dextromethorphan HBr 20 mg/10 mL and guaifenesin 200 mg/10 mL.

Clinical CLUE

Although multiple-dose containers can be used multiple times, they should be used for the same patient. There is a risk for cross-contamination when one container of medication is used for multiple patients. When opening a multiple-dose vial, the nurse should apply a label indicating the patient's name and date and time the vial was opened.

of doses or the number of milligrams in the container. Creams and ointments are sized by net weight (**Figure 5-6**). Weight should not be confused with dosage strength (medication weight per unit of measurement). **Unit dose** packages of medications contain enough medication for one (1) dose. When the unit dose package contains only one tablet (or other form of solid medication) the total number may be omitted, and the dosage strength is for the one tablet within the package.

Multiple-Dose and Single-Dose Packaging

A **multiple-dose**, or multiple-use, package contains enough medication for more than one dose (**Figure 5-7**). Medications in multiple-dose containers have preservatives, if necessary, to ensure each dose of medication is safe to administer as long as storage and expiration information on the label is followed.

Single-dose/single-use containers hold enough medication for a *typical* single dose (**Figure 5-8**). If a single-use container holds more than the dose ordered, the excess medication must be discarded. This is because the medication may not contain necessary preservatives or the container may not retain sterility that may be required for a subsequent dose. For example, it is not appropriate to save the unused tablet

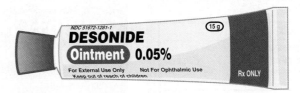

FIGURE 5-6   Desonide ointment net weight is 15 g, and dosage strength is 0.05% (0.05 g/100 g).

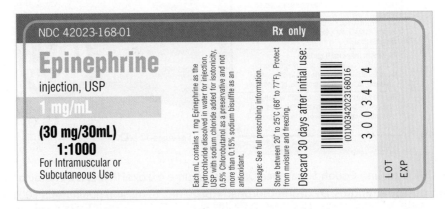

FIGURE 5-7   This multiple-dose vial of epinephrine may be used for more than one dose.

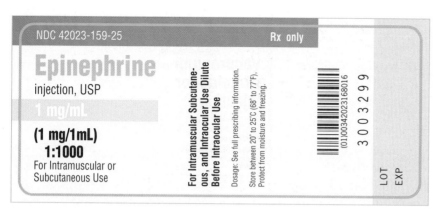

FIGURE 5-8   This single-dose vial of epinephrine may be used for only one dose.

from a single-dose packet that originally contained two tablets. However, it is appropriate to save the remaining tablets in a multiple-use bottle, providing the tablet used was removed correctly (using aseptic technique).

Route of Administration

The route, as mentioned in Chapter 3, is the bodily entry point for medication administration, leading to absorption into the bloodstream (**Figure 5-9**). Common routes include oral (PO), subcutaneous (subcut), intramuscular (IM), and intravenous (IV). Some other routes are ophthalmic (into the eye), otic (into the ear), nasal (into the nose), inhalation, topical, vaginal, rectal, intradermal (into the skin), and intraosseous

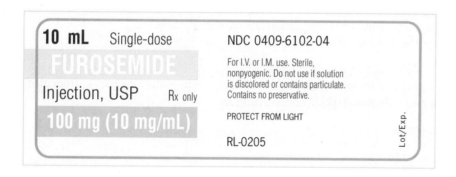

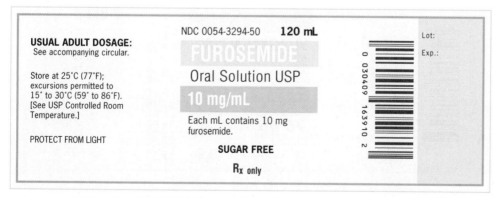

FIGURE 5-9   Both of these labels are for furosemide liquid 10 mg/mL, but one is for enteral administration (oral solution) and the other is for parenteral administration (injection, for IV or IM use).

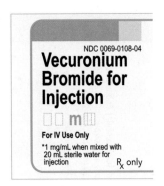

FIGURE 5-10   Dosage strength will be 1 mg/mL after reconstitution instructions are followed.

(into the bone). The route may be listed as part of the name, such as "nasal spray" or be listed separately such as "for IM or IV" use. It is assumed that tablets and capsules are enteral medications, unless another route is specified on the label. Suppositories are labeled with a phrase indicating rectal or vaginal route. Topical is the route for creams, ointments, and patches that are placed on the skin.

The importance of identifying the intended route cannot be overstated. Nurses have made fatal errors by administering medications through the wrong route, such as administering an oral solution intravenously. It should not be assumed that a medication delivered in a syringe can be given IV or IM. The nurse must always read the label to determine the route.

Reconstitution Instructions

Reconstitution is the process of reforming/transforming (changing form) a medication. Reconstitution instructions are mixing directions for liquefying a powdered (solid) medication (**Figures 5-10** and **5-11**). It is important to follow the manufacturer's direction for reconstitution. More details on reconstitution are provided in Chapter 9, "Parenteral Medication Dosage Calculations."

Warnings

The manufacturer may print **warnings** or alerts on the label to protect the patient from medication administration errors (**Figure 5-12**). Examples include:

- "Not for injection"

- "Package not child resistant"

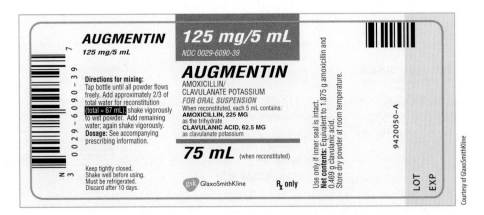

FIGURE 5-11   Directions for mixing Augmentin® oral suspension for PO administration.

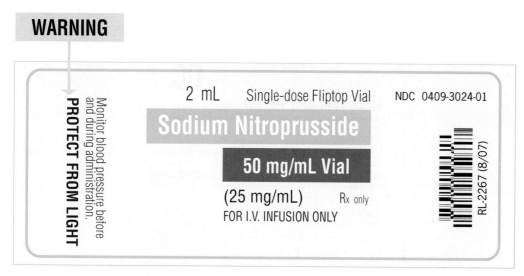

FIGURE 5-12   Warning on Sodium Nitroprusside.

- "Not for lock flush"

- "Protect from light"

  In addition, the pharmacist may attach warning labels, such as:

- "Shake well."

- "Do not drink alcohol while taking this medication."

  It is important to read all of the warnings on the label. Heeding warnings may prevent an error.

Controlled Substance Schedule

A **controlled substance** is a drug whose manufacturing or possession is regulated by the federal government. A **controlled substance schedule** differentiates controlled substances into five categories (schedules) according to their potential for abuse or addiction as follows (U.S. Drug Enforcement Administration, 2014):

- Schedule I—substances with most potential for abuse or addiction with no medicinal benefit (e.g., heroin)

- Schedule II—medications with the most potential for abuse or addiction (e.g., OxyContin®)

- Schedule III—medications with less abuse potential than schedule I or II, but abuse may lead to low to moderate physical dependence or high psychological dependence (e.g., Vicodin®)

- Schedule IV—medications with lower abuse potential than Schedule III (e.g., Valium®)

- Schedule V—substances with lowest potential for abuse or addiction, typically a combination medication in which the addictive substance has a low dosage strength (e.g., Robitussin AC®, which contains a small amount of codeine)

Controlled substances can be readily recognized with a large "C" on the medication label. The schedule number (I–V) is inserted in the center of the "C" as shown in **Figure 5-13**.

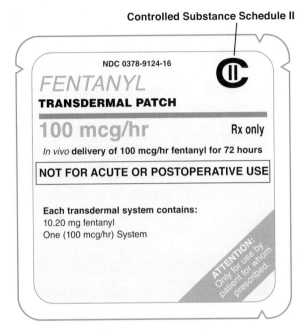

Controlled Substance Schedule II

NDC 0378-9124-16

FENTANYL

TRANSDERMAL PATCH

100 mcg/hr   Rx only

In vivo delivery of 100 mcg/hr fentanyl for 72 hours

NOT FOR ACUTE OR POSTOPERATIVE USE

Each transdermal system contains:
10.20 mg fentanyl
One (100 mcg/hr) System

ATTENTION: Only for use by patient for whom prescribed.

FIGURE 5-13 Fentanyl is a controlled substance schedule II medication.

Storage Information

The medication label will indicate the temperature range at which the medication should be stored. It also will provide other storage information if indicated, such as "protect from light" or "discard unused portion after 14 days" (**Figure 5-14**).

WARNING!

Do Not Misinterpret Schedule for Route

Use caution when interpreting the controlled substance schedule. Do not misinterpret schedule IV for the intravenous (IV) route of administration.

Manufacturing Information

The U.S. Food and Drug Administration (FDA) requires the following manufacturing information on every medication label (**Figure 5-15**):

- Pharmaceutical company—name of the company that manufactures the medication.

- **National Drug Code (NDC)**—a number that is a "universal product identifier for human drugs" (FDA, 2014). The NDC number is also called a **control number**. All medications and compounds that

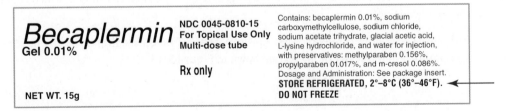

Becaplermin
Gel 0.01%

NDC 0045-0810-15
For Topical Use Only
Multi-dose tube

Rx only

NET WT. 15g

Contains: becaplermin 0.01%, sodium carboxymethylcellulose, sodium chloride, sodium acetate trihydrate, glacial acetic acid, L-lysine hydrochloride, and water for injection, with preservatives: methylparaben 0.156%, propylparaben 01.017%, and m-cresol 0.086%. Dosage and Administration: See package insert.
STORE REFRIGERATED, 2°–8°C (36°–46°F).
DO NOT FREEZE

FIGURE 5-14 The arrow is pointing to storage information on this becaplermin gel label.

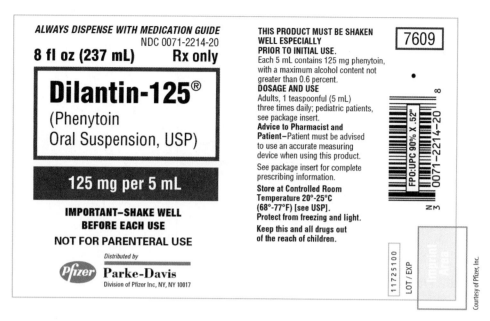

FIGURE 5-15   Manufacturer's information is printed on the label.

are manufactured for public distribution are registered with the FDA and given a three-part numeric code that is unique to the medication. The NDC Directory is maintained by the FDA. This directory lists product information by its NDC number. The old version was based on data provided on paper; the new version is based on electronically submitted information. In 2012 a process of merging the information from the old NDC Directory into the new version was started. The NDC Directory is now updated daily.

- Expiration date—the date past which the medication should not be administered.

- **Lot number**—a number identifying the batch and manufacturing plant. This number tracks medications made in the same lot, enabling them to be recalled if there is a problem with the medication.

- **Bar code**—a code required by the U.S. Department of Health and Human Services on the label of all human medications and biological agents. This provides the ability to *double-check* a medication (e.g., the nurse reads the drug name and scans the code), an approach that has been demonstrated to reduce medication errors. The bar code should never be used as the sole method of verifying the medication. More information on bar code scanning is provided in Chapter 6, "Elements of Safe Medication Administration."

WARNING!

Store Medications Per Label or Package Insert

Medications can lose potency and vaccines can be inactivated if not stored correctly. A California newspaper reported that the deaths of two people were linked to improper vaccine storage in a San Francisco bay area hospital. The vaccines were supposed to be refrigerated, but the temperature in the refrigerator was so low, they froze. The hospital pharmacist reported no one was assigned to check the temperature in the refrigerator (Mieszkowski, 2011). Nurses can prevent similar errors by always inspecting a medication prior to administration, and by *storing medications per label or package insert*.

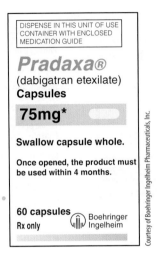

FIGURE 5-16   Pradaxa® label.

LEARNING ACTIVITY 5-1   Refer to **Figure 5-16** to answer the following questions.

1. What is the trade name?
2. What is the generic name?
3. What is the total number of capsules?
4. What is the dosage strength?
5. Can this capsule be opened?
6. How long can this medication be stored after opening?
7. What is the name of the manufacturer?

5-2   Information on a Medication Package Insert

In addition to the information listed on the medication label, the package insert provides detailed information for prescribing, storing, dispensing, and patient teaching. The package insert is designed to provide prescribers, pharmacists, and nurses necessary information to order, store, dispense, prepare, advise, and administer the medication safely. The package insert was reformatted in 2006 by the FDA (2009) to include highlights of significant information, a table of contents, a toll-free number, and Internet reporting information for reporting suspected side effects (**Figure 5-17**).

The typical components of a package insert include:

- *Indications and usage*—the medical conditions for which the preparation is intended and approved by the FDA to treat

- *Dosage and administration*—includes safe dosage range and intervals, dilution information (if required), route of administration, and rate of administration (if infused)

- *Dosage forms and strengths*—all of the available dosage forms and strengths, not just the enclosed form and strength as indicated on the label

- *Contraindications*—who and/or what conditions the medication *should not* be used to treat (e.g., people with allergies to the ingredients, people who have glaucoma, women who are nursing, or other reasons)

Nasonex® logo and image is reproduced with permission of Merck Sharp & Dohme Corp., Whitehouse Station, New Jersey, USA. All rights reserved.

HIGHLIGHTS OF PRESCRIBING INFORMA
These highlights do not include all the information needed to use NASONEX safely and effectively. See full prescribing information for NASONEX.

NASONEX® (mometasone furoate monohydrate) Nasal Spray, 50 mcg†
†calculated on the anhydrous basis
Initial U.S. Approval: 1997

------------------ **INDICATIONS AND USE** ------------------
NASONEX is a corticosteroid indicated for:
1. Treatment of Nasal Symptoms of Allergic Rhinitis in patients ≥2 years of age (1.1)
2. Treatment of Nasal Congestion Associated with Seasonal Allergic Rhinitis in patients ≥2 years of age (1.2)
3. Prophylaxis of Seasonal Allergic Rhinitis in patients ≥12 years of age (1.3)
4. Treatment of Nasal Polyps in patients ≥18 years of age (1.4)

------------------ **DOSAGE AND ADMINISTRATION** ------------------
For Intranasal Use Only
→ Treatment of Nasal Symptoms of Allergic Rhinitis (2.1)
  Adults & Adolescents (12 yrs. and older): 2 sprays in each nostril once daily
  Children (2-11 yrs.): 1 spray in each nostril once daily
→ Treatment of Nasal Congestion Associated with Seasonal Allergic Rhinitis (2.2)
  Adults & Adolescents (12 yrs. and older): 2 sprays in each nostril once daily
  Children (2-11 yrs.): 1 spray in each nostril once daily
→ Prophylaxis of Seasonal Allergic Rhinitis (2.3)
  Adults & Adolescents (12 yrs. and older): 2 sprays in each nostril once daily
→ Treatment of Nasal Polyps (2.4)

Adults (18 yrs. and older): 2 sprays in each nostril twice daily. 2 sprays in each nostril once daily may also be effective in some patients.

------------------ **DOSE FORMS AND STRENGTHS** ------------------
Nasal Spray: 50 mcg of mometasone furoate in each 100-microliter spray (3)

------------------ **CONTRAINDICATIONS** ------------------
Patients with known hypersensitivity to mometasone furoate or any of the ingredients of NASONEX. (4)

------------------ **WARNINGS AND PRECAUTIONS** ------------------
→ Epistaxis, nasal ulceration, Candida albicans infection, nasal septal perforation, impaired wound healing. Monitor patients periodically for signs of adverse effects on the nasal mucosa. Avoid use in patients with recent nasal ulcers, nasal surgery, or nasal trauma. (5.1)
→ Development of glaucoma or cataracts. Monitor patients closely with a change in vision or with a history of increased intraocular pressure, glaucoma, and/or cataracts. (5.2)
→ Potential worsening of existing tuberculosis; fungal, bacterial, viral, or parasitic infections; or ocular herpes simplex. More serious or even fatal course of chickenpox or measles in susceptible patients. Use caution in patients with the above because of the potential for worsening of these infections. (5.4)
→ Hypercorticism and adrenal suppression with higher than recommend dosages or at the regular dosage in susceptible individuals. If such changes occur, discontinue NASONEX Nasal Spray slowly. (5.5)
→ Potential reduction in growth velocity in children. Monitor growth routinely in pediatric patients receiving NASONEX Nasal Spray. (5.6, 8.4)

------------------ **ADVERSE REACTIONS** ------------------
The most common adverse reactions (≥5%) included headache, viral infection, pharyngitis, epistaxis and cough. (6)

To report SUSPECTED ADVERSE REACTIONS, contact Merck Sharp & Dohme Corp., a subsidiary of Merck & Co., Inc., at 1-877- 888-4231 or FDA 1-800-FDA-1088 or www.fda.gov/medwatch.

See 17 for PATIENT COUNSELING INFORMATION and FDA- approved patient labeling

FIGURE 5-17 Portion of Nasonex® package insert with revised format.

- *Warnings and precautions*—serious, possibly life-threatening conditions or reactions (side effects) that might occur if the medication is administered and how to administer or discontinue administering the medication if a reaction occurs

- *Adverse reactions*—less threatening reactions that have occurred during clinical trials (experiments prior to FDA approval) or after marketing for use by the general public

Clinical CLUE

If the package insert for a medication is not available, the nurse can view the package insert information online.

- *Drug interactions*—reactions of two types can occur:
  - Inside the body when a medication is administered while a different medication is still active in the body, there may be three possible reactions:
    - Increased potency of medication
    - Decreased potency of medication
    - New substance formation
  - Outside of the body, if two medications come in contact while mixing or infusing in an IV, generation of a new compound can form in the IV tubing, needle, or vial.
- *Use in specific populations*—reactions that occur within a specific group of patients, such as pregnant women, nursing mothers, children, the elderly, or patients with liver or kidney failure
- *Overdosage*—reactions/fatalities that have been observed after taking too much medication
- *Description*—chemical and physical description of the medication
- *Clinical pharmacology*—includes:
  - Action—how the drug works in the body, for example, "improves breathing by decreasing inflammation in the airways"
  - Pharmacodynamics—what the medication does on a cellular level, for example, promoting or blocking a process, such as occupying a receptor site to prevent transmission of chemical substance
  - Pharmacokinetics—effect of the body on the medication, for example, how it is absorbed, distributed, metabolized, and excreted
- *Nonclinical toxicology*—reports on animal studies indicating gene mutation, cancerous growths, or infertility and reports on the offspring of female animals that received the medication before and/or during pregnancy
- *Clinical studies*—controlled studies of the efficacy and safety of the medication when used to treat the conditions listed under *Indications*
- *How supplied/storage and handling*—describes the medication container, the total amount within the container, and total number of doses within the container; includes the NDC number and provides detailed storage information (**Figure 5-18**)
- *Patient counseling information*—information identifying, risks, usage instructions for best effect, how to handle a missed dose, and how to self-administer the medication (if applicable)

HOW SUPPLIED/STORAGE AND HANDLING

NASONEX (mometasone furoate monohydrate) Nasal Spray, 50 mcg is supplied in a white, high-density, polyethylene bottle fitted with a white metered-dose, manual spray pump, and blue cap. It contains 17 g of product formulation, 120 sprays, each delivering 50 mcg of mometasone furoate per actuation.

(NDC 0085-1288-01).

Store at 25°C (77°F); excursions permitted to 15-30°C (59-86°F) [see USP Controlled Room Temperature]. Protect from light. When NASONEX Nasal Spray, 50 mcg is removed from its cardboard container, prolonged exposure of the product to direct light should be avoided. Brief exposure to light, as with normal use, is acceptable.

SHAKE WELL BEFORE EACH USE.

Keep out of reach of children.

Nasonex® logo and image is reproduced with permission of Merck Sharp & Dohme Corp., Whitehouse Station, New Jersey, USA. All rights reserved.

FIGURE 5-18 How supplied/storage and handling section of Nasonex® package insert.

What's on a Label? ... Case Closure

Should the student nurse administer the otic solution into the eye? The label, stating "ofloxacin otic solution," not only contains the name of the medication, it also contains the route. The medication provided was the right drug, but the wrong route. The order called for ophthalmic (eye) drops, but the ofloxacin drops supplied were otic (ear) drops, so the student nurse should not administer this medication preparation. The correct preparation should have the following label:

ANTIBACTERIAL AGENT
Each mL contains ofloxacin 0.3% w/v (3 mg/mL) and benzalkonium chloride (0.005%) as preservative.

ADULT DOSAGE:
See package insert.

Store at room temperature 15-30°C (59-86°F). Discard 28 days after opening.

5 mL   STERILE

OFLOXACIN

Ofloxacin
Ophthalmic Solution USP

0.3% w/v

Apo-ofloxacin, ofloxacin ophthalmic solution (eye drops).

Chapter Summary

Learning Outcomes	Points to Remember
5-1 Differentiate information on a medication label.	• Generic name—chemical name; does not identify the manufacturer; listed in *United States Pharmacopeia—National Formulary (USP-NF)* • Trade/brand name—name specific to manufacturer, registered with U.S. Department of Commerce • Combination medication—lists the generic name of each medication and the dosage strength of each medication • Form—identified on label: solid (capsule, tablet, gelcap, suppository), liquid (oral liquid, injectable liquid, inhalant, drop, spray, mist), or other (topical cream, ointment, patch) • Dosage strength—amount of medication in each dosage unit (e.g., 325 mg per tablet, 80 mg per mL, 200 mcg per metered spray) • Total number, volume, or net weight—total number of solid medication units (e.g., tablets), total volume of liquid or total weight of ointment or cream per container (bottle, tube, etc.) • Multiple dose/multiple use—medication packaging containing more than one medication dose • Single dose—medication packaging that contains one typical medication dose • Single use—medication container designed to be used once and then discarded • Route of administration—bodily entry point for medication administration, leading to absorption into the bloodstream; may be implied in name (e.g., "nasal spray" implies nasal inhalation) • Reconstitution—process of mixing a medication (e.g., liquefying a powdered medication) • Warnings—alerts on the label to protect the patient from medication administration errors • Controlled substance schedule—classification of substances (Schedules I–V) that lead to physical or psychological dependence; schedule I (most potential for abuse) to schedule V (least potential for abuse); labeled with a "C" in which a Roman numeral schedule number is inserted in the center • Storage information—temperature range, lighting, shelf life • Manufacturing information—pharmaceutical company, NDC/control number, expiration date, lot number, bar code
5-2 Identify information on a medication package insert.	• The package insert is designed to provide prescribers, pharmacists, and nurses necessary information to order, store, dispense, prepare, advise, and administer the medication safely. • Highlights of prescriber information are included at the top of the insert followed by reporting information for suspected reactions. • Table of contents is given to provide easy navigation through document. • Some categories of information include indications and usage, dosage and administration, contraindications, precautions and warnings, adverse interactions, drug interactions, clinical studies, storage and handling, and patient counseling information.

Homework

For exercises 1–10, indicate if the statement is true or false. Correct false statements to make them true. (LO 5-1)

1. The *United States Pharmacopeia—National Formulary (USP-NF)* is a book that contains standards for medicines, dosage forms, drug substances, excipients, medical devices, and dietary supplements.

2. The generic name is registered with the U.S. Department of Commerce, Patent and Trademark Office by the manufacturer, so that no other pharmaceutical company can use the same name.

3. Dosage strength refers to the amount of medication in the container.

4. Reconstitution instructions are directions for liquefying a powdered medication.

5. All medications have a controlled schedule number.

6. There are five schedules for controlled substances; the first schedule is for highly addictive substances that have no medicinal benefit.

7. Only controlled schedule medications have a Roman numeral within the letter C on the medication label.

8. The package insert will provide more complete information about the drug than the label, including chemical and physical description, clinical pharmacology, indications and usage, contraindications, warnings, precautions, adverse reactions, overdosage, dosage and administration, preparation for administration, and manufacturer supply information.

9. The NDC number indicates the manufacturing batch, date, and location.

10. The route of administration may be indicated by the name of the medication.

For exercises 11–45, provide the information requested for each corresponding medication label that precedes it. (LO 5-1)

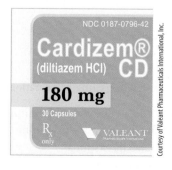

Courtesy of Valeant Pharmaceuticals International, Inc.

11. Generic name _____
12. Trade name _____
13. Total number of capsules _____
14. Dosage strength _____
15. Manufacturer _____

Rx only

NDC 10019-028-01

Midazolam C IV
Injection, USP

2 mg/2 mL
(1 mg/mL)

10 x 2 mL Vials

midazolam (as the hydrochloride)
FOR IM OR IV USE ONLY
CONTAINS BENZYL ALCOHOL

16. Generic name _____
17. Route of administration _____
18. Control schedule _____
19. Single-use or multi-use vial _____
20. NDC number _____

WARNING

Adult and Pediatric: Intravenous midazolam has been associated with respiratory depression and respiratory arrest, especially when used for sedation in noncritical care settings. In some cases, where this was not recognized promptly and treated effectively, death or hypoxic encephalopathy has resulted...

Neonates: Midazolam should not be administered by rapid injection in the neonatal population. Severe hypotension and seizures have been reported following rapid IV administration, particularly with concomitant use of fentanyl (see DOSAGE AND ADMINISTRATION for complete information).

21. To what conditions are neonates vulnerable when this medication is administered too rapidly?

NDC 0093-1075-78

CEFPROZIL
for Oral Suspension USP
125 mg/5 mL*

*Each 5 mL, when constituted according to directions, contains 125 mg anhydrous cefprozil.

℞ only

75 mL (when mixed)

TEVA

Courtesy of Teva USA.

22. Manufacturer _____
23. Route of administration _____
24. Dosage strength _____

25. Total volume after mixing _____

26. Trade name _____

27. NDC or Bar Code Number _____

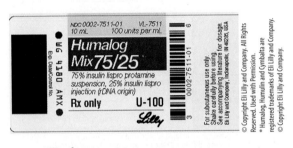

28. Trade name _____

29. Total volume _____

30. Dosage strength _____

31. Manufacturer _____

32. Where can you find the full prescribing information?

33. Is the number under the bar code the same as the NDC number?

34. Trade name _____

35. Is this a combination medication? If so, name the medications. _____

36. How many units are in 1 mL? _____

37. Total volume _____

38. Route of administration _____

39. Generic name _____

40. Net weight _____

41. Dosage strength _____

42. Route of administration _____

43. Can this medication be used in the eyes?

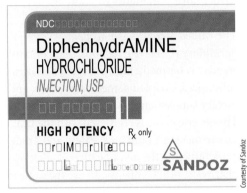

Label 1

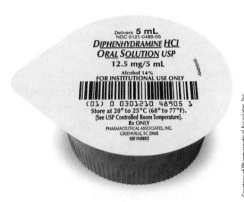

Label 2

44. Which label represents the medication form that should be used for the following order? "Diphenhydramine 25 mg PO q6h"

For questions 45–50, select the category (a–j) on the package insert where the requested information can be located. (LO 5-2)

    a. Indications and Usage/Use in Specific Populations

    b. Dosage and Administration

    c. Forms and Dosage Strength

    d. Contraindications

    e. Precautions and Warnings

    f. Adverse Reactions

    g. Drug Interactions

    h. Clinical Studies

    i. Storage and Handling

    j. Patient Counseling Information

45. Is the ordered dose safe to administer?

46. Is this medication safe to administer if the patient also has asthma?

47. Are there any increased risks if an elderly person takes this medication?
48. What should the nurse tell the patient about this medication?
49. Can this medication be administered if the patient is also taking iron?
50. Is this medication available in liquid form if the patient cannot swallow pills?

NCLEX-Style Review Questions

For questions 1–4, select the best response.

1. The prescriber orders: phenytoin 250 mg PO qid for 1 day. Which preparation should the nurse use?
   a. Phenytoin oral suspension 100 mg in a 4 mL single-dose container
   b. Phenytoin oral suspension 125 mg/5 mL in a 240 mL multiple-dose container
   c. Phenytoin ER 100 mg/capsule in a 180-capsule container
   d. Phenytoin injection 250 mg/5 mL in a 5 mL single-dose container

2. The medication label states: Protect from light. Store between 36–46°F (20–25°C). The nurse should:
   a. Place in a zip-lock bag and store at room temperature.
   b. Wrap in foil and store at room temperature.
   c. Place in a paper bag and store in the refrigerator.
   d. Wrap the vial in foil and store in the freezer.

3. The prescriber orders diazepam 5 mg PO, single dose, now. Which preparation should the nurse use?
   a. Diazepam inj 5 mg/mL single-dose container
   b. Diazepam oral solution 2 mg/5 mL single-dose container
   c. Diazepam 2 mg/tablet single-dose container
   d. Diazepam 5 mg/tablet multiple-dose container

4. The prescriber orders furosemide 10 mg IV bid. The nurse is supplied with furosemide with the following label. The nurse should:

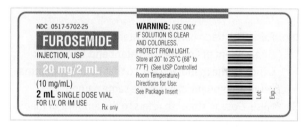

a. Call the pharmacist to deliver a different preparation.
b. Administer the contents and protect unused portion from light.
c. Administer the contents of the vial and discard.
d. Administer half of the contents and discard the remainder.

For questions 5 and 6, refer to the labels associated with the question and identify all information that can be found on the label. Select all that apply.

5.

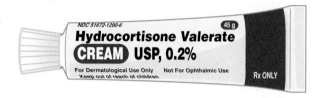

a. The dosage strength is 2 mg/g.
b. Requires a prescription.
c. To be applied in the eye.
d. Keep out of reach of children.
e. Net weight 20 grams.

6.

a. Store at room temperature.
b. May be administered subcut.
c. Protect from light.
d. Vial contains two 10 mL doses.
e. Solution should be clear.

REFERENCES

Mieszkowski, K. (2011). Medication storage error affects thousands of Kaiser patients. *The Bay Citizen*. Retrieved from http://www.baycitizen.org/health/story/medication-storage-error-affects-kaiser

U.S. Drug Enforcement Administration. (2014). *Controlled substance schedules.* Retrieved from http://www.deadiversion.usdoj.gov/schedules

U.S. Food and Drug Administration. (2009). *The FDA announces new prescription drug information format.* Retrieved from http://www.fda.gov/Drugs

/GuidanceComplianceRegulatoryInformation
/LawsActsandRules/ucm188665.htm

U.S. Food and Drug Administration. (2014). *National drug code directory, background information.* Retrieved from http://www.fda.gov/Drugs /InformationOnDrugs/ucm142438.htm

United States Pharmacopeia-National Formulary. (2014). USP-NF: An overview. Retrieved from http://www.usp.org/usp-nf

Chapter 5   ANSWER KEY

Learning Activity 5-1

1. Pradaxa®
2. dabigatran etexilate
3. 60 capsules per bottle
4. 75 mg per capsule
5. No, it must be swallowed whole.
6. 4 months
7. Boehringer Ingelheim Pharmaceuticals, Inc.

Homework

1. True
2. False. The trade name is registered with the U.S. Department of Commerce, Patent and Trademark Office by the manufacturer, so that no other pharmaceutical company can use the same name.
3. False. Dosage strength refers to the amount of medication per dosage unit.
4. True
5. False. Medications that are prone to physical or psychological abuse or dependence have a controlled schedule number.
6. True
7. True
8. True
9. False. The lot number indicates the manufacturing batch, date, and location.
10. True
11. diltiazem HCl
12. Cardizem® CD
13. 30 capsules
14. 180 mg/capsule
15. Valeant Pharmaceuticals International

16. midazolam HCl
17. IM/IV
18. IV
19. Multi-use, benzyl alcohol is a preservative
20. NDC 10019-028-01
21. Severe hypotension and seizures
22. Teva Pharmaceuticals USA
23. PO (oral; by mouth)
24. 125 mg/5 mL
25. 75 mL
26. There is no trade name. There is only a generic name, cefprozil.
27. 0093-1075-78
28. Dilantin-125
29. 237 mL
30. 125 mg/5 mL; 25 mg/mL
31. Pfizer/Parke-Davis
32. In the package insert
33. Yes
34. Humalog® Mix 75/25"
35. Yes, insulin lispro protamine suspension, and insulin lispro injection
36. 100 units
37. 10 mL
38. Subcut
39. Lidocaine HCl
40. 1 oz (28.3 g)
41. 3% or 3 g per 100 g
42. Topical
43. No, it is not for ophthalmic use.
44. Label 2
45. b (Dosage and administration)
46. d (Contraindications)
47. a (Use in specific populations)
48. j (Patient counseling information)
49. g (Drug interactions)
50. c (Forms and dosage strengths)

NCLEX-Style Review Questions

1. b
   Rationale: Phenytoin oral suspension 125 mg/5 mL in a multiple-dose container will provide enough medication for the ordered dose (250 mg is twice 125, so 10 mL could be obtained from the multiple-dose container).

2. c

    Rationale: 36–46°F is a refrigerated temperature; 32°F and below is freezing. Placing the medication in a paper bag will protect it from light.

3. d

    Rationale: In general, unless the patient has difficulty swallowing pills, tablets are used for oral doses rather than liquids. Single doses can be removed from multiple-dose containers, but a medication packaged as a single dose cannot be used for multiple doses.

4. d

    Rationale: The single-dose vial contains twice the dose required. Although 20 mg will be given over the course of the day, medication in a single-dose vial cannot be saved for subsequent doses. The nurse should discard the vial with remaining medication after removing 10 mg of furosemide.

5. a, b, d

    Rationale: The label information includes:
    a. USP, 0.2%.
    b. Rx ONLY.
    c. For Dermatological Use Only; Not for Opthalmic Use.
    d. Keep out of reach of children.
    e. Net weight 45 g.

6. a, c, e

    Rationale: The label states:
    a. Store between 68–77°F.
    b. For intravenous or intramuscular use.
    c. Protect from light.
    d. Discard unused portion; single-use vial.
    e. Use only if solution is clear and colorless.

© Forfunlife/Shutterstock

Chapter 6

Elements of Safe Medication Administration

CHAPTER OUTLINE

LEARNING OUTCOMES

Upon completion of the chapter, the student will be able to:

6-1 Explain the three medication label checks done during preparation for medication administration.

6-2 Differentiate the procedural and patient rights of medication administration.

6-3 Summarize the importance of patient assessment throughout the medication administration process.

6-4 Discuss the appropriate use of patient teaching as it relates to safe medication administration.

KEY TERMS

**Bar Code Medication
Administration (BCMA)**

high-alert medications

Institute of Medicine (IOM)

time-critical medications

workarounds

Case Consideration ... Drug Dilemma!

Over the course of several days, a staff nurse administered quinidine sulfate to a patient whose order was for quinine sulfate. Quinidine is classified as an antiarrhythmic medication (i.e., it is given to treat altered heart rhythms), while quinine is classified as an antimalarial medication, which, in the past, was also used to treat leg cramps. The patient had no documented history of heart problems. Because quinidine was the medication stocked in the patient's storage bin and was a typical medication administered on the medical unit in which the staff nurse worked, the assumption was made that quinidine was the right drug to administer. The nurse rationalized that quinine was an alternate drug name for quinidine. As a result of receiving the quinidine, the patient experienced a significant drop in blood pressure, one of the toxic side effects of this medication.

1. What went wrong?

2. How could this error have been avoided?

■ INTRODUCTION

Medication administration is a complex process that includes prescribing, transcribing, dispensing and administering drugs. Errors that occur when administering drugs account for 26–32% of all medication errors, and nurses administer most medications (Anderson & Townsend, 2010). The **Institute of Medicine (IOM)**, an independent organization that provides unbiased and authoritative advice to decision makers and the public, published a report entitled *To Err is Human: Building a Safer Health System*. This report revealed that "medication-related errors accounted for one out of every 131 outpatient deaths and one out of 854 inpatient deaths" (IOM, 1999). Because medication therapy is a primary treatment for many illnesses, it is imperative that nurses learn and embrace safe medication administration practices. This chapter focuses on the role of the nurse in safe medication administration.

6-1   Three Medication Label Checks

In order to ensure that the correct medication is about to be administered, the nurse should check the label three times. The medication should be checked *just prior* to medication preparation, *during* medication preparation, and *after* medication preparation.

Before Medication Preparation

The first medication label check occurs when retrieving the medication from the storage container. During this label check, the nurse should look at not only at the drug name, but also the expiration date.

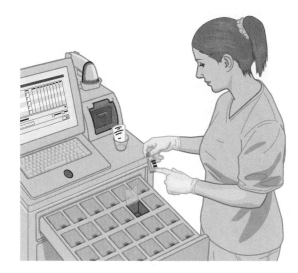

FIGURE 6-1   The first label check—the nurse looks at the medication label upon removing it from the Pyxis™ machine.

This label check occurs when the nurse removes a unit-dose medication from a storage unit such as the Pyxis MedStation®, which is a computer-controlled medication dispensing system (**Figure 6-1**). The first label check also occurs when the nurse retrieves refrigerated medications, such vaccines, antibiotics, or insulin. Stock-supplied medication—those available in multiple-dose containers, such as Maalox® or liquid Tylenol®—should also be checked when they are retrieved from their storage location.

During Medication Preparation

The second label check should occur while the medication is being prepared for administration and starts with matching the label to the medication administration record (MAR) or electronic medication administration record (eMAR) as shown in **Figure 6-2**. Examples of completion of the second label check include viewing the:

- Unit-dose medication label while placing it in a medicine cup

- Multiple-dose container label while pouring the medicine

- Label on the vial of injectable medication while drawing it up (**Figure 6-3**)

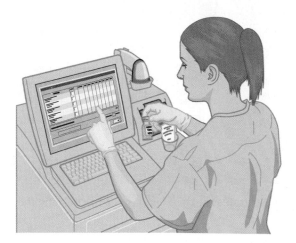

FIGURE 6-2   Matching the medication to the medication administration record or the patient medication list generated by the computerized dispensing system, the nurse demonstrates the second medication label check.

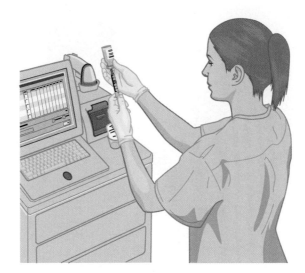

FIGURE 6-3 After matching the medication vial label to the eMAR, the nurse examines the vial label while withdrawing the medication, demonstrating the second medication label check.

After Medication Preparation

Once the nurse discerns that the medication is ready for administration, the third label check occurs just prior to administering the medication to the patient. This typically takes place at the bedside as depicted in **Figure 6-4**. Many healthcare agencies use **Bar Code Medication Administration (BCMA)** systems. BCMA systems require scanning bar codes of each medication prior to administration. Scanning the medication label bar code serves as an additional label check (**Figure 6-5**).

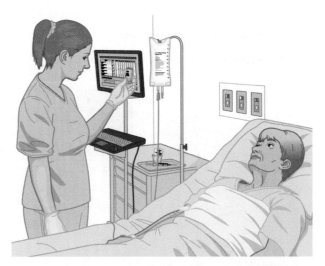

FIGURE 6-4 The nurse demonstrates the third label check by checking the medication label just prior to administration.

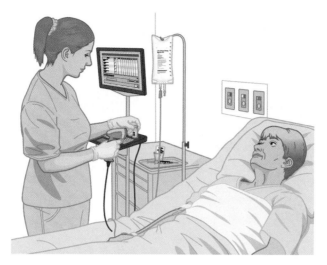

FIGURE 6-5   The nurse uses a bar code scanner to check the label of a prefilled syringe just before administration, demonstrating the third label check.

LEARNING ACTIVITY 6-1 Identify which label check (1st, 2nd, or 3rd) is demonstrated by the nurse in each scenario.

1.   The nurse draws up the regular insulin.
2.   The nurse scans the regular insulin vial at the patient's bedside.
3.   The nurse takes regular insulin out of the refrigerator.

6-2   Rights of Medication Administration

Safe medication administration is the responsibility of several members of the healthcare team:

- The prescriber must write a correct and complete order.

- The pharmacist must accurately fill the order.

- The nurse or other licensed personnel must safely administer the ordered medication(s).

The nurse can ensure safety when giving medication to patients by attending to the "Rights of Medication Administration." The "rights" are a set of safety checks that, when adhered to, will prevent a medication error. There are seven procedural rights and two additional patient rights. The Procedural Rights of Medication Administration are essential safety checks that must be performed with the administration of each and every medication. These rights indicate that **the *right patient* must receive the *right drug* in the *right dose* via the *right route* at the *right time* for the *right reason* followed by the *right documentation*.** The additional patient rights are those that enhance patient safety, and they indicate that patients have the:

- *Right to know* about their medications

- *Right to refuse* their medications

Right Patient

To ensure that the right patient is being medicated, the individual is checked by two identifiers. The first identifier is the patient's full name. The second identifier can be the date of birth (DOB), social security number (SSN), or medical record number (MRN). In a home care setting, the patient's address may be used as a second identifier. The name on the MAR must be exactly the same as the name of the patient.

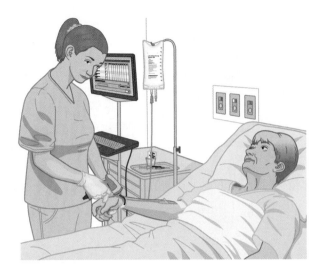

FIGURE 6-6   In addition to asking the patient to state his/her name and DOB, for proper patient identification, the nurse should visually inspect the patient's ID bracelet prior to scanning the bar code.

The nurse should ask the patient to state his or her full name and DOB and then check the patient's identification (ID) bracelet to ensure the information matches. If the patient is unable to state his or her name, the nurse should ask the parent or caregiver to state the patient's full name. In long-term care and outpatient facilities, the nurse may require photographic identification to ensure this basic right. In facilities that use BCMA, the patient's identification bracelet will be scanned after it is visually inspected by the nurse (**Figure 6-6**). Proper patient identification will ensure not only that the right patient is being medicated, but that the right MAR is being used for that patient.

Right Drug

To ensure that the patient receives the right drug, the nurse should perform three medication label checks during preparation for medication administration. Nurses should only administer medications that they themselves have prepared. With BCMA, the patient's ID band is scanned, and each medication is scanned and electronically checked against the eMAR. This process provides an *additional* safety check to ensure the right patient receives the right drug. The nurse should never rely solely on bar code scanning to identify the patient or the medication. Sometimes the nurse or the patient may not be familiar with the medication size, shape, or color. If the nurse or patient has any doubt about whether a medication is correct, the pharmacist should be contacted and the order should be rechecked. If a medication is ordered by a brand name, such as Tylenol®, and the pharmacy supplies the generic medication, acetaminophen, or a different brand (such as Paracetamol®), the nurse must verify that the drug supplied is the "right drug."

Clinical CLUE

The "right drug" check also includes checking the expiration date on the drug label. If the medication supplied is expired, the nurse should contact the pharmacist for an updated supply.

Right Dose

In order to administer the right dose, the nurse must look at the dosage strength of the medication that is supplied and perform a dosage calculation, if necessary. Nurses should use extreme caution with dosage calculations and pay close attention to decimal points. The nurse should approximate the amount to administer prior to performing a dosage calculation. Approximation prior to calculation will increase confidence that the calculated amount to administer is reasonable. Nurses should question unreasonable dosage calculation amounts. Because an alert is generated on the eMAR if an incorrect dose is scanned, the BCMA process helps to ensure that the correct dose is administered.

Clinical CLUE

It is the right and responsibility of the nurse to question orders thought to be inappropriate. Examples of questionable orders include:

- Orders yielding unusually large administration amounts, such as:

  - An order that requires the administration of more than 3 tablets for 1 dose

  - An order for a medication supplied in teaspoons requiring more than 3 t (15 mL)

  - An order for a medication supplied in ounces requiring more than 1 oz (30 mL)

- Orders for atypically high doses. To recognize unusual doses, nurses should become familiar with typical medication doses for the patient population they serve.

Right Route

Nurses must administer medications by the right route as indicated in the medication order. Drugs intended for one route may not be safe if administered by another route; for example, ear drops may not be safe to administer into the eye. The nurse should check that the route listed on the label is consistent with the ordered route. In addition, the nurse must be familiar with the right technique for medication administration via certain routes. Nurses who are not familiar with a particular route or technique should consult a reputable drug reference or their facility policy and procedure manual.

Right Time

The rule of thumb for the "right time" was that medications must be administered within 30 minutes of the scheduled time. Because this rule was difficult to follow, as was discovered by a 2008 study done by the Center for Medicare and Medicaid Services (CMS), the Institute for Safe Medication Practices (ISMP, 2011) established new guidelines for timely administration of medication, distinguishing **time-critical medications** from non-time-critical medications. Time-critical medications are those for which "early or late administration (30 minutes before or after scheduled time) might result in harm or negatively affect the patient's treatment" (Stokowski, 2012). Medications designated as time-critical are determined by each healthcare institution. Examples of time-critical medications include hormones, antibiotics, and cardiac medications. The ISMP (2011) has established the following guidelines for timely medication administration:

- Time-critical medications:

  - Medications ordered to be given at a specified time should be administered as close as possible to the ordered time. For example, insulin is often ordered to be given 30 minutes before breakfast, in which case, if breakfast comes at 0800, then the insulin should be given at 0730.

  - Other medications designated as time-critical should be administered within 30 minutes of scheduled administration time.

- Non-time-critical medications:

    - Daily, weekly, or monthly medications should be given within 2 hours of the scheduled time.

    - Medications ordered more than daily but not more than q4h should be administered within 60 minutes of scheduled time.

    - Medications ordered more than q4h should be given within 25% of the dosing interval, for example:
        - q3h medicine should be given within 45 minutes of the scheduled time
        - q2h medicine should be given within 30 minutes of the scheduled time
        - q1h medicine should be given within 15 minutes of the scheduled time

Medications ordered on a *prn* basis should be given within the frequency ordered, requiring the nurse to ensure that enough time has passed since the last dose before providing a subsequent dose. The *right time is the most frequently violated right of medication administration*, accounting for one-third of reported medication errors (Stokowski, 2012). Because an alert is generated on the eMAR if a medication is scanned at an unscheduled/inappropriate time, the BCMA process helps to ensure that a medication is administered at the right time.

Clinical CLUE

Depending on policy or orders, medications are sometimes held (not given) prior to procedures, such as dialysis, and then administered upon the patient's return.

Right Reason

The nurse must administer a medication for the right reason (Olin, 2012). This requires the nurse to know the rationale for each drug order. Knowing why a medication is ordered will inform the nurse as to when a medication should be withheld. For example, if a patient is receiving a medication for high blood pressure, the nurse will recognize the need to hold the medication and contact the prescriber if the blood pressure is low.

Clinical CLUE

High-alert medications are those that can cause significant harm if given in error. Prior to administration of most high-alert medications, it is recommended that two nurses independently check these six procedural rights: right patient, right drug, right dose, right route, right time, and right reason. More information regarding high-alert medications is included in Chapter 14.

Right Documentation

Medication administration should be followed by the right documentation. In health care, that which is not documented is considered not done. Lack of documentation of medication administration is particularly dangerous, because it could lead to the patient receiving a double dose of medication. Documentation on the MAR or eMAR should be done at the time the medication is administered. With BCMA, after the patient ID band and medication are scanned, the nurse administers the medication and then electronically signs off the medication as given (**Figure 6-7**).

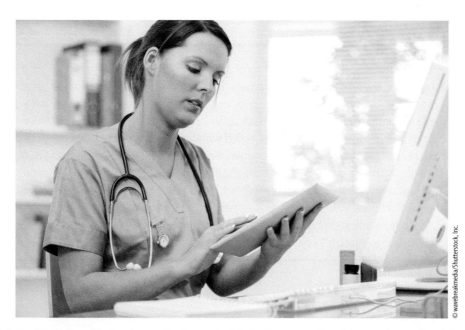

© wavebreakmedia/Shutterstock, Inc.

FIGURE 6-7   With the electronic medication administration record and bar code medication administration, the nurse can sign off a medication as given with a simple screen tap or click of a mouse.

Clinical CLUE

Just as important as documenting that a medication was given is the documentation of a medication that was intentionally not given. When a medication is not given, the nurse should also document the reason that the medication was not given, such as held for dialysis, patient vomiting, heart rate less than 60, or patient off the unit for procedure.

Right to Know

Patients have the right to know about the medications that they are receiving. They should be informed about the dose, schedule, reason, effect, and side effects of each medication. In addition, information regarding drug–drug interactions and drug–food interactions should be given in order to maximize the drugs' effects. Well informed patients promote medication administration safety. More information regarding the patient's right to know is covered in the Patient Teaching section of this chapter.

Right to Refuse

Patients have the right to refuse a medication and nurses must respect this right. The nurse should investigate a patient's reason for medication refusal and report it promptly to the prescriber. Medication refusal should be documented on the MAR/eMAR along with the reason for refusal.

LEARNING ACTIVITY 6-2 For the following medication order, identify the right as requested: Give David C. Smith (DOB 2/12/90) Synthroid® 0.1 mg PO 30 min ā breakfast (which is served at 0900).

1.   Right Route _____
2.   Right Dose _____ mcg
3.   Right Time _____ a.m.

WARNING!

Avoid Workarounds!

The BCMA system can improve patient safety by reducing medication errors, but only when used correctly by healthcare professionals. When a medication cannot be scanned, such as a medication with a damaged barcode label, a nurse might manually enter the medication information, bypassing the BCMA system. Omitted or unauthorized steps in the BCMA process are called **workarounds** and can place the patient at risk for medication error (LaDuke, 2009). Workarounds are sometimes called "overrides," because the BCMA process is overridden to continue with the medication administration process. In overriding the process, proper documentation may not occur, in which case the patient is exposed to the possibility of receiving an extra dose of medication. Other workarounds include neglecting to perform a visual five rights (patient, drug, dose, route, time) check and scanning medication bar codes after removing them from the packaging. In order to promote safe medication administration, nurses should avoid shortcuts and follow institutional BCMA guidelines.

6-3   Assessment

Assessment is an important component of safe medication administration. The nurse should assess the patient before, during, and after medication administration, because this enhances patient safety. **TABLE 6-1** provides examples of assessment parameters for each phase of medication administration.

LEARNING ACTIVITY 6-3 Cite assessments that should be made during each phase of medication administration for a patient that is scheduled to receive an intravenous pain medication.

1.   Before ＿＿＿＿＿＿＿＿＿＿
2.   During ＿＿＿＿＿＿＿＿＿＿
3.   After ＿＿＿＿＿＿＿＿＿＿

TABLE 6-1   Patient Observation Before, During, and After Medication Administration Enhances Patient Safety

Before	During	After
Check: • Allergies • Patient condition • Ability to use the prescribed route, for example: 　• Oral 　• IV site 　• Injection site 　• NGT placement	Observe that medication is received and retained, for example: • Did the patient swallow the pill(s)? • Was the suppository retained? • Did the medication infuse in its entirety?	Reassess: • Did the medication have the intended effect? For example, is the pain relieved? • Did the medication cause any side effects (e.g., rash, nausea)?

According to the National Council for Patient Information and Education (2013), "it is estimated that half of the 3.2 billion prescription medicines dispensed each year are not taken as prescribed." According to the Agency for Healthcare Research and Quality (2012), consistent evidence for education as an intervention for supporting medication adherence was found. Because patients have the right to know about the medications they are receiving, proper teaching should be provided to the patient. "Educating the patient before they leave the hospital reduces admissions, emergency department visits and saves money." (Leigh, 2009). If necessary, the caregiver, too, should receive medication information. Prior to teaching, the nurse needs to determine the knowledge and literacy level of the patient and caregiver. With attention to learning needs and literacy level, the nurse should provide the following information:

- Medication name—both brand and generic

- Where to obtain the medicine

- Purpose of the medication as it pertains to the patient's condition

- Dose and amount to administer

- Route and administration guidelines

- Scheduled times of administration

- Drug–drug interactions

- Adverse effects and when to contact the prescriber

    It is advisable to provide these instructions both verbally and in writing.

Clinical CLUE

Medicine is a very expensive component of healthcare treatment. When resources are limited, health insurance does not cover the cost or entire cost of medication, some patients will forgo their medications. Many companies that make prescription medicine have patient assistance programs (PAPs) to assist low-income patients in obtaining medications for free or at a reduced cost. Nurses should become aware and provide information to patients about resources available for patients with limited resources.

Effective patient medication teaching requires appropriate medication reference materials. *Nurse's Drug Handbook* is a comprehensive drug manual (**Figure 6-8**) that is updated annually and includes:

- Generic, trade, and alternate drug names

- Drug classification information

- Indications and dosages, as well as route, onset, peak, and duration information

- Incompatibilities and contraindications

- Interactions with drugs, food, and activities

- Adverse reactions, side effects, warnings, and precautions

- Nursing considerations, including key patient-teaching points

    Many other resources are available to nurses in print and online and should be accessible on all patient care units. Most electronic health records are linked to medication databases, making it convenient for the nurse to access information right from the patient's eMAR (**Figure 6-9**).

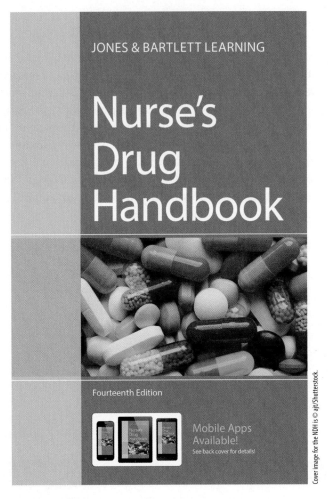

Cover image for the NDH is © ajt/Shutterstock.

FIGURE 6-8   A nursing drug handbook should be accessible on all patient care units. *Nurse's Drug Handbook* is a handy-sized, user-friendly reference.

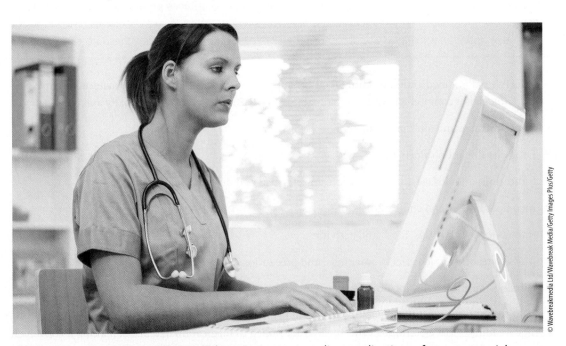

© Wavebreakmedia Ltd/Wavebreak Media/Getty Images Plus/Getty

FIGURE 6-9   This patient eMAR provides easy access to online medication reference materials.

WARNING!

Limit Distractions During Medication Administration!

An error reported to the ISMP more than a decade ago is still an excellent example of how easy it is to make an error when distracted and interrupted. A nurse who had just measured a dose of liquid chloral hydrate into a cup was interrupted by a pharmacist on her way to the patient's room. The conversation was social, and the nurse—who often had a cup of coffee in her hand—absentmindedly drank the medication, as if taking a sip of coffee! The nurse had to be driven home (ISMP, 2012).

LEARNING ACTIVITY 6-4 For the following medication order, indicate the information that should be provided to the patient for each specified category of patient teaching:

Amoxil® (amoxicillin 250 mg/5 mL), 5 mL PO q8h 1h ā meals or snacks

1.   Medication name _____
2.   Dose/amount to administer _____
3.   Schedule _____

Drug Dilemma ... Case Closure

When the nurse administered quinidine instead of quinine, the most obvious error was the violation of "right drug." The nurse should not have assumed quinine was another name for quinidine. Had the nurse clarified the drug name by consulting a drug manual, online site, or pharmacist, the error would have been avoided. The "right reason" for administering the medication was also violated, because quinidine was not indicated for this patient. If the nurse honored the patient's "right to know," and provided information on the purpose for quinidine, the patient might have recognized the wrong reason and exercised the "right to refuse." Instead, the rights of safe medication were ignored, and the patient suffered a drop in blood pressure, which could cause a fall or other harm, from a medication that was never ordered. The patient also did not receive the benefit of quinine, the prescribed drug.

Always perform the three checks and the rights of safe medication administration to prevent errors.

Chapter Summary

Learning Outcomes	Points to Remember
6-1 Explain the three medication label checks done during preparation for medication administration.	The medication label must be checked three times: • *Prior to medication preparation*—when retrieving from storage • *During medication preparation*—after matching the medication label to the MAR/eMAR, the label is viewed while placing unit dose medication in a medicine cup or while pouring medication from a multi-dose container or while drawing up medication for injection • *After medication preparation*—just prior to administration, usually at the patient bedside

6-2 Differentiate the procedural and patient rights of medication administration.	• The seven Procedural Rights of Medication Administration are: The *right patient* should receive the *right medication* in the *right dose* via the *right route* at the *right time* for the *right reason* followed by the *right documentation*. • Patient rights are: 　o *Right to know* 　o *Right to refuse* Note: The Bar Code Medication Administration (BCMA) process requires a visual inspection of the first five rights in addition to scanning the bar code of the patient's ID band and the bar codes of each medication. Omitting steps in the BCMA process is called a *workaround* and should be avoided.
6-3 Summarize the importance of patient assessment throughout the medication administration process.	• *Before* medication administration, check allergies, patient condition, and access to route. • *During* medication administration, check that the patient received and retained the medicine. • *After* medication administration check that the medication had the intended effect; observe for side effects.
6-4 Discuss the appropriate use of patient teaching as it relates to safe medication administration.	Teach the patient and/or caregiver: • Medication name and where to obtain it • Purpose, dose, route, schedule • Adverse effects and when to contact the prescriber Information for patient teaching can be obtained from *Nurse's Drug Handbook* or other medication references.

Homework

For exercises 1–5, indicate whether the statement is true or false. Correct the false statements. (LO 6-1)

1. To ensure that the right patient receives the right amount of medication, the medication label is to be checked three times.
2. For a multiple-dose container of liquid Tylenol®, the first label check occurs while pouring the medication.
3. By checking the label of ampicillin at the bedside, the nurse is demonstrating the third label check.
4. While drawing up the hepatitis B vaccine, the nurse checks the label, which demonstrates the second label check.
5. After retrieving the influenza vaccine from the refrigerator, the nurse matches the medication label to the eMAR, demonstrating the second label check.

For exercises 6–10, name the rights of medication administration that are also components of the medication order. (LO 6-2)

6. _____
7. _____
8. _____
9. _____
10. _____

For exercises 11–20, indicate whether or not the rights of medication administration are adhered to by stating, "Yes" or "No." State which right is violated or implemented. (LO 6-3)

11. A time-critical medication ordered q12h is given at 0800 and 2200.
12. A sublingual medication is placed between the cheeks and gums.
13. Acetaminophen 650 mg PO is ordered. Tylenol® 650 mg PO is given.
14. The nurse documents on the eMAR after medication administration.
15. The patient has an order for "Tylenol® 650 mg PO q4h prn fever greater than 101°F." The patient complains of back pain but does not have an order for pain medication. The nurse administers the Tylenol® per patient request.
16. A patient is refusing her medication. The nurse, knowing that the medication is needed for blood pressure regulation, crushes and mixes the medication with food and administers it to the patient.

17. The nurse questions an order for five capsules of Pancrease® prior to administration.
18. Stadol 2 mg IM stat is ordered. The nurse administers this medication via the intravenous line.
19. The label on the medication bottle states, "for optic use," and the medication is administered in the eyes.
20. Carlos S. Silva (DOB 4/7/43) receives medication ordered for Carol L. Silva (DOB 7/18/84).

For exercises 21–31, fill in the blanks. (LO 6-2)

21. The right _____ must receive the
22. Right _____ in the
23. Right _____ through the
24. Right _____ at the
25. Right _____ for the
26. Right _____ followed by the
27. Right _____.
28. The patient has the right to _____ about their medications.
29. The patient has the right to _____ their medications.
30. The _____ Rights of Medication Administration are essential to patient safety.
31. The _____ Rights of Medication Administration enhance patient safety.

For exercises 32–40, list the assessments that should be made during each phase of medication administration for a patient with the following orders *in italics*: (LO 6-3)

Tylenol 650 mg PR q4h prn fever greater than 38.6°C

32. Before: _____
_____

33. During: _____
_____

34. After: _____
_____

Digoxin 0.25 mg PO daily; hold for heart rate less than 60 beats per minute (bpm)

35. Before: _____
_____

36. During: _____
_____

37. After: _____
_____

Lorazepam 4 mg IM q4h prn for agitation

38. Before: _____
    _____

39. During: _____
    _____

40. After: _____
    _____

For exercises 41–45, indicate whether the statement is true or false and correct the false statements. (LO 6-4)

41. The nurse explains that diarrhea may occur after taking amoxicillin. This patient teaching is categorized as drug–drug interactions.

42. Where to obtain an ordered medication should be included with patient teaching.

43. Prior to patient teaching, the nurse should determine the patient's knowledge and literacy level.

44. The nurse should include the caregiver when providing medication teaching.

45. The patient should be instructed to discontinue a medication if any side effects occur.

For exercises 46–50, refer to the following order and indicate the information that should be provided to the patient for each specified category of patient teaching:

Humulin N NPH® U-100 30 units subcut daily 30 min ā breakfast

46. Medication name _____
    _____

47. Dose _____
    _____

48. Route _____
    _____

49. Schedule _____
    _____

50. Additional information _____
    _____

NCLEX-Style Review Questions

For questions 1–3, select the best response.

1. To ensure that a patient's medication is given at the right time, the nurse should:
   a. Check to be sure that at least 2 hours have passed since the last prn pain medicine.
   b. Administer time-critical medications within 30 minutes of the scheduled time.
   c. Administer q12h medications once in the morning and once in the evening.
   d. Give pc medications with meals.

2. Assessment during medication administration includes:
   a. Observing the patient swallowing the tablet
   b. Observing the medication reference materials
   c. Checking the patient's name band
   d. Checking the expiration date and lot number of the medication

3. The nurse ensures that the right patient is being medicated by asking the patient to state his name and date of birth (DOB) while scanning the patient identification band. If a patient is unable to state his name, the nurse should:
   a. Check the name on the door.
   b. Check the name on the bed.
   c. Ask the parent or caregiver to state the patient's name and DOB.
   d. Omit this step because the band will be scanned for identification.

For question 4–6, select all that apply.

4. Select the statements that should be included in a patient medication teaching plan.
   a. "The purpose of this medication is …"
   b. "This is how you administer this medicine …"
   c. "The *Nurse's Drug Handbook* classifies this medication as …"
   d. "Be alert to these side effects …"
   e. "You can obtain this medicine from …"
   f. "This medication can be crushed and …"
   g. "The manufacturer of this medication is …"
   h. "This medication interacts with these drugs …"

5. During medication preparation, the label should be checked:
   a. While scanning the patient's bar code
   b. When taking the medication from the storage container
   c. When pouring the liquid medication
   d. Just prior to administering the medication to the patient
   e. After the medication is administered to the patient

6. The BCMA process promotes which rights of medication administration?
   a. Right Patient
   b. Right Drug
   c. Right Dose
   d. Right Route
   e. Right Time
   f. Right Reason
   g. Right to Refuse
   h. Right to Know

REFERENCES

Agency for Healthcare Research and Quality. (2012). Closing the quality gap series: Medication adherence interventions: Comparative effectiveness. Retrieved from http://effectivehealthcare.ahrq.gov/search-for-guides-reviews-and-reports/?pageaction=displayproduct&productID=1248

Anderson, P., & Townsend, T. (2010). Medication errors: Don't let them happen to you. *American Nurse Today, 5*(3). Retrieved from http://www.americannursetoday.com/article.aspx?id=6356&fid=6276

Institute for Safe Medication Practices. (2011). Guidelines for timely medication administration: Response to the CMS 30-minute rule. *ISMP Medication Safety Alert!* Retrieved from https://www.ismp.org/newsletters/acutecare/articles/20110113.asp

Institute for Safe Medication Practices. (2012). Side tracks on the safety express: Interruptions lead to errors and unfinished … wait, what was I doing? *ISMP Medication Safety Alert!* Retrieved from https://www.ismp.org/Newsletters/acutecare/showarticle.aspx?id=37

Institute of Medicine. (1999). *To err is human: Building a safer health system.* Washington, DC: National Academy Press. Retrieved from https://www.iom.edu/~/media/Files/Report%20Files/1999/To-Err-is-Human/To%20Err%20is%20Human%201999%20%20report%20brief.pdf

LaDuke, Sharon, RN, BS. (May 2009). Playing it safe with bar code medication administration. *Nursing, 39*(5), 32–34. Retrieved from http://journals.lww.com/nursing/Fulltext/2009/05000/Playing_it_safe_with_bar_code_medication.17.aspx

Leigh, E. (2009). Teaching patients about their medications: The keys to decreasing non-compliance. The Center for Healthcare Communication Publication. Retrieved from http://www.communicatingwithpatients.com/articles/teaching_about_meds.html

National Council on Patient Information and Education. (2013). Accelerating progress in prescription medicine adherence: The adherence action agenda. Retrieved from http://www.bemedicinesmart.org/A3_Report.pdf

Olin, J. (March 13, 2012). The "rights" of medication administration. Retrieved from http://www.rncentral.com/blog/2012/the-rights-of-medication-administration/

Stokowski, L. A. (2012). Timely medication administration guidelines for nurses: Fewer wrong-time errors? *Medscape.* Retrieved from http://www.medscape.com/viewarticle/772501

Chapter 6   ANSWER KEY

Learning Activity 6-1
1. 2nd check
2. 3rd check
3. 1st check

Learning Activity 6-2
1. Oral, by mouth, PO
2. 100 mcg
3. 8:30 a.m.

Learning Activity 6-3
1. Check allergies, patient's pain level, IV site.
2. Check IV infusion; observe IV site.
3. Check if patient's pain was relieved; observe for side effects.

Learning Activity 6-4
1. The brand name is Amoxil®; the generic name is amoxicillin.
2. The dose is 250 mg; the amount to administer is 5 mL; explain how to measure 5 mL in a medicine cup or oral syringe.
3. The medication should be taken three times per day 8 hours apart 1 hour before meals or snacks (on an empty stomach), for example, at 0800, 1600, and 2400.

Homework

1. False. To ensure that the right medication is administered, the medication label is checked three times.
2. False. For a multiple-dose container of liquid Tylenol®, the first label check occurs when the medication is retrieved from the storage location.
3. True
4. True
5. False. Checking the label when retrieving the medication from the refrigerator is the first label check.
6. Right patient
7. Right drug
8. Right dose
9. Right route
10. Right time/frequency

11. No, the right time was violated. The correct times for administration are 0800 and 2000. Time-critical medications must be administered within 30 minutes of scheduled times.

12. No, the right route was violated. The medication should have been placed under the tongue. Buccal medications are administered between the cheek and gum.

13. Yes, right drug (acetaminophen is the generic name of Tylenol®).

14. Yes, right documentation

15. No, the right reason was violated. The nurse should contact the physician to get an order for pain medicine.

16. No, the right to refuse was violated. The nurse should respect the patient's right to refuse a medication. The nurse might try an alternate strategy, such as getting a family member to help convince the patient to take the medication.

17. Yes, right dose. Although this is a correct order, it is appropriate for the nurse to question an order for 5 capsules. The nurse should check a drug reference or consult the pharmacist regarding the appropriate dose and how it is supplied.

18. No, the right route was violated.

19. Yes, right route.

20. No, the right patient was violated.

21. Patient

22. Medication/drug

23. Dose/amount

24. Route

25. Time

26. Reason

27. Documentation

28. Know

29. Refuse

30. Procedural

31. Patient

32. Check allergies, check the patient's temperature to be certain that it is greater than 38.6°C, and check the rectal area (clean it, if necessary).

33. Check that the patient has retained the suppository.

34. Check the patient's temperature to determine if medication was effective; assess for side effects.

35. Check allergies, check the patient's heart rate to be sure that it is 60 bpm or higher, check that patient is able to take oral medications.

36. Check that the patient swallowed the medicine.

37. Assess the patient for medication effects and side effects.

38. Check allergies, determine if the patient is agitated, check the muscle site of injection, check the MAR for location of previous injections.

39. Check the injection site for redness or swelling.

40. Assess the patient for medication effects (i.e., decrease in agitation) and side effects.

41. False. This patient teaching is categorized as side effects.

42. True

43. True

44. True

45. False. The patient should be instructed about side effects to expect and when to contact the prescriber/provider.

46. Humulin N NPH®

47. 30 units; the patient should be taught how to draw up this dose/amount and the appropriate syringe to use.

48. Subcutaneous; the patient should be taught how to choose a subcutaneous site for injection and proper injection technique.

49. The patient should be taught that this medication should be given every day 30 minutes before breakfast.

50. Where to obtain the medicine, purpose of medication, drug–drug interactions, side effects, when to contact the prescriber/provider

NCLEX-Style Review Questions

1. b

   Rationale: Time-critical medications should be given within 30 minutes of the scheduled time unless they are ordered to be given at a specific time. PRN medications must be spaced out according to the frequency indicated in the order. Medications orders q12h should be given 12 hours apart. Medications ordered pc should be given after meals.

2. a

   Rationale: Assessment during medication administration includes observing whether or not the patient received and retained the medicine (e.g., observing the patient swallowing the tablet). Reviewing the medication reference materials will aid the nurse in preparing patient teaching. Checking the patient's name band is done prior to medication administration. Checking the expiration date and lot number should be done during medication preparation.

3. c

    Rationale: If a patient is unable to state his name and DOB during the patient identification process, the nurse should ask the parent or caregiver to state the patient's full name. The name labels on the door and/or bed are unofficial and should not be used for patient identification. If a caregiver or parent is not present, the nurse can match the patient's name and DOB or medical record number on the ID band with the corresponding information on the MAR/eMAR.

4. a, b, d, e, f, h

    Rationale: Patient teaching should include how to obtain the medication and the purpose, side effects, and instructions for administration of the medicine. Patient teaching does not require information regarding classification and manufacturer.

5. b, c, d

    Rationale: During medication preparation, the label should be checked when the medication is retrieved from its storage location, when pouring a multi-dose medication (or placing a unit-dose medication into a medicine cup or drawing up a medication from a vial), and just prior to administration. The medication label is not checked while scanning the patient's bar code or after the medication is administered.

6. a, b, c, e

    Rationale: By scanning both the patient's identification band and the medication label, the nurse ensures that the right patient is receiving the right medication. Because an alert is generated on the eMAR if an incorrect dose is scanned or a medication is scanned at an unscheduled/inappropriate time, the BCMA process also ensures the right dose and the right time.

© Forfunlife/Shutterstock

Chapter 7

Dosage Calculations

CHAPTER OUTLINE

LEARNING OUTCOMES

Upon completion of the chapter, the student will be able to:

7-1   Differentiate the dosage strength of the supplied medication from the ordered dose.

7-2   Apply the *CASE* approach to calculate dosages using ratio-proportion, the formula method, and dimensional analysis.

KEY TERMS

CASE approach

dimensional analysis

factor-label method

formula method

fractional ratio-proportion

linear ratio-proportion

Case Consideration ... Calculation Choices

After learning about each medication, the nursing student was ready to prepare the medications for administration. The patient needed an intravenous (IV) antibiotic, a liquid cough medicine, and several other medications that were dispensed as tablets and capsules. The student reviewed the medication administration record (MAR) and realized dosage calculations were indicated.

1. How is dosage calculation performed?

2. Is there one approach that can be used for all dosage calculations?

■ INTRODUCTION

When administering medications, each *case* should be considered separately. Because medications may be supplied in varying dosage strengths, varying amounts may be required to administer the same dosage of medication. For example, Paxil® CR is supplied as 12.5 mg tablets and 25 mg tablets. Administration of a 25 mg dose would require two 12.5 mg tablets or only one 25 mg tablet. Even though the dose is the same, the amount to administer is different.

The patient's needs may change; a patient who was able to take an oral dose of medication may be ordered to take nothing by mouth (NPO), and will then require a different form and route of medication. Medications should be ordered on a case-by-case basis; safe dosages vary depending on the patient's age, weight, kidney function, liver function, and individual response. The authorized prescriber will order the dosage and route, but the nurse will have to consider the individual patient and supplied medication prior to administration.

To ensure safety and accuracy with dosage calculations, use the **CASE approach**. *CASE* is an acronym for four steps of safe dosage calculation, which are:

- ■ **C**: *Convert*—convert to like units of measurement

- ■ **A**: *Approximate*—estimate the amount to administer

- ■ **S**: *Solve*—perform dosage calculation

- ■ **E**: *Evaluate*—check the dosage calculation and compare to approximated amount

The word *CASE* also reminds the nurse to consider the appropriateness of the medication and dose ordered in each individual case.

7-1   Comparing the Supply to the Ordered Dose

The first two steps of the *CASE* approach, **C**: *Convert* and **A**: *Approximate*, require the comparison of the dosage strength (referred to as "supply") to the ordered dose. For example, the ordered dose may be in grams (g), while the supply is in milligrams (mg). Step **C**: *Convert*, requires comparing the supply to the ordered dose and converting to the same unit of measurement, if they are different. If the supplied dosage strength and the ordered dose are in the same unit of measurement, the conversion step is not applicable (N/A).

Example:

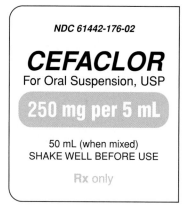

NDC 61442-176-02

CEFACLOR
For Oral Suspension, USP

250 mg per 5 mL

50 mL (when mixed)
SHAKE WELL BEFORE USE

Rx only

Ordered dose: 0.35 g

Supply: 250 mg/5 mL

Because the ordered dose is in grams and the supply is in milligrams, convert the ordered dose (0.35 g) to the unit of measurement in the supply, mg, using a ratio-proportion equivalency. To use ratio-proportion, set up the known equivalency $\frac{1\,g}{1,000\,mg}$ on the left against the unknown equivalency on the right:

$$\frac{1\ g}{1,000\ mg} = \frac{0.35\ g}{x\ mg}$$

$$x = 1,000 \times 0.35$$

$$x = 350\ mg$$

To convert grams to milligrams by dimensional analysis, use the conversion factor $\frac{1,000\,mg}{1\,g}$ to have mg in the final answer, allowing grams to be cancelled:

$$0.35\ \cancel{g} \times \frac{1,000\ mg}{1\ \cancel{g}} = 350\ mg$$

Both methods of conversion reveal the ordered dose, 0.35 g, is equivalent to 350 mg.

Step **A**: *Approximate*, requires approximating how much of the supplied medication to administer. To approximate, compare the supply to the ordered dose, and consider which is larger. In the previous example, the ordered dose, 350 mg, is larger than the supply of 250 mg, but less than twice the supply. Because the ordered dose is larger than the supply, it follows that the amount to administer will be larger than the supply dosage unit of 5 mL. Because it was determined that the ordered dose is less than twice the supply, it follows that the amount to administer will be less than 10 mL. Therefore, the amount to administer will be between 5–10 mL.

Example 1: Approximate the amount to administer.

Ordered dose: 500 mg

Supply: 250 mg/5 mL

To approximate the amount to administer, compare the supplied dosage of 250 mg to the ordered dosage of 500 mg. The ordered dose of 500 mg is twice as much as the supplied dosage of 250 mg, so the amount to administer needs to be proportionally larger (twice as much of the supply dosage unit). Because 250 mg are contained in the dosage unit of 5 mL, two times the dosage unit (i.e., 10 mL) will be required to administer a 500 mg dose.

Example 2:   Approximate the amount to administer.

Ordered dose: 75 mg

Supply: 150 mg/tablet

The ordered dose of 75 mg is half as large as the supplied dose of 150 mg, therefore the amount to administer will be proportionately smaller (half the dosage unit). Because the dosage unit is 1 tablet, ½ tablet will be needed.

When the ratio is not as clear, find measurable parameters, such as the ordered dose may be more than twice as much, but less than three times as much as the supplied dosage, or the ordered dose is less than half the supplied dosage strength but more than one-third.

Example 3:   Approximate the amount to administer.

Ordered dose: 210 mg

Supply: 125 mg/mL

The ordered dose is larger than the supplied dosage, but it is not twice as large, because 2 × 125 mg is 250 mg, and the ordered dose is 210. Therefore, more than 1 mL, but less than 2 mL will be required to administer 210 mg. This rough estimation will promote confidence in the calculated amount if it is between 1 and 2 mL.

WARNING!

Approximation Is Not a Substitute for Calculation

Approximation is a critical thinking step used to verify the correct equation was used and the calculation was performed accurately. The amount to administer should be calculated not approximated.

LEARNING ACTIVITY 7-1   Refer to the following labels to compare the ordered dose to the supply and determine steps *C* and *A* of the *CASE* approach. If the conversion step is not applicable, indicate N/A.

1.   Order: dantrolene 75 mg. Supply: See **Figure 7-1**.

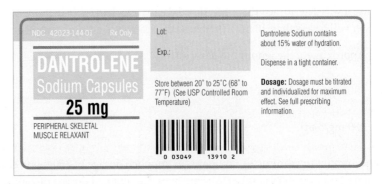

FIGURE 7-1

a.   **C**: *Convert*

b.   **A**: *Approximate*

2.   Order: tamsulosin 400 mcg. Supply: See **Figure 7-2**.

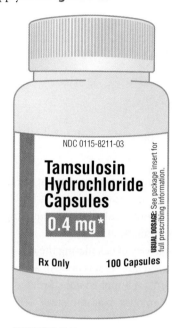

FIGURE 7-2

a.   **C**: *Convert*

b.   **A**: *Approximate*

3.   Order: diazepam 5 mg. Supply: See **Figure 7-3**.

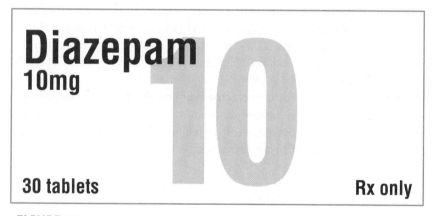

FIGURE 7-3

a.   **C**: *Convert*

b.   **A**: *Approximate*

7-2   Methods of Dosage Calculation

To perform step **S**: *Solve* of the *CASE* approach, three different methods of dosage calculation can be used, which are presented in this section: *ratio-proportion*, the *formula method*, and *dimensional analysis*. After performing the calculation, step **E**: *Evaluate*, is accomplished by comparing the answer to the approximated amount in step **A** and by checking (redoing) the calculation after replacing *x* with the calculated value.

To use ratio-proportion to solve basic dosage calculations, two equal fractions or ratios will be set up to compare the known supply to the ordered dose and unknown amount to administer:

- **Fractional ratio-proportion**:

$$\frac{\text{supplied dose}}{\text{dosage unit}} = \frac{\text{ordered dose}}{\text{amount to administer }(x)}$$

- **Linear ratio-proportion**:

$$\text{supplied dose : dosage unit} = \text{ordered dose : amount to administer }(x)$$

This method is most useful when the units of measurement are the same. If conversion of a unit of measurement is required, it is done as an additional step, prior to setting up the dosage calculation. Complex IV infusion calculations, or other calculations requiring multiple conversions, are not generally performed using the ratio-proportion method.

The **formula method** is a simple way of calculating the amount to administer. As with ratio-proportion, if a unit of measurement conversion is required, it is done in a separate step, prior to setting up the dosage calculation. With the formula method, the supplied dose, ordered dose, and the supplied dosage unit are placed in a formula to determine the amount to administer:

$$\frac{\text{ordered dose i.e., } \textbf{Desired dose }(D)}{\text{supplied dose i.e., dose on } \textbf{Hand }(H)} \times \text{dosage unit i.e., } \textbf{Quantity }(Q) = \text{amount to administer}(x)$$

Although this method is a quick way to perform dosage calculation, there is a tendency to eliminate the dosage unit in the dosage calculation because it is often 1 (e.g., 1 capsule, 1 tablet, 1 mL). When a dosage unit is a quantity other than 1, eliminating it in the calculation will yield an incorrect amount. To avoid error with the formula method, it is important to insert the dosage unit into every calculation. Additionally, different formulas are required for IV rate calculation. Implementing the wrong formula can result in medication errors.

Dimensional analysis, also known as the **factor-label method** (or conversion factor method, as referred to in Chapter 2), determines the amount to administer by multiplying a series of fractions. Dimensional analysis is a systematic method of converting units of measurement (dimensions). In other words, dimensions such as mg and mL in the dose and supply are multiplied by conversion factors to determine the amount to administer.

$$\text{amount to administer} = \overset{\textit{Supply}}{\frac{\text{dosage unit}}{\text{dose supplied}}} \times \overset{\textit{CF}}{\text{conversion factor}(s)} \times \overset{\textit{Order}}{\frac{\text{ordered dose}}{1}}$$

Compared to the other methods of dosage calculation, dimensional analysis is easier to remember, improves accuracy, and helps reduce medication errors (Cookson, 2013).

Dimensional analysis can be used for any dosage calculation. It is extremely useful when several conversions must be made to determine the amount to administer (e.g., converting minutes to hours, and grams to micrograms to determine the rate to administer certain IV medications). Using the *CASE* approach, the conversion step is used to identify the conversion factor(s) required, but the actual conversion(s) is performed during the calculation step. Because this is a very efficient way of performing multiple conversions, dimensional analysis is often used by critical care nurses. A research study done through Adelphi University examined the accuracy of dosage calculations done by students that used traditional methods versus dimensional analysis. Data analysis revealed that the dimensional analysis group performed with greater accuracy (Greenfield, Whelan, & Cohn, 2006). The current trend for nursing schools is to adopt dimensional analysis as the preferred method of dosage calculation.

Ratio-Proportion

A proportion compares two equivalent fractions or ratios. The fractional ratio-proportion compares two equivalent fractions and the linear ratio-proportion compares two equivalent ratios.

Fractional Ratio-Proportion

When preparing a fractional ratio-proportion, set the supplied dosage strength (supply) as the *known* equivalent on the left side of the equal sign, and the ordered dosage (order) as the *unknown* equivalent on the right side of the equal sign:

$$\frac{\text{supplied dose}}{\text{dosage unit}} = \frac{\text{ordered dose}}{\text{amount to administer } (x)}$$

Write the supplied dosage strength as a fraction with the supplied dose as the numerator and the dosage unit as the denominator. Write the ordered dose to administer as a fraction with the ordered dose as the numerator and the ordered amount to administer (usually x) as the denominator. Be sure to label all units of measurement, including x. The correct label for the answer will be the label attached to x.

Example 1:   Set up a fractional ratio-proportion equation in which x is the amount to administer.

  Order: digoxin 125 mcg PO daily

  Supply: See label.

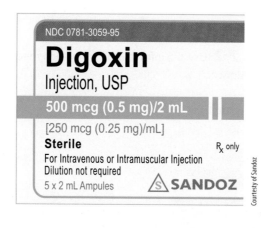

$$\overset{\textit{Supply}}{\frac{500 \text{ mcg}}{2 \text{ mL}}} = \overset{\textit{Order}}{\frac{125 \text{ mcg}}{x \text{ mL}}}$$

Example 2:   Set up a fractional ratio-proportion equation in which *x* is the amount to administer.

Order: bupropion HCl XR 300 mg PO daily

Supply: See label.

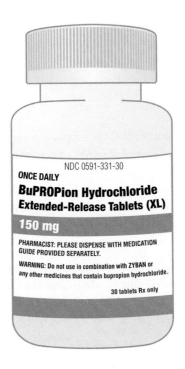

$$\underset{\text{Supply}}{\frac{150 \text{ mg}}{1 \text{ tab}}} = \underset{\text{Order}}{\frac{300 \text{ mg}}{x \text{ tab}}}$$

LEARNING ACTIVITY 7-2 Use the information from each medication label to set up a fractional ratio-proportion equation.

1.   **Order:** Benztropine mesylate 1 mg PO bid
      Supply: See label.

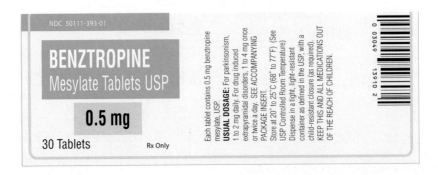

2.   **Order:** Zantac® 50 mg IV q8h

   Supply: See label.

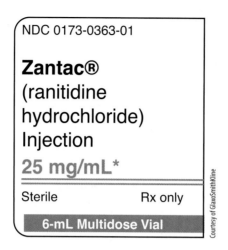

3.   **Order:** furosemide 40 mg PO daily

   Supply: See label.

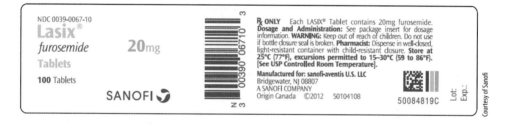

   For patient safety, when determining the amount of medication to administer using ratio-proportion, implement the *CASE* method.

Example 1:   Determine the number of capsules to administer, using ratio-proportion and the CASE method.

   Order: 0.5 g

   Supply: 250 mg per capsule

C: *Convert*—Convert ordered amount in grams to milligrams, using the equivalent 1 g = 1,000 mg

$$\frac{1\text{ g}}{1,000\text{ mg}} = \frac{0.5\text{ g}}{x\text{ mg}}$$

$$1 \times x = 1,000 \times 0.5$$

$$x = 500\text{ mg}$$

A: *Approximate*—Because the ordered dose is twice the supplied dose, two capsules will be needed.

S: *Solve*—Supply = 250 mg/1 cap; Order = 500 mg

- Set up the ratios, supply (known equivalent) = order (unknown equivalent):

$$\underset{\text{Supply}}{\frac{250 \text{ mg}}{1 \text{ cap}}} = \underset{\text{Order}}{\frac{500 \text{ mg}}{x \text{ cap}}}$$

- Cross-multiply: $250 \times x = 1 \times 500$
- Simplify: $250x = 500$
- Divide both sides by 250 to let x stand alone:

$$\frac{\cancel{250}x}{\cancel{250}} = \frac{500}{250}$$

$$x = 2 \text{ cap}$$

Because x cap is what is being solved, "cap" is the correct label for this answer.

E: *Evaluate*—Set up the ratio, replacing x cap with 2 cap and check the math:

$$\frac{250 \text{ mg}}{1 \text{ cap}} = \frac{500 \text{ mg}}{2 \text{ cap}}$$

$$250 \times 2 = 1 \times 500$$

$$500 = 500$$

Because the calculated amount forms a true statement and is consistent with the approximated amount, 2 cap, the answer is confirmed.

Example 2:   Determine the volume to administer, using ratio-proportion and the CASE method.

Order: 0.03 g

Supply: 15 mg/5 mL

C: *Convert*—Convert ordered amount in grams to milligrams, using the equivalent 1 g = 1,000 mg:

$$\frac{1 \text{ g}}{1,000 \text{ mg}} = \frac{0.03 \text{ g}}{x \text{ mg}}$$

$$1 \times x = 1,000 \times 0.03$$

$$x = 30 \text{ mg}$$

A: *Approximate*—Because the ordered dose is twice the dose supplied in 5 mL, 10 mL will be needed.

S: *Solve*—Supply = 15 mg/5 mL; Order = 30 mg

- Set up the ratios, supply (known equivalent) = order (unknown equivalent):

$$\begin{array}{cc} \textit{Supply} & \textit{Order} \\[4pt] \dfrac{15 \text{ mg}}{5 \text{ mL}} &= \dfrac{30 \text{ mg}}{x \text{ mL}} \end{array}$$

- Cross-multiply: $15 \times x = 5 \times 30$

- Simplify: $15x = 150$

- Divide both sides by 15 to let x stand alone:

$$\frac{\cancel{15}x}{\cancel{15}} = \frac{150}{15}$$
$$x = 10 \text{ mL}$$

E: *Evaluate*—Set up the ratio, replacing x mL with 10 mL and check the math:

$$\frac{15 \text{ mg}}{5 \text{ mL}} = \frac{30 \text{ mg}}{10 \text{ mL}}$$
$$15 \times 10 = 5 \times 30$$
$$150 = 150$$

Because the calculated amount forms a true statement and is consistent with the approximated amount, 10 mL, the answer is confirmed.

Example 3:

Order: 450 mg

Supply: 150 mg per tablet

C: *Convert*—Because the ordered dose and supplied dose are both measured in mg, no conversion is needed.

A: *Approximate*—Because the ordered dose is three times the supplied dose, three tablets will be needed.

S: *Solve*—Supply = 150 mg/1 tab; Order = 450 mg

- Set up the ratios, supply (known equivalent) = order (unknown equivalent):

$$\begin{array}{cc} \textit{Supply} & \textit{Order} \\[4pt] \dfrac{150 \text{ mg}}{1 \text{ tab}} &= \dfrac{450 \text{ mg}}{x \text{ tab}} \end{array}$$

- Cross-multiply: $150 \times x = 1 \times 450$

- Simplify: $150x = 450$

- Divide both sides by 150 to let x stand alone:

$$\frac{\cancel{150}x}{\cancel{150}} = \frac{450}{150}$$
$$x = 3 \text{ tab}$$

E: *Evaluate*—Set up the ratio, replacing *x* tab with 3 tab and check the math:

$$\frac{150 \text{ mg}}{1 \text{ tab}} = \frac{450 \text{ mg}}{3 \text{ tab}}$$
$$150 \times 3 = 1 \times 450$$
$$450 = 450$$

Because the calculated amount forms a true statement and is consistent with the approximated amount, 3 tab, the answer is confirmed.

LEARNING ACTIVITY 7-3 Using fractional ratio-proportion within the *CASE* approach, calculate the amount to administer for each ordered dose.

1.   Order: 2.5 mg; Supply: 5 mg/mL
2.   Order: 0.075 g; Supply: 25 mg per tablet
3.   Order: 1.45 mg; Supply 2 mg/5 mL

Linear Ratio-Proportion

When preparing a linear ratio-proportion, set the supplied dosage strength as a ratio on one side, and create a proportion using the ordered dosage and *x* as the unknown amount to administer:

supplied dosage strength (supply) = ordered amount to administer (order)

supplied dose : dosage unit = ordered dose : amount to administer (*x*)

Be sure to label all units of measurement, including *x*. The correct label for the answer will be the label attached to *x*. To solve a linear ratio-proportion, the product of the means (the two middle numbers) is equal to the product of the extremes (the two outer numbers).

Example 1:

Order: erythromycin delayed release 0.5 g PO bid

Supply: 250 mg per capsule

C: *Convert*—Convert ordered amount in grams to milligrams, using the equivalent 1 g = 1,000 mg

$$\frac{1 \text{ g}}{1,000 \text{ mg}} = \frac{0.5 \text{ g}}{x \text{ mg}}$$
$$1 \times x = 1,000 \times 0.5$$
$$x = 500 \text{ mg}$$

A: *Approximate*—Because the ordered dose is twice the supplied dose, two capsules will be needed.

S: *Solve*—Supply = 250 mg/1 cap; Order = 500 mg

■ Set up the ratios, supply = order:

Supply   *Order*

250 mg : 1 cap = 500 mg : *x* cap

Extremes   Means

- Set up the equation: $250 \times x = 1 \times 500$

- Simplify the equation: $250x = 500$

- Divide both sides by 250 to let x stand alone:

$$\frac{\cancel{250}x}{\cancel{250}} = \frac{500}{250}$$

$$x = 2 \text{ cap}$$

Because x cap is what is being solved, "cap" is the correct label for this answer.

E: Evaluate—Set up the ratio, replacing x cap with 2 cap and check the math:

$$250 \text{ mg} : 1 \text{ cap} = 500 \text{ mg} : 2 \text{ cap}$$

$$250 \times 2 = 1 \times 500$$

$$500 = 500$$

Because the calculated amount forms a true statement and is consistent with the approximated amount, 2 cap, the answer is confirmed.

Example 2:

  Order: 0.03 g

  Supply: 15 mg/5 mL

C: Convert—Convert ordered amount in grams to milligrams, using the equivalent 1 g = 1,000 mg

$$\frac{1 \text{ g}}{1,000 \text{ mg}} = \frac{0.03 \text{ g}}{x \text{ mg}}$$

$$1 \times x = 1,000 \times 0.03$$

$$x = 30 \text{ mg}$$

A: Approximate—Because the ordered dose is twice the dose supplied in 5 mL, 10 mL will be needed.

S: Solve—Supply = 15 mg/5; Order = 30 mg

- Set up the ratios, supply = order:

Supply   Order

$$15 \text{ mg} : 5 \text{ mL} = 30 \text{ mg} : x \text{ mL}$$

Extremes Means

- Set up the equation: $15 \times x = 5 \times 30$

- Simplify the equation: $15x = 150$

- Divide both sides by 15 to let x stand alone:

$$\frac{\cancel{15}x}{\cancel{15}} = \frac{150}{15}$$

$$x = 10 \text{ mL}$$

E: *Evaluate*—Set up the ratio, replacing *x* mL with 10 mL and check the math:

$$15 \text{ mg} : 5 \text{ mL} = 30 \text{ mg} : 10 \text{ mL}$$
$$15 \times 10 = 5 \times 30$$
$$150 = 150$$

Because the calculated amount forms a true statement and is consistent with the approximated amount, 10 mL, the answer is confirmed.

Example 3:

   Order: 450 mg

   Supply: 150 mg per tablet

C: *Convert*—Because the ordered dose and supplied dose are both measured in mg, no conversion is needed.

A: *Approximate*—Because the ordered dose is three times the supplied dose, three tablets will be needed.

S: *Solve*—Supply = 150 mg/1 tab; Order = 450 mg

- Set up the ratios, supply = order:

$$\underset{\textit{Supply}}{} \qquad \underset{\textit{Order}}{}$$
$$150 \text{ mg} : 1 \text{ tab} = 450 \text{ mg} : x \text{ tab}$$

$$\underset{\textit{Extremes}}{} \quad \underset{\textit{Means}}{}$$

- Set up the equation: $150 \times x = 1 \times 450$
- Simplify the equation: $150x = 450$
- Divide both sides by 150 to let *x* stand alone:

$$\frac{\cancel{150}x}{\cancel{150}} = \frac{450}{150}$$
$$x = 3 \text{ tab}$$

E: *Evaluate*—Set up the ratio, replacing *x* tab with 3 tab and check the math:

$$150 \text{ mg} : 1 \text{ tab} = 450 \text{ mg} : 3 \text{ tab}$$
$$150 \times 3 = 1 \times 450$$
$$450 = 450$$

Because the calculated amount forms a true statement and is consistent with the approximated amount, 3 tab, the answer is confirmed.

LEARNING ACTIVITY 7-4 Using the linear ratio-proportion method within the *CASE* approach, calculate the amount to administer for each ordered dose.

1.   Order: 5 mg; Supply: 2 mg/tab
2.   Order: 0.5 g; Supply: 100 mg/15 mL
3.   Order: 0.25 g; Supply 125 mg/cap

Formula Method

The formula method uses the following formula to calculate the amount to administer:

$$\frac{\text{ordered dose i.e., } \textbf{Desired dose } (D)}{\text{supplied dose i.e., dose on } \textbf{Hand } (H)} \times \text{dosage unit i.e., } \textbf{Quantity}\,(Q) = \text{amount to administer}(x)$$

$$\frac{D}{H} \times Q = x$$

Example 1:

Ordered Dose: 0.5 g

Supply: 250 mg per capsule

C: *Convert*—Convert the ordered dose from grams to milligrams, using the conversion factor $\frac{1,000\ \text{mg}}{1\ \text{g}}$.

$$0.5\ \cancel{\text{g}}\ \times\ \frac{1,000\ \text{mg}}{1\ \cancel{\text{g}}} = 500\ \text{mg}$$

A: *Approximate*—Because the ordered dose is twice the supplied dose, two capsules will be needed.

S: *Solve*—$D = 500$ mg; $H = 250$ mg; $Q = 1$ cap

$$\frac{500\ \cancel{\text{mg}}}{250\ \cancel{\text{mg}}} \times 1\ \text{cap} = x\ (\text{cap})$$

$$2 \times 1\ \text{cap} = x$$

$$2\ \text{cap} = x$$

E: *Evaluate*—Replace x with 2 cap and check the math:

$$\frac{500\ \cancel{\text{mg}}}{250\ \cancel{\text{mg}}} \times 1\ \text{cap} = 2\ \text{cap}$$

$$2 \times 1\ \text{cap} = 2\ \text{cap}$$

Because the calculated amount forms a true statement and is consistent with the approximated amount, 2 cap, the answer is confirmed.

> **NOTE:** Because the dose is supplied in capsules, the unit of measurement for x must be capsules. This reminds the nurse that after all units of measurement cancel out, cap should remain. If after performing the calculations for x, mg remains, the nurse knows the equation was set up incorrectly.

Example 2:

Ordered Dose: 0.03 g

Supply: 15 mg/5 mL

C: *Convert*—Convert the ordered dose from grams to milligrams, using the conversion factor $\frac{1,000 \text{ mg}}{1 \text{ g}}$.

$$0.03 \ \cancel{\text{g}} \times \frac{1,000 \text{ mg}}{1 \ \cancel{\text{g}}} = 30 \text{ mg}$$

A: *Approximate*—Because the ordered dose is twice the supplied dose, twice the volume (10 mL) will be needed.

S: *Solve*—*D* = 30 mg; *H* = 15 mg; *Q* = 5 mL

$$\frac{30 \ \cancel{\text{mg}}}{15 \ \cancel{\text{mg}}} \times 5 \text{ mL} = x \text{ (mL)}$$

$$2 \times 5 \text{ mL} = x$$

$$10 \text{ mL} = x$$

E: *Evaluate*—Replace *x* with 10 mL and check the math:

$$\frac{30 \ \cancel{\text{mg}}}{15 \ \cancel{\text{mg}}} \times 5 \text{ mL} = 10 \text{ mL}$$

$$2 \times 5 \text{ mL} = 10 \text{ mL}$$

Because the calculated amount forms a true statement and is consistent with the approximated amount, 10 mL, the answer is confirmed.

Example 3:

Ordered Dose: 450 mg

Supply: 150 mg per tablet

C: *Convert*—Because the ordered dose and supplied dose are both measured in mg, no conversion is needed.

A: *Approximate*—Because the ordered dose three times the supplied dose, three tablets will be needed.

S: *Solve*—*D* = 450 mg; *H* = 150 mg; *Q* = 1 tab

$$\frac{450 \ \cancel{\text{mg}}}{150 \ \cancel{\text{mg}}} \times 1 \text{ tab} = x \text{ (tab)}$$

$$3 \times 1 \text{ tab} = x$$

$$3 \text{ tab} = x$$

E: *Evaluate*—Replace *x* with 3 tab and check the math:

$$\frac{450 \ \cancel{\text{mg}}}{150 \ \cancel{\text{mg}}} \times 1 \text{ tab} = 3 \text{ tab}$$

$$3 \times 1 \text{ tab} = 3 \text{ tab}$$

Because the calculated amount forms a true statement and is consistent with the approximated amount, 3 tab, the answer is confirmed.

LEARNING ACTIVITY 7-5 Using the formula method within the *CASE* approach, calculate the amount to administer for each ordered dose.

1.   Ordered Dose: 0.45 g; Supply: 150 mg/tab
2.   Ordered Dose: 0.2 mg; Supply: 100 mcg/mL
3.   Ordered Dose: 20 mg; Supply 100 mg/5 mL

Dimensional Analysis

Dimensional analysis links known quantities to an unknown quantity through a series of conversion factors (CF). For example, to determine the number of seconds in 1 week, a series of conversion factors will be set up in an equation in order that all factor labels (units of measurement) will cancel out except seconds and week:

$$x \text{ (seconds/week)} = \frac{60 \text{ seconds}}{1 \text{ minute}} \times \frac{60 \text{ minutes}}{1 \text{ hour}} \times \frac{24 \text{ hours}}{1 \text{ day}} \times \frac{7 \text{ days}}{1 \text{ week}} = 604,800 \text{ seconds/week}$$

Notice in the above example, that seconds/week is the amount to be determined, so seconds is placed in the numerator of the first fraction, and week is placed in the denominator of the final fraction. Small, known conversion factors form a bridge between seconds and weeks. To avoid error, it is important that the conversion factors are for 1 unit of measurement (i.e., 1 minute or 1 hour or 1 day, in the previous example). Although it is possible to use larger conversion factors such as 3,600 seconds/60 minutes, this factor is error-prone. After all of the labels (units of measurement) are cancelled, seconds/week remains. Unit of measurement cancellation is an important aspect of dimensional analysis.

To apply dimensional analysis to dosage calculation, set up the equation as follows:

$$\text{amount to administer} = \overset{Supply}{\frac{\text{dosage unit}}{\text{dose supplied}}} \times \overset{CF}{\text{conversion factor}(s)} \times \overset{Order}{\frac{\text{ordered dose}}{1}}$$

Multiple conversions can be included in one equation, and dimensional analysis can be used to determine dosage in complex IV equations. For example, to determine how many mcg are administered over 1 minute, if a solution containing 2.4 g/L is infusing IV at 5 mL/h, the equation would be set up as:

$$x \text{ (mcg/min)} = \overset{CF}{\frac{1,000 \text{ mcg}}{1 \text{ mg}}} \times \overset{CF}{\frac{1,000 \text{ mg}}{1 \text{ g}}} \times \overset{Supply}{\frac{2.4 \text{ g}}{1 \text{ L}}} \times \overset{CF}{\frac{1 \text{ L}}{1,000 \text{ mL}}} \times \overset{Order}{\frac{5 \text{ mL}}{1 \text{ h}}} \times \overset{CF}{\frac{1 \text{ h}}{60 \text{ min}}}$$

Although this complex calculation may look intimidating and difficult, it will be covered and simplified in Chapter 15, "Critical Care Calculations." For safety and accuracy, the *CASE* approach should be employed when using dimensional analysis.

Example 1:

Ordered Dose: 0.5 g

Supply: 250 mg per capsule

C: *Convert*—To cancel grams, use the conversion factor $\frac{1,000 \text{ mg}}{1 \text{ g}}$.

A: Approximate—Mentally convert 0.5 g to 500 mg to determine the ordered dose is twice the supplied dose, therefore, two capsules will be needed.

S: Solve—Supply = 1 cap/250 mg; Conversion factor = 1,000 mg/1g; Order = 0.5 g/1

$$x \, (\text{cap}) = \frac{1 \, \text{cap}}{250 \, \cancel{\text{mg}}} \times \frac{1,000 \, \cancel{\text{mg}}}{1 \, \cancel{\text{g}}} \times \frac{0.5 \, \cancel{\text{g}}}{1}$$

$$x = \frac{500 \, \text{cap}}{250}$$

$$x = 2 \, \text{cap}$$

E: Evaluate—Replace *x* with 2 cap and check the math:

$$2 \, \text{cap} = \frac{1 \, \text{cap}}{250 \, \cancel{\text{mg}}} \times \frac{1,000 \, \cancel{\text{mg}}}{1 \, \cancel{\text{g}}} \times \frac{0.5 \, \cancel{\text{g}}}{1}$$

$$2 \, \text{cap} = \frac{500 \, \text{cap}}{250}$$

$$2 \, \text{cap} = 2 \, \text{cap}$$

Because the calculated amount forms a true statement and is consistent with the approximated amount, 2 cap, the answer is confirmed.

> **NOTE:** Because the dose is supplied in capsules, the unit of measurement for *x* must be capsules. This reminds the nurse to place cap in the numerator. After all units of measurement cancel out, cap should remain. If after performing the calculations for *x*, mg remains, the nurse knows the equation was set up incorrectly.

Example 2:

Ordered Dose: 0.03 g

Supply: 15 mg/5 mL

C: Convert—To cancel grams, use the conversion factor $\frac{1,000 \, \text{mg}}{1 \, \text{g}}$.

A: Approximate—Mentally convert 0.03 g to 30 mg to determine the ordered dose is twice the supplied dose, therefore, twice the supply volume, or 10 mL, will be needed.

S: Solve—Supply = 5 mL/15 mg; Conversion factor = 1,000 mg/1 g; Order = 0.03 g/1

$$x \left(\text{mL} \right) = \frac{5 \, \text{mL}}{15 \, \cancel{\text{mg}}} \times \frac{1,000 \, \cancel{\text{mg}}}{1 \, \cancel{\text{g}}} \times \frac{0.03 \, \cancel{\text{g}}}{1}$$

$$x = \frac{150 \, \text{mL}}{15}$$

$$x = 10 \, \text{mL}$$

E: *Evaluate*—Replace *x* with 10 mL and check the math:

$$10 \text{ mL} = \frac{5 \text{ mL}}{15 \cancel{\text{ mg}}} \times \frac{1,000 \cancel{\text{ mg}}}{1 \cancel{\text{ g}}} \times \frac{0.03 \cancel{\text{ g}}}{1}$$

$$10 \text{ mL} = \frac{150 \text{ mL}}{15}$$

$$10 \text{ mL} = 10 \text{ mL}$$

Because the calculated amount forms a true statement and is consistent with the approximated amount, 10 mL, the answer is confirmed.

Example 3:

Ordered Dose: 450 mg

Supply: 150 mg per tablet

C: *Convert*—Because the ordered dose and supplied dose are both measured in mg, no conversion factor is needed.

A: *Approximate*—Because the ordered dose is three times the supplied dose, three tablets will be needed.

S: *Solve*—Supply = 1 tab/150 mg; Order = 450 mg/1

$$x \left(\text{tab} \right) = \frac{1 \text{ tab}}{150 \cancel{\text{ mg}}} \times \frac{450 \cancel{\text{ mg}}}{1}$$

$$x = \frac{450 \text{ tab}}{150}$$

$$x = 3 \text{ tab}$$

E: *Evaluate*—Replace *x* with 3 tab and check the math:

$$3 \text{ tab} = \frac{1 \text{ tab}}{150 \text{ mg}} \times \frac{450 \text{ mg}}{1}$$

$$3 \text{ tab} = \frac{450 \text{ tab}}{150}$$

$$3 \text{ tab} = 3 \text{ tab}$$

Because the calculated amount forms a true statement and is consistent with the approximated amount, 3 tab, the answer is confirmed.

LEARNING ACTIVITY 7-6 Using dimensional analysis within the *CASE* approach, calculate the amount to administer for each ordered dose.

1.   Ordered Dose: 2 g; Supply: 100 mg/mL
2.   Ordered Dose: 150 mcg; Supply: 0.25 mg/2 mL
3.   Ordered Dose: 1 mg; Supply 2 mg/5 mL

Calculation Choices ... Case Closure

The *CASE* approach should be implemented to prevent calculation errors. Any of the three methods (ratio-proportion, formula, or dimensional analysis) may be used to solve basic calculations. However, when multiple conversions are necessary, as in complex IV rate calculations, ratio-proportion is generally not used. Several different formulas are needed to perform all types of dosage calculation by the formula method. Many find it difficult to memorize and recall the various formulas, which may result in dosage calculation errors.

Dimensional analysis can be used when no conversion is needed, but it is particularly useful when multiple conversions are needed to calculate the dose. All dosage calculations can be performed using dimensional analysis. Because dimensional analysis is less error-prone, it is the preferred calculation method of many institutions.

Chapter Summary

Learning Outcomes	Points to Remember
7-1 Differentiate the dosage strength of the supplied medication from the ordered dose.	Dosage strength $= \frac{dose\ supplied}{dosage\ unit}$; for example, the dosage strength of 250 mg tablets $= \frac{250\ mg}{1\ tab}$ To compare the supplied dosage strength to the ordered dose, use the first two steps of the *CASE* approach, **C**: *Convert* and **A**: *Approximate*: **C**: *Convert*—Convert ordered dose and supplied dose to the same unit of measurement (if necessary). **A**: *Approximate*—Approximate the number of dosage units to administer by comparing the ordered dose to the supplied dose. Example: Order: 0.45 g Supply: 225 mg per tablet **C**: *Convert*—0.45 g to 450 mg **A**: *Approximate*—Because the ordered dose, 450 mg, is twice the supplied dose of 225 mg per tablet, two tablets are needed.

7-2 Apply the *CASE* approach to calculate dosages using ratio-proportion, the formula method, and dimensional analysis.

After performing **C**: *Convert* and **A:** *Approximate* as shown in the previous example, execute the final two steps, **S:** *Solve* and **E:** *Evaluate:*

S: *Solve*—Determine the amount to administer by using any of the following methods:

Ratio-Proportion:

- Fractional ratio-proportion

$$\underset{\text{SUPPLY}}{\frac{\text{supplied dose}}{\text{dosage unit}}} = \underset{\text{ORDER}}{\frac{\text{ordered dose}}{\text{amount to administer (or } x)}}$$

Example: $\dfrac{225 \text{ mg}}{1 \text{ tab}} = \dfrac{450 \text{ mg}}{x \text{ tab}}$

- Linear ratio-proportion

supplied dose : dosage unit = ordered dose : amount to administer (x)

Example: 225 mg : 1 tab = 450 mg : x tab

Formula:

$$\frac{\text{ordered dose or } \textbf{D}\text{esired dose } (D)}{\text{supplied dose or dose on } \textbf{H}\text{and } (H)} \times \text{dosage unit or } \textbf{Q}\text{uantity} (Q)$$
$$= \text{amount to administer } (x)$$

Example: $\dfrac{450 \text{ \sout{mg}}}{225 \text{ \sout{mg}}} \times 1 \text{ tab} = x \text{ (tab)}$

Dimensional Analysis:

amount to administer $(x) =$

$$\frac{\text{dosage unit}}{\text{supplied dose}} \times \text{conversion factor} (s) \times \frac{\text{ordered dose}}{1}$$

$$x \text{ (tab)} = \frac{1 \text{ tab}}{225 \text{ \sout{mg}}} \times \frac{1{,}000 \text{ \sout{mg}}}{1 \text{ \sout{g}}} \times \frac{0.45 \text{ \sout{g}}}{1}$$

$$x = 2 \text{ tab}$$

E: *Evaluate*—Evaluate the accuracy of the result by replacing x with the answer and checking the math; also compare the answer to the approximated answer to confirm the result. Because 2 tab is consistent with the approximated answer, the answer for this example is confirmed.

Homework

For exercises 1–10, refer to the following labels to compare the ordered dose to the supply and determine steps *C* and *A* of the *CASE* method. (LO 7-1)

1. **Order:** levothyroxine 0.075 mg PO daily
   Supply:

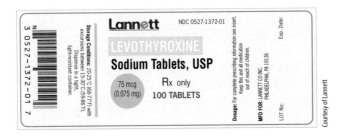

a. *C*: *Convert*
b. *A*: *Approximate*

2. **Order:** Cymbalta® 60 mg PO daily
   Supply:

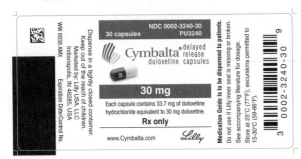

a. *C*: *Convert*
b. *A*: *Approximate*

3. **Order:** amiodarone 400 mg PO daily
   Supply:

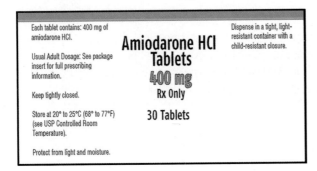

a. *C*: *Convert*
b. *A*: *Approximate*

4. **Order:** clonazepam 500 mcg PO bid
   Supply:

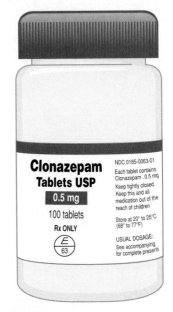

a. *C*: *Convert*
b. *A*: *Approximate*

5. **Order:** methotrexate 0.025 g IM weekly
   Supply:

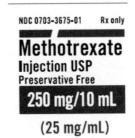
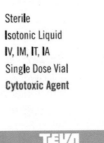

a. *C*: *Convert*
b. *A*: *Approximate*

6. Order: methadone HCl 15 mg GT daily
Supply:

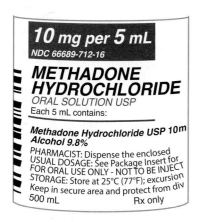

a. *C*: Convert
b. *A*: Approximate

7. Order: docusate sodium 100 mg PO nightly
Supply:

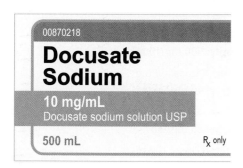

a. *C*: Convert
b. *A*: Approximate

8. Order: cefaclor 0.25 g PO bid
Supply:

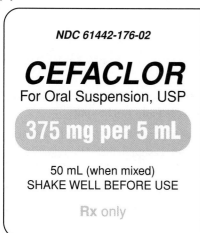

a. *C*: Convert
b. *A*: Approximate

9. Order: ondansetron HCl 8 mg PO bid
Supply:

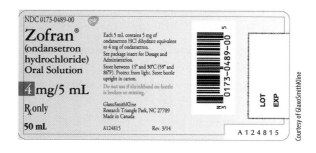

a. *C*: Convert
b. *A*: Approximate

10. Order: Epogen® 1,200 units subcut 3 times per week
Supply:

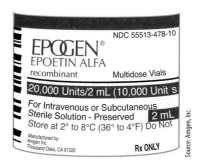

a. *C*: Convert
b. *A*: Approximate

For questions 11–20, use fractional ratio-proportion within the *CASE* approach to determine the amount to administer. Assume all tablets are scored and can be split. (LO 7-2)

11. Ordered Dose: 2.25 g
Supply: 750 mg/cap

12. Ordered Dose: 375 mg
Supply: 250 mg/tablet

13. Ordered Dose: 0.325 g
Supply: 250 mg/5 mL

14. Ordered Dose: 0.25 g
Supply: 125 mg/tab

15. Ordered Dose: 0.75 g
Supply: 1 g/10 mL

16. Ordered Dose: 450 mcg
Supply: 1 mg/10 mL

17. Ordered Dose: 125 mg
Supply: 50 mg/tab

18. Ordered Dose: 300 mcg
Supply: 0.15 mg/tab

19. **Ordered Dose:** 750 mg
    Supply: 300 mg/5 mL

20. **Ordered Dose:** 30 mEq
    Supply: 20 mEq/15 mL

For questions 21–30, use linear ratio-proportion within the *CASE* approach to determine the amount to administer. Assume all tablets are scored and can be split. (LO 7-2)

21. **Ordered Dose:** 1.5 g
    Supply: 750 mg/cap

22. **Ordered Dose:** 125 mg
    Supply: 250 mg/tablet

23. **Ordered Dose:** 1.25 g
    Supply: 250 mg/5 mL

24. **Ordered Dose:** 375 mg
    Supply: 125 mg/tab

25. **Ordered Dose:** 1 g
    Supply: 750 mg/10 mL

26. **Ordered Dose:** 375 mcg
    Supply: 1 mg/10 mL

27. **Ordered Dose:** 650 mg
    Supply: 325 mg/tab

28. **Ordered Dose:** 250 mcg
    Supply: 0.5 mg/tab

29. **Ordered Dose:** 750 mg
    Supply: 375 mg/cap

30. **Ordered Dose:** 40 mEq
    Supply: 20 mEq/15 mL

For questions 31–40, use the formula method within the *CASE* approach to determine the amount to administer. Assume all tablets are scored and can be split. (LO 7-2)

31. **Ordered Dose:** 1.5 g
    Supply: 500 mg/cap

32. **Ordered Dose:** 300 mg
    Supply: 250 mg/5 mL

33. **Ordered Dose:** 0.75 g
    Supply: 250 mg/5 mL

34. **Ordered Dose:** 75 mg
    Supply: 150 mg/tab

35. **Ordered Dose:** 0.32 g
    Supply: 80 mg/10 mL

36. **Ordered Dose:** 50 mg
    Supply: 10 mg/5 mL

37. **Ordered Dose:** 375 mg
    Supply: 125 mg/cap

38. **Ordered Dose:** 200 mg
    Supply: 0.6 g/12 mL

39. **Ordered Dose:** 1,500 mg
    Supply: 750 mg/10 mL

40. **Ordered Dose:** 0.5 g
    Supply: 250 mg/50 mL

For questions 41–50, use dimensional analysis within the *CASE* approach to determine the amount to administer. Assume all tablets are scored and can be split. (LO 7-2)

41. **Ordered Dose:** 450 mg
    Supply: 150 mg/cap

42. **Ordered Dose:** 0.5 g
    Supply: 250 mg/tablet

43. **Ordered Dose:** 0.625 g
    Supply: 250 mg/5 mL

44. **Ordered Dose:** 175 mg
    Supply: 70 mg/tab

45. **Ordered Dose:** 1 g
    Supply: 500 mg/10 mL

46. **Ordered Dose:** 60 mg
    Supply: 40 mg/20 mL

47. **Ordered Dose:** 12.5 mg
    Supply: 25 mg/tab

48. **Ordered Dose:** 100 mg
    Supply: 20 mg/5 mL

49. **Ordered Dose:** 0.12 g
    Supply: 60 mg/15 mL

50. **Ordered Dose:** 10 mEq
    Supply: 20 mEq/15 mL

NCLEX-Style Review Questions

For questions 1–4, select the best response. Assume all tablets are scored and can be split.

1. The prescriber orders 345 mg of a medication. The medication is supplied as 230 mg tablets. The nurse should administer:
   a. 2½ tablets
   b. 2 tablets
   c. 1½ tablets
   d. 1 tablet

2. The prescriber orders 3.75 mg of a corticosteroid. The dosage strength is 2.5 mg/tab. The nurse should administer:
  a. ½ tab
  b. 1½ tab
  c. 2 tab
  d. 2½ tab

3. The order calls for 50 mg. Which dosage strength should the nurse choose?
  a. 12.5 mg/tab
  b. 25 mg/tab
  c. 75 mg/tab
  d. 100 mg/tab

4. The prescriber orders 200 mg of an anti-infective medication. The dosage strength is 50 mg in 5 mL. The nurse should administer:
  a. 4 mL
  b. 10 mL
  c. 20 mL
  d. 40 mL

For questions 5–6, select all that apply.

5. The prescriber orders 160 mg of an antipyretic. The dosage strength is 80 mg/teaspoon. The nurse should administer:
  a. 2.5 mL
  b. 5 mL
  c. 7.5 mL
  d. 10 mL
  e. ½ t
  f. 2 t

6. The prescriber orders 750 mg of cough syrup. The dosage strength is 250 mg/10 mL. The nurse advises the patient to take:
  a. 1 T
  b. 1 oz
  c. 2 T
  d. 6 t
  e. 30 mL
  f. 0.33 mL

REFERENCES

Cookson, K. L. (2013). Dimensional analysis: Calculate dosages the easy way. *Nursing, 43*(6), 57–62. Lippincott Williams, & Wilkins.

Greenfield, S., Whelan, B., & Cohn, E. (2006). Use of dimensional analysis to reduce medication errors. *Journal of Nursing Education, 45*(2), 91–94. Retrieved from http://www.ncbi.nlm.nih.gov/pubmed/16496864

Chapter 7   ANSWER KEY

Learning Activity 7-1

1. a. N/A
    b. The ordered amount is triple the supply, so 3 capsules are needed to deliver the ordered dose.

2. a. Convert 0.4 mg to mcg.

$$\frac{1\,mg}{1,000\,mcg} = \frac{0.4\,mg}{x\,mcg}$$

$$1x = 1,000 \times 0.4 = 400\,mcg$$

or

$$x(mcg) = \frac{1,000\,mcg}{1\,\cancel{mg}} \times 0.4\,\cancel{mg} = 400\,mcg$$

   b. The ordered amount is equivalent to the supplied dosage, so 1 cap is needed to deliver the ordered dose.

3. a. N/A
    b. The ordered dose is less than the supplied dosage strength by half, so ½ tab is needed to deliver the ordered amount.

Learning Activity 7-2

1. $\dfrac{0.5\,mg}{1\,tab} = \dfrac{1\,mg}{x\,tab}$

2. $\dfrac{25\,mg}{1\,mL} = \dfrac{50\,mg}{x\,mL}$

3. $\dfrac{20\,mg}{1\,tab} = \dfrac{40\,mg}{x\,tab}$

Learning Activity 7-3

1. **C:** N/A
    A: Ordered amount is half of the supplied amount; half the supply volume, or 0.5 mL, is needed to deliver the ordered amount.

    S:
$$\frac{5\,mg}{1\,mL} = \frac{2.5\,mg}{x\,mL}$$

$$5x = 2.5$$

$$\frac{\cancel{5}x}{\cancel{5}} = \frac{2.5}{5}$$

$$x = 0.5\,mL$$

E:

$$\frac{5 \text{ mg}}{1 \text{ mL}} = \frac{2.5 \text{ mg}}{0.5 \text{ mL}}$$

$$5 \times 0.5 = 1 \times 2.5$$

Because the calculated amount forms a true statement when inserted into the equation and is consistent with the approximated amount, 0.5 mL, the answer is confirmed.

2. **C:** Convert 0.075 g to 75 mg.
   A: Order is greater than the supply by three times, so 3 tablets are needed to deliver the ordered amount.

S:

$$\frac{25 \text{ mg}}{1 \text{ tab}} = \frac{75 \text{ mg}}{x \text{ tab}}$$

$$25x = 75$$

$$x = 3 \text{ tab}$$

E:

$$\frac{25 \text{ mg}}{1 \text{ tab}} = \frac{75 \text{ mg}}{3 \text{ tab}}$$

$$25 \times 3 = 1 \times 75$$

Because the calculated amount forms a true statement when inserted into the equation and is consistent with the approximated amount, 3 tablets, the answer is confirmed.

3. **C:** N/A
   A: The order is less than the supply, therefore less than 5 mL will be needed to deliver the ordered amount.

S:

$$\frac{2 \text{ mg}}{5 \text{ mL}} = \frac{1.45 \text{ mg}}{x \text{ mL}}$$

$$2x = 5 \times 1.45$$

$$\frac{2x}{2} = \frac{7.25}{2}$$

$$x = 3.625 \text{ mL, which rounds to 3.6 mL}$$

E:

$$\frac{2 \text{ mg}}{5 \text{ mL}} = \frac{1.45 \text{ mg}}{3.625 \text{ mL}}$$

$$2 \times 3.625 = 5 \times 1.45$$

Because the calculated amount forms a true statement when inserted into the equation and is consistent with the approximated amount, less than 5 mL, the answer is confirmed.

Learning Activity 7-4

1. **C:** N/A
   A: Ordered amount is more than two times the supplied amount, so more than 2 tabs are needed to deliver the ordered amount.

S:

$$2 \text{ mg} : 1 \text{ tab} = 5 \text{ mg} : x \text{ tab}$$

$$2x = 1 \times 5$$

$$\frac{2x}{2} = \frac{5}{2}$$

$$x = 2\frac{1}{2} \text{ tab}$$

E:

$$2 \text{ mg} : 1 \text{ tab} = 5 \text{ mg} : 2\frac{1}{2} \text{ tab}$$

$$2 \times 2\frac{1}{2} = 1 \times 5$$

Because the calculated amount forms a true statement when inserted into the equation and is consistent with the approximated amount, more than 2 tablets, the answer is confirmed.

2. **C:** Convert 0.5 g to 500 mg.
   A: Order is five times greater than the supply, so five times the supply volume, or 75 mL, is needed to deliver the ordered amount.

S:

$$100 \text{ mg} : 15 \text{ mL} = 500 \text{ mg} : x \text{ mL}$$

$$100x = 15 \times 500$$

$$\frac{100x}{100} = \frac{7,500}{100}$$

$$x = 75 \text{ mL}$$

E:

$$100 \text{ mg} : 15 \text{ mL} = 500 \text{ mg} : 75 \text{ mL}$$

$$100 \times 75 = 15 \times 500$$

Because the calculated amount forms a true statement when inserted into the equation and is consistent with the approximated amount, 75 mL, the answer is confirmed.

3. **C:** Convert 0.25 g to 250 mg.
   A: Order is two times the supplied amount, so 2 capsules are needed to deliver the ordered amount.

S:

$$125 \text{ mg} : 1 \text{ cap} = 250 \text{ mg} : x \text{ cap}$$

$$125x = 1 \times 250$$

$$\frac{125x}{125} = \frac{250}{125}$$

$$x = 2 \text{ cap}$$

E:

$$125 \text{ mg} : 1 \text{ cap} = 250 \text{ mg} : 2 \text{ cap}$$

$$125 \times 2 = 1 \times 250$$

Because the calculated amount forms a true statement when inserted into the equation and is consistent with the approximated amount, 2 cap, the answer is confirmed.

Learning Activity 7-5

1. **C:** Convert 0.45 g to 450 mg.

   A: Order is three times the supplied amount, so 3 capsules are needed to deliver the ordered amount.

   S:
   $$\frac{450 \text{ mg}}{150 \text{ mg}} \times 1 \text{ tab} = x \text{ (tab)}$$
   $$3 \text{ tab} = x$$

   E:
   $$\frac{450 \text{ mg}}{150 \text{ mg}} \times 1 \text{ tab} = 3 \text{ tab}$$

   Because the calculated amount forms a true statement when inserted into the equation and is consistent with the approximated amount, 3 tab, the answer is confirmed.

2. **C:** Convert 0.2 mg to 200 mcg.

   A: Order is two times the supplied amount, so 2 mL are needed to deliver the ordered amount.

   S:
   $$\frac{200 \text{ mcg}}{100 \text{ mcg}} \times 1 \text{ mL} = x \text{ (mL)}$$
   $$2 \text{ mL} = x$$

   E:
   $$\frac{200 \text{ mcg}}{100 \text{ mcg}} \times 1 \text{ mL} = 2 \text{ mL}$$

   Because the calculated amount forms a true statement when inserted into the equation and is consistent with the approximated amount, 2 mL, the answer is confirmed.

3. **C:** N/A

   A: The ordered amount is one-fifth of the supplied amount, so one-fifth of the supply volume, or 1 mL, is needed to deliver the ordered amount.

   S:
   $$\frac{20 \text{ mg}}{100 \text{ mg}} \times 5 \text{ mL} = x \text{ (mL)}$$
   $$1 \text{ mL} = x$$

   E:
   $$\frac{20 \text{ mg}}{100 \text{ mg}} \times 5 \text{ mL} = 1 \text{ mL}$$

   Because the calculated amount forms a true statement when inserted into the equation and is consistent with the approximated amount, 1 mL, the answer is confirmed.

Learning Activity 7-6

1. **C:** Use the conversion factor 1,000 mg/1 g.

   A: Mentally convert 2 g to 2,000 mg and determine that the ordered amount is 20 times larger than the supplied amount, so 20 times the supply volume, or 20 mL, is needed to deliver the ordered amount.

   S:
   $$x\,(\text{mL}) = \frac{1 \text{ mL}}{100 \text{ mg}} \times \frac{1{,}000 \text{ mg}}{1 \text{ g}} \times \frac{2 \text{ g}}{1}$$
   $$x = \frac{2{,}000}{100} = 20 \text{ mL}$$

   E:
   $$20 \text{ mL} = \frac{1 \text{ mL}}{100 \text{ mg}} \times \frac{1{,}000 \text{ mg}}{1 \text{ g}} \times \frac{2 \text{ g}}{1}$$

   Because the calculated amount forms a true statement when inserted into the equation and is consistent with the approximated amount, 20 mL, the answer is confirmed.

2. **C:** Convert using the conversion factor 1 mg/1,000 mcg.

   A: Mentally convert 150 mcg to 0.15 mg to determine the ordered amount is less than the supplied amount, so less than 2 mL are needed to deliver the ordered amount.

   S:
   $$x\,(\text{mL}) = \frac{2 \text{ mL}}{0.25 \text{ mg}} \times \frac{1 \text{ mg}}{1{,}000 \text{ mcg}} \times \frac{150 \text{ mcg}}{1}$$
   $$x = \frac{300 \text{ mL}}{250} = 1.2 \text{ mL}$$

   E:
   $$1.2 \text{ mL} = \frac{2 \text{ mL}}{0.25 \text{ mg}} \times \frac{1 \text{ mg}}{1{,}000 \text{ mcg}} \times \frac{150 \text{ mcg}}{1}$$

   Because the calculated amount forms a true statement when inserted into the equation and is consistent with the approximated amount, less than 2 mL, the answer is confirmed.

3. **C:** N/A

   A: The ordered amount is half the supplied amount, so half the supply volume, or 2.5 mL, is needed to deliver the ordered amount.

   S:
   $$x\,(\text{mL}) = \frac{5 \text{ mL}}{2 \text{ mg}} \times \frac{1 \text{ mg}}{1}$$
   $$x = \frac{5 \text{ mL}}{2} = 2.5 \text{ mL}$$

E:

$$2.5 \text{ mL} = \frac{5 \text{ mL}}{2 \text{ mg}} \times \frac{1 \text{ mg}}{1}$$

Because the calculated amount forms a true statement when inserted into the equation and is consistent with the approximated amount, 2.5 mL, the answer is confirmed.

Homework

1. **C:** Convert 0.075 mg to 75 mcg.
    A: Because the amount ordered equals the amount in 1 tablet, 1 tablet is needed to provide the ordered dose.
2. **C:** N/A
    A: Because the amount ordered is twice the supplied dose, 2 capsules are needed to provide the ordered dose.
3. **C:** N/A
    A: Because the ordered dose is the same as the supplied dose, 1 tablet is needed to provide the ordered dose.
4. **C:** Convert 500 mcg to 0.5 mg or use the conversion factor 1 mg/1,000 mcg.
    A: Because the ordered dose equals the supplied dose, 1 tablet is needed to provide the ordered dose.
5. **C:** Convert 0.025 g to 25 mg or use the conversion factor 1,000 mg/1 g.
    A: Because the ordered dose equals the supplied dose, 1 mL is needed to provide the ordered dose.
6. **C:** N/A
    A: Because the ordered dose is one and one-half (1½) the dose supplied in 5 mL, 7.5 mL are needed to provide the ordered dose.
7. **C:** N/A
    A: Because the ordered dose is 10 times the supplied dose, 10 times the supply volume, or 10 mL, is needed to provide the ordered dose.
8. **C:** Convert 0.25 g to 250 mg or use the conversion factor 1,000 mg/1 g.
    A: Because the ordered dose is less than the supplied dose, less than the supply volume of 5 mL is needed to provide the ordered dose.
9. **C:** N/A
    A: Because the ordered dose is twice the supplied dose, two times the supply volume, or 10 mL, is needed to provide the ordered dose.

10. **C:** N/A
    A: Because the ordered dose is less than ½ of the dose supplied in 2 mL, less than 1 mL is needed to provide the ordered dose. (Note: For a more accurate estimate, the supplied amount could be further reduced to ⅛ of the dose supplied in 2 mL. Therefore, the amount to administer will be less than 0.25 mL.)
11. **C:** Convert 2.25 g to 2,250 mg.
    A: Because the amount ordered is approximately three times the supplied dose, about 3 capsules are needed to provide the ordered dose.

    S:
    $$\frac{750 \text{ mg}}{1 \text{ cap}} = \frac{2,250 \text{ mg}}{x \text{ cap}}$$
    $$750x = 2,250$$
    $$x = 3 \text{ cap}$$

    E:
    $$\frac{750 \text{ mg}}{1 \text{ cap}} = \frac{2,250 \text{ mg}}{3 \text{ cap}}$$
    $$750 \times 3 = 1 \times 2,250$$
    $$2,250 = 2,250$$

    Because the calculated amount forms a true statement when inserted into the equation and is consistent with the approximated amount, 3 capsules, the answer is confirmed.
12. **C:** N/A
    A: Because the ordered dose is 1½ times the supplied dose, 1½ tablets are needed to provide the ordered dose.

    S:
    $$\frac{250 \text{ mg}}{1 \text{ tab}} = \frac{375 \text{ mg}}{x \text{ tab}}$$
    $$250x = 375$$
    $$x = 1\frac{1}{2} \text{ tab}$$

    E:
    $$\frac{250 \text{ mg}}{1 \text{ tab}} = \frac{375 \text{ mg}}{1\frac{1}{2} \text{ tab}}$$
    $$250 \times 1\frac{1}{2} = 1 \times 375$$
    $$375 = 375$$

    Because the calculated amount forms a true statement when inserted into the equation and is consistent with the approximated amount, 1½ tablets, the answer is confirmed.

13. **C:** Convert 0.325 g to 325 mg.
 A: Because the ordered dose is more than one times but less than twice the supply, more than 5 mL but less than 10 mL are needed to provide the ordered dose.

S:
$$\frac{250\ mg}{5\ mL} = \frac{325\ mg}{x\ mL}$$
$$250x = 5 \times 325$$
$$x = 6.5\ mL$$

E:
$$\frac{250\ mg}{5\ mL} = \frac{325\ mg}{6.5\ mL}$$
$$250 \times 6.5 = 5 \times 325$$

Because the calculated amount forms a true statement when inserted into the equation and is consistent with the approximated amount, 5 to 10 mL, the answer is confirmed.

14. **C:** Convert 0.25 g to 250 mg.
 A: Because the ordered dose is twice the dose supplied in 1 tablet, 2 tablets are needed to provide the ordered dose.

S:
$$\frac{125\ mg}{1\ tab} = \frac{250\ mg}{x\ tab}$$
$$125x = 250$$
$$x = 2\ tab$$

E:
$$\frac{125\ mg}{1\ tab} = \frac{250\ mg}{2\ tab}$$
$$125 \times 2 = 1 \times 250$$

Because the calculated amount forms a true statement when inserted into the equation and is consistent with the approximated amount, 2 tablets, the answer is confirmed.

15. **C:** N/A
 A: Because the ordered amount is less than the supply, less than 10 mL are needed to provide the ordered dose.

S:
$$\frac{1\ g}{10\ mL} = \frac{0.75\ g}{x\ mL}$$
$$x = 10 \times 0.75$$
$$x = 7.5\ mL$$

E:
$$\frac{1\ g}{10\ mL} = \frac{0.75\ g}{7.5\ mL}$$
$$1 \times 7.5 = 10 \times 0.75$$

Because the calculated amount forms a true statement when inserted into the equation and is

consistent with the approximated amount, less than 10 mL, the answer is confirmed.

16. **C:** Convert 450 mcg to 0.45 mg.
 A: Because the ordered dose is less than half the supply, less than half of 10 mL is needed to provide the ordered dose.

S:
$$\frac{1\ mg}{10\ mL} = \frac{0.45\ mg}{x\ mL}$$
$$x = 10 \times 0.45$$
$$x = 4.5\ mL$$

E:
$$\frac{1\ mg}{10\ mL} = \frac{0.45\ mg}{4.5\ mL}$$
$$1 \times 4.5 = 10 \times 0.45$$

Because the calculated amount forms a true statement when inserted into the equation and is consistent with the approximated amount, less than 5 mL, the answer is confirmed.

17. **C:** N/A
 A: The ordered dose is more than twice the supply, so more than 2 tabs are needed to provide the ordered dose.

S:
$$\frac{50\ mg}{1\ tab} = \frac{125\ mg}{x\ tab}$$
$$50x = 125$$
$$x = 2\frac{1}{2}\ tab$$

E:
$$\frac{50\ mg}{1\ tab} = \frac{125\ mg}{2\frac{1}{2}\ tab}$$
$$50 \times 2\frac{1}{2} = 1 \times 125$$

Because the calculated amount forms a true statement when inserted into the equation and is consistent with the approximated amount, more than 2 tablets, the answer is correct.

18. **C:** Convert 0.15 mg to 150 mcg.
 A: Because the ordered dose is 2 times the dose supplied, 2 tablets are needed to provide the ordered dose.

S:
$$\frac{150\ mcg}{1\ tab} = \frac{300\ mcg}{x\ tab}$$
$$150x = 300$$
$$x = 2\ tab$$

E:

$$\frac{150 \text{ mcg}}{1 \text{ tab}} = \frac{300 \text{ mcg}}{2 \text{ tab}}$$

$$150 \times 2 = 1 \times 300$$

Because the calculated amount forms a true statement when inserted into the equation and is consistent with the approximated amount, 2 tablets, the answer is confirmed.

19. **C:** N/A

A: Because the ordered dose is more than twice the supply, more than 10 mL are needed to provide the ordered dose.

S:

$$\frac{300 \text{ mg}}{5 \text{ mL}} = \frac{750 \text{ mg}}{x \text{ mL}}$$

$$300x = 3,750$$

$$x = 12.5 \text{ mL}$$

E:

$$\frac{300 \text{ mg}}{5 \text{ mL}} = \frac{750 \text{ mg}}{12.5 \text{ mL}}$$

$$300 \times 12.5 = 5 \times 750$$

Because the calculated amount forms a true statement when inserted into the equation and is consistent with the approximated amount, greater than 10 mL, the answer is confirmed.

20. **C:** N/A

A: Because the ordered dose is 1½ times the dose supplied in 15 mL, more than 15 mL, but less than 30 mL, are needed to provide the ordered dose.

S:

$$\frac{20 \text{ mEq}}{15 \text{ mL}} = \frac{30 \text{ mEq}}{x \text{ mL}}$$

$$20x = 450$$

$$x = 22.5 \text{ mL}$$

E:

$$\frac{20 \text{ mEq}}{15 \text{ mL}} = \frac{30 \text{ mEq}}{22.5 \text{ mL}}$$

$$20 \times 22.5 = 15 \times 30$$

Because the calculated amount forms a true statement when inserted into the equation and is consistent with the approximated amount, 15 to 30 mL, the answer is correct.

21. **C:** Convert 1.5 g to 1,500 mg.

A: Because the ordered dose is twice the supplied dose, 2 capsules are needed to provide the ordered dose.

S: 750 mg : 1 cap = 1,500 mg : x cap

$$750x = 1,500$$

$$x = 2 \text{ cap}$$

E: 750 mg : 1 cap = 1,500 mg : 2 cap

$$750 \times 2 = 1 \times 1,500$$

Because the calculated amount forms a true statement when inserted into the equation and is consistent with the approximated amount, 2 capsules, the answer is correct.

22. **C:** N/A

A: Because the ordered dose is half as much as the supplied dose, ½ tablet is needed to provide the ordered dose.

S: 250 mg : 1 tab = 125 mg : x tab

$$250x = 125$$

$$x = \frac{1}{2} \text{ tab}$$

E: 250 mg : 1 tab = 125 mg : $\frac{1}{2}$ tab

$$250 \times \frac{1}{2} = 1 \times 125$$

Because the calculated amount forms a true statement when inserted into the equation and is consistent with the approximated amount, ½ tablet, the answer is confirmed.

23. **C:** Convert 1.25 g to 1,250 mg.

A: Because the ordered dose is five times as large as the supply, five times the supply volume, or 25 mL, is needed to provide the ordered dose.

S: 250 mg : 5 mL = 1,250 mg : x mL

$$250x = 6,250$$

$$x = 25 \text{ mL}$$

E: 250 mg : 5 mL = 1,250 mg : 25 mL

$$250 \times 25 = 5 \times 1,250$$

Because the calculated amount forms a true statement when inserted into the equation and is consistent with the approximated amount, 25 mL, the answer is confirmed.

24. **C:** N/A

A: Because the ordered dose is three times the dose supplied in 1 tablet, 3 tablets are needed to provide the ordered dose.

S: 125 mg : 1 tab = 375 mg : x tab

$125x = 375$

$x = 3$ tab

E: 125 mg : 1 tab = 375 mg : 3 tab

$125 \times 3 = 1 \times 375$

Because the calculated amount forms a true statement when inserted into the equation and is consistent with the approximated amount, 3 tablets, the answer is confirmed.

25. **C:** Convert 1 g to 1,000 mg.

A: Because the ordered amount is greater than the dose supplied in 10 mL, more than 10 mL are needed to provide the ordered dose.

S: 750 mg : 10 mL = 1,000 mg : x mL

$750x = 10,000$

$x = 13.3333$ mL or 13.3 mL

E: 750 mg : 10 mL = 1,000 mg : 13.33 mL

$750 \times 13.3333 \cong 10 \times 1,000$

Because the calculated amount forms a true statement when inserted into the equation and is consistent with the approximated amount, greater than 10 mL, the answer is confirmed.

26. **C:** Convert 1 mg to 1,000 mcg.

A: Because the ordered dose is less than half of the dose supplied in 10 mL, less than 5 mL are needed to provide the ordered dose.

S: 1,000 mcg : 10 mL = 375 mcg : x mL

$1,000x = 3,750$

$x = 3.75$ rounded to 3.8 mL

E: 1,000 mcg : 10 mL = 375 mcg : 3.75 mL

$1,000 \times 3.75 = 10 \times 375$

Because the calculated amount forms a true statement when inserted into the equation and is consistent with the approximated amount, less than 5 mL, the answer is confirmed.

27. **C:** N/A

A: The ordered dose is twice the supplied dose, so 2 tablets are needed to provide the ordered dose.

S: 325 mg : 1 tab = 650 mg : x tab

$325x = 650$

$x = 2$ tab

E: 325 mg : 1 tab = 650 mg : 2 tab

$325 \times 2 = 1 \times 650$

Because the calculated amount forms a true statement when inserted into the equation and is consistent with the approximated amount, 2 tablets, the answer is confirmed.

28. **C:** Convert 0.5 mg to 500 mcg.

A: Because the ordered dose is half of the dose supplied in 1 tablet, ½ tablet is needed to provide the ordered dose.

S: 500 mcg : 1 tab = 250 mg : x tab

$500x = 250$

$x = \dfrac{1}{2}$ tab

E: 500 mcg : 1 tab = 250 mg : $\dfrac{1}{2}$ tab

$500 \times \dfrac{1}{2} = 1 \times 250$

Because the calculated amount forms a true statement when inserted into the equation and is consistent with the approximated amount, ½ tablet, the answer is confirmed.

29. **C:** N/A

A: Because the ordered dose is twice the dose supplied in 1 capsule, 2 capsules are needed to provide the ordered dose.

S: 375 mg : 1 cap = 750 mg : x cap

$375x = 750$

$x = 2$ cap

E: 375 mg : 1 cap = 750 mg : 2 cap

$375 \times 2 = 1 \times 750$

Because the calculated amount forms a true statement when inserted into the equation and is consistent with the approximated amount, 2 capsules, the answer is confirmed.

30. **C:** N/A

A: Because the ordered dose is twice the dose supplied in 15 mL, twice the supply volume, or 30 mL, are needed to provide the ordered dose.

S: 20 mEq : 15 mL = 40 mEq : x mL

$20x = 600$

$x = 30$ mL

E: 20 mEq : 15 mL = 40 mEq : 30 mL

$$20 \times 30 = 15 \times 40$$

Because the calculated amount forms a true statement when inserted into the equation and is consistent with the approximated amount, 30 mL, the answer is confirmed.

31. **C:** Convert 1.5 g to 1,500 mg.

   A: Because the ordered dose is three times the supplied dose, 3 capsules are needed to provide the ordered dose.

S: $\dfrac{1,500 \text{ mg}}{500 \text{ mg}} \times 1 \text{ cap} = x \text{ (cap)}$

$$3 \text{ cap} = x$$

E: $\dfrac{1,500 \text{ mg}}{500 \text{ mg}} \times 1 \text{ cap} = 3 \text{ cap}$

Because the calculated amount forms a true statement when inserted into the equation and is consistent with the approximated amount, 3 capsules, the answer is correct.

32. **C:** N/A

   A: Because the ordered dose is more than one times but less than twice as much as the supplied dose, between 5 and 10 mL are needed to provide the ordered dose.

S: $\dfrac{300 \text{ mg}}{250 \text{ mg}} \times 5 \text{ mL} = x \text{ (mL)}$

$$6 \text{ mL} = x$$

E: $\dfrac{300 \text{ mg}}{250 \text{ mg}} \times 5 \text{ mL} = 6 \text{ mL}$

Because the calculated amount forms a true statement when inserted into the equation and is consistent with the approximated amount, between 5 and 10 mL, the answer is confirmed.

33. **C:** Convert 0.75 g to 750 mg.

   A: Because the ordered dose is three times larger than the dose supplied in 5 mL, three times the supply volume, or 15 mL, is needed to provide the ordered dose.

S: $\dfrac{750 \text{ mg}}{250 \text{ mg}} \times 5 \text{ mL} = x \text{ (mL)}$

$$15 \text{ mL} = x$$

E: $\dfrac{750 \text{ mg}}{250 \text{ mg}} \times 5 \text{ mL} = 15 \text{ mL}$

Because the calculated amount forms a true statement when inserted into the equation and is consistent with the approximated amount, 15 mL, the answer is confirmed.

34. **C:** N/A

   A: Because the ordered dose is half as large as the dose supplied in 1 tablet, ½ tablet is needed to provide the ordered dose.

S: $\dfrac{75 \text{ mg}}{150 \text{ mg}} \times 1 \text{ tab} = x \text{ (tab)}$

$$\dfrac{1}{2} \text{ tab} = x$$

E: $\dfrac{75 \text{ mg}}{150 \text{ mg}} \times 1 \text{ tab} = \dfrac{1}{2} \text{ tab}$

Because the calculated amount forms a true statement when inserted into the equation and is consistent with the approximated amount, ½ tab, the answer is confirmed.

35. **C:** Convert 0.32 g to 320 mg.

   A: Because the ordered amount is four times greater than the dose supplied in 10 mL, four times the supply volume, or 40 mL, is needed to provide the ordered dose.

S: $\dfrac{320 \text{ mg}}{80 \text{ mg}} \times 10 \text{ mL} = x \text{ (mL)}$

$$40 \text{ mL} = x$$

E: $\dfrac{320 \text{ mg}}{80 \text{ mg}} \times 10 \text{ mL} = 40 \text{ mL}$

Because the calculated amount forms a true statement when inserted into the equation and is consistent with the approximated amount, 40 mL, the answer is confirmed.

36. **C:** N/A

   A: Because the ordered dose is five times larger than the dose supplied in 5 mL, five times the supply volume, or 25 mL, are needed to provide the ordered dose.

S: $\dfrac{50 \text{ mg}}{10 \text{ mg}} \times 5 \text{ mL} = x \text{ (mL)}$

$$25 \text{ mL} = x$$

E: $\dfrac{50 \text{ mg}}{10 \text{ mg}} \times 5 \text{ mL} = 25 \text{ mL}$

Because the calculated amount forms a true statement when inserted into the equation and is consistent with the approximated amount, 25 mL, the answer is confirmed.

37. **C:** N/A

    A: The ordered dose is three times the supplied dose, so 3 capsules are needed to provide the ordered dose.

    S:
    $$\frac{375 \text{ mg}}{125 \text{ mg}} \times 1 \text{ cap} = x \text{ (cap)}$$
    $$3 \text{ cap} = x$$

    E:
    $$\frac{375 \text{ mg}}{125 \text{ mg}} \times 1 \text{ cap} = 3 \text{ cap}$$

    Because the calculated amount forms a true statement when inserted into the equation and is consistent with the approximated amount, 3 cap, the answer is confirmed.

38. **C:** Convert 0.6 g to 600 mg.

    A: Because the ordered dose is ⅓ of the dose supplied in 12 mL, ⅓ of the supply volume, or 4 mL, is needed to provide the ordered dose.

    S:
    $$\frac{200 \text{ mg}}{600 \text{ mg}} \times 12 \text{ mL} = x \text{ (mL)}$$
    $$4 \text{ mL} = x$$

    E:
    $$\frac{200 \text{ mg}}{600 \text{ mg}} \times 12 \text{ mL} = 4 \text{ mL}$$

    Because the calculated amount forms a true statement when inserted into the equation and is consistent with the approximated amount, 4 mL, the answer is confirmed.

39. **C:** N/A

    A: Because the ordered dose is twice the dose supplied in 10 mL, twice the supply volume, or 20 mL, is needed to provide the ordered dose.

    S:
    $$\frac{1,500 \text{ mg}}{750 \text{ mg}} \times 10 \text{ mL} = x \text{ (mL)}$$
    $$20 \text{ mL} = x$$

    E:
    $$\frac{1,500 \text{ mg}}{750 \text{ mg}} \times 10 \text{ mL} = 20 \text{ mL}$$

    Because the calculated amount forms a true statement when inserted into the equation and is consistent with the approximated amount, 20 mL, the answer is confirmed.

40. **C:** Convert 0.5 g to 500 mg.

    A: Because the ordered dose is twice the dose supplied in 50 mL, twice the supply volume, or 100 mL, is needed to provide the ordered dose.

    S:
    $$\frac{500 \text{ mg}}{250 \text{ mg}} \times 50 \text{ mL} = x \text{ (mL)}$$
    $$100 \text{ mL} = x$$

    E:
    $$\frac{500 \text{ mg}}{250 \text{ mg}} \times 50 \text{ mL} = 100 \text{ mL}$$

    Because the calculated amount forms a true statement when inserted into the equation and is consistent with the approximated amount, 100 mL, the answer is confirmed.

41. **C:** N/A

    A: Because the ordered dose is three times the supplied dose, 3 capsules are needed to provide the ordered dose.

    S:
    $$x \text{ (cap)} = \frac{1 \text{ cap}}{150 \text{ mg}} \times \frac{450 \text{ mg}}{1}$$
    $$x = 3 \text{ cap}$$

    E:
    $$3 \text{ cap} = \frac{1 \text{ cap}}{150 \text{ mg}} \times \frac{450 \text{ mg}}{1}$$

    Because the calculated amount forms a true statement when inserted into the equation and is consistent with the approximated amount, 3 capsules, the answer is confirmed.

42. **C:** Use the conversion factor 1,000 mg/1 g to cancel grams.

    A: Mentally convert 0.5 g to 500 mg to determine the ordered dose is twice the supplied dose, so 2 tablets are needed to provide the ordered dose.

    S: $x \text{ (tab)} = \dfrac{1 \text{ tab}}{250 \text{ mg}} \times \dfrac{1,000 \text{ mg}}{1 \text{ g}} \times \dfrac{0.5 \text{ g}}{1}$
    $$x = 2 \text{ tab}$$

    E: $2 \text{ tab} = \dfrac{1 \text{ tab}}{250 \text{ mg}} \times \dfrac{1,000 \text{ mg}}{1 \text{ g}} \times \dfrac{0.5 \text{ g}}{1}$

    Because the calculated amount forms a true statement when inserted into the equation and is consistent with the approximated amount, 2 tab, the answer is confirmed.

43. **C:** Use the conversion factor 1,000 mg/1 g to cancel grams.

    A: Mentally convert 0.625 g to 625 mg to determine the ordered dose is more than twice as large as the dose supplied in 5 mL, therefore, more than 10 mL are needed to provide the ordered dose.

    S: $x \text{ (mL)} = \dfrac{5 \text{ mL}}{250 \text{ mg}} \times \dfrac{1,000 \text{ mg}}{1 \text{ g}} \times \dfrac{0.625 \text{ g}}{1}$
    $$x = 12.5 \text{ mL}$$

E: $12.5 \text{ mL} = \dfrac{5 \text{ mL}}{250 \text{ mg}} \times \dfrac{1{,}000 \text{ mg}}{1 \text{ g}} \times \dfrac{0.625 \text{ g}}{1}$

Because the calculated amount forms a true statement when inserted into the equation and is consistent with the approximated amount, the answer, 12.5 mL, is confirmed.

44. **C:** N/A

A: Because the ordered dose is more than twice the dose supplied in 1 tablet, more than 2 tablets are needed to provide the ordered dose.

S: $x \left(\text{tab} \right) = \dfrac{1 \text{ tab}}{70 \text{ mg}} \times \dfrac{175 \text{ mg}}{1}$

$x = 2\dfrac{1}{2} \text{ tab}$

E: $2\dfrac{1}{2} \text{ tab} = \dfrac{1 \text{ tab}}{70 \text{ mg}} \times \dfrac{175 \text{ mg}}{1}$

Because the calculated amount forms a true statement when inserted into the equation and is consistent with the approximated amount, the answer, 2½ tablets, is confirmed.

45. **C:** Use the conversion factor 1,000 mg/1 g to cancel grams.

A: Mentally convert 1 g to 1,000 mg to determine the ordered amount is twice the dose supplied in 10 mL, therefore, twice the supply volume, or 20 mL, is needed to provide the ordered dose.

S: $x \left(\text{mL} \right) = \dfrac{10 \text{ mL}}{500 \text{ mg}} \times \dfrac{1{,}000 \text{ mg}}{1 \text{ g}} \times \dfrac{1 \text{ g}}{1}$

$x = 20 \text{ mL}$

E: $20 \text{ mL} = \dfrac{10 \text{ mL}}{500 \text{ mg}} \times \dfrac{1{,}000 \text{ mg}}{1 \text{ g}} \times \dfrac{1 \text{ g}}{1}$

Because the calculated amount forms a true statement when inserted into the equation and is consistent with the approximated amount, 20 mL, the answer is confirmed.

46. **C:** N/A

A: Because the ordered dose is 1½ times the dose supplied in 20 mL, more than 20 mL but less than 40 mL are needed to provide the ordered dose.

S: $x \left(\text{mL} \right) = \dfrac{20 \text{ mL}}{40 \text{ mg}} \times \dfrac{60 \text{ mg}}{1}$

$x = 30 \text{ mL}$

E: $30 \text{ mL} = \dfrac{20 \text{ mL}}{40 \text{ mg}} \times \dfrac{60 \text{ mg}}{1}$

Because the calculated amount forms a true statement when inserted into the equation and is consistent with the approximated amount, 20–40 mL, the answer is confirmed.

47. **C:** N/A

A. The ordered dose is half the supplied dose, so ½ tablet is needed to provide the ordered dose.

S: $x \left(\text{tab} \right) = \dfrac{1 \text{ tab}}{25 \text{ mg}} \times \dfrac{12.5 \text{ mg}}{1}$

$x = \dfrac{1}{2} \text{ tab}$

E: $\dfrac{1}{2} \text{ tab} = \dfrac{1 \text{ tab}}{25 \text{ mg}} \times \dfrac{12.5 \text{ mg}}{1}$

Because the calculated amount forms a true statement when inserted into the equation and is consistent with the approximated amount, ½ tablet, the answer is confirmed.

48. **C:** N/A

A: Because the ordered dose is five times the dose supplied in 5 mL, five times the supply volume, or 25 mL, is needed to provide the ordered dose.

S: $x \left(\text{mL} \right) = \dfrac{5 \text{ mL}}{20 \text{ mg}} \times \dfrac{100 \text{ mg}}{1}$

$x = 25 \text{ mL}$

E: $25 \text{ mL} = \dfrac{5 \text{ mL}}{20 \text{ mg}} \times \dfrac{100 \text{ mg}}{1}$

Because the calculated amount forms a true statement when inserted into the equation and is consistent with the approximated amount, 25 mL, the answer is confirmed.

49. **C:** Use the conversion factor 1,000 mg/1 g to cancel grams.

A: Mentally convert 0.12 g to 120 mg to determine that the ordered dose is twice the dose supplied in 15 mL, so twice the supply volume, or 30 mL, is needed to provide the ordered dose.

S: $x \left(\text{mL} \right) = \dfrac{15 \text{ mL}}{60 \text{ mg}} \times \dfrac{1{,}000 \text{ mg}}{1 \text{ g}} \times \dfrac{0.12 \text{ g}}{1}$

$x = 30 \text{ mL}$

E: $30 \text{ mL} = \dfrac{15 \text{ mL}}{60 \text{ mg}} \times \dfrac{1{,}000 \text{ mg}}{1 \text{ g}} \times \dfrac{0.12 \text{ g}}{1}$

Because the calculated amount forms a true statement when inserted into the equation and is consistent with the approximated amount, 30 mL, the answer is confirmed.

50. **C:** N/A

   A: Because the ordered dose is half the dose supplied in 15 mL, half the supply volume, or 7.5 mL, is needed to provide the ordered dose.

   S: $x\,(\text{mL}) = \dfrac{15\text{ mL}}{20\text{ mEq}} \times \dfrac{10\text{ mEq}}{1}$

   $x = 7.5\text{ mL}$

   E: $7.5\text{ mL} = \dfrac{15\text{ mL}}{20\text{ mEq}} \times \dfrac{10\text{ mEq}}{1}$

   Because the calculated amount forms a true statement when inserted into the equation and is consistent with the approximated amount, 7.5 mL, the answer is confirmed.

NCLEX-Style Review Questions

1. c

   Rationale: $x = \dfrac{1\text{ tab}}{230\text{ mg}} \times \dfrac{345\text{ mg}}{1} = 1\dfrac{1}{2}\text{ tab}$

2. b

   Rationale: $x = \dfrac{1\text{ tab}}{2.5\text{ mg}} \times \dfrac{3.75\text{ mg}}{1} = 1\dfrac{1}{2}\text{ tab}$

3. b

   Rationale: The nurse should give the fewest whole tablets; therefore, the nurse should give two 25 mg tablets. If half-tablets are needed, the tablet should be scored (see Chapter 8).

4. c

   Rationale: $x = \dfrac{5\text{ mL}}{50\text{ mg}} \times \dfrac{200\text{ mg}}{1} = 20\text{ mL}$

5. d, f

   Rationale: $x = \dfrac{1\text{ t}}{80\text{ mg}} \times \dfrac{160\text{ mg}}{1} = 2\text{ t} = 10\text{ mL}$

6. b, c, d, e

   Rationale:

   $x = \dfrac{10\text{ mL}}{250\text{ mg}} \times \dfrac{750\text{ mg}}{1} = 30\text{ mL} = 2\text{ T} = 1\text{ oz} = 6\text{ t}$

© Forfunlife/Shutterstock

Chapter 8

Enteral Medication Dosage Calculations

CHAPTER OUTLINE

8-1 Solid Enteral Medications
- A. Tablets
- B. Capsules
- C. Dosage Calculations with Tablets and Capsules

8-2 Liquid Enteral Medications
- A. Types of Liquid Medications
- B. Dosage Calculations with Liquid Medications
  1. Calculating Daily Doses

LEARNING OUTCOMES

Upon completion of the chapter, the student will be able to:

8-1 Calculate dosages for solid enteral medications.

8-2 Calculate dosages for liquid enteral medications.

KEY TERMS

buccal
caplet
capsule
elixir
enteric-coated
gastrostomy tube

gelcap
jejunal tube
nasogastric
nasojejunal
reconstitution
scored
Spansule

suppository
sublingual
suspension
sustained-release
syrup
tablet

Case Consideration ... Shifty Shortcut

After learning the various methods of dosage calculations, the nursing student tells her peer, "I do not understand why the instructor makes this material so complicated! Calculating dosages is simple ... you take the ordered dose (*D*) and divide it by the supply amount (*H*) and that's all there is to it!" For example, if the physician orders 650 mg of acetaminophen and the supply is 325 mg tablets, the calculation is: 650 mg ÷ 325 mg/tablet = 2 tablets."

In the clinical setting, the nursing student applied this "simple" approach to dosage calculations to the following medication order:

Give 650 mg of acetaminophen PO now from a supply dose of 80 mg/2.5 mL.

650 mg ÷ 80 mg = 8.1 mL

1. What went wrong?

2. How could this error be avoided?

■ INTRODUCTION

This chapter applies the methods of dosage calculations to enteral medication administration. As described in Chapter 3, enteral medications are absorbed through the gastrointestinal tract. Enteral medications are most commonly given via the oral (by mouth, or PO) route. When the oral route is unavailable, medications may be given through a tube:

- **Nasogastric** (NG)/NGT—A tube inserted through the nose into the gastric (stomach) region (**Figure 8-1**)

- **Nasojejunal** (NJ)/NJT—A tube inserted through the nose into the jejunum (the middle section of the small intestine, as shown in **Figure 8-2**)

- **Gastrostomy tube/jejunal tube** (GT/J-tube)—A tube inserted directly through the abdomen into the stomach or jejunum (**Figure 8-3**)

Enteral medications may also be given through the rectum. A **suppository** is a solid, bullet-shaped medication, usually composed of glycerin, that is designed for easy insertion into the rectum. Most enteral medications are supplied in the form of tablets, capsules, or liquids.

8-1　Solid Enteral Medications

Tablets

Solid enteral medications given orally or via enteral tube are supplied in the form of tablets and capsules. Solid medications that can be administered through tubes must be crushed and mixed with fluid. **Tablets** are compressed powdered medications that are available in a variety of types, shapes, and sizes:

- **Caplets** (**Figure 8-4**) are oval-shaped tablets with a smooth coating to make them tamper resistant.

- **Scored** tablets are marked with indentations that facilitate dividing the dose in halves or quarters as marked (**Figure 8-5**). In order to cut tablets evenly, they should be divided with the aid of a tablet-splitter (**Figure 8-6**). Because medication may not be evenly distributed throughout an unscored tablet, it is improper to divide and administer tablets that are not scored (Wesdyk, 2012).

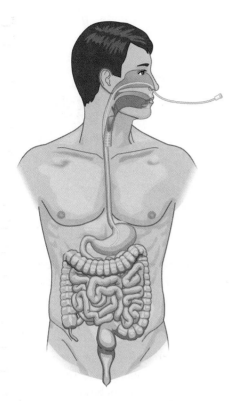

FIGURE 8-1   Nasogastric tube.

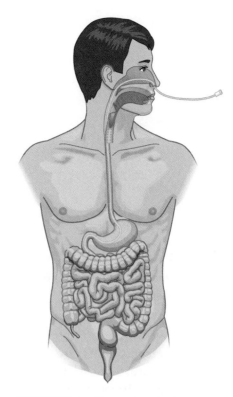

FIGURE 8-2   Naso jejunal tube.

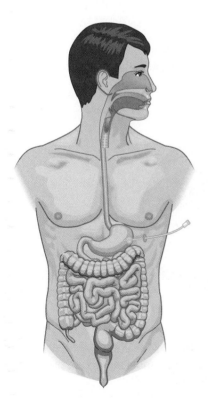

FIGURE 8-3   This gastrostomy tube is also called a G-tube. A percutaneous tube threaded into the jejunum is called a J-tube.

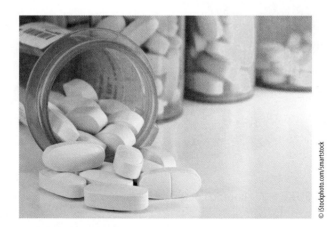

FIGURE 8-4   Caplets.

© iStockphoto.com/smartstock

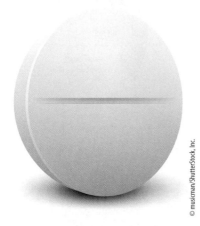

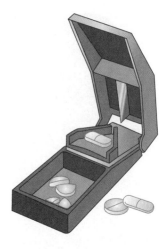

FIGURE 8-5   When a partial (half) dose is needed, if a tablet is scored, it can be cut along the indentation.

FIGURE 8-6   This device, called a tablet (or pill) splitter, is used to divide scored tablets.

- **Enteric-coated** tablets (**Figure 8-7**) have an outer coating designed to withstand gastric juice, causing the tablet to pass through the stomach and dissolve in the small intestine. The coating prevents the medication from irritating the stomach lining. Enteric-coated tablets should not be crushed.

- **Sublingual** tablets (**Figure 8-8**) are designed to be placed under the tongue for rapid absorption into the bloodstream. Sublingual tablets should not be swallowed because this will interfere with the desired rapid effect.

- **Buccal** tablets (**Figure 8-9**) are placed between the gum and the cheek, and, like sublingual tablets, they should not be swallowed because they are designed to dissolve through the mucous membranes of the mouth to rapidly enter the bloodstream.

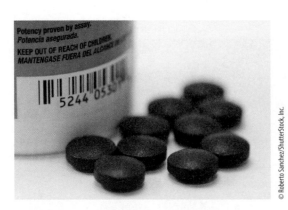

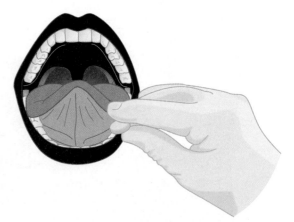

FIGURE 8-7   Enteric-coated tablets.

FIGURE 8-8   Sublingual tablets are placed under the tongue.

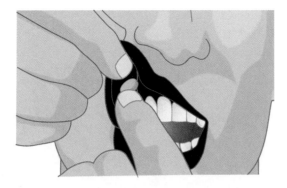

FIGURE 8-9   Buccal tablets are placed between the gums and the cheek.

Clinical CLUE

Some tablets and caplets may be crushed and mixed with liquid for oral administration or administration through an enteral feeding tube. Tablets and caplets that cannot be crushed include buccal and sublingual tablets, time-released pills, and enteric-coated pills. The Institute for Safe Medication Practice (ISMP) publishes a list of medications that are not safe for crushing (Mitchell, 2013). Nurses should always check a reputable drug reference before crushing solid medication.

Capsules

An oval or round gelatinous container filled with powder or liquid medication is called a **capsule** (**Figure 8-10**). Capsules are not divided or crushed, but are administered whole to achieve the desired effect. Some capsules may be opened and mixed with food for ease of administration. Nurses should always check a drug reference to determine which capsules may be opened and mixed with food. Capsules come in a variety of colors, sizes, and types:

- **Spansules** are timed-release (also known as **sustained-release**) capsules containing tiny beads of medicine (**Figure 8-11**) that dissolve at spaced intervals designed for long-acting medications. Spansules may be opened and mixed with food but the medicine beads should not be crushed.

- **Gelcaps** are gelatin shells that usually contain liquid medication (**Figure 8-12**). Gelcaps should not be crushed or opened.

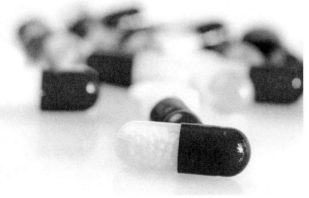

© Gayvoronskaya_Yana/ShutterStock, Inc.

FIGURE 8-10   Capsules.

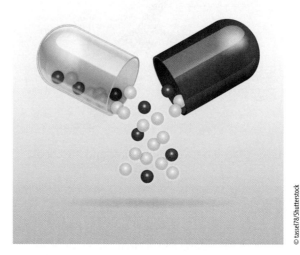

© tassel78/Shutterstock

FIGURE 8-11   Because the beads inside the spansule release medication over time, they should be administered whole and should not be crushed or opened.

Dosage Calculations with Tablets and Capsules

When administering solid oral medication, the nurse must calculate the number tablets or capsules. To calculate the number of tablets or capsules to administer, first determine, by looking at the drug label, the dosage strength (also called "supply dosage" or "supply"), which is the amount of drug in each tablet or capsule. The nurse also needs to know which solid medications cannot be divided and which capsules should be swallowed whole. This information can be obtained from a drug reference manual or a pharmacist. Once the necessary information is obtained, a dosage calculation is performed by applying the *CASE* approach to one of the three methods, as outlined in Chapter 7.

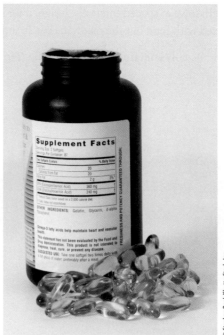

© Stephen Bonk/ShutterStock, Inc.

FIGURE 8-12   Gelcaps.

Example 1:   Determine the amount to administer for the following order and supply.

   Order: famotidine 40 mg PO at bedtime

Supply: See **Figure 8-13**.

C: *Convert*—Because the order is in milligrams (mg) and the supply is in milligrams, there is no conversion.

A: *Approximate*—The ordered dose, 40 mg, is twice the supply amount of 20 mg. Therefore, twice the 1 tablet supply (i.e., 2 tablets) will be needed to administer the ordered dose.

S: *Solve*

Ratio-Proportion

$$\frac{20 \text{ mg}}{1 \text{ tab}} = \frac{40 \text{ mg}}{x \text{ tab}} \text{ or}$$

$$20 \text{ mg} : 1 \text{ tab} = 40 \text{ mg} : x \text{ tab}$$

$$20x = 40$$

$$\frac{20x}{20} = \frac{40}{20}$$

$$x = 2 \text{ tab}$$

Formula Method

$$\frac{40 \text{ mg}}{20 \text{ mg}} \times 1 \text{ tab} = x \text{ (tab)}$$

$$\frac{40 \text{ tab}}{20} = x$$

$$2 \text{ tab} = x$$

Dimensional Analysis

$$x \text{ (tab)} = \frac{1 \text{ tab}}{20 \text{ mg}} \times \frac{40 \text{ mg}}{1}$$

$$x = \frac{40 \text{ tab}}{20}$$

$$x = 2 \text{ tab}$$

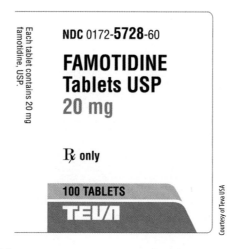

NDC 0172-**5728**-60

FAMOTIDINE
Tablets USP
20 mg

Each tablet contains 20 mg famotidine, USP.

℞ only

100 TABLETS

TEVA

Courtesy of Teva USA

FIGURE 8-13   Famotidine tablets.

E: *Evaluate*

Ratio-Proportion	Formula Method
$$\frac{20\ mg}{1\ tab} = \frac{40\ mg}{2\ tab}\ \text{or}$$ 20 mg : 1 tab = 40 mg : 2 tab $20 \times 2 = 1 \times 40$ $40 = 40$	$$\frac{40\ \cancel{mg}}{20\ \cancel{mg}} \times 1\ tab = 2\ tab$$ $$\frac{40\ tab}{20} = 2\ tab$$ 2 tab = 2 tab

Dimensional Analysis	
$$2\ tab = \frac{1\ tab}{20\ \cancel{mg}} \times \frac{40\ \cancel{mg}}{1}$$ $$2\ tab = \frac{40\ tab}{20}$$ 2 tab = 2 tab	

Because the calculated amount accurately completes the equation, and is consistent with the approximate amount, 2 tab, the answer is confirmed.

Example 2:   Determine the amount to administer for the following order and supply.

Order: Tylenol® 0.75 g PO q6h prn headache

Supply: Tylenol 500 mg capsules

C: *Convert*—Using the equivalent 1 g = 1,000 mg, convert the ordered amount 0.75 g to 750 mg. For dimensional analysis, use the conversion factor 1,000 mg/1 g.

A: *Approximate*—The ordered dose, 750 mg, is 1½ times the supply of 500 mg; therefore, approximately 1½ caplets will be needed to administer the ordered dose.

S: *Solve*

Ratio-Proportion	Formula Method
$$\frac{500\ mg}{1\ cap} = \frac{750\ mg}{x\ cap}\ \text{or}$$ 500 mg : 1 cap = 750 mg : *x* cap $500x = 750$ $$\frac{500x}{500} = \frac{750}{500}$$ $$x = 1\frac{1}{2}\ cap$$	$$\frac{750\ \cancel{mg}}{500\ \cancel{mg}} \times 1\ cap = x\ (cap)$$ $$\frac{750\ cap}{500} = x$$ $$1\frac{1}{2}\ cap = x$$

Dimensional Analysis

$$x \, (\text{cap}) = \frac{1 \, \text{cap}}{500 \, \cancel{\text{mg}}} \times \frac{1,000 \, \cancel{\text{mg}}}{1 \, \cancel{\text{g}}} \times \frac{0.75 \, \cancel{\text{g}}}{1}$$

$$x = \frac{750 \, \text{cap}}{500}$$

$$x = 1\frac{1}{2} \, \text{cap}$$

E: *Evaluate*

Ratio-Proportion	**Formula Method**
$\dfrac{500 \, \text{mg}}{1 \, \text{cap}} = \dfrac{750 \, \text{mg}}{1.5 \, \text{cap}}$ or	$\dfrac{750 \, \cancel{\text{mg}}}{500 \, \cancel{\text{mg}}} \times 1 \, \text{cap} = 1\dfrac{1}{2} \, \text{cap}$
$500 \, \text{mg} : 1 \, \text{cap} = 750 \, \text{mg} : 1.5 \, \text{cap}$	$\dfrac{750 \, \text{cap}}{500} = 1\dfrac{1}{2} \, \text{cap}$
$500 \times 1.5 = 1 \times 750$	
$750 = 750$	$1\dfrac{1}{2} \, \text{cap} = 1\dfrac{1}{2} \, \text{cap}$

Dimensional Analysis

$$1\frac{1}{2} \, \text{cap} = \frac{1 \, \text{cap}}{500 \, \cancel{\text{mg}}} \times \frac{1,000 \, \cancel{\text{mg}}}{1 \, \cancel{\text{g}}} \times \frac{0.75 \, \cancel{\text{g}}}{1}$$

$$1\frac{1}{2} \, \text{cap} = \frac{750 \, \text{cap}}{500}$$

$$1\frac{1}{2} \, \text{cap} = 1\frac{1}{2} \, \text{cap}$$

Because the calculated amount accurately completes the equation and is consistent with the approximated amount, 1½ cap, the answer is confirmed.

Clinical CLUE

If the Tylenol® caplets in Example 2 are not scored, the pharmacist should be contacted to obtain an alternate form of this medication, such as elixir, suspension, or scored tablet, because only scored tablets or caplets can be divided.

Example 3:   Determine the amount to administer for the following order and supply.

Order: clomipramine 100 mg PO at bedtime

Supply: clomipramine 75 mg capsules

C: *Convert*—Because the order is in milligrams and the supply is in milligrams, there is no conversion.

A: *Approximate*—Because the ordered dose is more than the supply amount, but less than two times the supply amount, more than one capsule, but less than two capsules, will be needed. Because capsules cannot be divided, the pharmacist should be contacted to determine if the medication is available in alternate dosage strengths or forms.

S: *Solve*

Ratio-Proportion	Formula Method
$\dfrac{75\ mg}{1\ cap} = \dfrac{100\ mg}{x\ cap}$ or	$\dfrac{100\ \cancel{mg}}{75\ \cancel{mg}} \times 1\ cap = x\ (cap)$
$75\ mg : 1\ cap = 100\ mg : x\ cap$	$\dfrac{100\ cap}{75} = x$
$75x = 100$	$1\dfrac{1}{3}\ cap = x$
$\dfrac{75x}{75} = \dfrac{100}{75}$	
$x = 1\dfrac{1}{3}\ cap$	

Dimensional Analysis	
$x\ (cap) = \dfrac{1\ cap}{75\ \cancel{mg}} \times \dfrac{100\ \cancel{mg}}{1}$	
$x = \dfrac{100\ cap}{75}$	
$x = 1\dfrac{1}{3}\ cap$	

E: *Evaluate*

Ratio-Proportion	Formula Method
$\dfrac{75\ mg}{1\ cap} = \dfrac{100\ mg}{1\dfrac{1}{3}\ cap}$ or	$\dfrac{100\ \cancel{mg}}{75\ \cancel{mg}} \times 1\ cap = 1\dfrac{1}{3}\ cap$
$75\ mg : 1\ cap = 100\ mg : 1\dfrac{1}{3}\ cap$	$\dfrac{100\ cap}{75} = 1\dfrac{1}{3}\ cap$
$75 \times \dfrac{4}{3} = 1 \times 100$	$1\dfrac{1}{3}\ cap = 1\dfrac{1}{3}\ cap$
$\dfrac{300}{3} = 100$	

> **Dimensional Analysis**
>
> $$1\frac{1}{3} \text{ cap} = \frac{1 \text{ cap}}{75 \text{ mg}} \times \frac{100 \text{ mg}}{1}$$
>
> $$1\frac{1}{3} \text{ cap} = \frac{100 \text{ cap}}{75}$$
>
> $$1\frac{1}{3} \text{ tab} = 1\frac{1}{3} \text{ cap}$$

Because the calculated amount includes a partial capsule and this information is consistent with the approximated amount in Step 2, the amount is confirmed, but the medication in this form (capsule) cannot be administered as ordered. Therefore, the prescriber should be contacted to order this medication in a different form, because capsules cannot be divided.

LEARNING ACTIVITY 8-1 For each order and supply, apply the *CASE* approach and use one of the three methods of dosage calculation to determine the amount to administer. If the *Convert* step is not needed, indicate N/A (not applicable). For the *Approximate* step, identify whether more or less than the supply is needed. For the *Solve* step, set up the equation using a preferred method of dosage calculation. For the *Evaluate* step, check your result by inserting the obtained answer into the equation and compare to the approximated value.

1. **Order:** pioglitazone 0.045 g PO daily
    Supply: pioglitazone 15 mg tablets
    C: _____ A: _____ S: _____ E: _____
    Administer: _____ tab

2. **Order:** pravastatin 40 mg PO nightly
    Supply: pravastatin 20 mg tablets
    C: _____ A: _____ S: _____ E: _____
    Administer: _____ tab

3. **Order:** fluoxetine 15 mg PO daily
    Supply: fluoxetine 10 mg scored tablets
    C: _____ A: _____ S: _____ E: _____
    Administer: _____ tab

8-2   Liquid Enteral Medications

Types of Liquid Medications

Enteral medication that is available in liquid form may be given orally or through a tube placed into the stomach or intestines. Liquid medications are prepared in various forms:

- **Elixir**—A liquid that contains water, alcohol, and a sweetener (**Figure 8-14**)

- **Suspension**—A thick, sweetened liquid that contains fine particles of a drug that cannot be dissolved and must be stirred or shaken prior to administration to evenly disperse the particles (see **Figure 8-15**)

- **Syrup**—A liquid that contains water, concentrated sugar, and dissolved medication (see **Figure 8-16**)

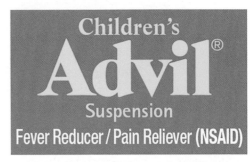

Do Not Use If breakable ring on bottle cap
is separated or missing.

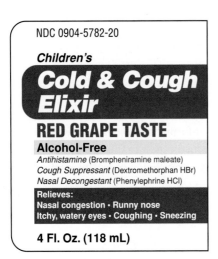

NDC 0904-5782-20

Children's

Cold & Cough Elixir

RED GRAPE TASTE

Alcohol-Free

Antihistamine (Brompheniramine maleate)
Cough Suppressant (Dextromethorphan HBr)
Nasal Decongestant (Phenylephrine HCl)

Relieves:
Nasal congestion • Runny nose
Itchy, watery eyes • Coughing • Sneezing

4 Fl. Oz. (118 mL)

Children's

Advil®

Suspension

Fever Reducer / Pain Reliever (NSAID)

Active ingredient (in each 5 mL)............. Ibuprofen 100 mg
Uses temporarily reduces fever, relieves minor aches and
pains due to the common cold, flu, sore throat, headaches
and toothaches

Grape-Flavored Liquid
4 FL OZ (120 mL)

Courtesy of Pfizer

FIGURE 8-14 Although many elixirs
contain alcohol, this elixir is alcohol-free.

FIGURE 8-15 Shaking Children's Advil® prior to
administration will evenly suspend the undissolved
particles of medication.

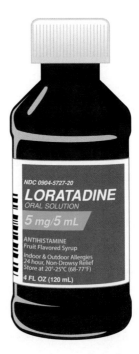

NDC 0904-5727-20
LORATADINE
ORAL SOLUTION
5 mg/5 mL

ANTIHISTAMINE
Fruit Flavored Syrup

Indoor & Outdoor Allergies
24 hour, Non-Drowsy Relief
Store at 20°-25°C (68-77°F)

4 FL OZ (120 mL)

FIGURE 8-16 Many children's medications, such as Loratadine®, are available in a syrup.

WARNING!

Shake well

A 35-year-old patient was hospitalized for evaluation and treatment of a seizure disorder. The patient was receiving carbamazepine suspension. Daily drug serum levels consistently fell below the therapeutic range, leading the physician to gradually increase the dose. On the seventh day, the patient became stuporous and unresponsive. The lab tests revealed a toxic level of carbamazepine. Investigation of this incident revealed that failure to shake the suspension prior to administration resulted in dilute initial doses while the remaining solution used for the later doses contained toxic doses of carbamazepine (Flynn, 2003). Remember to shake all suspensions well prior to administration.

Some enteral medications are available in powder form and must be mixed just prior to administration. **Reconstitution**, or the mixing of powdered medication, is typically done by a pharmacist. When necessary, the nurse may reconstitute a powdered medication by following the instructions on the drug label or package insert.

Liquid medications contain a certain amount of medication in a given volume. For example, Loratadine® syrup (Figure 8-16) contains 5 mg of medication in every 5 mL of liquid, therefore, the supply (dosage strength) of Loratadine is expressed as 5 mg/5 mL. Once the order and supply are determined, a dosage calculation may be performed. If the supply is expressed in teaspoons, it can be converted to milliliters, using the conversion 1 tsp = 5 mL.

Dosage Calculations with Liquid Medication

Example 1: After contacting the provider regarding the order for clomipramine that resulted in the need for 1½ capsules (in Example 3 of the previous section), the provider changed the order to clomipramine oral liquid.

Determine the amount to administer for the following order and supply.

Order: clomipramine 100 mg PO at bedtime

Supply: clomipramine 10 mg/mL

C: *Convert*—Because the order is in milligrams and the supply is in milligrams, there is no conversion.

A: *Approximate*—The ordered dose, 100 mg, is 10 times the supply amount of 10 mg, therefore, 10 times the supply (1 mL) volume (i.e., 10 mL) will be needed.

S: *Solve*

Ratio-Proportion	Formula Method
$\dfrac{10 \text{ mg}}{1 \text{ mL}} = \dfrac{100 \text{ mg}}{x \text{ mL}}$ or 10 mg : 1 mL = 100 mg : x mL $10x = 100$ $\dfrac{10x}{10} = \dfrac{100}{10}$ $x = 10$ mL	$\dfrac{100 \text{ mg}}{10 \text{ mg}} \times 1 \text{ mL} = x \text{ (mL)}$ $\dfrac{100 \text{ mL}}{10} = x$ $10 \text{ mL} = x$

Dimensional Analysis

$$x \text{ (mL)} = \frac{1 \text{ mL}}{10 \text{ mg}} \times \frac{100 \text{ mg}}{1}$$

$$x = \frac{100 \text{ mL}}{10}$$

$$x = 10 \text{ mL}$$

E: *Evaluate*

Ratio-Proportion

$$\frac{10 \text{ mg}}{1 \text{ mL}} = \frac{100 \text{ mg}}{10 \text{ mL}} \text{ or}$$

10 mg: 1 mL = 100 mg: 10 mL

$$10 \times 10 = 1 \times 100$$

$$100 = 100$$

Formula Method

$$\frac{100 \text{ mg}}{10 \text{ mg}} \times 1 \text{ mL} = 10 \text{ mL}$$

$$\frac{100 \text{ mL}}{10} = 10 \text{ mL}$$

$$10 \text{ mL} = 10 \text{ mL}$$

Dimensional Analysis

$$10 \text{ mL} = \frac{1 \text{ mL}}{10 \text{ mg}} \times \frac{100 \text{ mg}}{1}$$

$$10 \text{ mL} = \frac{100 \text{ mL}}{10}$$

$$10 \text{ mL} = 10 \text{ mL}$$

Because the calculated amount accurately completes the equation and is consistent with the approximated amount, 10 mL, the answer is confirmed.

Example 2: Determine the amount to administer for the following order and supply.

Order: loratadine 10 mg PO daily

Supply: loratadine 5 mg/5 mL

C: *Convert*—Because the order is in milligrams and the supply is in milligrams, there is no conversion.

A: *Approximate*—The ordered dose, 10 mg, is twice the supply amount of 5 mg, therefore, twice the supply volume of 5 mL (i.e., 10 mL) will be needed to administer the ordered dose.

S: *Solve*

Ratio-Proportion	Formula Method
$\dfrac{5\ mg}{5\ mL} = \dfrac{10\ mg}{x\ mL}$ or	$\dfrac{10\ \cancel{mg}}{5\ \cancel{mg}} \times 5\ mL = x\ (mL)$
$5\ mg : 5\ mL = 10\ mg : x\ mL$	
$5x = 50$	$\dfrac{50\ mL}{5} = x$
$\dfrac{5x}{5} = \dfrac{50}{5}$	$10\ mL = x$
$x = 10\ mL$	

Dimensional Analysis

$$x\ (mL) = \dfrac{5\ mL}{5\ \cancel{mg}} \times \dfrac{10\ \cancel{mg}}{1}$$

$$x = \dfrac{50\ mL}{5}$$

$$x = 10\ mL$$

E: *Evaluate*

Ratio-Proportion	Formula Method
$\dfrac{5\ mg}{5\ mL} = \dfrac{10\ mg}{10\ mL}$ or	$\dfrac{10\ \cancel{mg}}{5\ \cancel{mg}} \times 5\ mL = 10\ mL$
$5\ mg : 5\ mL = 10\ mg : 10\ mL$	
$5 \times 10 = 5 \times 10$	$\dfrac{50\ mL}{5} = 10\ mL$
$50 = 50$	$10\ mL = 10\ mL$

Dimensional Analysis

$$10\ mL = \dfrac{5\ mL}{5\ \cancel{mg}} \times \dfrac{10\ \cancel{mg}}{1}$$

$$10\ mL = \dfrac{50\ mL}{5}$$

$$10\ mL = 10\ mL$$

Because the calculated amount accurately completes the equation and is consistent with the approximated amount, 10 mL, the answer is confirmed. This volume of medication can be administered with a medication cup, oral syringe, or calibrated medication spoon.

Rounding RULE

- When a dosage calculation yields a volume that requires rounding, the volume should be rounded according the calibration of equipment used to administer the medication. When more than one device is available to administer a medication, the device selected should be one that minimizes the need for rounding. For example, if a dosage calculation yields a volume of 8.15 mL, the nurse should round the quantity to 8.2 mL and deliver it in an oral syringe calibrated to tenths instead of a medicine cup that is calibrated to whole milliliters.

Example 3: Determine the amount to administer for the following order and supply.

Order: cefaclor 0.433 g PO qid

Supply: cefaclor 375 mg/5 mL

C: *Convert*—Using the equivalent 1 g = 1,000 mg, convert the ordered amount 0.433 g to 433 mg. For dimensional analysis, use the conversion factor 1,000 mg/1 g.

A: *Approximate*—The ordered dose, 433 mg, is more than the supply amount of 375 mg, but less than twice the supply. Therefore, more than the supply volume of 5 mL, but less than 10 mL, will be needed to administer the ordered dose.

S: *Solve*

Ratio-Proportion	Formula Method
$\dfrac{375 \text{ mg}}{5 \text{ mL}} = \dfrac{433 \text{ mg}}{x \text{ mL}}$ or	$\dfrac{433 \text{ mg}}{375 \text{ mg}} \times 5 \text{ mL} = x \text{ (mL)}$
375 mg : 5 mL = 433 mg: x mL	
$375x = 2,165$	$\dfrac{2,165 \text{ mL}}{375} = x$
$\dfrac{375x}{375} = \dfrac{2,165}{375}$	$5.773 \text{ mL} = x$
$x = 5.773$	Round to 5.8 mL
Round to 5.8 mL	

Dimensional Analysis

$$x \text{ (mL)} = \frac{5 \text{ mL}}{375 \text{ mg}} \times \frac{1,000 \text{ mg}}{1 \text{ g}} \times \frac{0.433 \text{ g}}{1}$$

$$x = \frac{2,165 \text{ mL}}{375}$$

$$x = 5.773 \text{ mL}$$

Round to 5.8 mL

E: *Evaluate*

Ratio-Proportion	Formula Method
$\dfrac{375 \text{ mg}}{5 \text{ mL}} = \dfrac{433 \text{ mg}}{5.773 \text{ mL}}$ or 375 mg: 5 mL = 433 mg: 5.773 mL $375 \times 5.773 = 5 \times 433$ $2{,}165 = 2{,}165$	$\dfrac{433 \text{ mg}}{375 \text{ mg}} \times 5 \text{ mL} = 5.773 \text{ mL}$ $\dfrac{2{,}165 \text{ mL}}{375} = 5.773 \text{ mL}$ 5.773 mL = 5.773 mL

Dimensional Analysis

$$5.773 \text{ mL} = \frac{5 \text{ mL}}{375 \text{ mg}} \times \frac{1{,}000 \text{ mg}}{1 \text{ g}} \times \frac{0.433 \text{ g}}{1}$$

$$5.773 \text{ mL} = \frac{2{,}165 \text{ mL}}{375}$$

$$5.773 \text{ mL} = 5.773 \text{ mL}$$

Because the calculated amount, 5.773 mL, accurately completes the equation and is consistent with the approximated amount, 5–10 mL, the answer is confirmed. This volume should be rounded to 5.8 mL and administered using a 10 mL oral syringe. Because the medicine cup and medication spoon do not have a 5.8 mL calibration, these devices would not be appropriate for accurate administration of this medication order.

Calculating Daily Doses

Most dosage calculations are done to determine the amount to administer for a single dose. Periodically, the nurse may need to calculate a daily dose, which is accomplished by multiplying the ordered dose by the number of times the patients is scheduled to receive the medication. Using the previous example, the daily dose for cefaclor 0.433 g PO qid, would be calculated as follows:

$$\frac{0.433 \text{ g}}{\text{dose}} \times 4 \text{ doses}/\text{day} = 1.732 \text{ g per day or } 1{,}732 \text{ mg per day}$$

Clinical CLUE

Procedure for Administration of Medications via Enteral Tube

1. Follow the guidelines for safe medication administration outlined in Chapter 6.

2. Measure liquid medications in separate devices, or, after checking a drug reference to determine that a solid medication can be crushed, do the following:

   a. Crush solid medication with a pill crusher.

   b. Dissolve in at least 20 mL of water.

   c. Mix each solid medication separately.

3. If the enteral tube is an NGT, check tube placement to be sure it is in the stomach by withdrawing 2 mL of stomach contents via syringe and testing the aspirate with pH litmus paper; aspirates at pH 5.5 or less will indicate correct placement.

4. Raise the head of the bed so that the patient is sitting upright.

5. Administer medications using one of these methods:

   a. Remove bulb or barrel (Chapter 3, Figure 3-15) from large syringe and use as a funnel to pour medications through, one at a time, allowing them to flow into the tube by gravity or:

   b. Inject medications by depressing the plunger (Chapter 3, Figure 3-16), one at a time, through a Luer lock syringe into a Luer lock adapter.

6. Flush medications through the tube by instilling an additional 5 to 30 mL of water, using small flush volumes for children. When giving multiple medications, give a flush between each medication.

7. Have patient sit upright for 10 minutes after medication administration.

LEARNING ACTIVITY 8-2 Apply the *CASE* approach and use one of the three methods of dosage calculation to determine the amount to administer and calculate the daily dose.

1. **Order:** guaifenesin 50 mg PO q4h
    Supply: guaifenesin 100 mg/5 mL
    C: _____ A: _____ S: _____ E: _____
    Administer: _____ mL
    Administer: _____ t
    Daily Dose: _____ mg

2. **Order:** docusate sodium 100 mg via NGT bid
    Supply: docusate sodium 150 mg/15 mL
    C: _____ A: _____ S: _____ E: _____
    Administer: _____ mL, _____ t
    Daily Dose: _____ mg

3. **Order:** aluminum hydroxide 1.2 g PO qid
    Supply: aluminum hydroxide 600 mg/5 mL
    C: _____ A: _____ S: _____ E: _____
    Administer: _____ t
    Daily Dose: _____ g, _____ mg

Shifty Shortcut ... Case Closure

The student did not follow any of the accepted methods of dosage calculation. When using the formula method to perform dosage calculations for solid enteral medications, the supply amount (Q) is typically *one* tablet or capsule. After performing several $\frac{D}{H} \times Q$ calculations with a Q of 1, some students try to shortcut the formula by dropping the Q. The danger in dropping the Q is that a dosage error occurs when the supply amount is not 1, which is most often the case for enteral liquid medications, such as Tylenol:

Order: Tylenol 650 mg PO now

Supply: Tylenol 80 mg/2.5 mL

Calculation: $\frac{650 \text{ mg}}{80 \text{ mg}} \times 2.5 \text{ mL} = 20.3 \text{ mL}$

Elimination of the Q in this example would lead to an insufficient dosage administration:
$\frac{650 \text{ mg}}{80 \text{ mg}} = 8.1 \text{ mL}$

To avoid this type of error, always perform Step 4 of the CASE approach, *Evaluate,* by inserting the values into the equation, $\frac{D}{H} \times Q = x$, and comparing the calculated answer to the approximated answer.

D = 650 mg, H = 80 mg, Q = 2.5 mL, x = 8.1 m, thus:

$$\frac{650 \ \cancel{mg}}{80 \ \cancel{mg}} \times 2.5 \ mL \neq 8.1 \ mL$$

Performing the *Evaluate* step will help the nurse discover this error and prompt this calculation correction:

$$\frac{650 \ \cancel{mg}}{80 \ \cancel{mg}} \times 2.5 \ mL = 20.3 \ mL$$

This error could have been avoided had the student followed the *CASE* approach. The approximation step would have revealed the amount ordered is more than eight times larger than the supply amount, therefore the volume to administer should be more than eight times the supply volume.

Chapter Summary

Learning Outcomes	Points to Remember
8-1 Calculate dosages for solid enteral medications.	*Nasogastric/nasojejunal tube*—tube inserted through the nose into the stomach or jejunum
	Gastrostomy/jejunal tube—tube inserted through the abdomen into the stomach or jejunum
	Solid enteral medication preparations include:
	• *Suppository*—solid bullet-shaped medication inserted into the rectum
	• *Tablets*—compressed powdered medications
	• *Caplets*—oval-shaped tablets with a smooth coating
	• *Scored tablets*—indented to facilitate dividing tabs
	• *Enteric-coated tablets*—have an outer coating to prevent irritation of the stomach lining; should not be crushed
	• *Sublingual/buccal tablets*—placed under the tongue/between the cheek and gum for rapid absorption into the bloodstream
	• *Capsule*—an oval or round gelatinous container filled with powder or liquid medication; not divided or crushed
	• *Spansules* –capsules containing tiny beads of medicine that dissolve at spaced intervals for a sustained-release effect
	• *Gelcaps*—gelatin shells that usually contain liquid medication; should not be crushed or opened
	Example:
	Order: ampicillin 1 g PO now
	Supply: ampicillin 500 mg tablets
	D = 1 g, H = 500 mg, Q = 1 tab

C: *Convert*—Convert 1 g to 1,000 mg; for dimensional analysis, use conversion factor $\frac{1,000 \text{ mg}}{1 \text{ g}}$

A: *Approximate*—Because the ordered dose is twice the supply, two tablets will be needed.

S: *Solve*

Methods of Calculation:

- Ratio-proportion: supply dose = ordered dose/x

$$\frac{500 \text{ mg}}{1 \text{ tab}} = \frac{1,000 \text{ mg}}{x \text{ tab}}$$

$$500x = 1,000$$

$$x = 2 \text{ tab}$$

- Formula method: $\frac{D}{H} \times Q = x$

$$\frac{1,000 \text{ mg}}{500 \text{ mg}} \times 1 \text{ tab} = x \text{ (tab)}$$

$$2 \text{ tab} = x$$

- Dimensional analysis:

$$x = \text{supply} \times \text{conversion factor} \times \frac{\text{ordered dose}}{1}$$

$$x \text{ (tab)} = \frac{1 \text{ tab}}{500 \text{ mg}} \times \frac{1,000 \text{ mg}}{1 \text{ g}} \times \frac{1 \text{ g}}{1}$$

$$x = \frac{1,000 \text{ tab}}{500} = 2 \text{ tab}$$

E: *Evaluate:* Replace x with 2 tab to check calculation and compare to approximated amount for consistency.

8-2 Calculate dosages for liquid enteral medications.

Liquid enteral medication preparations include:
- *Elixir*—a sweetened liquid that contains water, alcohol
- *Suspension*—a thick, sweetened liquid that must be shaken prior to administration to evenly disperse the particles
- *Syrup*—concentrated sugar water with dissolved medication

Some medications are supplied in powder form and require reconstitution (mixing with liquid, usually water)

Example:

Order: ampicillin 1 g PO now

Supply: ampicillin 250 mg/5mL

$D = 1$g, $H = 250$ mg, $Q = 5$ mL

C: *Convert*—Convert 1 g to 1,000 mg; for dimensional analysis, use conversion factor $\frac{1,000 \text{ mg}}{1 \text{ g}}$

A: *Approximate*—Because the ordered dose is four times the supply, four times 5 mL (20 mL) will be needed.

S: *Solve:*

Methods of calculation:

- Ratio-proportion: supply dose = ordered dose/x

$$\frac{250 \text{ mg}}{5 \text{ mL}} = \frac{1{,}000 \text{ mg}}{x \text{ mL}}$$

$$250x = 5{,}000$$

$$x = 20 \text{ mL}$$

- Formula method: $\frac{D}{H} \times Q = x$

$$\frac{1{,}000 \text{ mg}}{250 \text{ mg}} \times 5 \text{ mL} = x \text{ (mL)}$$

$$20 \text{ mL} = x$$

- Dimensional analysis:

$$x = \text{supply} \times \text{conversion factor} \times \frac{\text{ordered dose}}{1}$$

$$x \text{ (mL)} = \frac{5 \text{ mL}}{250 \text{ mg}} \times \frac{1{,}000 \text{ mg}}{1 \text{ g}} \times \frac{1 \text{ g}}{1}$$

$$x = \frac{5{,}000 \text{ mL}}{250} = 20 \text{ mL}$$

E: *Evaluate*—Replace *x* with 20 mL to check calculation and compare to approximated amount for consistency.

Homework

For exercises 1–10, use the *CASE* approach with a preferred method of dosage calculation. Determine the amount to administer and the daily dose of medication. (LO 8-1)

1. **Order:** Wellbutrin XL® 0.45 g PO daily
   Supply: Wellbutrin XL 150 mg tablets
   C: _____ A: _____
   S: _____ E: _____
   Administer: _____ tab
   Daily Dose: _____ mg

2. **Order:** Buspirone® 7.5 mg PO bid
   Supply: Buspirone 5 mg scored tablets
   C: _____ A: _____
   S: _____ E: _____
   Administer: _____ tab
   Daily Dose: _____ mg

3. **Order:** glipizide 20 mg PO daily
   Supply: glipizide 10 mg tablets
   C: _____ A: _____
   S: _____ E: _____
   Administer: _____ tab
   Daily Dose: _____ g

4. **Order:** hydralazine 0.05 g PO qid
   Supply: hydralazine 25 mg tablets
   C: _____ A: _____
   S: _____ E: _____
   Administer: _____ tab
   Daily Dose: _____ mg, _____ g

5. **Order:** methylprednisolone 10 mg PO now
   Supply: methylprednisolone 4 mg scored tablets
   C: _____ A: _____
   S: _____ E: _____
   Administer: _____ tab
   Daily Dose: _____ g

6. **Order:** spironolactone 0.075 g PO daily
   Supply: spironolactone 50 mg scored tablets
   C: _____ A: _____
   S: _____ E: _____
   Administer: _____ tab
   Daily Dose: _____ mg

7. **Order:** cephalexin 250 mg PO q6h
   Supply: cephalexin 500 mg capsules
   C: _____ A: _____
   S: _____ E: _____
   Administer: _____ cap
   Daily Dose: _____ mg, _____ g

8. **Order:** propanolol 20 mg PO qid
   Supply: propanolol 10 mg tablets
   C: _____ A: _____
   S: _____ E: _____
   Administer: _____ tab
   Daily Dose: _____ mg

9. **Order:** dexamethasone 3,750 mcg PO bid
   Supply: dexamethasone 1.5 mg scored tablets
   C: _____ A: _____
   S: _____ E: _____
   Administer: _____ tab
   Daily Dose: _____ mg, _____ mcg

10. **Order:** ibuprofen 300 mg PO q6h prn
    Supply: ibuprofen 200 mg enteric-coated tablets
    C: _____ A: _____
    S: _____ E: _____
    Administer: _____ tab
    Daily Dose: _____ mg

For exercises 11–20, calculate the amount to administer, using one of the three methods of dosage calculations. (LO 8-2)

11. **Order:** guaifenesin 2 teaspoon PO q4h prn for cough
    Supply: guaifenesin 100 mg/5 mL
    C: _____ A: _____
    S: _____ E: _____
    Administer: _____ mL
    Daily Dose: _____ t, _____ mg

12. **Order:** docusate sodium 50 mg PO bid
    Supply: docusate sodium 150 mg/15 mL
    C: _____ A: _____
    S: _____ E: _____
    Administer: _____ mL
    Administer: _____ tsp
    Daily Dose: _____ mg

13. **Order:** aluminum hydroxide 800 mg PO qid
    Supply: aluminum hydroxide 600 mg/5 mL
    C: _____ A: _____
    S: _____ E: _____
    Administer: _____ mL
    Daily Dose: _____ mg, _____ g

14. **Order:** phenytoin oral suspension 75 mg per NGT tid
    Supply: phenytoin oral suspension 125 mg/5 mL
    C: _____ A: _____
    S: _____ E: _____

Administer: _____ mL

Daily Dose: _____ mg

15. Order: penicillin V potassium oral solution 0.5 g PO q8h

Supply: penicillin V potassium oral solution 125 mg/5 mL

C: _____ A: _____

S: _____ E: _____

Administer: _____ mL

Daily Dose: _____ mg, _____ g

16. Order: furosemide 60 mg via GT q12h

Supply: furosemide 40 mg/t

C: _____ A: _____

S: _____ E: _____

Administer: _____ t, _____ mL

Daily Dose: _____ mg

17. Order: amoxicillin 0.375 g PO qid

Supply: amoxicillin 400 mg/5 mL

C: _____ A: _____

S: _____ E: _____

Administer: _____ mL

Daily Dose: _____ g, _____ mg

18. Order: alprazolam 250 mcg per GT tid

Supply: alprazolam 1 mg/mL

C: _____ A: _____

S: _____ E: _____

Administer: _____ mL

Daily Dose: _____ mcg, _____ mg

19. Order: acetaminophen 400 mg PO q4h prn for fever

Supply: acetaminophen 80 mg/½ t

C: _____ A: _____

S: _____ E: _____

Administer: _____ t, _____ mL

Daily Dose: _____ mg, _____ g

20. Order: amitriptyline 75 mg PO daily

Supply: amitriptyline 25 mg/5 mL

C: _____ A: _____

S: _____ E: _____

Administer: _____ mL, _____ t, _____ T

Daily Dose: _____ g

For questions 21–50, use the medication label provided and one of the three methods of dosage calculations to determine the amount to administer. Be sure to label answers appropriately. (LO 8-1, 8-2)

NOTE: Although it is no longer required to write out each step, continue to use the *CASE* approach.

21. Order: metoprolol 0.1 g PO daily

Supply:

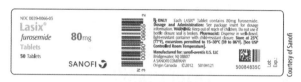

NDC 0781-1223-01

Metoprolol Tartrate Tablets, USP

50mg

Rx only

100 tablets

Each tablet contains: Metroprolol Tartrate, USP 50mg **Usual Dosage:** See package insert. Store at 20°–25°C (68°–77°F) (see USP Controlled Room Temperature). Dispense in a tight, light-resistant container. **KEEP THIS AND ALL DRUGS OUT OF REACH OF CHILDREN.**

Administer: _____

22. Order: Lasix® 40 mg PO bid

Supply:

NDC 0039-0066-05

Lasix®

furosemide   80 mg

Tablets

50 Tablets

SANOFI

Rx ONLY   Each LASIX® Tablet contains 80mg. furosemide. **Dosage and Administration:** See package insert for dosage information. **WARNING:** Keep out of reach of children. Do not use if bottle closure seal is broken. **Pharmacist:** Dispense in well-closed, light-resistant container with child-resistant closure. **Store at 25°C (77°F), excursions permitted to 15–30°C (59 to 86°F). [see USP Controlled Room Temperature].** Manufactured for: sanofi-aventis U.S. LLC Bridgewater, NJ 08807 A SANOFI COMPANY Origin Canada   ©2012   50104121   50084835C

Courtesy of Sanofi

Administer: _____

23. Order: dexamethasone 2 mg PO bid

Supply:

NDC 0603-1147-56

DEXAMETHASONE ELIXIR, USP

0.5 mg/5 mL

Rx only

8 FL OZ (237 mL)

Qualitest®

EACH 5 mL (TEASPOONFUL) CONTAINS: Dexamethasone, USP .... 0.5mg Also contains: Benzoic Acid, USP (as preservative) .... 0.1% w/v Alcohol .... 5.1% v/v **USUAL ADULT DOSAGE:** See accompanying package insert. **WARNINGS: KEEP THIS AND ALL DRUGS OUT OF THE REACH OF CHILDREN.** In case of accidental overdose, seek professional assistance or contact a Poison Control Center immediately. **STORE at 20° to 25°C (68° to 77°F) [see USP Controlled Room Temperature].** **KEEP TIGHTLY CLOSED** **AVOID FREEZING** DISPENSE in a tight container as defined in the USP. Manufactured by: QUALITEST PHARMACEUTICALS HUNTSVILLE, AL 35811 Rev. 3/15 R1 8062890 1145

Courtesy of Endo

Administer: _____

24. Order: nitroglycerin 600 mcg SL stat

Supply:

Warning: To prevent loss of potency, keep these tablets in the original container. Close tightly immediately after each use. Keep this and all drugs out of reach of children. Store up to 25°C (77°F). Protect from moisture. Usual Dosage: See package insert.

NDC 68462-147-01

NITROGLYCERIN TABLETS, USP

Rx Only

0.6 mg

(1/100 gr)

100 Sublingual Tablets

Administer: _____

25. **Order:** lovastatin 40 mg PO bid
Supply:

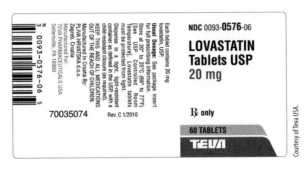

Administer: _____

26. **Order:** levofloxacin 750 mg via NGT daily
Supply:

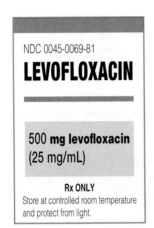

NDC 0045-0069-81

LEVOFLOXACIN

500 mg levofloxacin
(25 mg/mL)

Rx ONLY
Store at controlled room temperature
and protect from light.

Administer: _____

27. **Order:** Plavix® 0.3 g PO loading dose now
Supply:

List No. 1171-50   NDC 63653-1171-5
500 Tablets

Plavix®
(clopidogrel bisulfate)

75 mg

Dispense with
Medication Guide

Rx only

Usual adult dosage: See package insert
DISPENSE IN TIGHT, LIGHT-RESISTANT CONTAINER.
Each tablet contains 97.875 mg of clopidogrel
bisulfate equivalent to 75 mg of clopidogrel base.
Store at 25° C (77° F); excursions permitted to
15°–30° C (59°–86° F) [see USP Controlled
Room Temperature]

Courtesy of Sanofi

Administer: _____

28. **Order:** Xanax® 500 mcg PO tid
Supply:

Pfizer   NDC 0009-0029-01

Xanax® **C IV**

alprazolam
tablets, USP

0.25 mg

100 Tablets   **Rx only**

Courtesy of Pfizer, Inc.

Administer: _____

29. **Order:** Zofran® oral solution 8 mg per NGT q12h
Supply:

NDC 0173-0489-00
Zofran®
(ondansetron
hydrochloride)
Oral Solution
4 mg/5 mL
Rx only
50 mL

Each 5 mL contains 5 mg of
ondansetron HCl dihydrate equivalent
to 4 mg of ondansetron.
See package insert for Dosage and
Administration.
Store between 15° and 30°C (59° and
86°F). Protect from light. Store bottle
upright in carton.
Do not use if shrinkband on bottle
is broken or missing.

GlaxoSmithKline
Research Triangle Park, NC 27709
Made in Canada

A124815   Rev. 3/14   A 1 2 4 8 1 5

LOT
EXP

Courtesy of GlaxoSmithKline

Administer: _____

30. **Order:** digoxin 125 mcg PO daily
Supply:

100 Tablets   NDC 0173-0249-55
DIGOXIN
Tablets, USP
Each scored tablet contains
250 mcg (0.25 mg)
Rx only

See prescribing information for dosage information.
Store at 25°C (77°F) in a dry place (see insert).
Dispense in tight container as defined in the USP.
Do not use if printed safety seal under cap
is broken or missing.

Lot/Exp.

Courtesy of GlaxoSmithKline

Administer: _____

31. Order: cephalexin 1 g PO q6h
Supply:

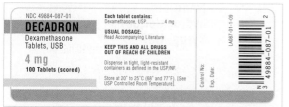

NDC 0093-**3147**-01

CEPHALEXIN
Capsules USP
500 mg*

℞ only

E 10/2009

100 CAPSULES

TEVA

* Each capsule contains cephalexin monohydrate equivalent to 500 mg cephalexin.
Usual Adult Dosage: 250 mg every six hours. For more severe infections, dose may be increased, not to exceed 4 g a day. See literature.

Courtesy of Teva USA

Administer: _____

32. Order: Decadron® 2 mg PO daily
Supply:

NDC 49884-087-01

DECADRON
Dexamethasone
Tablets, USB

4 mg
100 Tablets (scored)

Each tablet contains:
Dexamethasone, USP............4 mg

USUAL DOSAGE:
Read Accompanying Literature

KEEP THIS AND ALL DRUGS OUT OF REACH OF CHILDREN

Dispense in tight, light-resistant containers as defined in the USP/NF.

Store at 20° to 25°C (68° and 77°F). [See USP Controlled Room Temperature].

LA087-01-1-09

Control No:
Exp. Date:

3 49884-087-01 2

Decadron® logo and image is reproduced with permission of Merck Sharp & Dohme Corp., Whitehouse Station, New Jersey, USA. All rights reserved.

Administer: _____

33. Order: captopril 25 mg PO q12h
Supply:

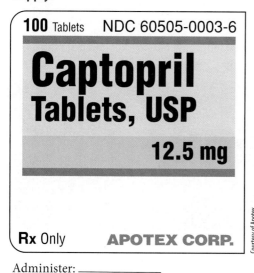

100 Tablets   NDC 60505-0003-6

Captopril
Tablets, USP

12.5 mg

Rx Only   **APOTEX CORP.**

Courtesy of Apotex

Administer: _____

34. Order: Augmentin® suspension 0.5 g PO qid
Supply:

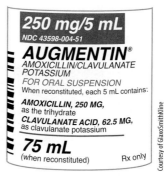

250 mg/5 mL
NDC 43598-004-51

AUGMENTIN®
AMOXICILLIN/CLAVULANATE
POTASSIUM
FOR ORAL SUSPENSION
When reconstituted, each 5 mL contains:

AMOXICILLIN, 250 MG,
as the trihydrate
CLAVULANATE ACID, 62.5 MG,
as clavulanate potassium

75 mL
(when reconstituted)   Rx only

Courtesy of GlaxoSmithKline

Administer: _____

35. Order: diphenhydramine elixir 50 mg nightly
Supply:

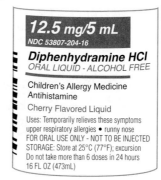

12.5 mg/5 mL
NDC 53807-204-16

Diphenhydramine HCl
ORAL LIQUID - ALCOHOL FREE

Children's Allergy Medicine
Antihistamine

Cherry Flavored Liquid

Uses: Temporarily relieves these symptoms upper respiratory allergies • runny nose
FOR ORAL USE ONLY - NOT TO BE INJECTED
STORAGE: Store at 25°C (77°F); excursion
Do not take more than 6 doses in 24 hours
16 FL OZ (473mL)

Administer: _____

36. Order: Lanoxin® 0.25 mg PO daily
Supply:

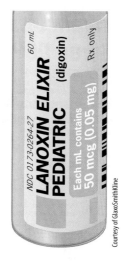

60 mL

Rx only

NDC 0173-0264-27

LANOXIN ELIXIR
PEDIATRIC
(digoxin)

Each mL contains
50 mcg (0.05 mg)

Courtesy of GlaxoSmithKline

Administer: _____

37. Order: Advil® 250 mg PO tid
Supply:

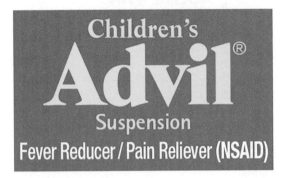

Do Not Use If breakable ring on bottle cap is separated or missing.

Children's
Advil®
Suspension
Fever Reducer / Pain Reliever (NSAID)

Active ingredient (in each 5 mL) .... Ibuprofen 100 mg
Uses temporarily reduces fever, relieves minor aches and pains due to the common cold, flu, sore throat, headaches and toothaches

**Grape-Flavored Liquid
4 FL OZ (120 mL)**

Courtesy of Pfizer

Administer: _____

38. Order: oxybutynin syrup 15 mg PO daily
Supply:

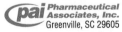

NDC 0121-0671-16

**Oxybutynin Chloride
Syrup USP**

5 mg/5 mL

Each teaspoonful (5 mL) contains:
5 mg oxybutynin chloride.

Rx ONLY

16 fl oz (473 mL)

pai *Pharmaceutical
Associates, Inc.*
Greenville, SC 29605

Courtesy of Pharmaceutical Associates

Administer: _____

39. Order: carbamazepine 200 mg via GT bid
Supply:

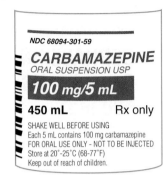

NDC 68094-301-59

CARBAMAZEPINE
ORAL SUSPENSION USP
100 mg/5 mL
450 mL   Rx only

SHAKE WELL BEFORE USING
Each 5 mL contains 100 mg carbamazepine
FOR ORAL USE ONLY - NOT TO BE INJECTED
Store at 20°-25°C (68-77°F)
Keep out of reach of children.

Administer: _____

40. Order: Zantac® syrup 100 mg PO bid
Supply:

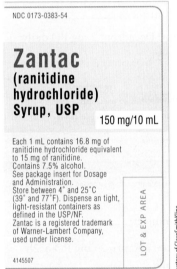

NDC 0173-0383-54

**Zantac
(ranitidine
hydrochloride)
Syrup, USP**

150 mg/10 mL

Each 1 mL contains 16.8 mg of
ranitidine hydrochloride equivalent
to 15 mg of ranitidine.
Contains 7.5% alcohol.
See package insert for Dosage
and Administration.
Store between 4° and 25°C
(39° and 77°F). Dispense an tight,
light-resistant containers as
defined in the USP/NF.
Zantac is a registered trademark
of Warner-Lambert Company,
used under license.

4145507

LOT & EXP AREA

Courtesy of GlaxoSmithKline

Administer: _____

41. Order: ibuprofen 600 mg PO q8h prn pain
Supply:

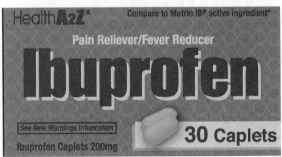

HealthA2Z®   Compare to Motrin IB® active ingredient*

Pain Reliever/Fever Reducer

Ibuprofen

See New Warnings Information

Ibuprofen Caplets 200mg

30 Caplets

Courtesy of Allegiant Health

Administer: _____

42. Order: Vistaril® 12.5 mg via NGT qid
Supply:

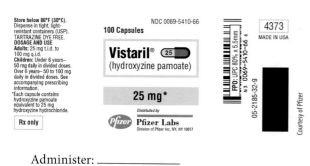

Administer: _____

43. Order: Vasotec® 7.5 mg PO bid
Supply:

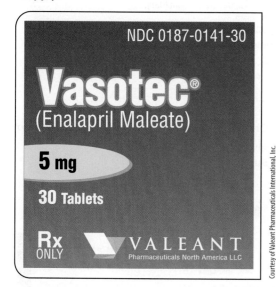

Administer: _____

44. Order: Synthroid® 0.15 mg PO q am
Supply:

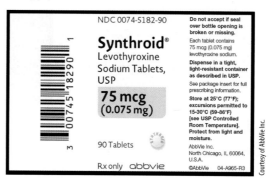

Administer: _____

45. Order: valproic acid 350 mg via NGT bid
Supply:

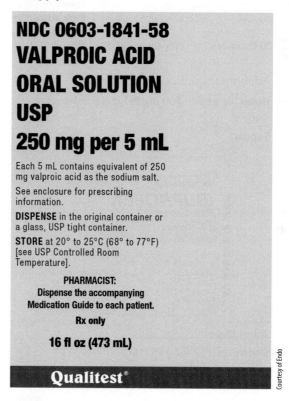

Administer: _____

46. Order: DiaBeta® 5 mg PO daily

Supply:

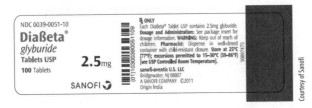

Administer: _____

47. Order: Altace® 2,500 mcg PO bid

Supply:

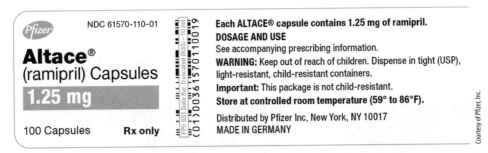

Administer: _____

48. Order: ibuprofen 400 mg PO q6h prn for fever
> 102°F

Supply:

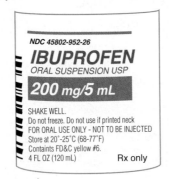

Administer: _____

49. Order: cefaclor 0.2 g PO tid

Supply:

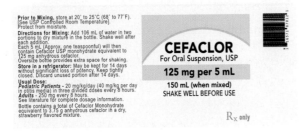

Administer: _____

50. Order: Nystatin® 200,000 units swish and swallow qid

Supply:

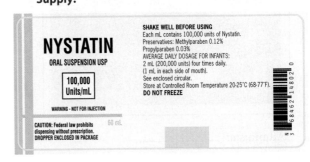

Administer: _____

NCLEX-Style Review Questions

For questions 1–4, select the best response.

1. A patient is to receive 75 mg of Biaxin® (clarithromycin). Biaxin suspension is supplied as 125 mg/5 mL. The nurse should:

   a. Measure 8.3 mL into a calibrated spoon.

   b. Draw up ½ t into an oral syringe.

   c. Measure 3 mL into a medication cup.

   d. Draw up 3 mL into an oral syringe.

2. The physician orders 162 mg of Ecotrin° (enteric-coated aspirin) PO daily. The medication available on the unit is 325 mg enteric-coated aspirin tablets and 325 mg scored aspirin tablets. The nurse should:

   a. Divide the enteric-coated tablet in quarters and give ½ tablet.

   b. Contact the pharmacist and request a different dosage strength.

   c. Administer 2 tablets PO daily.

   d. Divide the scored tablet in quarters and give ½ tablet.

3. The physician's order reads alprazolam 0.25 mg PO now. The available supply is alprazolam 1 mg/mL. To correctly measure this dose of alprazolam, the nurse will use a:

   a. 1 mL syringe

   b. 3 mL syringe

   c. Calibrated spoon

   d. Medication cup

4. To administer to an adult Lactulose 20 g from a supply of 10 g/15 mL, the nurse should:

   a. Draw up 7.5 mL into a 10 mL syringe.

   b. Pour 1 ounce into a calibrated medicine cup.

   c. Give 30 mL with an oral syringe.

   d. Measure 6 t into a calibrated teaspoon.

For questions 5–6, select all that apply.

5. When administering enteral medications, the nurse should:

   a. Perform a dosage calculation to determine the correct number of tablets to administer.

   b. Use a pill-splitter to evenly divide tablets, caplets, and capsules.

   c. Administer sublingual medications with a large cup of water to assist the patient in swallowing the tablets.

   d. Vigorously shake suspensions to ensure even distribution of the medication.

   e. Administer gelcaps under the tongue to promote rapid absorption.

   f. Crush enteric-coated tablets prior to administration.

   g. Use a calibrated device to administer liquid medications.

6. The nurse must administer medications through a feeding tube to a patient who is unable to swallow. The nurse should:

   a. Check a drug reference to determine which medications can be crushed.

   b. Contact the provider to obtain an alternate form of medication for enteric-coated tablets.

   c. Check the tube placement prior to administration of medication.

   d. Liquefy all solid medications.

   e. Have the pharmacist convert all ordered solid medications to liquids, if available.

REFERENCES

Flynn, E. A. (2003). *Shake well*. Retrieved from http://www.webmm.ahrq.gov/printviewCase.aspx?caseID=26

Mitchell, J. F. (2013). *Oral dosage forms that should not be crushed*. Retrieved from https://www.ismp.org/tools/DoNotCrush.pdf

Wesdyk, R. (2012). *Tablet scoring: Discussion Guidance and compendial development*. Retrieved from http://www.fda.gov/downloads/AdvisoryCommittees/CommitteesMeetingMaterials/Drugs/AdvisoryCommitteeforPharmaceuticalScienceandClinicalPharmacology/UCM315770.pdf

Chapter 8　ANSWER KEY

Learning Activity 8-1

1. **C**: Use conversion factor 1,000 mg/1 g;
   A: Three times the supply of 1 tab is needed;
   S: x (tab) $= \frac{1\,tab}{15\,mg} \times \frac{1,000\,mg}{1\,g} \times \frac{0.045\,g}{1}$;
   E: 3 Tab $= \frac{1\,tab}{15\,mg} \times \frac{1,000\,mg}{1\,g} \times \frac{0.045\,g}{1}$; This statement is true and is consistent with the approximated amount and, therefore, is confirmed. Administer: 3 tab.

2. **C**: N/A; **A**: Two times the supply of 1 tab is needed;
   S: x (tab) $= \frac{1\,tab}{20\,mg} \times \frac{40\,mg}{1}$;
   E: 2 tab $= \frac{1\,tab}{20\,mg} \times \frac{40\,mg}{1}$; This statement is true and is consistent with approximated amount and, therefore, is confirmed. Administer: 2 tab.

3. **C**: N/A, **A**: More than the supply of 1 tab is needed;
   S: x (tab) $= \frac{1\,tab}{10\,mg} \times \frac{15\,mg}{1}$;
   E: $1\frac{1}{2}$ tab $= \frac{1\,tab}{10\,mg} \times \frac{15\,mg}{1}$; This statement is true and is consistent with approximated amount and, therefore, is confirmed. Administer: 1½ (scored) tab.

Learning Activity 8-2

1. **C**: N/A; **A**: Half the supply of 5 mL is needed;
   S: x (mL) $= \frac{5\,mL}{100\,mg} \times \frac{50\,mg}{1}$;
   E: 2.5 mL $= \frac{5\,mL}{100\,mg} \times \frac{50\,mg}{1}$; This statement is true

and is consistent with approximated amount and, therefore, is confirmed. Administer: 2.5 mL, ½ t; Daily dose: 300 mg.

2. **C:** N/A; **A:** Less than the supply of 15 mL is needed; **S:** $x \text{ (mL)} = \frac{15 \text{ mL}}{150 \text{ mg}} \times \frac{100 \text{ mg}}{1}$;

   E: $10 \text{ mL} = \frac{15 \text{ mL}}{150 \text{ mg}} \times \frac{100 \text{ mg}}{1}$; This statement is true and is consistent with approximated amount and, therefore, is confirmed. Administer: 10 mL, 2 t; Daily dose: 200 mg.

3. **C:** Use conversion factors 1,000 mg/1 g, 1 t/5 mL; **A:** Two times the supply of 5 mL is needed; **S:** $x \text{ (t)} = \frac{1 \text{ t}}{5 \text{ mL}} \times \frac{5 \text{ mL}}{600 \text{ mg}} \times \frac{1,000 \text{ mg}}{1 \text{ g}} \times \frac{1.2 \text{ g}}{1}$;

   E: $2 \text{ t} = \frac{1 \text{ t}}{5 \text{ mL}} \times \frac{5 \text{ mL}}{600 \text{ mg}} \times \frac{1,000 \text{ mg}}{1 \text{ g}} \times \frac{1.2 \text{ g}}{1}$; This statement is true and is consistent with approximated amount and, therefore, is confirmed. Administer: 2 t; Daily dose: 4.8 g, 4,800 mg.

Homework

1. **C:** Use conversion factor 1,000 mg/1g;
   A: Three times the supply of 1 tab is needed;
   S: $x \text{ (tab)} = \frac{1 \text{ tab}}{150 \text{ mg}} \times \frac{1,000 \text{ mg}}{1 \text{ g}} \times \frac{0.45 \text{ g}}{1}$;

   E: $3 \text{ tab} = \frac{1 \text{ tab}}{150 \text{ mg}} \times \frac{1,000 \text{ mg}}{1 \text{ g}} \times \frac{0.45 \text{ g}}{1}$; This statement is true and is consistent with approximated amount and, therefore, is confirmed. Administer: 3 tab; Daily dose: 450 mg.

2. **C:** N/A; **A:** More than the supply of 1 tab is needed; **S:** $x \text{ (tab)} = \frac{1 \text{ tab}}{5 \text{ mg}} \times \frac{7.5 \text{ mg}}{1}$;

   E: $1\frac{1}{2} \text{ tab} = \frac{1 \text{ tab}}{5 \text{ mg}} \times \frac{7.5 \text{ mg}}{1}$; This statement is true and is consistent with approximated amount and, therefore, is confirmed. Administer: 1½ (scored) tab; Daily dose: 15 mg.

3. **C:** N/A; **A:** Two times the supply of 1 tab is needed; **S:** $x \text{ (tab)} = \frac{1 \text{ tab}}{10 \text{ mg}} \times \frac{20 \text{ mg}}{1}$;

   E: $2 \text{ tab} = \frac{1 \text{ tab}}{10 \text{ mg}} \times \frac{20 \text{ mg}}{1}$; This statement is true and is consistent with approximated amount and, therefore, is confirmed. Administer: 2 tab; Daily dose: 0.02 g.

4. **C:** Use conversion factor 1,000 mg/1 g;
   A: Two times the supply of 1 tab is needed; **S:** $x \text{ (tab)} = \frac{1 \text{ tab}}{25 \text{ mg}} \times \frac{50 \text{ mg}}{1}$;

   E: $2 \text{ tab} = \frac{1 \text{ tab}}{25 \text{ mg}} \times \frac{50 \text{ mg}}{1}$; This statement is true and is consistent with approximated amount and, therefore, is confirmed. Administer: 2 tab; Daily dose: 200 mg, 0.2 g.

5. **C:** N/A; **A:** More than two times the supply of 1 tab is needed; **S:** $x \text{ (tab)} = \frac{1 \text{ tab}}{4 \text{ mg}} \times \frac{10 \text{ mg}}{1}$;

6. **C:** Use conversion factor 1,000 mg/1 g; **A:** More than the supply of 1 tab, but less than 2 tabs is needed; **S:** $x \text{ (tab)} = \frac{1 \text{ tab}}{50 \text{ mg}} \times \frac{1,000 \text{ mg}}{1 \text{ g}} \times \frac{0.075 \text{ g}}{1}$;

   E: $1\frac{1}{2} \text{ tab} = \frac{1 \text{ tab}}{50 \text{ mg}} \times \frac{1,000 \text{ mg}}{1 \text{ g}} \times \frac{0.075 \text{ g}}{1}$; This statement is true and is consistent with approximated amount and, therefore, is confirmed. Administer: 1½ (scored) tab; Daily dose: 75 mg.

7. **C:** N/A; **A:** Half the supply of 1 capsule is needed; **S:** $x \text{ (cap)} = \frac{1 \text{ cap}}{500 \text{ mg}} \times \frac{250 \text{ mg}}{1}$;

   E: $\frac{1}{2} \text{ cap} = \frac{1 \text{ cap}}{500 \text{ mg}} \times \frac{250 \text{ mg}}{1}$; This statement is true and is consistent with approximated amount and, therefore, is confirmed. Do not administer: ½ cap—contact authorized prescriber as capsules cannot be divided; Daily dose: 1,000 mg, 1 g.

8. **C:** N/A; **A:** Two times the supply of 1 tablet is needed; **S:** $x \text{ (tab)} = \frac{1 \text{ tab}}{10 \text{ mg}} \times \frac{20 \text{ mg}}{1}$;

   E: $2 \text{ tab} = \frac{1 \text{ tab}}{10 \text{ mg}} \times \frac{20 \text{ mg}}{1}$; This statement is true and is consistent with approximated amount and, therefore, is confirmed. Administer: 2 tab; Daily dose: 80 mg.

9. **C:** Use conversion factor 1 mg/1,000 mcg; **A:** More than two times the supply of 1 tab is needed; **S:** $x \text{ (tab)} = \frac{1 \text{ tab}}{1.5 \text{ mg}} \times \frac{1 \text{ mg}}{1,000 \text{ mcg}} \times \frac{3,750 \text{ mcg}}{1}$;

   E: $2\frac{1}{2} \text{ tab} = \frac{1 \text{ tab}}{1.5 \text{ mg}} \times \frac{1 \text{ mg}}{1,000 \text{ mcg}} \times \frac{3,750 \text{ mcg}}{1}$; This statement is true and is consistent with approximated amount and, therefore, is confirmed. Administer: 2½ tab; Daily dose: 7.5 mg, 7,500 mcg.

10. **C:** N/A; **A:** More than the supply of 1 tab, but less than 2 tabs is needed; **S:** $x \text{ (tab)} = \frac{1 \text{ tab}}{200 \text{ mg}} \times \frac{300 \text{ mg}}{1}$;

    E: $1\frac{1}{2} \text{ tab} = \frac{1 \text{ tab}}{200 \text{ mg}} \times \frac{300 \text{ mg}}{1}$; Although this statement is true and consistent with approximated amount, the provider should be contacted for an alternate drug form because enteric-coated tablets cannot be divided. Do not administer. If alternate form is available, daily dose will be 1,200 mg.

11. **C:** Use conversion factor 1 t/5 mL; **A:** Two times the supply volume of 5 mL; **S:** $x \text{ (mL)} \frac{5 \text{ mL}}{1 \text{ t}} \times \frac{2 \text{ t}}{1}$;

    E: $10 \text{ mL} = \frac{5 \text{ mL}}{1 \text{ t}} \times \frac{2 \text{ t}}{1}$; This statement is true and is consistent with approximated amount and, therefore, is confirmed. Administer: 10 mL (200 mg); Daily dose: 12 t; 1,200 mg.

12. **C:** N/A; **A:** One-third of the supply of 15 mL is needed; **S:** $x \text{ (mL)} = \frac{15 \text{ mL}}{150 \text{ mg}} \times \frac{50 \text{ mg}}{1}$;

E: 5 mL = $\frac{15\text{ mL}}{150\text{ mg}} \times \frac{50\text{ mg}}{1}$; This statement is true and is consistent with approximated amount and, therefore, is confirmed. Administer: 5 mL, 1 t; Daily dose: 100 mg.

13. **C:** N/A; **A:** More than the supply of 5 mL, but less than 10 mL is needed; **S:** x (mL) = $\frac{5\text{ mL}}{600\text{ mg}} \times \frac{800\text{ mg}}{1}$; **E:** 6.7 mL $\cong \frac{5\text{ mL}}{600\text{ mg}} \times \frac{800\text{ mg}}{1}$; This statement is true and is consistent with approximated amount and, therefore, is confirmed. Administer: 6.7 mL; Daily dose: 3,200 mg, 3.2 g.

14. **C:** N/A; **A:** Less than the supply of 5 mL is needed; **S:** x (mL) = $\frac{5\text{ mL}}{125\text{ mg}} \times \frac{75\text{ mg}}{1}$; **E:** 3 mL = $\frac{5\text{ mL}}{125\text{ mg}} \times \frac{75\text{ mg}}{1}$; This statement is true and is consistent with approximated amount and, therefore, is confirmed. Administer: 3 mL; Daily dose: 225 mg.

15. **C:** Use conversion factor 1,000 mg/1 g; **A:** Four times the supply of 5 mL is needed; **S:** x (mL) = $\frac{5\text{ mL}}{125\text{ mg}} \times \frac{1,000\text{ mg}}{1\text{ g}} \times \frac{0.5\text{ g}}{1}$; **E:** 20 mL = $\frac{5\text{ mL}}{125\text{ mg}} \times \frac{1,000\text{ mg}}{1\text{ g}} \times \frac{0.5\text{ g}}{1}$; This statement is true and is consistent with approximated amount and, therefore, is confirmed. Administer: 20 mL; Daily dose: 1,500 mg, 1.5 g.

16. **C:** N/A; **A:** More than the supply of 1 t, but less than 2 t, is needed; **S:** x (t) = $\frac{1\text{ t}}{40\text{ mg}} \times \frac{60\text{ mg}}{1}$; **E:** $1\frac{1}{2}$ t = $\frac{1\text{ t}}{40\text{ mg}} \times \frac{60\text{ mg}}{1}$; This statement is true and is consistent with approximated amount and, therefore, is confirmed. Administer: 1½ t, 7.5 mL; Daily dose: 120 mg.

17. **C:** Use conversion factor 1,000 mg/1 g; **A:** Less than the supply of 5 mL is needed; **S:** x (mL) = $\frac{5\text{ mL}}{400\text{ mg}} \times \frac{1,000\text{ mg}}{1\text{ g}} \times \frac{0.375\text{ g}}{1}$; **E:** 4.7 mL $\cong \frac{5\text{ mL}}{400\text{ mg}} \times \frac{1,000\text{ mg}}{1\text{ g}} \times \frac{0.375\text{ g}}{1}$; This statement is true and is consistent with approximated amount and, therefore, is confirmed. Administer: 4.7 mL; Daily dose: 1.5 g, 1,500 mg.

18. **C:** Use conversion factor 1 mg/1,000 mcg; **A:** Less than the supply of 1 mL is needed; **S:** x (mL) = $\frac{1\text{ mL}}{1\text{ mg}} \times \frac{1\text{ mg}}{1,000\text{ mcg}} \times \frac{250\text{ mcg}}{1}$; **E:** 0.25 mL = $\frac{1\text{ mL}}{1\text{ mg}} \times \frac{1\text{ mg}}{1,000\text{ mcg}} \times \frac{250\text{ mcg}}{1}$; This statement is true and is consistent with approximated amount and, therefore, is confirmed. Administer: 0.25 mL; Daily dose: 750 mcg, 0.75 mg.

19. **C:** N/A; **A:** Five times the supply of ½ t is needed; **S:** x (t) = $\frac{\frac{1}{2}\text{ t}}{80\text{ mg}} \times \frac{400\text{ mg}}{1}$;

20. **E:** $2\frac{1}{2}$ t = $\frac{\frac{1}{2}\text{ t}}{80\text{ mg}} \times \frac{400\text{ mg}}{1}$; This statement is true and is consistent with approximated amount and, therefore, is confirmed. Administer: 2½ t, 12.5 mL; Daily dose: 2,400 mg, 2.4 g.

20. **C:** N/A; **A:** three times the supply of 5 mL is needed; **S:** x (mL) = $\frac{5\text{ mL}}{25\text{ mg}} \times \frac{75\text{ mg}}{1}$; **E:** 15 mL = $\frac{5\text{ mL}}{25\text{ mg}} \times \frac{75\text{ mg}}{1}$; this statement is true and is consistent with approximated amount and, therefore, is confirmed. Administer: 15 mL, 3 t, 1 T; Daily dose: 0.075 g.

21. 2 tab
22. ½ (scored) tab
23. 20 mL
24. 1 tab
25. 2 tab
26. 30 mL
27. 4 tab; NOTE: The nurse should question this order because a dose of 4 tablets is more than the typical number of tablets to administer.
28. 2 tab
29. 10 mL
30. ½ tab; NOTE: Tablet should be scored.
31. 2 cap
32. ½ (scored) tab
33. 2 tab
34. 10 mL
35. 20 mL
36. 5 mL
37. 12.5 mL (Use a medicine cup, because it has a 12.5 mL calibration and the capacity to hold 12.5 mL ($2\frac{1}{2}$ t).)
38. 15 mL
39. 10 mL
40. 6.7 mL
41. 3 tab
42. Do not administer. Partial capsules cannot be given. Contact provider for liquid preparation to be administered via NGT.
43. 1½ (scored) tab
44. 2 tab
45. 7 mL
46. 2 tab
47. 2 tab Capsules
48. 10 mL
49. 8 mL
50. 2 mL

NCLEX-Style Review Questions

1. d

   Rationale: The correct volume to administer, 3 mL, must be measured in a syringe because there is no 3 mL calibration on a medication cup.

2. b

   Rationale: Enteric-coated tablets cannot be divided, therefore the nurse must contact the pharmacist (or prescriber) to obtain an alternate dosage strength. Scored aspirin tablets cannot replace the ordered enteric-coated tablets.

3. a

   Rationale: The correct volume to administer, 0.25 mL, must be measured in a 1 mL syringe because there is no 0.25 mL calibration on a 3 mL syringe, calibrated spoon, or medication cup.

4. b

   Rationale: The correct volume to administer, 30 mL, is the equivalent of 1 fluid ounce and can be measured in a calibrated medicine cup. Although 30 mL and 6 t are correct volumes, it would be impractical to administer these volumes using an oral syringe or calibrated teaspoon, because these devices have a maximum capacity of 10 mL.

5. a, d, g

   Rationales: Answers b, c, e, and f are incorrect because: (1) Capsules should not be divided. (2) Sublingual medications are not to be swallowed so they are absorbed rapidly by the blood vessels under the tongue. (3) Gelcaps must be swallowed. (4) Enteric-coated tablets must not be crushed.

6. a, b, c, e

   Rationale: Answer d is incorrect because not all solid medications can be crushed for liquification.

© Forfunlife/Shutterstock

Chapter 9

Parenteral Medication Dosage Calculations

CHAPTER OUTLINE

LEARNING OUTCOMES

Upon completion of the chapter, the student will be able to:

9-1   Perform calculations for injectable medications.

9-2   Round calculated dosages to the appropriate syringe calibration.

9-3   Perform calculations for reconstitution of medications.

9-4   Convert the dosage strength from a percentage or ratio to milligrams per milliliter (mg/mL).

9-5   Determine the amount of medication in a given volume when the dosage strength is given as a percentage or ratio.

KEY TERMS

concentration	maximum dilution	solvent
diluent	minimum concentration	strength
dosage strength	minimum dilution	supply volume
maximum concentration	reconstitution	
	solute	

Case Consideration ... Concentrate on the Concentration!

The patient was experiencing ventricular tachycardia, a life-threatening heart rhythm. The physician prescribed lidocaine 100 mg IV. The hospital unit was supplied with lidocaine concentrations of 1%, 2%, and 10%. Thinking, $10 \times 10 = 100$, the nurse administered lidocaine 10%, 10 mL IV over 2 minutes.

1. What went wrong?

2. How could this error have been avoided?

■ INTRODUCTION

Medications administered by the parenteral route are administered by any route outside of the gastrointestinal (GI) tract (enteral route). However, parenteral commonly refers to medications administered by injection, with a needle piercing the skin. Common parenteral routes include intravenous (IV), intramuscular (IM), and subcutaneous (subcut). Of these three routes, the IV route provides the fastest absorption as the medication goes directly into the blood stream. The IM route allows injected medications to enter the circulatory system through blood vessels in the muscles. The subcutaneous route provides a slow, sustained rate of medication absorption as the medication is inserted into the adipose tissue below the skin. A less common injection route, the intradermal (ID) route, is mainly used for skin testing. There are other injection routes used in specialty areas such as the intraosseous (into the bone), epidural (into the epidural space of the spinal column), and intrathecal (into the arachnoid space of the brain or spinal column) routes. Other routes of medication administration, such as inhalation or transdermal, are technically considered parenteral because they are administered outside the enteral route. However, in general and in this text, the term *parenteral* refers to injection routes. When preparing parenteral medications, it is extremely important to use the appropriate **concentration** (**dosage strength** or **strength**), which is the amount of medication *per* dosage unit. Medications that are too concentrated can irritate the vein or other tissue at the administration site, so they should not be used. Medications that are too dilute may deliver the required dose in too large a volume for the patient or administration site to tolerate. In order to administer the prescribed dose of medication, the nurse must select the appropriate concentration in addition to performing dosage calculation.

9-1   Injectable Solution Calculations

The methods of dosage calculation for liquid medications, as explained in Chapter 7, are used to calculate volumes of medication to inject.

Example 1:   Determine the amount to administer for the following order and supply.

  Order: diphenhydramine 100 mg IM now

  Supply: See **Figure 9-1**.

C: *Convert*—Because the dose is ordered and supplied in milligrams, no conversion is required.

A: *Approximate*—The ordered dose, 100 mg, is twice the amount supplied in 1 mL. Therefore, 2 mL are needed to administer the ordered dose.

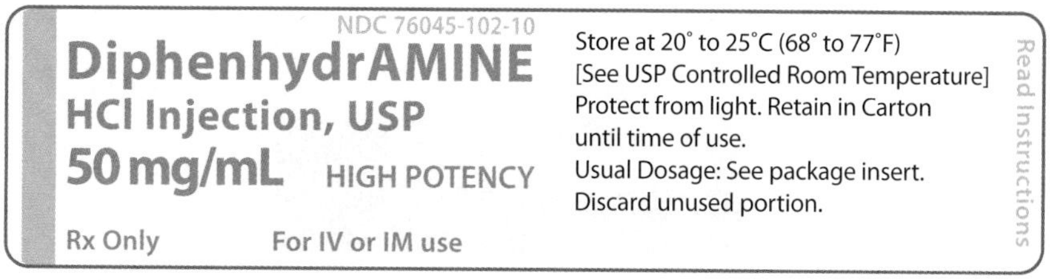

NDC 76045-102-10

DiphenhydrAMINE
HCl Injection, USP
50 mg/mL   HIGH POTENCY

Rx Only   For IV or IM use

Store at 20° to 25°C (68° to 77°F)
[See USP Controlled Room Temperature]
Protect from light. Retain in Carton
until time of use.
Usual Dosage: See package insert.
Discard unused portion.

Read Instructions

FIGURE 9-1

S: *Solve*

Ratio-Proportion

$$\frac{50 \text{ mg}}{1 \text{ mL}} = \frac{100 \text{ mg}}{x \text{ mL}} \text{ or}$$

$$50 \text{ mg} : 1 \text{ mL} = 100 \text{ mg} : x \text{ mL}$$

$$50x = 100$$

$$\frac{50x}{50} = \frac{100}{50}$$

$$x = 2 \text{ mL}$$

Formula Method

$$\frac{100 \text{ mg}}{50 \text{ mg}} \times 1 \text{ mL} = x \text{ (mL)}$$

$$\frac{100 \text{ mL}}{50} = x$$

$$2 \text{ mL} = x$$

Dimensional Analysis

$$x \text{ (mL)} = \frac{1 \text{ mL}}{50 \text{ mg}} \times \frac{100 \text{ mg}}{1}$$

$$x = \frac{100 \text{ mL}}{50}$$

$$x = 2 \text{ mL}$$

E: *Evaluate*

Ratio-Proportion

$$\frac{50 \text{ mg}}{1 \text{ mL}} = \frac{100 \text{ mg}}{2 \text{ mL}} \text{ or}$$

$$50 \text{ mg} : 1 \text{ mL} = 100 \text{ mg} : 2 \text{ mL}$$

$$50 \times 2 = 1 \times 100$$

$$100 = 100$$

Formula Method

$$\frac{100 \text{ mg}}{50 \text{ mg}} \times 1 \text{ mL} = 2 \text{ mL}$$

$$\frac{100 \text{ mL}}{50} = 2 \text{ mL}$$

$$2 \text{ mL} = 2 \text{ mL}$$

Dimensional Analysis

$$2 \text{ mL} = \frac{1 \text{ mL}}{50 \text{ mg}} \times \frac{100 \text{ mg}}{1}$$

$$2 \text{ mL} = \frac{100 \text{ mL}}{50}$$

$$2 \text{ mL} = 2 \text{ mL}$$

Because the calculated volume accurately completes the equation and is consistent with the approximated volume, 2 mL, the answer is confirmed.

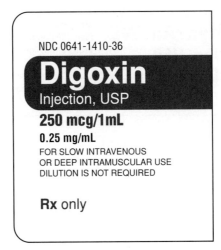

FIGURE 9-2

Example 2:   Determine the amount to administer for the following order and supply.

Order: digoxin 500 mcg IM stat

Supply: See **Figure 9-2**.

C: *Convert*—Convert 0.25 mg to 250 mcg. For dimensional analysis (DA), use the conversion factor 1 mg/1,000 mcg. (Refer to Chapter 2 on metric conversion for information on converting units of measurement.)

A: *Approximate*—The ordered dose, 500 mcg, is twice the amount supplied in 1 mL. Therefore, 2 mL will be needed to administer the ordered dose.

S: *Solve*

Ratio-Proportion	Formula Method
$\dfrac{250 \text{ mcg}}{1 \text{ mL}} = \dfrac{500 \text{ mcg}}{x \text{ mL}}$ or 250 mcg : 1 mL = 500 mcg : x mL $250x = 500$ $\dfrac{250x}{250} = \dfrac{500}{250}$ $x = 2$ mL	$\dfrac{500 \text{ mcg}}{250 \text{ mcg}} \times 1 \text{ mL} = x \text{ (mL)}$ $\dfrac{500 \text{ mL}}{250} = x$ $2 \text{ mL} = x$

Dimensional Analysis

$$x \text{ (mL)} = \frac{1 \text{ mL}}{0.25 \text{ mg}} \times \frac{1 \text{ mg}}{1,000 \text{ mcg}} \times \frac{500 \text{ mcg}}{1}$$

$$x = \frac{500 \text{ mL}}{250}$$

$$x = 2 \text{ mL}$$

E: *Evaluate*

Ratio-Proportion	Formula Method
$\dfrac{250 \text{ mcg}}{1 \text{ mL}} = \dfrac{500 \text{ mcg}}{2 \text{ mL}}$ or	$\dfrac{500 \text{ mcg}}{250 \text{ mcg}} \times 1 \text{ mL} = 2 \text{ mL}$
250 mcg: 1 mL = 500 mcg: 2 mL	$\dfrac{500 \text{ mL}}{250} = 2 \text{ mL}$
$250 \times 2 = 1 \times 500$	
500 = 500	2 mL = 2 mL

Dimensional Analysis

$$2 \text{ mL} = \frac{1 \text{ mL}}{0.25 \text{ mg}} \times \frac{1 \text{ mg}}{1,000 \text{ mcg}} \times \frac{500 \text{ mcg}}{1}$$

$$2 \text{ mL} = \frac{500 \text{ mL}}{250}$$

$$2 \text{ mL} = 2 \text{ mL}$$

Because the calculated volume accurately completes the equation and is consistent with the approximated volume, 2 mL, the answer is confirmed.

Example 3: Determine the amount to administer for the following order and supply.

Order: furosemide 30 mg IM daily

Supply: See **Figure 9-3**.

C: *Convert*—Because the dose is ordered and supplied in milligrams, no conversion is required.

A: *Approximate*—The ordered dose, 30 mg, is three times greater than the amount supplied in 1 mL. Therefore, 3 mL are needed to administer the ordered dose.

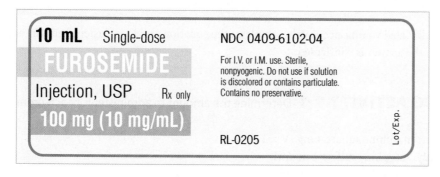

FIGURE 9-3

S: *Solve*

Ratio-Proportion	Formula Method
$\dfrac{10\ mg}{1\ mL} = \dfrac{30\ mg}{x\ mL}$ or 10 mg : 1 mL = 30 mg : x mL $10x = 30$ $\dfrac{10x}{10} = \dfrac{30}{10}$ $x = 3$ mL	$\dfrac{30\ \cancel{mg}}{10\ \cancel{mg}} \times 1\ mL = x\ (mL)$ $\dfrac{30\ mL}{10} = x$ $3\ mL = x$

Dimensional Analysis

$x\ (mL) = \dfrac{1\ mL}{10\ \cancel{mg}} \times \dfrac{30\ \cancel{mg}}{1}$

$x = \dfrac{30\ mL}{10}$

$x = 3$ mL

E: *Evaluate*

Ratio-Proportion	Formula Method
$\dfrac{10\ mg}{1\ mL} = \dfrac{30\ mg}{3\ mL}$ or 10 mg : 1 mL = 30 mg : 3 mL $10 \times 3 = 1 \times 30$ $30 = 30$	$\dfrac{30\ \cancel{mg}}{10\ \cancel{mg}} \times 1\ mL = 3\ mL$ $\dfrac{30\ mL}{10} = 3\ mL$ $3\ mL = 3\ mL$

Dimensional Analysis

$3\ mL = \dfrac{1\ mL}{10\ \cancel{mg}} \times \dfrac{30\ \cancel{mg}}{1}$

$3\ mL = \dfrac{30\ mL}{10}$

$3\ mL = 3\ mL$

Because the calculated volume accurately completes the equation and is consistent with the approximated volume, 3 mL, the answer is confirmed.

LEARNING ACTIVITY 9-1 Determine the amount to administer for each order and supply.

1. **Order:** morphine sulfate 4 mg IV × 1 dose
   Supply: morphine sulfate 2 mg/mL
2. **Order:** methyldopa 350 mg IV q6h
   Supply: methyldopa 250 mg/5 mL in 10 mL vial

3.　　**Order:** ketorolac 15 mg IV q6h
　　　Supply: ketorolac 30 mg/mL in 1 mL prefilled syringe

9-2　Rounding According to Appropriate Syringe Calibration

Rounding quantities is always done according to the equipment used. For example, if a scale is calibrated to tenths, then weights are recorded in amounts rounded to tenths. Likewise, with dosage calculations, volumes are rounded according to the equipment that will be used to measure the medication. Syringes used to administer parenteral medications are available in various sizes and calibrations. Large syringes are calibrated to whole numbers or tenths, while the smallest syringe is calibrated to hundredths. Because injection volumes tend to be small quantities, calculated amounts are generally rounded to tenths or hundredths.

Clinical CLUE

To prevent catheter rupture, certain intravenous access lines (e.g., peripherally inserted central catheter [PICC]) require the use of a 10 mL syringe to administer IV medications or flush solutions. This is because the lumen size of the barrel of the 10 mL syringe exerts less pressure than smaller volume syringes with narrower lumens. Some syringe companies manufacture prefilled 3 mL and 5 mL syringes for flushing PICC lines that have a lumen the diameter of a 10 mL syringe. However, the nurse should not use these to measure medications, because they are not designed for this use and have 0.5 mL calibrations. For these catheters, use the syringe with the most accurate calibrations to measure the amount of medication to administer. Then transfer the medication to another device, by further diluting in a larger syringe or IV bag.

Syringe Selection

Injectable medications are available as premixed solution or dry powder. A premixed solution contains a specified amount of medication diluted within a specified volume of solution that forms a concentration known as the dosage strength or strength. Medications that are not stable for long periods of time when mixed are marketed as powdered medications that require **reconstitution** (reformation as a liquid). Some medications are available as powders that will need a certain volume of **diluent** (**solvent**, liquid that dilutes) added to achieve the specified dosage strength. All medications must be in liquid form to be administered via the injection route.

Medication administration sites, as well as age of the patient and size of the muscle, affect the volume that can be administered, as indicated in **TABLE 9-1**. The volume of medication that is required to deliver the prescribed dose determines the size of the syringe to be used for administering the dose. Calibrations on the syringe vary by syringe size as shown in **TABLE 9-2**. The nurse will round the amount to administer, based on the calibration of the syringe required to administer the correct volume of medication. For example, if the amount to administer is less than 1 mL, then a 1 mL syringe can be used. The 1 mL syringe is calibrated by hundredths, so the volume to administer will be rounded to hundredths. The 3 mL syringe, however, is calibrated to tenths, so amounts larger than 1 mL will be administered in a 3 mL syringe and will be rounded to tenths (**TABLE 9-3**).

Three (3) mL is the maximal volume that can be injected through a parenteral route, other than IV; therefore, most calculations for injections, other than IV, will yield quantities of 3 mL or less. If more than 3 mL are needed to deliver the ordered dose intramuscularly, divide the amount to administer equally between two syringes for administration into separate IM sites.

Rules for Rounding

When a dosage calculation yields a volume other than the calibration of the appropriate syringe, the volume must be rounded. Rounding rules are summarized in Table 9-3.

TABLE 9-1 Maximum Injection Volumes for Administration Sites	
Administration Route/Site	**Maximum Volume**
Intradermal (ID)	0.1 mL
Subcutaneous (subcut)	1 mL—adult 0.5—child
Intramuscular (IM) Adult:	
Vastus lateralis	3 mL
Ventrogluteal	3 mL
Deltoid	1 mL
Child:	
Vastus lateralis	
6 to 12 years	2 mL
0 to 5 years	1 mL
Premature infant	0.5 mL

Rounding RULE!

Round the amount to administer to the calibration of the appropriate syringe.

Example 1: For the following order and supply, determine amount to administer and the appropriate syringe for administration.

Order: thiamine 75 mg IM tid

Supply: thiamine 100 mg/mL

TABLE 9-2 Syringe Sizes and Calibrations	
Syringe Size (Volume)	**Calibration**
0.5 mL tuberculin syringe	Hundredth (0.01 mL)
1 mL tuberculin syringe	Hundredth (0.01 mL)
3 mL (standard syringe)	Tenth (0.1 mL)
5 mL (large volume syringe)	Two-tenths (0.2 mL)
10 mL (large volume syringe)	Two-tenths (0.2 mL)
20 to 60 mL (large volume syringes)	Whole number (1 mL)

TABLE 9-3 Rules Based on Syringe Selection		
Volume to Be Administered	**Syringe Size**	**Rounding Rules**
Less than 1 mL and does not calculate evenly to tenths — e.g., 0.432 mL	1 mL or smaller Calibrated in hundredths — Use 1 mL syringe or 0.5 mL syringe.	Round to the nearest hundredth. — Round to 0.43 mL.
Less than 1 mL, but *greater* than or *equal* to 0.5 mL, and volume calculates exactly in tenths — e.g., 0.9 mL	1 mL or smaller (calibrated in hundredths) *or* 3 mL (calibrated in tenths) — Use 1 mL syringe or 3 mL syringe.	*Do not round.* Volume can be accurately measured in tenths—no rounding needed. — Do not round.
1 mL to 3 mL — e.g., 1.432 mL	3 mL (calibrated in tenths) — Use 3 mL syringe.	Round to the nearest tenth. — Round to 1.4 mL.

C: *Convert*—Because the dose is ordered and supplied in milligrams, no conversion is required.

A: *Approximate*—The ordered dose, 75 mg, is $\dfrac{3}{4}$ of the amount supplied in 1 mL. Therefore, 0.75 mL will be needed to administer the ordered dose.

S: *Solve*

Ratio-Proportion

$$\frac{100 \text{ mg}}{1 \text{ mL}} = \frac{75 \text{ mg}}{x \text{ mL}} \text{ or}$$

$$100 \text{ mg}: 1 \text{ mL} = 75 \text{ mg}: x \text{ mL}$$

$$100x = 75$$

$$\frac{100x}{100} = \frac{75}{100}$$

$$x = 0.75 \text{ mL}$$

Formula Method

$$\frac{75 \text{ mg}}{100 \text{ mg}} \times 1 \text{ mL} = x \text{ (mL)}$$

$$\frac{75 \text{ mL}}{100} = x$$

$$0.75 \text{ mL} = x$$

Dimensional Analysis

$$x \text{ (mL)} = \frac{1 \text{ mL}}{100 \text{ mg}} \times \frac{75 \text{ mg}}{1}$$

$$x = \frac{75 \text{ mL}}{100}$$

$$x = 0.75 \text{ mL}$$

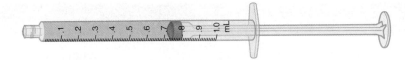

FIGURE 9-4 One (1) mL syringe containing 0.75 mL.

E: *Evaluate*

Ratio-Proportion	Formula Method
$\dfrac{100 \text{ mg}}{1 \text{ mL}} = \dfrac{75 \text{ mg}}{0.75 \text{ mL}}$ or 100 mg : 1 mL = 75 mg : 0.75 mL $100 \times 0.75 = 1 \times 75$ $75 = 75$	$\dfrac{75 \text{ mg}}{100 \text{ mg}} \times 1 \text{ mL} = 0.75 \text{ mL}$ $\dfrac{75 \text{ mL}}{100} = 0.75 \text{ mL}$ 0.75 mL = 0.75 mL

Dimensional Analysis

$$0.75 \text{ mL} = \frac{1 \text{ mL}}{100 \text{ mg}} \times \frac{75 \text{ mg}}{1}$$

$$0.75 \text{ mL} = \frac{75 \text{ mL}}{100}$$

$$0.75 \text{ mL} = 0.75 \text{ mL}$$

Because the calculated volume accurately completes the equation and is consistent with the approximated volume, 0.75 mL, the answer is confirmed.

The volume needed to administer a 75 mg dose is less than 1 mL and does not calculate evenly to tenths, so a 1 mL syringe is appropriate for administering the dose (**Figure 9-4**).

Example 2: Determine amount to administer for the following order and supply.

Order: diazepam 10 mg IM stat

Supply: diazepam 5 mg/mL

C: *Convert*—Because the dose is ordered and supplied in milligrams, no conversion is required.

A: *Approximate*—The ordered dose, 10 mg, is twice the amount supplied in 1 mL. Therefore, 2 mL will be needed to administer the ordered dose.

S: *Solve*

Ratio-Proportion	Formula Method
$\dfrac{5\text{ mg}}{1\text{ mL}} = \dfrac{10\text{ mg}}{x\text{ mL}}$ or $\quad$ 5 mg : 1 mL = 10 mg : x mL $\quad\quad$ $5x = 10$ $\quad\quad\quad$ $\dfrac{5x}{5} = \dfrac{10}{5}$ $\quad\quad\quad\quad$ $x = 2$ mL	$\dfrac{10\text{ }\cancel{\text{mg}}}{5\text{ }\cancel{\text{mg}}} \times 1\text{ mL} = x\text{ (mL)}$ $\quad\quad\quad$ $\dfrac{10\text{ mL}}{5} = x$ $\quad\quad\quad\quad$ $2\text{ mL} = x$

Dimensional Analysis
$x\text{ (mL)} = \dfrac{1\text{ mL}}{5\text{ }\cancel{\text{mg}}} \times \dfrac{10\text{ }\cancel{\text{mg}}}{1}$ $\quad\quad$ $x = \dfrac{10\text{ mL}}{5}$ $\quad\quad$ $x = 2\text{ mL}$

E: *Evaluate*

Ratio-Proportion	Formula Method
$\dfrac{5\text{ mg}}{1\text{ mL}} = \dfrac{10\text{ mg}}{2\text{ mL}}$ or $\quad$ 5 mg : 1 mL = 10 mg : 2 mL $\quad$ $5 \times 2 = 1 \times 10$ $\quad$ $10 = 10$	$\dfrac{10\text{ }\cancel{\text{mg}}}{5\text{ }\cancel{\text{mg}}} \times 1\text{ mL} = 2\text{ mL}$ $\quad\quad\quad$ $\dfrac{10\text{ mL}}{5} = 2\text{ mL}$ $\quad\quad\quad\quad$ $2\text{ mL} = 2\text{ mL}$

Dimensional Analysis
$2\text{ mL} = \dfrac{1\text{ mL}}{5\text{ }\cancel{\text{mg}}} \times \dfrac{10\text{ }\cancel{\text{mg}}}{1}$ $\quad\quad$ $2\text{ mL} = \dfrac{10\text{ mL}}{5}$ $\quad\quad$ $2\text{ mL} = 2$

Because the calculated volume accurately completes the equation and is consistent with the approximated volume, 2 mL, the answer is confirmed.

The volume needed to administer a 10 mg dose is greater than 1 mL, so a 3 mL syringe is appropriate for administering the dose (**Figure 9-5**).

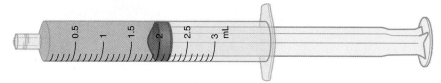

FIGURE 9-5   3 mL syringe containing 2 mL.

Example 3:   Determine amount to administer for the following order and supply.

Order: gentamicin 65 mg IM q8h

Supply: gentamicin 40 mg/mL

C: *Convert*—Because the dose is ordered and supplied in milligrams, no conversion is required.

A: *Approximate*—The ordered dose, 65 mg, is greater than the amount supplied in 1 mL, but less than the amount supplied in 2 mL. Therefore, between 1 and 2 mL will be needed to administer the ordered dose.

S: *Solve*

Ratio-Proportion	Formula Method
$\dfrac{40 \text{ mg}}{1 \text{ mL}} = \dfrac{65 \text{ mg}}{x \text{ mL}}$ or $40 \text{ mg}: 1 \text{ mL} = 65 \text{ mg}: x \text{ mL}$ $40x = 65$ $\dfrac{40x}{40} = \dfrac{65}{40}$ $x = 1.625$ round to 1.6 mL	$\dfrac{65 \text{ mg}}{40 \text{ mg}} \times 1 \text{ mL} = x \text{ (mL)}$ $\dfrac{65 \text{ mL}}{40} = x$ $1.625 \text{ mL} = x$ round to 1.6 mL

Dimensional Analysis	
$x \text{ (mL)} = \dfrac{1 \text{ mL}}{40 \text{ mg}} \times \dfrac{65 \text{ mg}}{1}$ $x = \dfrac{65 \text{ mL}}{40}$ $x = 1.625 \text{ mL}$ round to 1.6 mL	

E: *Evaluate*

Ratio-Proportion	Formula Method
$\dfrac{40 \text{ mg}}{1 \text{ mL}} = \dfrac{65 \text{ mg}}{1.625 \text{ mL}}$ or $40 \text{ mg}: 1 \text{ mL} = 65 \text{ mg}: 1.625 \text{ mL}$ $40 \times 1.625 = 1 \times 65$ $65 = 65$	$\dfrac{65 \text{ mg}}{40 \text{ mg}} \times 1 \text{ mL} = 1.625 \text{ mL}$ $\dfrac{65 \text{ mL}}{40} = 1.625 \text{ mL}$ $1.625 \text{ mL} = 1.625 \text{ mL}$ round to 1.6 mL

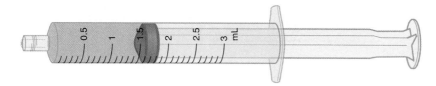

FIGURE 9-6   3 mL syringe containing 1.6 mL.

Dimensional Analysis

$$1.625 \text{ mL} = \frac{1 \text{ mL}}{40 \text{ mg}} \times \frac{65 \text{ mg}}{1}$$

$$1.625 \text{ mL} = \frac{65 \text{ mL}}{40}$$

$$1.625 \text{ mL} = 1.625 \text{ mL}$$

round to 1.6 mL

Because the calculated amount, 1.6 mL, accurately completes the equation and is consistent with the approximated amount, between 1 and 2 mL, the answer is confirmed.

The volume needed to administer a 65 mg dose is greater than 1 mL, so a 3 mL syringe is appropriate for administering the dose (**Figure 9-6**).

Example 4:   Determine amount to administer for the following order and supply.

Order: lorazepam 1 mg IM one time dose, 2 h before surgery

Supply: lorazepam 2 mg/mL

C: *Convert*—Because the dose is ordered and supplied in milligrams, no conversion is required.

A: *Approximate*—The ordered dose, 1 mg, is half the amount supplied in 1 mL. Therefore, 0.5 mL, will be needed to administer the ordered dose.

S: *Solve*

Ratio-Proportion	Formula Method
$\dfrac{2 \text{ mg}}{1 \text{ mL}} = \dfrac{1 \text{ mg}}{x \text{ mL}}$ or	$\dfrac{1 \text{ mg}}{2 \text{ mg}} \times 1 \text{ mL} = x \text{ (mL)}$
2 mg : 1 mL = 1 mg : x mL	
$2x = 1$	$\dfrac{1 \text{ mL}}{2} = x$
$\dfrac{2x}{2} = \dfrac{1}{2}$	$0.5 \text{ mL} = x$
$x = 0.5 \text{ mL}$	

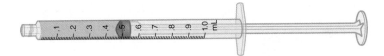

FIGURE 9-7 One (1) mL syringe containing 0.5 mL.

Dimensional Analysis

$$x \, (\text{mL}) = \frac{1 \, \text{mL}}{2 \, \cancel{\text{mg}}} \times \frac{1 \, \cancel{\text{mg}}}{1}$$

$$x = \frac{1 \, \text{mL}}{2}$$

$$x = 0.5 \, \text{mL}$$

E: *Evaluate*

Ratio-Proportion

$$\frac{2 \, \text{mg}}{1 \, \text{mL}} = \frac{1 \, \text{mg}}{0.5 \, \text{mL}} \quad \text{or}$$

2 mg : 1 mL = 1 mg : 0.5 mL

$$2 \times 0.5 = 1 \times 1$$

$$1 = 1$$

Formula Method

$$\frac{1 \, \cancel{\text{mg}}}{2 \, \cancel{\text{mg}}} \times 1 \, \text{mL} = 0.5 \, \text{mL}$$

$$\frac{1 \, \text{mL}}{2} = 0.5 \, \text{mL}$$

$$0.5 \, \text{mL} = 0.5 \, \text{mL}$$

Dimensional Analysis

$$0.5 \, \text{mL} = \frac{1 \, \text{mL}}{2 \, \cancel{\text{mg}}} \times \frac{1 \, \cancel{\text{mg}}}{1}$$

$$0.5 \, \text{mL} = \frac{1 \, \text{mL}}{2}$$

$$0.5 \, \text{mL} = 0.5 \, \text{mL}$$

Because the calculated volume accurately completes the equation and is consistent with the approximated volume, 0.5 mL, the answer is confirmed.

The volume needed to administer a 1 mg dose is less than 1 mL and calculates evenly to the tenths, so both a 1 mL syringe (**Figure 9-7**) and a 3 mL syringe (**Figure 9-8**) are appropriate for administering the dose.

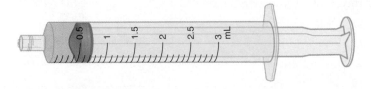

FIGURE 9-8 3 mL syringe containing 0.5 mL.

LEARNING ACTIVITY 9-2 For each order and supply, determine the volume to administer and mark the appropriate syringe with that volume.

1.   **Order:** 25 mg **Supply:** 50 mg/mL Volume to administer:_____

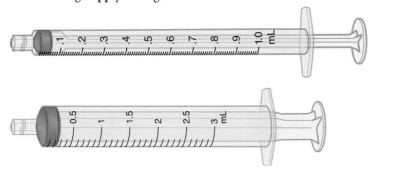

2.   **Order:** 12 mg **Supply:** 22 mg/mL Volume to administer:_____

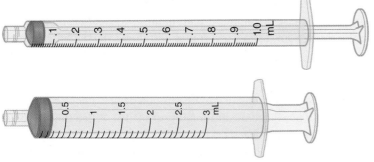

3.   **Order:** 30 mg **Supply:** 20 mg/mL Volume to administer:_____

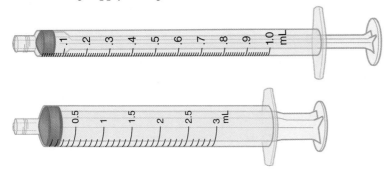

9-3   Reconstitution Calculations

Either the nurse or pharmacist must reconstitute powdered medications for parenteral administration (**Figure 9-10**, **Figure 9-11**, and **Figure 9-12**). Powdered medications, referred to as **solutes**, are reconstituted into a liquid by dissolving the powder in a solvent (diluent). Common diluents are bacteriostatic water, sterile water, and sterile normal saline (**Figure 9-9**). Lidocaine, a medication added to numb the injection site, is sometimes listed as a diluent but requires a specific order by the prescriber.

WARNING!

Lidocaine Is a Medication!

Lidocaine may be listed as a diluent, but always requires a specific order for use. Use other diluents, such as 0.9% NaCl or bacteriostatic water, as directed by the manufacturer, unless lidocaine is prescribed!

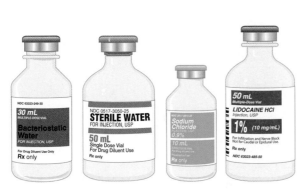

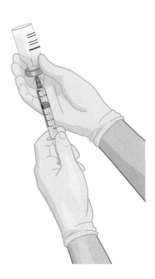

FIGURE 9-9 Bacteriostatic water, sterile water, and sterile normal saline are common diluents. Lidocaine is used occasionally to numb the site of administration but requires an order.

FIGURE 9-10 After cleansing the rubber diaphragm with alcohol and injecting air, the nurse withdraws the diluent.

Intravenous medications can be reconstituted with a reconstitution device, a device that connects an IV solution (**Figure 9-13**) to a vial of powdered medication (**Figure 9-14**). When this device is used, the IV solution becomes the diluent. The device produces a closed system between the medication vial and the IV bag (**Figures 9-15** and **9-16**). Because the IV bag will then contain the entire contents of the medication vial, reconstitution devices are only used when the entire vial is needed for the ordered dose. For this reason, no dosage calculation is required when a reconstitution device is used.

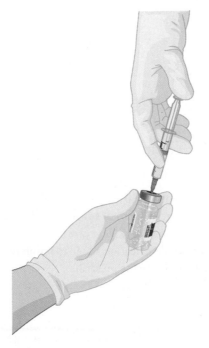

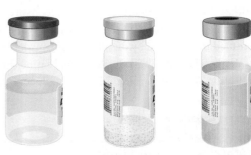

FIGURE 9-11 After cleansing the rubber diaphragm with alcohol, the nurse injects the diluent into the vial of powdered medication.

FIGURE 9-12 The reconstituted medication is now ready for use.

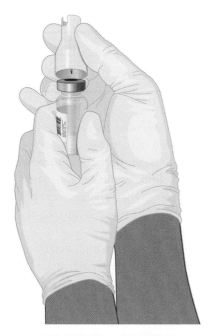

FIGURE 9-13   The medication vial is attached to the reconstitution device using aseptic technique.

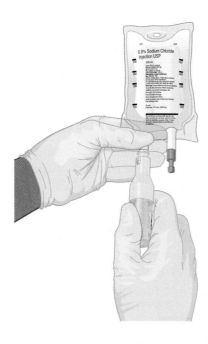

FIGURE 9-14   The medication vial is attached to the IV bag.

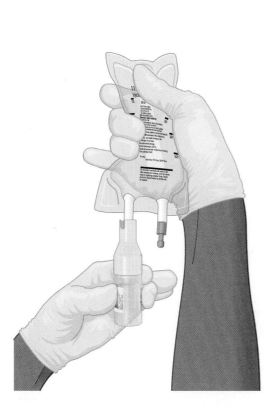

FIGURE 9-15   The IV fluid is squeezed into the vial and then drains back into the IV bag.

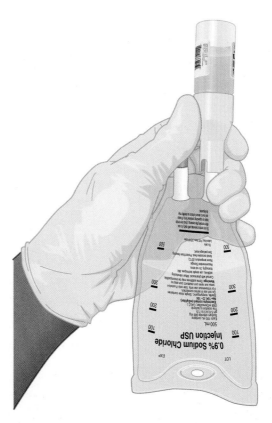

FIGURE 9-16   All solution from the medication vial has been displaced into the IV bag, and the reconstituted medication is now ready for use.

WARNING!

Device Devised for Full Doses!

Reconstitution devices are to be used only when the full dose of medication in the vial is ordered.

The medication package insert, and often the label, will provide directions for reconstitution. Reconstitution directions are also found in many drug guides. Included in these directions are the acceptable diluent, the required volume of diluent, and the resulting dosage strength (**Figure 9-17**). The volume of the reconstituted medication may be larger than the volume of diluent added due to expansion of the powdered medication. Therefore, the nurse must refer to the package insert or label for the new dosage strength and not calculate strength based on the volume injected into the vial of medication.

The reconstituted medication should be labeled if the dose is not immediately withdrawn from the vial. The label should include the preparation date and time, dosage strength, storage information, discard date, and preparer's initials (**Figure 9-18**).

WARNING!

Manufacturer's Recommendations for Reconstitution Rule!

Some powdered medications may expand significantly after reconstituting with a diluent. For example, 1 gram of powdered medication may result in a dosage strength of 100 mg/mL (1,000 mg/10 mL) after only

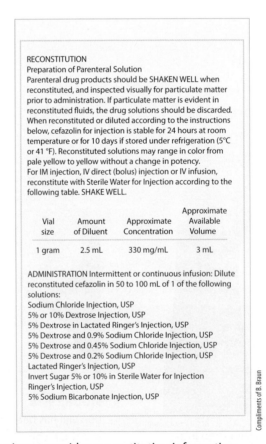

RECONSTITUTION
Preparation of Parenteral Solution
Parenteral drug products should be SHAKEN WELL when reconstituted, and inspected visually for particulate matter prior to administration. If particulate matter is evident in reconstituted fluids, the drug solutions should be discarded. When reconstituted or diluted according to the instructions below, cefazolin for injection is stable for 24 hours at room temperature or for 10 days if stored under refrigeration (5°C or 41 °F). Reconstituted solutions may range in color from pale yellow to yellow without a change in potency.
For IM injection, IV direct (bolus) injection or IV infusion, reconstitute with Sterile Water for Injection according to the following table. SHAKE WELL.

Vial size	Amount of Diluent	Approximate Concentration	Approximate Available Volume
1 gram	2.5 mL	330 mg/mL	3 mL

ADMINISTRATION Intermittent or continuous infusion: Dilute reconstituted cefazolin in 50 to 100 mL of 1 of the following solutions:
Sodium Chloride Injection, USP
5% or 10% Dextrose Injection, USP
5% Dextrose in Lactated Ringer's Injection, USP
5% Dextrose and 0.9% Sodium Chloride Injection, USP
5% Dextrose and 0.45% Sodium Chloride Injection, USP
5% Dextrose and 0.2% Sodium Chloride Injection, USP
Lactated Ringer's Injection, USP
Invert Sugar 5% or 10% in Sterile Water for Injection
Ringer's Injection, USP
5% Sodium Bicarbonate Injection, USP

Compliments of B. Braun

FIGURE 9-17 The package insert provides reconstitution information.

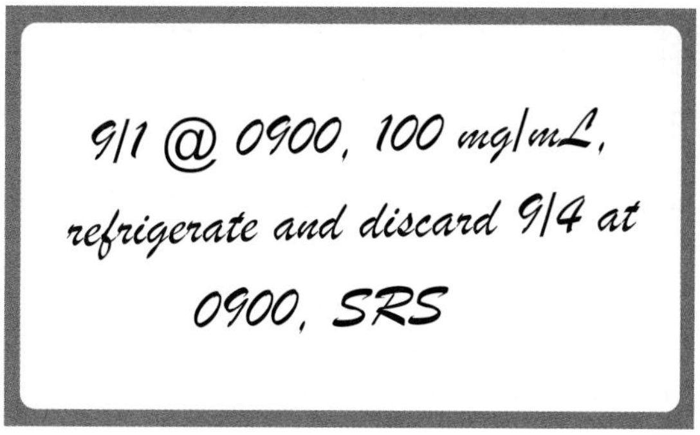

9/1 @ 0900, 100 mg/mL,
refrigerate and discard 9/4 at
0900, SRS

FIGURE 9-18   After reconstituting a medication, the nurse applies a label indicating date and time of reconstitution, dosage strength, storage instructions, discard date, and initials.

8 mL of diluent are added. Always follow the manufacturer's recommendations for the type and amount of diluent, as well as the resulting dosage strength.

Single Reconstitution Options

Many powdered injectable medications have only one reconstitution option. In other words, the manufacturer provides instructions for adding only one volume of diluent, which results in only one dosage strength. The diluent amount will always be proportional to the medication amount. For example, a vial containing nafcillin sodium powder for injection reveals:

■ 1.7 mL of diluent is added to a 0.5 g vial

■ 3.4 mL of diluent is added to a 1 g vial

■ 6.8 mL of diluent is added to a 2 g vial

Each of these reconstitutions yields a dosage strength of 250 mg/mL when mixed.

Clinical CLUE

To determine the number of doses in a multiple-dose vial, divide the total amount of medication in the vial by the dose ordered. For example, to determine the number of 500 mg doses of nafcillin in each of these vials:

▪ 0.5 g vial: 500 ~~mg~~/vial ÷ 500 ~~mg~~/dose = 1 dose/vial

▪ 1 g vial: 1,000 ~~mg~~/vial ÷ 500 ~~mg~~/dose = 2 doses/vial

▪ 2 g vial: 2,000 ~~mg~~/vial ÷ 500 ~~mg~~/dose = 4 doses/vial

Remember: A single-dose/single-use vial contains no more than one (1) dose.

When reconstituting single-strength medications follow these steps:

1. Determine the type and amount of diluent to instill and the resulting dosage strength.

2. Calculate the amount of reconstituted medication needed to administer the prescribed dose.

3. Determine the number of doses in the vial.

4. Prepare a label, if using a multi-dose vial.

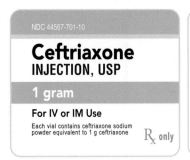

FIGURE 9-19

Example 1: For the following order and supply, determine the necessary information to perform each requested step, *1–4 (in italics),* in the reconstitution process. Use the package insert/medication label as needed.

Order: ceftriaxone sodium 0.5 g IV bid

Supply: See **Figure 9-19**.

1. *Determine the type and amount of diluent to instill and the resulting dosage strength.* Instill 9.6 mL of any of the following diluents: 0.9% NaCl, sterile water for injection, D₅W, or bacteriostatic water plus 0.9% benzyl alcohol. The resulting dosage strength is 100 mg/mL.

2. *Calculate the amount of reconstituted medication needed to administer the prescribed dose.*

C: *Convert*—Because the order is in grams and the supply is reconstituted to milligrams, convert 0.5 g to 500 mg. For DA, use the conversion factor 1,000 mg/1 g.

A: *Approximate*—The ordered dose, 500 mg, is five times the amount supplied in 1 mL. Therefore, 5 mL will be needed to administer the ordered dose.

S: *Solve*

Ratio-Proportion	Formula Method
$\dfrac{100 \text{ mg}}{1 \text{ mL}} = \dfrac{500 \text{ mg}}{x \text{ mL}}$ or	$\dfrac{500 \text{ mg}}{100 \text{ mg}} \times 1 \text{ mL} = x \text{ (mL)}$
$100 \text{ mg} : 1 \text{ mL} = 500 \text{ mg} : x \text{ mL}$	
$100x = 500$	$\dfrac{500 \text{ mL}}{100} = x$
$\dfrac{100x}{100} = \dfrac{500}{100}$	$5 \text{ mL} = x$
$x = 5 \text{ mL}$	

Dimensional Analysis

$$x\,(mL) = \frac{1\,mL}{100\,\cancel{mg}} \times \frac{1{,}000\,\cancel{mg}}{1\,\cancel{g}} \times \frac{0.5\,\cancel{g}}{1}$$

$$x = \frac{500\,mL}{100}$$

$$x = 5\,mL$$

E: *Evaluate*

Ratio-Proportion

$$\frac{100\,mg}{1\,mL} = \frac{500\,mg}{5mL} \text{ or}$$

100 mg : 1 mL = 500 mg : 5mL

$100 \times 5 = 1 \times 500$

$500 = 500$

Formula Method

$$\frac{500\,\cancel{mg}}{100\,\cancel{mg}} \times 1\,mL = 5\,mL$$

$$\frac{500\,mL}{100} = 5\,mL$$

$$5\,mL = 5\,mL$$

Dimensional Analysis

$$5\,mL = \frac{1\,mL}{100\,\cancel{mg}} \times \frac{1{,}000\,\cancel{mg}}{1\,\cancel{g}} \times \frac{0.5\,\cancel{g}}{1}$$

$$5\,mL = \frac{500\,mL}{100}$$

$$5\,mL = 5\,mL$$

Because the calculated volume accurately completes the equation and is consistent with the approximated volume, 5 mL, the answer is confirmed.

3. *Determine the number of doses in the vial.*

$$1{,}000\,\cancel{mg}\ (1\,g)/vial \div 500\,\cancel{mg}/dose = 2\,doses/vial$$

4. *Prepare a label, if using a multi-dose vial.* A reconstitution label should include date and time prepared, 100 mg/mL, expiration date (24 h from the time of preparation), room temperature storage, and preparer's initials.

Example 2: For the following order and supply, determine the necessary information to perform each requested step, *1–4 (in italics),* in the reconstitution process. Use the package insert/medication label as needed.

Order: acyclovir 0.35 g IV q8h

Supply: See **Figure 9-20**.

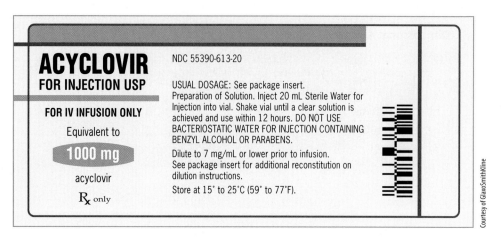

FIGURE 9-20

1. *Determine the type and amount of diluent to instill and the resulting dosage strength.* Instill 20 mL of sterile water. The dosage strength is 50 mg/mL.

2. *Calculate the amount of reconstituted medication needed to administer the prescribed dose.*

C: *Convert*—Because the order is in grams and the supply is reconstituted to milligrams, convert 0.35 g to 350 mg; for DA, use the conversion factor 1000 mg/1 g.

A: *Approximate*—The ordered dose, 350 mg, is seven times the amount supplied in 1 mL. Therefore, 7 mL will be needed to administer the ordered dose.

S: *Solve*

Ratio-Proportion	Formula Method
$\dfrac{50\text{ mg}}{1\text{ mL}} = \dfrac{350\text{ mg}}{x\text{ mL}}$ or $50\text{ mg} : 1\text{ mL} = 350\text{ mg} : x\text{ mL}$ $50x = 350$ $\dfrac{50x}{50} = \dfrac{350}{50}$ $x = 7\text{ mL}$	$\dfrac{350\ \cancel{\text{mg}}}{50\ \cancel{\text{mg}}} \times 1\text{ mL} = x\text{ (mL)}$ $\dfrac{350\text{ mL}}{50} = x$ $7\text{ mL} = x$

Dimensional Analysis

$$x \, (\text{mL}) = \frac{1 \, \text{mL}}{50 \, \text{mg}} \times \frac{1000 \, \text{mg}}{1 \, \text{g}} \times \frac{0.35 \, \text{g}}{1}$$

$$x = \frac{350 \, \text{mL}}{50}$$

$$x = 7 \, \text{mL}$$

E: *Evaluate*

Ratio-Proportion

$$\frac{50 \, \text{mg}}{1 \, \text{mL}} = \frac{350 \, \text{mg}}{7 \text{mL}} \quad \text{or}$$

$$50 \, \text{mg} : 1 \, \text{mL} = 350 \, \text{mg} : 7 \text{mL}$$

$$50 \times 7 = 1 \times 350$$

$$350 = 350$$

Formula Method

$$\frac{350 \, \text{mg}}{50 \, \text{mg}} \times 1 \, \text{mL} = 7 \, \text{mL}$$

$$\frac{350 \, \text{mL}}{50} = 7 \, \text{mL}$$

$$7 \, \text{mL} = 7 \, \text{mL}$$

Dimensional Analysis

$$7 \, \text{mL} = \frac{1 \, \text{mL}}{50 \, \text{mg}} \times \frac{1000 \, \text{mg}}{1 \, \text{g}} \times \frac{0.35 \, \text{g}}{1}$$

$$7 \, \text{mL} = \frac{350 \, \text{mL}}{50}$$

$$7 \, \text{mL} = 7 \, \text{mL}$$

Because the calculated amount accurately completes the equation and the answer is consistent with the approximated volume, 7 mL, the answer is confirmed.

3. *Determine the number of doses in the vial.*

$$1000 \, \text{mg/vial} \div 350 \, \text{mg/dose} = 2.9 \, \text{doses}$$

The vial contains two full doses to be used within 12 hours of preparation, with the second dose due 8 hours after the first dose.

4. *Prepare a label, if using a multi-dose vial.* Reconstitution label should include date and time prepared, 50 mg/mL, expiration date (12 h from the time of preparation), room temperature storage, and preparer's initials.

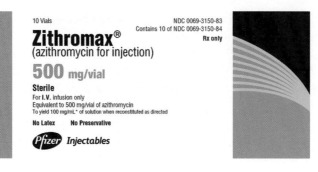

FIGURE 9-21

LEARNING ACTIVITY 9-3 For the following order and supply, determine the necessary information to perform each requested step in the reconstitution process. Use the package insert/medication label as needed.

Order: Zithromax® (azithromycin for injection) 500 mg IV daily

Supply: See **Figure 9-21**.

1. Determine the type and amount of diluent to instill and the resulting dosage strength.
2. Calculate the amount of reconstituted medication needed to administer the prescribed dose.
3. Determine the number of doses in the vial.
4. Prepare a label if using a multi-dose vial; identify required information.

Multiple Reconstitution Options

Some powdered medications can be reconstituted to different dosage strengths. The manufacturer provides instructions for creating different concentrations by adding different amounts of diluent to the same vial of medication, as illustrated in **Figure 9-22**.

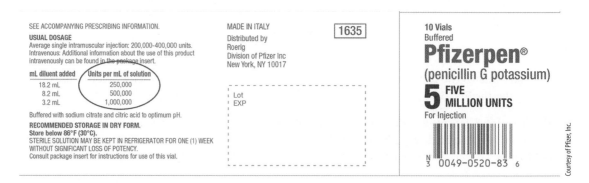

FIGURE 9-22 Pfizerpen® has three different concentrations listed on the label.

The **maximum concentration**, also referred to as **minimum dilution**, uses the least amount of diluent. The maximum concentration would be indicated for administration routes requiring smaller volumes, such as IM. The **minimum concentration** or **maximum dilution** uses the greatest amount of diluent. This would be indicated for administration routes that could accommodate larger volumes, such as the IV route. Figure 9-22 indicates that the addition of 3.2 mL of diluent to the vial would yield a dosage strength of 1,000,000 units/mL. This is the maximum concentration (minimum dilution) suggested by the manufacturer. The minimum concentration (maximum dilution), 250,000 units/mL, results from adding 18.2 mL of diluent to the vial. There may be a concentration between the minimum and maximum concentration that is appropriate for the patient.

WARNING!

Reconstitute for the Right Route!

The amount of diluent needed to reconstitute the same medication may vary depending upon route!

Medications that can be reconstituted for IM or IV use often have directions specific to the route (**Figure 9-23**). In general, the medication reconstituted for IM administration will require less diluent than for IV administration. When preparing to reconstitute a powdered medication with multiple dosage strength options, approximate the volume to administer for each dosage strength. To determine which dosage strength to use, the nurse should take into consideration the guidelines for multiple reconstitution options (see Clinical Clue).

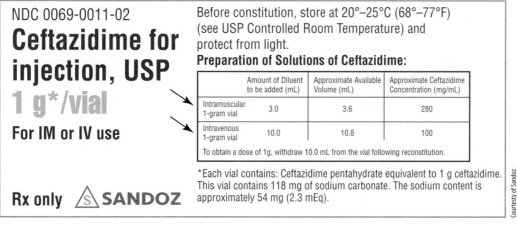

NDC 0069-0011-02

Ceftazidime for injection, USP

1 g*/vial

For IM or IV use

Rx only   S SANDOZ

Before constitution, store at 20°–25°C (68°–77°F) (see USP Controlled Room Temperature) and protect from light.
Preparation of Solutions of Ceftazidime:

	Amount of Diluent to be added (mL)	Approximate Available Volume (mL)	Approximate Ceftazidime Concentration (mg/mL)
Intramuscular 1-gram vial	3.0	3.6	280
Intravenous 1-gram vial	10.0	10.8	100

To obtain a dose of 1g, withdraw 10.0 mL from the vial following reconstitution.

*Each vial contains: Ceftazidime pentahydrate equivalent to 1 g ceftazidime. This vial contains 118 mg of sodium carbonate. The sodium content is approximately 54 mg (2.3 mEq).

Courtesy of Sandoz

FIGURE 9-23   The nurse must recognize the difference between IM and IV reconstitution instructions on this medication label.

Clinical CLUE

Multiple Reconstitution Option Guidelines

After approximating injection volume for all dosage strength options, the nurse will decide which option is best, giving consideration to these guidelines:

1. Consider the route:

   - If the route is IM, consider maximum injection amounts (i.e., 3 mL for adults, 1 mL for children, 1 mL for infants).

   - If the route is IV and the medication will be further diluted in a mini-bag (as discussed in Chapter 10), the maximum concentration (minimum volume) is often used.

2. Do not choose the maximum volume (minimum concentration) if there is a reasonable smaller volume option.

3. Do not choose the minimum volume (maximum concentration) if there is another reasonable option.

4. Do not choose an option that requires rounding if there is an option that does not require rounding. A quantity that is not rounded is more precise.

Example 1: For the following order and supply, calculate the amount to administer for the most reasonable dosage strength option indicated on the label.

    Order: penicillin G potassium 250,000 units IM q6h

  Supply: See **Figure 9-24**.

C: *Convert*—Because the order is in units and the supply, when mixed, is in units, there is no conversion.

A: *Approximate*—Each dosage strength compares to the ordered amount, 250,000 units, as follows:

- 250,000 units/mL (when diluted with 18.2 mL)—The ordered amount, 250,000 units, is the same as the amount supplied in 1 mL, so the **supply volume** of 1 mL is needed.

- 500,000 units/mL (when diluted with 8.2 mL)—The ordered amount, 250,000 units, is half of amount supplied in 1 mL, so 0.5 mL is needed.

- 1,000,000 units/mL (when diluted with 3.2 mL)—The ordered amount, 250,000 units, is 1/4 the amount supplied in 1 mL, so the supply volume of 0.25 mL is needed.

After approximating the volume to administer for each dosage strength, the nurse will apply the Multiple Option Reconstitution Guidelines:

- The maximum IM injection volume is 3 mL for adults and 1 mL for children, therefore all concentrations can be administered to adults and children.

- The most concentrated dosage strength, 1,000,000 units/mL (which would be the most irritating) should be avoided because other reasonable options exist.

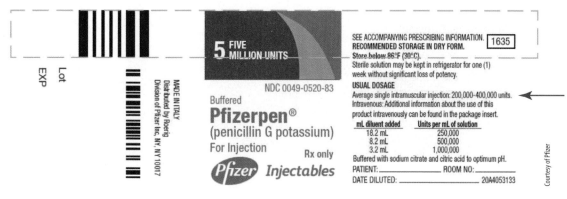

FIGURE 9-24

- Only 0.5 mL is needed to deliver the ordered dose if reconstituted to the 500,000 units/mL dosage strength. Following the guidelines, this is the most reasonable option, and the injection volume is appropriate for IM injection in children and adults.

- The 250,000 units/mL dosage strength is also appropriate because the injection volume for this strength is 1 mL and the greater dilution volume will make it less irritating. For an adult, this would be the most reasonable option, because it is the least irritating and is only 1/3 of the maximal injection volume.

S: *Solve*—For this example, the adult dosage strength of 250,000 units/mL will be used.

Ratio-Proportion	Formula Method
$\dfrac{250{,}000 \text{ units}}{1 \text{ mL}} = \dfrac{250{,}000 \text{ units}}{x \text{ mL}}$ or	$\dfrac{250{,}000 \text{ units}}{250{,}000 \text{ units}} \times 1 \text{ mL} = x \text{ (mL)}$
$250{,}000 \text{ units} : 1 \text{ mL} = 250{,}000 \text{ units} : x \text{ mL}$	$\dfrac{250{,}000 \text{ mL}}{250{,}000} = x$
$250{,}000x = 250{,}000$	$1 \text{ mL} = x$
$\dfrac{250{,}000x}{250{,}000} = \dfrac{250{,}000}{250{,}000}$	
$x = 1 \text{ mL}$	

Dimensional Analysis

$$x \text{ (mL)} = \frac{1 \text{ mL}}{250,000 \cancel{\text{ units}}} \times \frac{250,000 \cancel{\text{ units}}}{1}$$

$$x = \frac{250,000 \text{ mL}}{250,000}$$

$$x = 1 \text{ mL}$$

E: *Evaluate*

Ratio-Proportion

$$\frac{250,000 \text{ units}}{1 \text{ mL}} = \frac{250,000 \text{ units}}{1 \text{ mL}} \quad \text{or}$$

$$250,000 \text{ units} : 1 \text{ mL} = 250,000 \text{ units} : 1 \text{ mL}$$

$$250,000 \times 1 = 1 \times 250,000$$

$$250,000 = 250,000$$

Formula Method

$$\frac{250,000 \cancel{\text{ units}}}{250,000 \cancel{\text{ units}}} \times 1 \text{ mL} = 1 \text{ mL}$$

$$\frac{250,000 \text{ mL}}{250,000} = 1 \text{ mL}$$

$$1 \text{ mL} = 1 \text{ mL}$$

Dimensional Analysis

$$1 \text{ mL} = \frac{1 \text{ mL}}{250,000 \cancel{\text{ units}}} \times \frac{250,000 \cancel{\text{ units}}}{1}$$

$$1 \text{ mL} = \frac{250,000 \text{ mL}}{250,000}$$

$$1 \text{ mL} = 1 \text{ mL}$$

Because the calculated volume accurately completes the equation and is consistent with the approximated volume, 1 mL, the answer is confirmed.

Example 2:   For the following order and supply, calculate the amount to administer for the most reasonable dosage strength option indicated on the label.

Order: penicillin G potassium 750,000 units IV q6h.

Supply: See **Figure 9-25**.

C: *Convert*—Because the order is in units and the supply, when mixed, is in units, there is no conversion.

A: *Approximate*—Each dosage strength compares to the ordered amount, 750,000 units, as follows:

- 250,000 units/mL (when diluted with 18.2 mL)—The ordered amount, 750,000 units, is three times larger than amount supplied in 1 mL, so 3 mL are needed.

- 500,000 unit/mL (when diluted with 8.2 mL)—The ordered amount, 750,000 units, is 1½ times amount supplied in 1 mL, so 1.5 mL are needed.

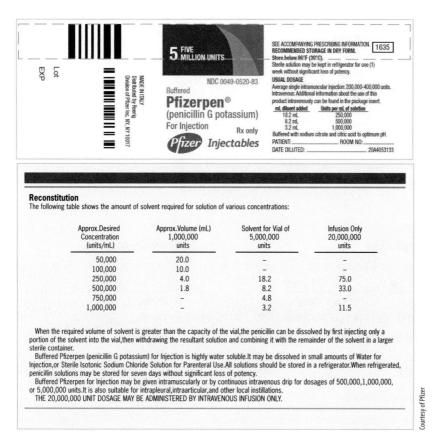

FIGURE 9-25

- 750,000 units/mL (when diluted with 4.8 mL)—The ordered amount, 750,000 units/mL, is the same amount supplied in 1 mL, so 1 mL is needed

- 1,000,000 units/mL (when diluted with 3.2 mL)—The ordered amount, 750,000 units, is 3/4 the amount supplied in 1 mL, so 0.75 mL is needed.

After approximating the volume to administer for each dosage strength, the nurse will apply the Multiple Option Reconstitution Guidelines. Because the route is IV, the nurse will determine that the most concentrated dosage strength, 1,000,000 units/mL, should be used because the medication will be further diluted in an IV mini-bag for IV administration.

S: *Solve*

Ratio-Proportion	Formula Method
$\dfrac{1{,}000{,}000 \text{ units}}{1 \text{ mL}} = \dfrac{750{,}000 \text{ units}}{x \text{ mL}}$ or	$\dfrac{750{,}000 \text{ units}}{1{,}000{,}000 \text{ units}} \times 1\,\text{mL} = x \text{ (mL)}$
$1{,}000{,}000 \text{ units} : 1 \text{ mL} = 750{,}000 \text{ units} : x \text{ mL}$	$\dfrac{750{,}000 \text{ mL}}{1{,}000{,}000} = x$
$1{,}000{,}000x = 750{,}000$	$0.75 \text{ mL} = x$
$\dfrac{1{,}000{,}000x}{1{,}000{,}000} = \dfrac{750{,}000}{500{,}000}$	
$x = 0.75 \text{ mL}$	

Dimensional Analysis

$$x \text{ (mL)} = \frac{1 \text{ mL}}{1{,}000{,}000 \text{ units}} \times \frac{750{,}000 \text{ units}}{1}$$

$$x = \frac{750{,}000 \text{ mL}}{1{,}000{,}000}$$

$$x = 0.75 \text{ mL}$$

E: *Evaluate*

Ratio-Proportion

$$\frac{1{,}000{,}000 \text{ units}}{1 \text{ mL}} = \frac{750{,}000 \text{ units}}{0.75 \text{ mL}} \quad \text{or}$$

$$1{,}000{,}000 \text{ units} : 1 \text{ mL} = 750{,}000 \text{ units} : 0.75 \text{ mL}$$

$$1{,}000{,}000 \times 0.75 = 1 \times 750{,}000$$

$$750{,}000 = 750{,}000$$

Formula Method

$$\frac{750{,}000 \text{ units}}{1{,}000{,}000 \text{ units}} \times 1 \text{ mL} = 0.75 \text{ mL}$$

$$\frac{750{,}000 \text{ mL}}{1{,}000{,}000} = 0.75 \text{ mL}$$

$$0.75 \text{ mL} = 0.75 \text{ mL}$$

Dimensional Analysis

$$0.75 \text{ mL} = \frac{1 \text{ mL}}{1{,}000{,}000 \text{ units}} \times \frac{750{,}000 \text{ units}}{1}$$

$$0.75 \text{ mL} = \frac{750{,}000 \text{ mL}}{1{,}000{,}000}$$

$$0.75 \text{ mL} = 0.75 \text{ mL}$$

Because the calculated volume accurately completes the equation and is consistent with the approximated volume, 0.75 mL, the answer is confirmed. Note: Because of the ease of withdrawing 1 mL, and because no calculation is required, preparing the dosage strength 750,000 units/mL is also appropriate for mixing this IV dose.

LEARNING ACTIVITY 9-4 For the following order and supply:

A. Identify the diluent(s) that should be used to reconstitute the medication.
B. Determine the volume of diluent to use.
C. Determine the resulting dosage strength.

1. **Order:** acyclovir 400 mg IV q8h for 7 days

    Supply: See **Figure 9-26**.

2. **Order:** Azactam® 500 mg IM q12h

    Supply: See **Figure 9-27**.

3. **Order:** ceftriaxone 500 mg IV q6h

    Supply: See **Figure 9-28**.

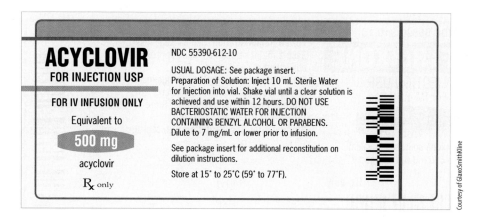

FIGURE 9-26

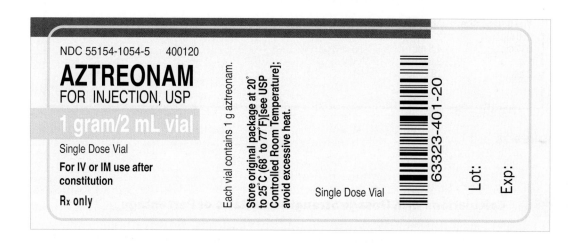

For intramuscular injection: For each gram of aztreonam add at least 3 mL of Sterile Water for Injections or 0.9% Sodium Chloride Injection BP and shake well.

FIGURE 9-27

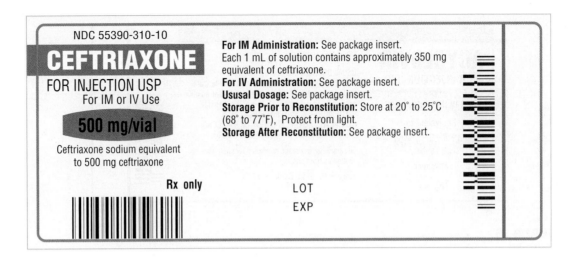

FIGURE 9-28

| 9-4 | **Calculations with Dosage Strength as a Ratio or Percentage** |

Sometimes dosage strength is expressed as a percentage (per 100), meaning grams (g) per 100 mL. For example, dextrose 50% contains 50 g of dextrose in every 100 mL of solution. The concentration of a medication may also be expressed as a ratio of grams to milliliters. For example, epinephrine 1:1,000 contains 1 g in 1,000 mL of solution, which is the equivalent of 1 mg/1 mL.

Clinical CLUE

The dosage strength can be written as a ratio or percentage. Remember the units of measurements for each:

Percentage	grams per 100 milliliters
	g/100 mL
Ratio	grams per milliliters
	g:mL

Calculating Dosage of Percent and Ratio Strength Medications

It is important to remember the units of measurement that are implied when medications are labeled with a dosage strength expressed as a percentage or ratio. When ratio or percentage dosage strengths are written as a fraction, the numerator will be *grams* and the denominator will be *milliliters*. To perform a dosage calculation with a medication that is supplied as a percent or ratio:

1. Convert the concentration to a fraction:

   a. Percent = g/100 mL
   b. Ratio = g/mL

2. Convert the concentration to mg/mL.

Example 1:   Convert the dosage strength to mg/mL from the following supply.

   Supply: 500 mL bottle of Mannitol 20%

1. Convert 20% to a fraction g/100 mL:
   20% = 20 g/100 mL

2. Convert 20 g to mg using the conversion factor 1,000 mg/1 g:

$$x \text{ (mg)} = \frac{1{,}000 \text{ mg}}{1 \text{ g}} \times \frac{20 \text{ g}}{1} = 20{,}000 \text{ mg}$$

3. Determine the number of mg in 1 mL:

$$\frac{20{,}000 \text{ mg}}{100 \text{ mL}} = \frac{x \text{ mg}}{1 \text{ mL}}$$
$$100x = 20{,}000$$
$$\frac{100x}{100} = \frac{20{,}000}{100}$$
$$x = 200 \text{ mg}$$

   A 20% mannitol solution contains 200 mg of mannitol per mL.

Example 2:   Convert the dosage strength to mg/mL from the following supply.

   Supply: 10 mL prefilled syringe of Xylocaine 1%

1. Convert 1% to a fraction g/100 mL:
   1% = 1 g/100 mL

2. Convert 1 g to mg using the conversion factor 1,000 mg/1 g:

$$x \text{ (mg)} = \frac{1{,}000 \text{ mg}}{1 \text{ g}} \times \frac{1 \text{ g}}{1} = 1{,}000 \text{ mg}$$

3. Determine the number of mg in 1 mL:

$$\frac{1,000\ \text{mg}}{100\ \text{mL}} = \frac{x\ \text{mg}}{1\ \text{mL}}$$

$$100x = 1,000$$

$$\frac{100x}{100} = \frac{1,000}{100}$$

$$x = 10\ \text{mg}$$

1% Xylocaine solution has 10 mg of Xylocaine per mL.

Example 3:   Convert the dosage strength to mg/mL from the following supply.

   Supply: 10 mL prefilled syringe of epinephrine 1:10,000

1. Convert 1:10,000 to a fraction g/mL:
1:10,000 = 1 g/10,000 mL

2. Convert 1 g to mg using the conversion factor 1,000 mg/1 g:

$$x\ (\text{mg}) = \frac{1,000\ \text{mg}}{1\ \text{g}} \times \frac{1\ \text{g}}{1} = 1,000\ \text{mg}$$

3. Determine the number of mg in 1 mL:

$$\frac{1,000\ \text{mg}}{10,000\ \text{mL}} = \frac{x\ \text{mg}}{1\ \text{mL}}$$

$$10,000x = 1,000$$

$$\frac{10,000x}{10,000} = \frac{1,000}{10,000} = \frac{1}{10} = 0.1$$

$$x = 0.1\ \text{mg}$$

A 1:10,000 epinephrine solution has 0.1 mg of epinephrine per mL.

Clinical CLUE

To prevent medication errors, medications are also labeled with the amount of medication in 1 mL. Look for this, especially when the medication is labeled as a percentage or ratio.

LEARNING ACTIVITY 9-5 Convert the dosage strength to mg/mL from the following supplies.

1.   **Supply:** epinephrine 1:1000
2.   **Supply:** Dextran 6%
3.   **Supply:** albumin 25%

Determining the Amount of Medication in a Given Volume When the Dosage Strength Is a Percentage or Ratio

On occasion, the nurse will be given a volume to administer and must be able to calculate the number of grams of medication within that volume:

- For ratio-proportion (RP), the strength of the solution or supply, $\frac{g}{100\ mL}$, is the first ratio. The unknown quantity, x g, is the numerator of the second ratio, and the ordered volume is the denominator of the second ratio:

$$\frac{g}{100\ mL} = \frac{x\ g}{ordered\ mL} \quad or\ g\ :\ 100\ mL = x\ g\ :\ ordered\ mL$$

- For the formula method (FM), the formula is:

$$\frac{(ordered\ volume)\ \cancel{mL}}{(supply\ volume)\ 100\ \cancel{mL}} \times (supply)\ g = x\ (g)$$

For DA, to determine x g, the first factor is the supply (percent solution), $\frac{g}{100\ mL}$:

$$x\ (g) = \frac{g}{100\ \cancel{mL}} \times \frac{supply\ \cancel{mL}}{1}$$

Example: Determine how many mg are in 50 mL of mannitol 10% (i.e., 10 g/100 mL).

C: *Convert*—Convert 10 grams to 10,000 mg; for DA, use the conversion factor 1,000 mg/1 g.

A: *Approximate*—The given volume, 50 mL, is ½ of the supply volume, 100 mL. Therefore, ½ of the 10,000 mg supply amount (i.e., 5,000 mg) is the amount of mannitol present in 50 mL.

S: *Solve*

Ratio-Proportion	Formula Method
$\frac{10,000\ mg}{100\ mL} = \frac{x\ mg}{50\ mL}$ or $10,000\ mg: 100\ mL = x\ mg: 50\ mL$ $100x = 500,000$ $\frac{100x}{100} = \frac{500,000}{100}$ $x = 5,000\ mg$	$\frac{50\ \cancel{mL}}{100\ \cancel{mL}} \times 10,000\ mg = x\ (mg)$ $\frac{500,000\ mg}{100} = x$ $5,000\ mg = x$

Dimensional Analysis

$$x\ (mg) = \frac{1,000\ mg}{1\ \cancel{g}} \times \frac{10\ \cancel{g}}{100\ \cancel{mL}} \times \frac{50\ \cancel{mL}}{1}$$

$$x = \frac{500,000\ mg}{100}$$

$$x = 5,000\ mg$$

E: *Evaluate*

Ratio-Proportion	Formula Method
$\dfrac{10,000\ mg}{100\ mL} = \dfrac{5,000\ mg}{50\ mL}$ or $10,000\ mg : 100\ mL = 5,000\ mg : 50\ mL$ $10,000 \times 50 = 100 \times 5,000$ $500,000 = 500,000$	$\dfrac{50\ \cancel{mL}}{100\ \cancel{mL}} \times 10,000\ mg = 5,000\ mg$ $\dfrac{500,000\ mg}{100} = 5,000\ mg$ $5,000\ mg = 5,000\ mg$

Dimensional Analysis

$$5,000\ mg = \frac{1,000\ mg}{1\ \cancel{g}} \times \frac{10\ \cancel{g}}{100\ \cancel{mL}} \times \frac{50\ \cancel{mL}}{1}$$

$$5,000\ mg = \frac{500,000\ mg}{100}$$

$$5,000\ mg = 5,000\ mg$$

Because the calculated number of grams accurately completes the equation and is consistent with the approximated amount, 5000 mg, the answer is confirmed.

LEARNING ACTIVITY 9-6 Determine the milligrams of medication in the following supplies and volumes:

1. 50 mL of dextrose 50%
2. 12 mL of Fluorouracil 5%
3. 10 mL of epinephrine 1:10,000

Concentrate on the Concentration ... Case Closure

The patient was prescribed lidocaine 100 mg IV, but was administered 1,000 mg of lidocaine. The nurse used 10 mL of the wrong concentration of lidocaine. A drug reference would have indicated that lidocaine 10%—that is, 10 g/100 mL (10,000 mg/100 mL)—is too concentrated for direct IV push. To prevent this type of error, labels now additionally list the dosage strength per 1 mL. Had the nurse noted the concentration was 10 times greater than intended, or had the nurse understood that a percentage concentration represented the number of grams in 100 mL, this error could have been avoided.

Chapter Summary

Learning Outcomes	Points to Remember
9-1 Perform calculations for injectable medications.	Ratio-proportion (RP): $\dfrac{\text{supply amt}}{\text{supply mL}} = \dfrac{\text{ordered amt}}{x \text{ (ordered) mL}}$ Formula method (FM): $\dfrac{\text{ordered } \cancel{\text{amt}}}{\text{supply } \cancel{\text{amt}}} \times \text{supply mL} = x \text{ (mL)}$ Dimensional analysis (DA): $x \text{ (mL)} = \dfrac{\text{supply mL}}{\text{supply } \cancel{\text{amt}}} \times \dfrac{\text{ordered } \cancel{\text{amt}}}{1}$
9-2 Round calculated dosages to the appropriate syringe calibration.	Syringe selection: • Volumes less than 1 mL, use 1 mL syringe or smaller • Volumes between 0.5 mL and 1 mL that calculate evenly to the tenth, use 1 mL syringe or 3 mL syringe • Volumes 1 mL or greater, use 3 mL syringe or larger if indicated Rounding rules—round to calibration of required syringe: • Round to the nearest hundredth when using 1 mL syringe or smaller • Round to the nearest tenth when using 3 mL syringe
9-3 Perform calculations for reconstitution of medications.	Refer to the medication label, package insert, or drug guide for reconstitution information. Example: *Order:* ampicillin 0.125 g IM q6h *Supply:* 500 mg vial *Label:* Add 1.8 mL SW or NS; resulting supply 250 mg/mL; stable at room temperature for 24 h For this example, the nurse will add 1.8 mL diluent to the 500 mg vial and perform this dosage calculation: **C:** *Convert:* Convert 0.125 g to 125 mg; for DA, use CF $\frac{1{,}000 \text{ mg}}{1 \text{ g}}$. **A:** *Approximate:* Because the ordered dose is half the supply dose, half the supply volume or 0.5 mL is needed.

S: *Solve:*

RP:	**FM:**
$\dfrac{250 \text{ mg}}{1 \text{ mL}} = \dfrac{125 \text{ mg}}{x \text{ mL}}$ $x = 0.5 \text{ mL}$	$\dfrac{125 \text{ mg}}{250 \text{ mg}} \times 1 \text{ mL} = x \text{ (mL)}$ $0.5 \text{ mL} = x$

DA:

$$x \text{ (mL)} = \frac{1 \text{ mL}}{250 \text{ mg}} \times \frac{1,000 \text{ mg}}{1 \text{ g}} \times \frac{0.125 \text{ g}}{1}$$

$$x = \frac{125 \text{ mL}}{250} = 0.5 \text{ mL}$$

E: *Evaluate:* Replace **x** with 0.5 mL to check calculation and compare to approximated amount for consistency.

If a reconstituted medication comes from a multi-dose vial, the nurse must create a reconstitution label. To determine the number of doses in the vial:

$$500 \text{ mg/vial} \div 125 \text{ mg/dose} = 4 \text{ doses/vial}$$

A reconstitution label (with initials, date and time of preparation, supply, discard date, storage info) is needed for the remaining doses.

9-4 Convert the dosage strength from a percentage or ratio to mg/mL.

- Convert the concentration to a fraction:
  - Percent = g/100 mL
  - Ratio = g : mL
- Convert the grams to mg and determine the number of mg in 1 mL (divide the number of mg by the number of mL in the concentration).

9-5 Determine the amount of medication in a given volume when the dosage strength is given as a percentage or ratio.

- Ratio-proportion:

$$\frac{g}{100 \text{ mL}} = \frac{x \text{ g}}{\text{ordered mL}} \quad \text{or g: 100 mL} = x \text{ g : ordered mL}$$

- Formula method:

$$\frac{\text{(ordered volume) mL}}{\text{(supply volume)100 mL}} \times \text{(supply) g} = x \text{ (g)}$$

- Dimensional analysis:

$$x \text{ (g)} = \frac{g}{100 \text{ mL}} \times \frac{\text{supply mL}}{1}$$

Homework

For exercises 1–10, determine the amount to administer for each order and supply. (LO 9-1)

1. Order: metoprolol 5 mg IV q2min for 3 doses
   Supply:

2. Order: metoclopramide 10 mg IV × 1 dose
   Supply:

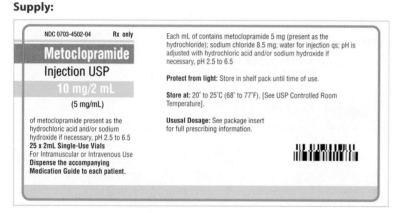

3. Order: hydromorphone 1.5 mg IV q3h
   Supply:

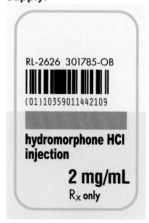

4. Order: haloperidol 2 mg IV q4h prn agitation
   Supply:

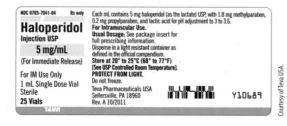

5. **Order:** flumazenil 200 mcg IV stat
   Supply:

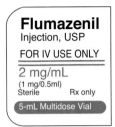

> **Flumazenil**
> Injection, USP
> FOR IV USE ONLY
> 2 mg/mL
> (1 mg/0.5ml)
> Sterile   Rx only
> 5-mL Multidose Vial

6. **Order:** fentanyl 0.1 mg IM 30 min before surgery
   Supply:

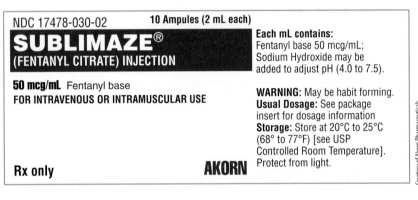

> NDC 17478-030-02   **10 Ampules (2 mL each)**
>
> **SUBLIMAZE®**
> **(FENTANYL CITRATE) INJECTION**
>
> **50 mcg/mL** Fentanyl base
> **FOR INTRAVENOUS OR INTRAMUSCULAR USE**
>
> **Rx only**   **AKORN**
>
> **Each mL contains:**
> Fentanyl base 50 mcg/mL;
> Sodium Hydroxide may be
> added to adjust pH (4.0 to 7.5).
>
> **WARNING:** May be habit forming.
> **Usual Dosage:** See package
> insert for dosage information
> **Storage:** Store at 20°C to 25°C
> (68° to 77°F) [see USP
> Controlled Room Temperature].
> Protect from light.

Courtesy of Akorn Pharmaceuticals

7. **Order:** atropine 0.5 mg IV stat
   Supply:

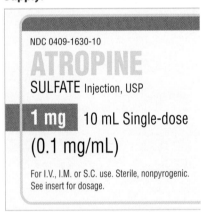

> NDC 0409-1630-10
> **ATROPINE**
> SULFATE Injection, USP
> **1 mg** 10 mL Single-dose
> **(0.1 mg/mL)**
> For I.V., I.M. or S.C. use. Sterile, nonpyrogenic.
> See insert for dosage.

8. Order: bumetanide 500 mcg IV daily
Supply:

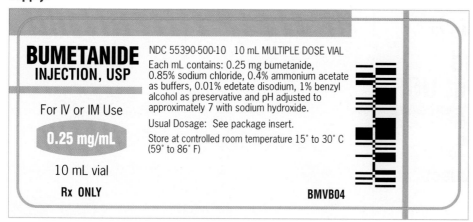

9. Order: butorphanol 1.5 mg q4h prn
Supply:

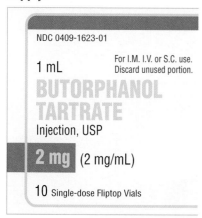

10. Order: furosemide 40 mg IV bid
Supply:

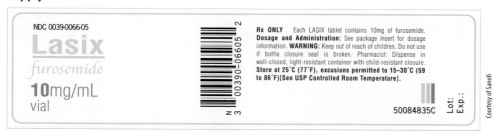

For exercises 11–20, determine the amount to administer for each order and supply. Use Rounding Rules when necessary and mark the appropriate syringe with the ordered volume. (LO 9-2)

11. **Order:** isoniazid 300 mg IM every third day

Supply:

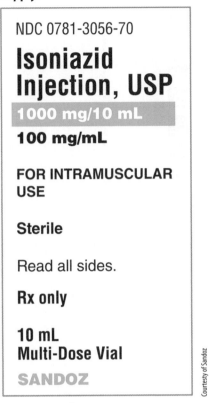

NDC 0781-3056-70

Isoniazid Injection, USP

1000 mg/10 mL

100 mg/mL

FOR INTRAMUSCULAR USE

Sterile

Read all sides.

Rx only

10 mL Multi-Dose Vial

SANDOZ

Courtesy of Sandoz

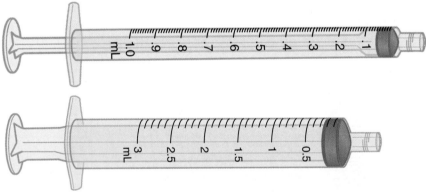

12. **Order:** haloperidol 1.25 mg IV q2h prn agitation

Supply:

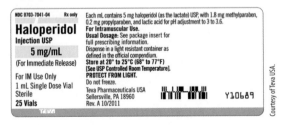

NDC 0703-7041-04　　Rx only

Haloperidol
Injection USP

5 mg/mL

(For Immediate Release)

For IM Use Only
1 mL Single Dose Vial
Sterile
25 Vials

TEVA

Each mL contains 5 mg haloperidol (as the lactate) USP, with 1.8 mg methylparaben, 0.2 mg propylparaben, and lactic acid for pH adjustment to 3 to 3.6.
For Intramuscular Use.
Usual Dosage: See package insert for full prescribing information.
Dispense in a light resistant container as defined in the official compendium.
Store at 20° to 25°C (68° to 77°F)
[See USP Controlled Room Temperature].
PROTECT FROM LIGHT.
Do not freeze.
Teva Pharmaceuticals USA
Sellersville, PA 18960
Rev. A 10/2011

Y10689

Courtesy of Teva USA.

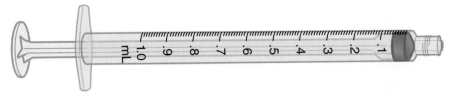

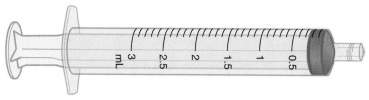

13. Order: methylergonovine 200 mcg q4h × 24 hours
Supply:

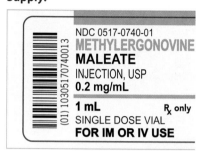

NDC 0517-0740-01
**METHYLERGONOVINE
MALEATE**
INJECTION, USP
0.2 mg/mL

1 mL   Rx only
SINGLE DOSE VIAL
FOR IM OR IV USE

(01) 1030517074013

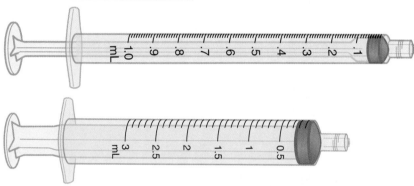

14. Order: midazolam 1.325 mg IV × 1 dose
Supply:

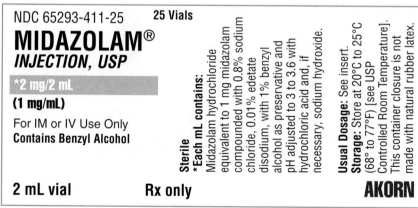

NDC 65293-411-25   **25 Vials**

MIDAZOLAM®
INJECTION, USP

*2 mg/2 mL
(1 mg/mL)

For IM or IV Use Only
Contains Benzyl Alcohol

Sterile
*Each mL contains:
Midazolam hydrochloride equivalent to 1 mg midazolam compounded with 0.8% sodium chloride, 0.01% edetate disodium, with 1% benzyl alcohol as preservative and pH adjusted to 3 to 3.6 with hydrochloric acid and, if necessary, sodium hydroxide.

Usual Dosage: See insert.
Storage: Store at 20°C to 25°C (68° to 77°F) [see USP Controlled Room Temperature]. This container closure is not made with natural rubber latex.

2 mL vial   **Rx only**

AKORN

Courtesy of Akorn Pharmaceuticals

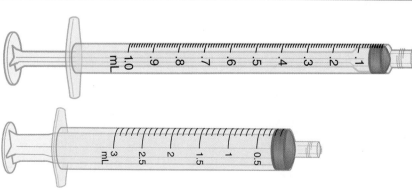

15. Order: orphenadrine 60 mg IV q12h

Supply:

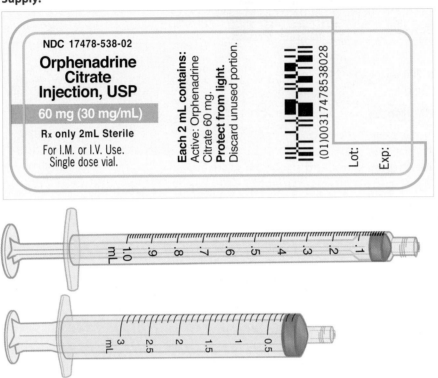

NDC 17478-538-02

Orphenadrine Citrate Injection, USP

60 mg (30 mg/mL)

Rx only 2mL Sterile

For I.M. or I.V. Use.
Single dose vial.

Each 2 mL contains:
Active: Orphenadrine Citrate 60 mg.
Protect from light.
Discard unused portion.

Lot:

Exp:

16. Order: oxymorphone 0.5 mg subcut q4h prn pain

Supply:

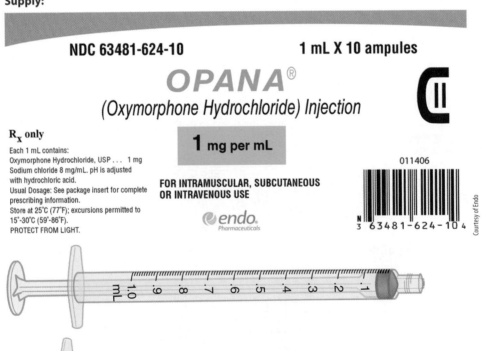

NDC 63481-624-10

1 mL X 10 ampules

OPANA®

(Oxymorphone Hydrochloride) Injection

1 mg per mL

C II

R_x only

Each 1 mL contains:
Oxymorphone Hydrochloride, USP . . . 1 mg
Sodium chloride 8 mg/mL. pH is adjusted
with hydrochloric acid.
Usual Dosage: See package insert for complete
prescribing information.
Store at 25°C (77°F); excursions permitted to
15°-30°C (59°-86°F).
PROTECT FROM LIGHT.

**FOR INTRAMUSCULAR, SUBCUTANEOUS
OR INTRAVENOUS USE**

endo.
Pharmaceuticals

011406

3 63481-624-10 4

Courtesy of Endo

17. Order: oxytocin 10 units IM stat
Supply:

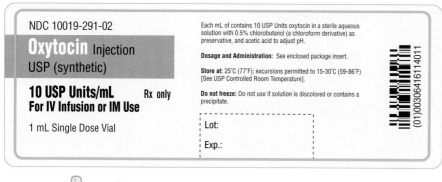

NDC 10019-291-02

Oxytocin Injection
USP (synthetic)

10 USP Units/mL   Rx only
For IV Infusion or IM Use

1 mL Single Dose Vial

Each mL of contains 10 USP Units oxytocin in a sterile aqueous solution with 0.5% chlorobutanol (a chloroform derivative) as preservative, and acetic acid to adjust pH.

Dosage and Administration: See enclosed package insert.

Store at: 25°C (77°F); excursions permitted to 15-30°C (59-86°F) [See USP Controlled Room Temperature].

Do not freeze: Do not use if solution is discolored or contains a precipitate.

Lot:

Exp.:

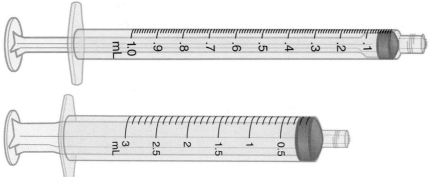

18. Order: phenobarbital 40 mg IM q8h
Supply:

NDC 0641-0476-25

Phenobarbital
Sodium Injection, USP

65 mg/mL   Rx only
FOR IM OR SLOW IV USE
25 x 1 mL DOSETTE Vials

DO NOT USE IF DISCOLORED
OR CONTAINS A PRECIPITATE

Each mL contains Phenobarbital sodium 65 mg, alcohol 0.1 mL propylene glycol 0.578 mL and butyl alcohol 0.015 mL in Water for injection pH 9.2-10.2 hydrochloric acid added, if needed for pH adjustment.

Usual Dosage: See package insert.

Store at: 20°-25°C (44°-77°F); [See USP Controlled Room Temperature].

Lot:

Exp.:

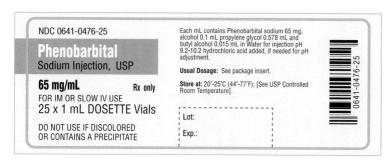

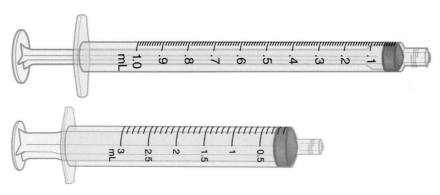

19. **Order:** thiamine 75 mg IM tid
    Supply:

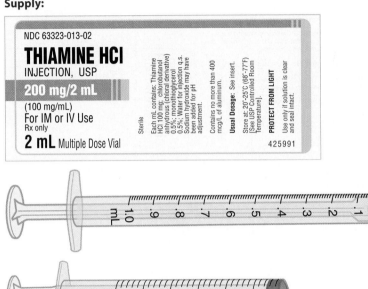

20. **Order:** cyanocobalamin subcut 300 mcg/day
    × 5 days
    Supply:

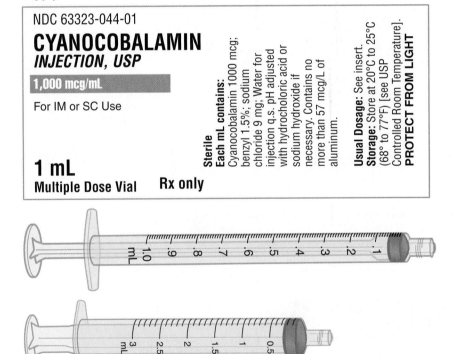

For exercises 21–25, determine the answers for a–c for each order and supply. (LO 9-3)

a. Determine the type and amount of diluents to instill.

b. Determine the resulting dosage strength.

c. Calculate the amount of reconstituted medication needed to administer the prescribed dose.

21. Order: levothyroxine 75 mcg IV daily

Supply:

NDC 63323-647-10

LEVOTHYROXINE SODIUM
FOR INJECTION

200 mcg/vial

For Intravenous Use
Single Use Vial
Discard any unused portion.

Rx only

Sterile, Lyophilized Preservative Free
Each vial contains:
Levothyroxine sodium 200 mcg; inactive ingredients: see carton label.
Usual Dosage: See insert.
Storage: Store at 20°C to 25°C (68° to 77°F) [see USP Controlled Room Temperature].
PROTECT FROM LIGHT
Reconstituion Directions:
Reconstitute the lyophilized levothyroxine sodium by aseptically adding 5 mL of 0.9% Sodium Chloride Injection, USP. Shake vial to ensure complete mixing. The resultant solution will have a final concentration of 40 mcg/mL. Use immediately after reconstitution. Discard any unused portion.

22. Order: acetazolamide 250 mg IV daily

Supply:

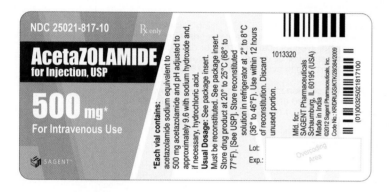

Courtesy of Sagent Pharmaceuticals

NDC 25021-817-10   R only

AcetaZOLAMIDE
for Injection, USP

500 mg*
For Intravenous Use

SAGENT

***Each vial contains:** acetazolamide sodium equivalent to 500 mg acetazolamide and pH adjusted to approximately 9.6 with sodium hydroxide and, if necessary, hydrochloric acid.
Usual Dosage: See package insert. Must be reconstituted. See package insert. Store drug product at 20° to 25°C (68° to 77°F). [See USP]. Store reconstituted solution in refrigerator at 2° to 8°C (36° to 46°F). Use within 12 hours of reconstitution. Discard unused portion.

1013320

Mfd. for:
SAGENT Pharmaceuticals
Schaumburg, IL 60195 (USA)
Made in India
Code No.: KR/DRUGS/KTK/28/284/2009
(01)00032502181710

Lot:
Exp.:   Overcoding Area

DOSAGE AND ADMINISTRATION

Preparation and Storage of Parenteral Solution
Each 500 mg vial containing sterile acetazolamide sodium should be reconstituted with at least 5 mL of Sterile Water for Injection prior to use. Store drug product at 20° to 25°C (68° to 77°F). [See USP Controlled Room Temperature.] Reconstituted solutions retain their physical and chemical properties for 3 days under refrigeration at 2° - 8°C (36° - 46°F), or 12 hours at room temperature 20° to 25°C (68° to 77°F). CONTAINS NO PRESERVATIVE. The direct intravenous route of administration is preferred.

Intramuscular administration is not recommended.

23. Order: acyclovir 750 mg IV q8h for 10 days

Supply:

ACYCLOVIR
FOR INJECTION USP

For IV INFUSION ONLY

Equivalent to

1000 mg

acyclovir

Rx ONLY

NDC 55390-613-20

Usual Dosage: See package insert.
Preparation of Solution:
Inject 20 mL Sterile Water for Injection into vial. Shake vial until a clear solution is achieved and use within 12 hours. DO NOT USE BACTERIOSTATIC WATER FOR INJECTION CONTAINING BENZYL ALCOHOL OR PARABENS.

Dilute to 7 mg/mL or lower prior to infusion. See package insert for additional reconstitution and dilution instructions.
Storage: Store at 20°C to 25°C (68° to 77°F)

24. **Order:** allopurinol 200 mg IV daily

    Supply:

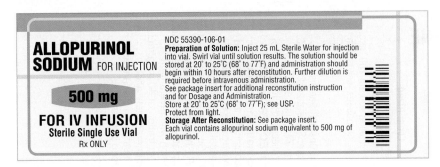

25. **Order:** Basiliximab 20 mg IV 2h before transplant

    Supply:

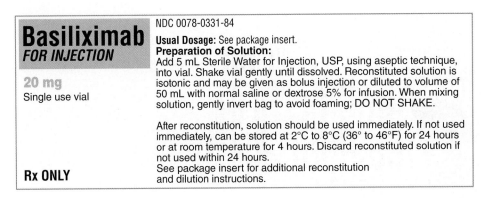

For exercises 26–30, determine the answer for a–d for each order and supply (LO 9-3):

a. Determine the number of vials needed to administer the dose.

b. Determine the type and amount of diluents to instill.

c. Determine the resulting dosage strength.

d. Calculate the amount of reconstituted medication needed to administer the prescribed dose.

26. Order: azacitidine 25 mg subcut daily × 7 days

   Supply:

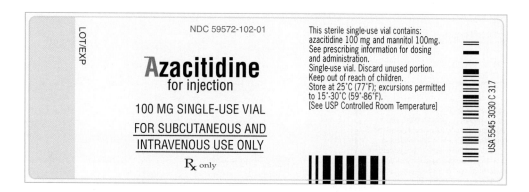

| **Features and properties of azacitidine** |

Instructions for Subcutaneous Administration

Azacitidine should be reconstituted aseptically with 4 mL sterile water for injection. The diluent should be injected slowly into the vial. Vigorously shake or roll the vial until a uniform suspension is achieved. The suspension will be cloudy. The resulting suspension will contain azacitidine 25 mg/mL. Do not filter the suspension after reconstitution. Doing so could remove the active substance.

27. **Order:** cephalexin 0.5 g IM q8h × 24 h
    Supply:

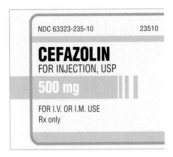

Not Cephalexin
Call pharmacy

RECONSTITUTION
Preparation of Parenteral Solution
Parenteral drug products should be SHAKEN WELL when reconstituted, and inspected visually for particulate matter prior to administration. If particulate matter is evident in reconstituted fluids, the drug solutions should be discarded. When reconstituted or diluted according to the instructions below, cefazolin for injection is stable for 24 hours at room temperature or for 10 days if stored under refrigeration (5°C or 41 °F). Reconstituted solutions may range in color from pale yellow to yellow without a change in potency
For IM injection, IV direct (bolus) injection or IV infusion, reconstitute with Sterile Water for Injection according to the following table. SHAKE WELL.

Vial size	Amount of Diluent	Approximate Concentration	Approximate Available Volume
1 gram	2.5 mL	330 mg/mL	3 mL

ADMINISTRATION
Intermittent or continuous infusion: Dilute reconstituted cefazolin in 50 to 100 mL of 1 of the following solutions:
Sodium Chloride Injection, USP
5% or 10% Dextrose Injection, USP
5% Dextrose in Lactated Ringer's Injection, USP
5% Dextrose and 0.9% Sodium Chloride Injection, USP
5% Dextrose and 0.45% Sodium Chloride Injection, USP
5% Dextrose and 0.2% Sodium Chloride Injection, USP
Lactated Ringer's Injection, USP
Invert Sugar 5% or 10% in Sterile Water for Injection
Ringer's Injection, USP
5% Sodium Bicarbonate Injection, USP

Courtesy of Hospira

28. Order: Vfend® 240 mg IV q 12 h

Supply:

1 Vial

Vfend® I.V.
(voriconazole) for injection

200 mg*
200 mg* of voriconazole

Sterile Single Use Vial

For I.V. Infusion Only

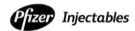 **Injectables**

Store at controlled room temperature, 15° to 30°C (59° to 86°F).

DOSAGE AND USE:
Reconstitute with 19 mL of Water for Injection to give a clear solution containing 10 mg/mL Vfend and an extractable volume of 20 mL. **Must be further diluted before use.** For administration, the required volume of the reconstituted solution is added to a recommended compatible infusion solution to provide a final Vfend solution containing 0.5-5 mg/mL. For appropriate diluents and storage recommendations, refer to prescribing information.

FOR INTRAVENOUS ADMINISTRATION

* With reconstitution each mL contains 10 mg voriconazole and 160 mg sulfobutyl ether ß-cyclodextrin sodium (SBECD)

Reconstitution
The powder is reconstituted with 19 mL of Water For Injection to obtain an extractable volume of 20 mL of clear concentrate containing 10 mg/mL of voriconazole. It is recommended that a standard 20 mL (non-automated) syringe be used to ensure that the exact amount (19.0 mL) of Water for Injection is dispensed. Discard the vial if a vacuum does not pull the diluent into the vial. Shake the vial until all the powder is dissolved.

Dilution
VFEND must be infused over 1-2 hours, at a concentration of 5 mg/mL or less. Therefore, the required volume of the 10 mg/mL VFEND concentrate should be further diluted as follows (appropriate diluents listed below):
1. Calculate the volume of 10 mg/mL VFEND concentrate required based on the patient's weight (see Table 2).
2. In order to allow the required volume of VFEND concentrate to be added, withdraw and discard at least an equal volume of diluent from the infusion bag or bottle to be used. The volume of diluent remaining in the bag or bottle should be such that when the 10 mg/mL VFEND concentrate is added, the final concentration is not less than 0.5 mg/mL nor greater than 5 mg/mL.
3. Using a suitable size syringe and aseptic technique, withdraw the required volume of VFEND concentrate from the appropriate number of vials and add to the infusion bag or bottle. **Discard Partially Used Vials.**
The final VFEND solution must be infused over 1-2 hours at a maximum rate of 3 mg/kg per hour.

Courtesy of Pfizer, Inc.

29. **Order:** Visudyne® 10 mg IV × 1 dose

    Supply:

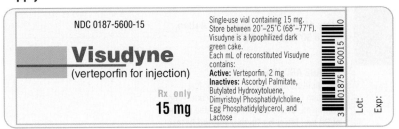

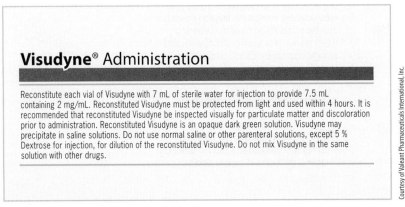

Courtesy of Valeant Pharmaceuticals International, Inc.

30. **Order:** pantoprazole 40 mg IV daily

    Supply:

NDC 0008-0923-51

Contains 1 mg edetate disodium.
Reconstitution needed.
Usual Dosage: See package insert.
Preparation of Solution:
Add 10 mL of 0.9% Sodium Chloride Injection, USP; further dilute (admix) with 100 mL of 5% Dextrose Injection, USP, 0.9% Sodium Chloride Injection, USP, or Lactated Ringer's Injection, USP, to final concentration of approx. 0.4 mg/mL.

Reconstituted solution may be stored for up to 6 hours at room temperature prior to further dilution. Admixed solution may be stored at room temperature and must be used within 24 hours from the time of initial reconstitution.

See package insert for additional reconstitution and dilution instructions.

PROTONIX I.V.
(pantoprazole sodium)
for injection

Equivalent to
40 mg
pantoprazole per vial
For I.V. infusion only.

Rx ONLY

For exercises 31–40, convert the dosage strength to mg/mL. (LO 9-4)

31. mannitol 15%

32. albumin 5%

33. Plasbumin® 25%

34. sodium chloride 3%

35. Dextran 6%

36. Fluorouracil 5%

37. Osmitrol® 25%

38. Resectisol® 20%

39. epinephrine 1:10,000

40. sodium chloride 5%

For exercises 41–50, determine the amount of medication for each supply and volume. (LO 9-5)

41. 300 mL of mannitol 15%

42. 250 mL of albumin 5%

43. 3.5 mL of lidocaine 10%

44. 35 mL of dextrose 50%
45. 6 mL of epinephrine 1:1,000
46. 7.4 mL of epinephrine 1:10,000
47. 4 mL of lidocaine 2%
48. 20 mL of lidocaine 1%
49. 8 mL of DigiFab® 1:100
50. 15 mL of albumin 25%

NCLEX-Style Review Questions

For questions 1–4, select the best response.

1. The prescriber orders amikacin 375 mg IM q8h. The nurse has a supply of amikacin 250 mg/mL. How many mL of the supply should the nurse administer? (LO 9-1)
   a. 0.5 mL
   b. 0.75 mL
   c. 1.5 mL
   d. 1.8 mL

2. The prescriber orders ketorolac 20 mg IV q6h. The nurse is supplied with ketorolac 30 mg/mL. Which syringe(s) should the nurse use to administer this dose? (LO 9-2)
   a. 0.5 mL tuberculin syringe
   b. 1 mL tuberculin syringe
   c. 3 mL standard syringe
   d. 1 mL or 3 mL syringe

3. The patient exhibits signs of ventricular fibrillation. The prescriber orders epinephrine 1 mg IV stat. The nurse should administer: (LO 9-4)
   a. 1 mL of epinephrine 1:1,000
   b. 1 mL of epinephrine 1:10,000
   c. 10 mL of epinephrine 1:1,000
   d. 10 mL of epinephrine 1:10,000

4. The prescriber orders 100 mL of magnesium sulfate 10% IV. How much magnesium will the nurse administer with this dose? (LO 9-4)
   a. 10 mg
   b. 100 mg
   c. 1,000 mg
   d. 10,000 mg

For questions 5–6, select all that apply.

5. The prescriber orders Pfizerpen® 333,340 units IM for a 5-year-old child.
   Supply:

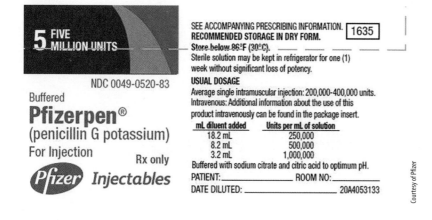

   a. The maximum volume IM is 3 mL.
   b. Can be refrigerated for 7 days
   c. Buffered for optimal pH
   d. Dilute with 8.2 mL.
   e. Dilute with 3.2 mL.
   f. Inject into the deltoid muscle.
6. The prescriber orders ciprofloxacin 200 mg IV q12h.
   Supply:

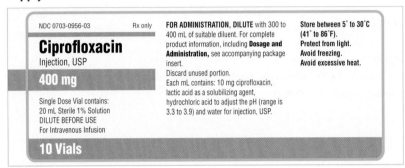

   a. For intravenous infusion.
   b. Vial holds 2 doses.
   c. Dilute with 300 to 400 mL.
   d. Store in refrigerator.
   e. Protect from light.

REFERENCES

Berman, A., Snyder, S., & Jackson, C. (2009). *Skills in clinical nursing* (6th ed.). Upper Saddle River, NJ: Pearson Education.

Deglin, J. H., & Vallerand, A. H. (2009). *Davis's drug guide for nurses* (11th ed.). Philadelphia, PA: F. A. Davis Company.

Gahart, G. L., & Nazareno, A. R. (2011). *2011 intravenous medications* (27th ed.). St. Louis, MO: Mosby.

Institute for Safe Medicine Practices. (2004). Safety issues with adding lidocaine to IV potassium infusions. *Acute Care ISMP Medication Safety Alert!*. Retrieved from www.ismp.org/Newsletters/acutecare/articles/20040212_2 .asp

Jones & Bartlett Learning. (2015). *2014 Nurse's Drug Handbook* (14th ed.). Burlington, MA: Author.

Chapter 9   ANSWER KEY

Learning Activity 9-1
1. 2 mL
2. 7 mL
3. 0.5 mL

Learning Activity 9-2
1. 0.5 mL

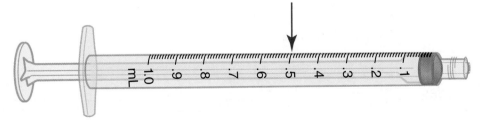

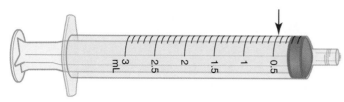

2.   0.55 mL

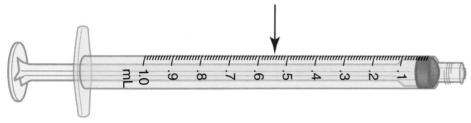

3.   1.5 mL

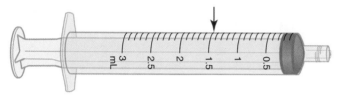

Learning Activity 9-3
1.   Sterile water, 4.8 mL; 100 mg/mL
2.   5 mL
3.   1 dose
4.   No label is needed.

Learning Activity 9-4
1.   a. Sterile water
     b. 10 mL
     c. 500 mg/10 mL or 50 mg/mL
2.   a. Sterile water
     b. At least 3 mL
     c. 1000 mg/5 mL or 200 mg/mL
3.   a. D5W or NS
     b. 4.8 mL
     c. 100 mg/mL

Learning Activity 9-5
1.   1 mg/mL
2.   60 mg/mL
3.   250 mg/mL

Learning Activity 9-6
1.   25,000 mg
2.   600 mg
3.   1 mg

Homework

1. 5 mL
2. 2 mL
3. 0.75 mL
4. 0.4 mL
5. 0.1 mL
6. 2 mL
7. 5 mL
8. 2 mL
9. 0.75 mL
10. 4 mL
11. 3 mL

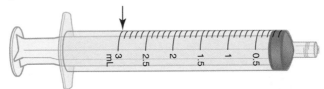

12. 0.25 mL

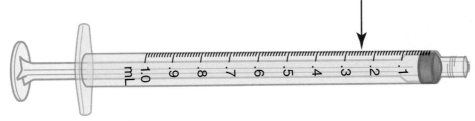

13. 1 mL

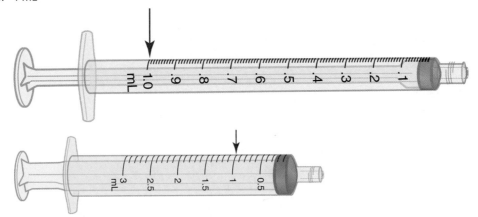

14. 1.325 mL rounds to 1.3 mL

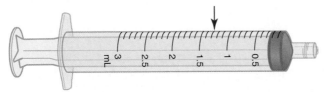

15. 2 mL

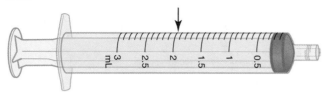

16. 0.5 mL

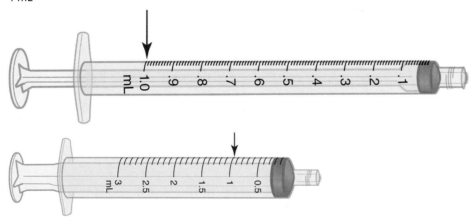

17. 1 mL

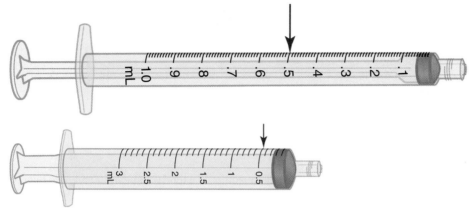

18. 0.615 mL rounds to 0.62 mL.

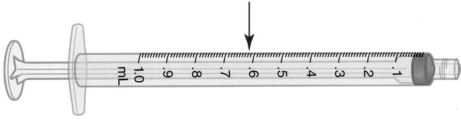

19. 0.75 mL

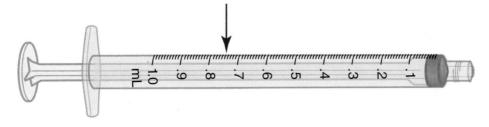

20. 0.3 mL

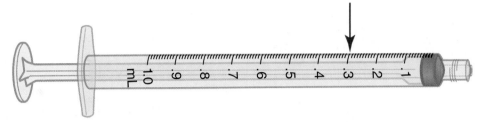

21. 5 mL NS; 40 mcg/mL; 1.87 mL rounded to 1.9 mL
22. 5 mL SW; 500 mg/5 mL or 100 mg/mL; 2.5 mL
23. 20 mL SW; 1,000 mg/20 mL or 50 mg/mL; 15 mL
24. 25 mL SW; 500 mg/25 mL or 20 mg/mL; 10 mL
25. 5 mL SW; 20 mg/5 mL or 4 mg/mL; 5 mL
26. 1; 4 mL sterile water; 25 mg/mL; 1 mL
27. 1; 1.25 mL (drawn up using a 1 mL and 3 mL syringe) NS or D5W or other IV solution listed; 330 mg/mL; 1.5 mL
28. 2; 19 mL SW in each vial; 10 mg/mL; 24 mL
29. 1; 7 mL SW; 2 mg/mL; 5 mL
30. 1; 10 mL NS; 40 mg/10 mL or 4 mg/mL; 10 mL (then further dilute/admix to a total volume of 100 mL, and final concentration of 0.4 mg/mL)
31. 150 mg/mL
32. 50 mg/mL
33. 250 mg/mL
34. 30 mg/mL
35. 60 mg/mL
36. 50 mg/mL
37. 250 mg/mL
38. 200 mg/mL
39. 0.1 mg/mL
40. 50 mg/mL
41. 45 g; 45,000 mg
42. 12.5 g; 12,500 mg
43. 0.35 g; 350 mg
44. 17.5 g; 17,500 mg
45. 0.006 g; 6 mg
46. 0.00074 g; 0.74 mg
47. 0.08 g; 80 mg
48. 0.2 g; 200 mg
49. 0.08 g; 80 mg
50. 3.75 g; 3,750 mg

NCLEX-Style Review Questions

1. c
   Rationale: $\dfrac{250 \text{ mg}}{1 \text{ mL}} = \dfrac{375 \text{ mg}}{1.5 \text{ mL}}$; $\dfrac{375 \text{ mg}}{250 \text{ mg}} \times 1 \text{ mL} = 1.5 \text{ mL}$; $1.5 \text{ mL} = \dfrac{1 \text{ mL}}{250 \text{ mg}} \times \dfrac{375 \text{ mg}}{1}$

2. b
   Rationale: Because the dose is less than 1 mL and does not calculate evenly to the tenths, the nurse will round the quantity 0.666 to 0.67 and draw up into a 1 mL syringe.

3. a
   Rationale: $1{:}1{,}000 = \dfrac{1 \text{ g}}{1{,}000 \text{ mL}} = \dfrac{1{,}000 \text{ mg}}{1{,}000 \text{ mL}} = \dfrac{1 \text{ mg}}{1 \text{ mL}}$; draw up 1 mL for a 1 mg dose

4. d

    Rationale: 10 g/100 mL = 10,000 mg

5. b, c, d

    Rationale: The maximum volume IM for a 5-year-old child is 1 mL. Medication can be stored in refrigerator for 1 week (b) and is buffered (c). 8.2 mL yields a concentration of 500,000 units/mL resulting in 0.67 mL injection (d); 3.2 mL results in a very concentrated injection of 0.33 mL injection. The vastus lateralis is used for 5-year-old children.

6. a, c, e

    Rationale: This medication is for intravenous infusion (a). This is a single-dose vial. (b) Must be further diluted with 300-400 mL of suitable diluent per package insert. (c). Store at room temperature (41–86° F). Protect from light (e).

© Forfunlife/Shutterstock

Chapter 10

Infusion Therapy and Calculations

LEARNING OUTCOMES

Upon completion of the chapter, the student will be able to:

10-1 Differentiate solutions used for infusion therapy.

10-2 Identify equipment used for infusion therapy.

10-3 Calculate infusion therapy flow rates.

10-4 Calculate infusion time and volume.

10-5 Cite important observations to be made during infusion therapy.

KEY TERMS

back-prime
cannula
central line
controllers
distal port
drop factor
extravasation
heparin lock
hypertonic
hypodermoclysis
hypotonic
implantable subcutaneous
   infusion port
infiltration
in-line filter
intravenous piggyback (IVPB)

isotonic
IV push/bolus medication
KVO
lumen
maintenance fluids
microemboli
osmolality
osmolarity
patient-controlled analgesia
   (PCA) pump
peripheral venous catheter
peripherally inserted central
   catheter (PICC) line
phlebitis
primary line
prime
proximal port

port
prehydration
replacement fluids
saline lock
secondary line
smart pump
syringe pump
time tape
TKO
tonicity
total parenteral nutrition
   (TPN)
vesicant
volume-control sets
Y-tubing

Case Consideration ... Intravenous Incident!

After delivery of a healthy newborn, a mother is receiving intravenous (IV) fluids at 125 mL/h via infusion pump to replace fluid lost during childbirth. The nurse, upon transferring the woman from the labor and delivery suite to the patient care unit, removed the infusion pump in order to use it for another labor patient, at which point the IV solution continued to infuse manually. When making rounds, the instructor asked the nursing student, "At how many drops per minute is the

IV infusing?" The student stated, "I'm not sure, but I know the rate is 125 mL/h." The instructor assessed the flow rate and determined that the IV was actually infusing faster than the ordered rate and manually adjusted the rate accordingly.

1. How can a nurse be sure a manually regulated IV is infusing on time?

2. Why it is important to assess IV flow rate?

■ INTRODUCTION

Infusion therapy refers to all aspects of solution and medication infusion, typically administered via the IV route that are infused directly through a vein. The subcutaneous route, though less common, can also be used for infusion therapy. Subcutaneous infusion of fluids is called **hypodermoclysis** (HDC) or clysis. Solutions are ordered to infuse continuously or intermittently. An intermittent infusion is one that maintains venous or subcutaneous access, keeping the route open and available with an access device, in order to administer medications and supplemental fluids. A continuous infusion may be prescribed for various reasons, including:

- Rehydration—When a patient has lost bodily fluids due to an event such as surgery or an episode of sweating, vomiting, diarrhea, or hemorrhage, rehydration can be accomplished by infusing fluids to replenish fluid volume, often referred to as **replacement fluids**.

- **Prehydration**—To prevent dehydration, fluids may be infused in advance of an event that causes dehydration, such as chemotherapy.

- Maintenance of fluid and electrolyte balance—Fluids that are given to maintain normal levels of fluid and electrolytes are called **maintenance fluids**.

Nurses must be able to perform calculations to determine correct infusion rates. After ordered by the provider, nurses initiate and monitor infusion therapy. This nursing responsibility requires the ability to differentiate solutions, manipulate infusion equipment, perform infusion calculations, and monitor infusion therapy.

10-1   Solutions

Components

Solutions vary by components and concentration of components. There are two major categories of infusion therapy solutions, differentiated by the size of the particles that make them up—crystalloid (small particles that form crystals) and colloid (large particles that do not break down in water). This chapter focuses on crystalloid solutions, because they are routinely administered intravenous solutions. Two major components of crystalloid solutions are dextrose (D) and sodium chloride (NaCl). Sodium chloride solutions are also called saline solutions and are available in various concentrations, distinguished by fractions or percentages (**TABLE 10-1**). Normal saline (NS) is 0.9% sodium chloride and is termed "normal" because the **osmolarity**, or particles per liter, is approximately the same as plasma. Dextrose solutions are available in 5%, 10%, 20%, and 50% concentrations, denoted by a number, often written as a subscript, in the solution name, for example, D_5W. Dextrose 5% is typically combined with saline, as shown in Table 10-1. Another common crystalloid, Lactated Ringer's solution (LR), is a combination of fluid and electrolytes.

TABLE 10-1	Commonly Prescribed Intravenous Solutions		
Classification	**Solution**	**Description**	**Other Uses**
Replacement fluids Replace fluid lost from the circulatory system (volume expanders)	Normal saline (NS) (**Figure 10-1**)	0.9% sodium chloride (0.9% NaCl)	Replaces NaCl Infused with blood transfusions
	Lactated Ringer's (LR) (**Figure 10-2**)	NS plus potassium (K), calcium (Ca), and lactate (a buffer)	Replaces Na, Cl, K, and Ca Buffers serum pH
Maintenance fluids Maintain fluid balance of cells (fluid shifts out from circulatory system)	¼ normal saline (¼ NS) (**Figure 10-3**)	0.225% NaCl	Pediatric maintenance fluid Replaces NaCl
	5% dextrose ¼ normal saline (D_5 ¼ NS) (**Figure 10-4**)	5% dextrose and 0.225% NaCl	Pediatric maintenance fluid Adds calories and replaces NaCl
	½ normal saline (½ NS) (**Figure 10-5**)	0.45% NaCl	Adult maintenance fluid Replaces small amounts of NaCl
	5% dextrose ½ normal saline (D_5½ NS) (**Figure 10-6**)	5% dextrose and 0.45% NaCl	Adult maintenance fluid Adds calories and replaces small amounts of NaCl

Tonicity

A crystalloid solution is categorized by its **tonicity**, also known as **osmolality**, which is the number of particles (osmoles) in a kilogram of fluid. Body fluids are often measured by weight, so the term *osmolality* is used to refer to the body fluids. Infusion fluid is measured by volume, so the term *osmolarity* is used to refer to infusion fluids. However, because the density of water is 1 kg/L (1 liter of water weighs 1 kg), the term *osmolality* is often used interchangeably with *osmolarity* (David, 2007). There are three tonicities:

- **Isotonic**—Isotonic solutions are used to expand intravascular volume. These solutions have the same osmolarity as plasma (270–300 milli-osmoles per liter [mOsm/L]). Therefore, they do not promote the shift of fluid into or out of cells (tissue), and the IV solution remains in the blood vessels longer than maintenance fluids. Patients with normal electrolyte levels are likely to receive isotonic solutions. Mainly isotonic solutions are used for hypodermoclysis.

- **Hypotonic**—Hypotonic solutions are used as maintenance fluids. These solutions have fewer particles than plasma, producing a pressure gradient that causes fluid to move from the vascular bed (circulatory system) into the cells. As a result, hypotonic solutions hydrate cells.

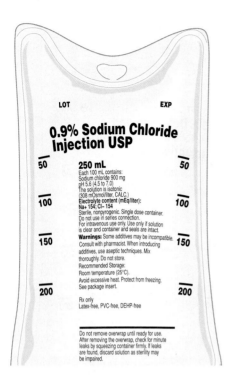

FIGURE 10-1   Normal saline (NS) is 0.9% sodium chloride solution.

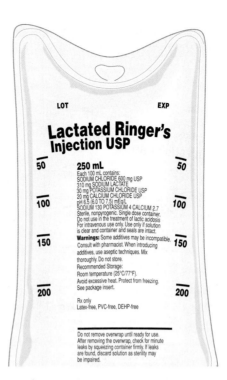

FIGURE 10-2   Abbreviated LR and also known as Ringer's lactate (RL) or Hartmann's solution, Lactated Ringer's solution is the most physiologically adaptable fluid because its electrolyte content is most closely related to the composition of the body's serum and plasma.

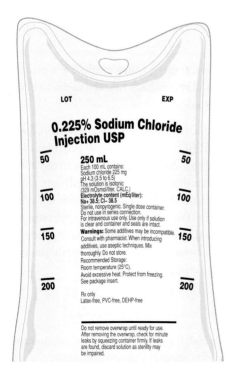

FIGURE 10-3   Because 0.225% is one-fourth of 0.9%, 0.225% sodium chloride is called ¼ NS.

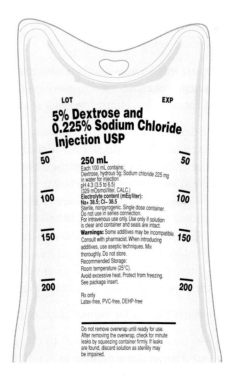

FIGURE 10-4   Dextrose 5% in 0.225% sodium chloride, is called D₅¼ NS.

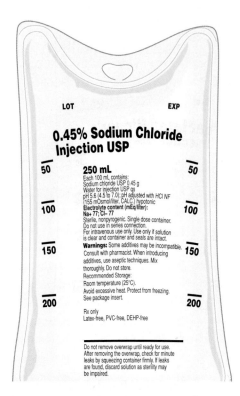

FIGURE 10-5   Because 0.45% sodium chloride is half of 0.9%, 0.45% sodium chloride is called ½ NS.

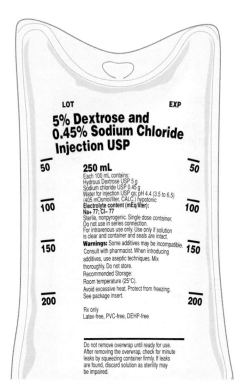

FIGURE 10-6   The addition of dextrose 5% provides calories and free water to the hypotonic solution of 0.45% sodium chloride, making D_5½ NS a good choice for maintenance fluids.

Hypotonic solutions are also used to dilute the blood when serum levels of an electrolyte or glucose become too high.

- **Hypertonic**—These solutions have more particles than plasma, therefore they produce a pressure gradient that causes fluid to move from the cells and interstitial spaces back into the vascular bed. Patients with low electrolyte levels are likely to receive hypertonic solutions.

The dextrose in 5% dextrose in water (D_5W) can be easily metabolized by the average person, leaving the equivalent of distilled water in the bloodstream (Metheny, 2012). Therefore, D_5W provides a hypotonic effect, liberating water from the bloodstream to the cells. Higher concentrations of dextrose are not metabolized as quickly and therefore provide a hypertonic effect (pulling fluid from the cells into the vascular space). Normal serum osmolarity is approximately 300 mOsm/L (David, 2007). The normal range for tonicity of an IV solution is 240 to 340 mOsm/L (Kee, Paulanka, Polek, 2010). Although the osmolarity of D_5¼ NS is 331 mOsm/L, D_5¼ NS acts like a hypotonic solution. The effect of the solution is primarily determined by the tonicity of the solution to which D_5W is added. Because ¼ NS is a hypotonic solution, adding the equivalent of distilled water (D_5W) heightens the hypotonic effect.

Other less commonly used intravenous solutions are:

- Dextrose 5% in 0.3% sodium chloride (D_5 ⅓ NS) is sometimes used as maintenance fluid.

- 3% sodium chloride (3% NaCl) and 5% sodium chloride (5% NaCl) are very hypertonic solutions used to raise the serum sodium or to pull fluid back into the vascular space.

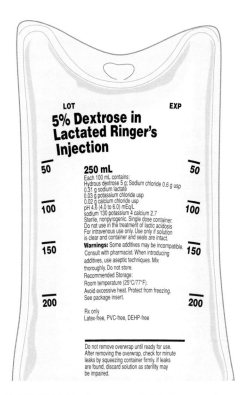

FIGURE 10-7   Dextrose 5% in Lactated Ringer's solution, D₅LR, is a replacement fluid and can be used to correct acidosis (except lactic acidosis) because lactate, when metabolized, converts to bicarbonate, thereby acting as a buffer (acid neutralizer).

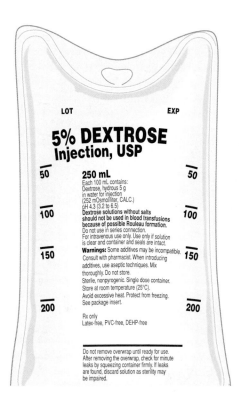

FIGURE 10-8   Dextrose 5% in water, D₅W, has an initial osmolarity similar to that of intravascular fluid (isotonic), but this concentration of dextrose is rapidly metabolized, changing the osmolality of the solution (to hypotonic).

- Ringer's solution, an isotonic solution like LR but without lactate, is used in a similar fashion to LR, but does not act as a buffering agent.

- 5% dextrose in Lactated Ringer's (D₅LR) adds calories to LR (**Figure 10-7**).

- 5% dextrose in water (D₅W) is a hypotonic solution used to lower serum sodium levels (**Figure 10-8**).

- 10% dextrose in water (D₁₀W) is a hypertonic solution used to provide calories and to maintain blood sugar levels.

Solution Additives

Some IV solutions are available, premixed by the manufacturer, with additives such as medications or electrolytes. **Figure 10-9** shows an IV solution premixed with potassium chloride (KCl), a commonly prescribed additive for IV maintenance fluids. **Figure 10-10** shows an IV solution premixed with heparin, a medication that decreases the clotting ability of the blood. Premixed additives are clearly marked on IV solution bags. As shown in **Figure 10-11**, additives can also be inserted by the nurse or pharmacist into an IV solution through an injection port on the solution container, after which a label should be applied, indicating the name and amount of additive, date, time, and signature of the person mixing the IV. If the solution is to be stored, the expiration date and storage information are also written on the label.

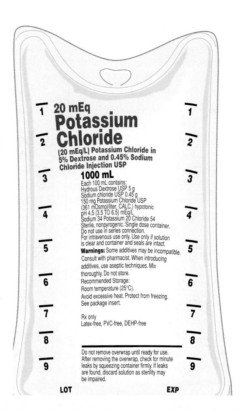

FIGURE 10-9 This premixed liter bag of D₅½ NS + 20 mEq KCl shows the additive, KCl, clearly marked in red.

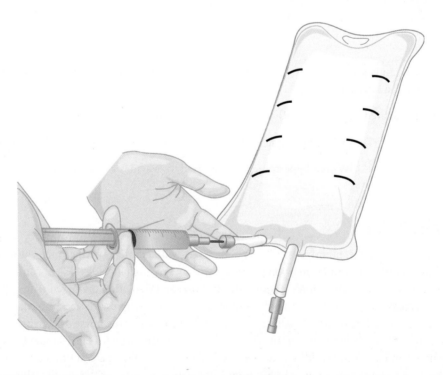

FIGURE 10-10 IV solution bags have injection ports on the front or bottom of the bag. The nurse is injecting a medication into the injection port at the bottom of this IV solution container.

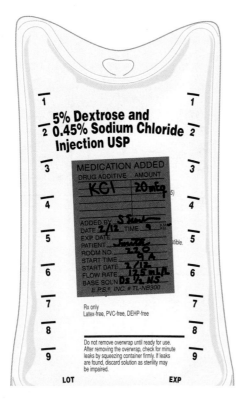

FIGURE 10-11   When the nurse inserts an IV solution additive, a label clearly indicating the name and amount of additive must be applied to the solution container.

LEARNING ACTIVITY 10-1 Define the term and identify one solution with the corresponding tonicity and effect.

1.   Isotonic
2.   Hypotonic
3.   Hypertonic

10-2   Equipment for Infusion Therapy

Solution Containers

Although some intravenous solutions are available in glass bottles, most are supplied in plastic bags (**Figure 10-12**). Solution containers come in various sizes, including 1,000 mL, 500 mL, 250 mL, 100 mL, 50 mL, and 25 mL. Larger solution containers are typically used for continuous infusions, while the smaller bags, sometimes called "mini-bags," and are used for intermittent IV medication administration.

Tubing

Prescribed solutions and medications are infused by way of tubing that connects the solution container to the patient's vein for IV infusion or butterfly needle device inserted into subcutaneous tissue for HDC infusion. The nurse must attach appropriate tubing and then **prime**, or clear the air from the tubing, by running the solution through it. Tubing is primed by following the manufacturer instructions on the tubing package.

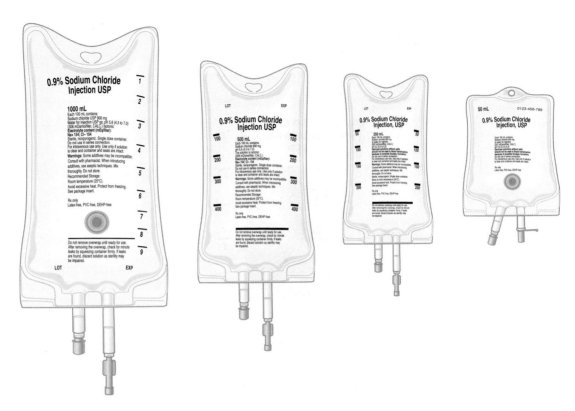

FIGURE 10-12 Intravenous solutions are available in bags of various sizes.

Primary and Secondary Tubing

The main solution, typically the continuous infusion and referred to as the **primary line**, is connected to the patient with primary (long) tubing (**Figure 10-13**). Intermittent infusions, usually medications, are often infused by way of secondary (short) tubing (**Figure 10-14**) connected to the primary line. Most primary tubing is equipped with:

- A spike at the top of the tubing used to pierce the solution container
- A drip chamber used to count drops per minute for manually regulated infusions
- A one-way valve that prevents backflow of fluid from an infusion that is connected to the primary line

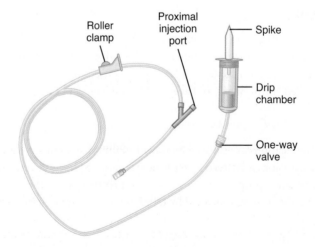

FIGURE 10-13 Primary IV tubing.

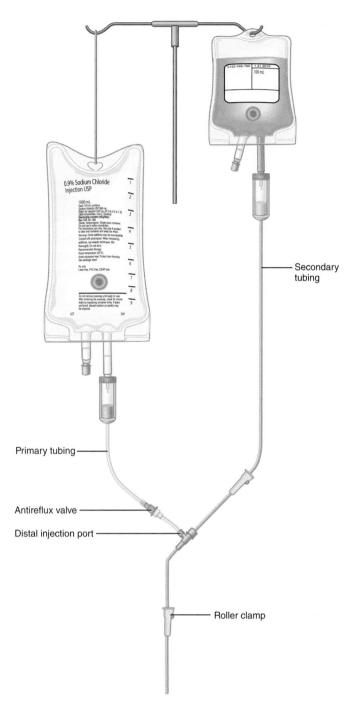

FIGURE 10-14   Medications infused via IVPB must hang higher than the primary solution as gravity will cause the higher solution to infuse first.

- A roller clamp used to regulate the number of drops per minute

- One or more injection ports:

  - The **distal port** (port farthest from the patient insertion site) is the connection point for the **secondary line** used for the infusion of **intravenous piggyback (IVPB)** medications—medications in mini-bags that are connected (piggybacked) to the primary line through secondary (short) tubing.

- The middle port may be used as a connection point to run additional compatible IV primary solutions/medications.

- The **proximal port** (port closest to the patient insertion site) is used for administration of medications that can be directly injected, also called **"IV push"** or **"IV bolus" medications**.

Secondary tubing, much shorter than primary tubing, lacks an injection port and a one-way valve. The absence of a one-way valve allows secondary tubing to be **back-primed** (primed from the bottom to the top of the tubing using backflow from the primary IV solution) once it is attached to the distal injection port on the primary tubing.

Clinical CLUE

For infection control purposes, IV tubing and solutions are changed on a regular basis, in accordance with agency policy. Common practice is to change tubing every 72 to 96 hours (Centers for Disease Control and Prevention, 2011), along with IV site change. Solution changes are generally required every 24 hours.

Blood Transfusion Tubing

The administration of blood and blood products is commonly done with special tubing, called **Y-tubing** (**Figure 10-15**) which has two spikes that are y-connected, to pierce two solution containers, and an **in-line filter**. The y-connected tubing allows normal saline and the blood or blood product to be connected to the same tubing. NS is used to flush the IV tubing before and after the transfusion. The filter removes **microemboli** (small clots) and particles from the blood before it is infused into the patient. Blood transfusions are regulated in the same way as any intravenous infusion.

In-Line Filters

Besides blood and blood products, some intravenous solutions require the use of a filter attached to the primary line (**Figure 10-16**). The main purpose of an in-line filter is to remove particulate matter, such as crystals (which precipitate), from the IV solution.

Monitoring Equipment

Infusion orders include a specific volume of fluid to be infused over a specified period of time. Nurses calculate infusion flow rates in milliliters per hour (mL/h) or drops per minute (gtt/min) and are responsible for establishing, monitoring, and maintaining a prescribed infusion. Infusions can be regulated manually by counting the number of drops per minute that fall in the drip chamber or electronically using an infusion device.

Infusion Pumps

Various types of electronic devices are available to regulate intravenous fluid and/or medication infusions, including the following:

- Traditional infusion pump—Also known as a large-volume infusion device because it is capable of delivering volumes as large as 999 mL in 1 hour

- **Syringe pump**—Also known as a small-volume infusion device because it delivers fluids and medications directly from a syringe; often used in pediatric and critical care settings

- **Patient-controlled analgesia (PCA) pump**—A device that allows the patient to self-administer intravenous pain medication with the press of a button

- **Smart pump**—A computerized infusion pump equipped with medication error–prevention software that alarms when infusion settings exceed best practice guidelines

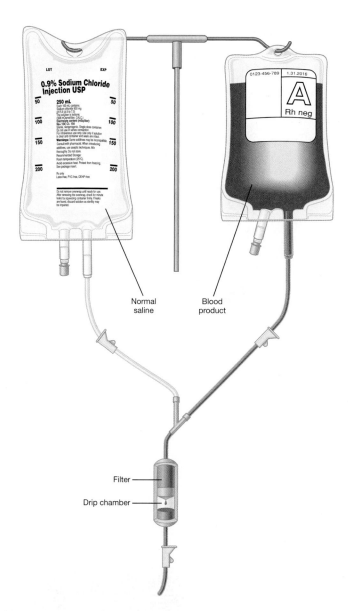

FIGURE 10-15   Y-tubing, used for the administration of blood and blood products, allows for easy access to NS, used to flush a line after a transfusion.

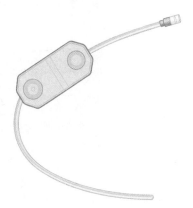

FIGURE 10-16   To infuse highly concentrated IV solutions, the nurse should attach an in-line filter to the primary line.

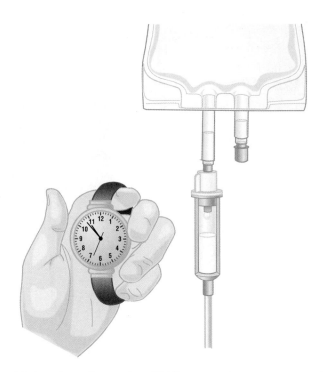

FIGURE 10-17   To establish a manually regulated IV flow rate, the nurse counts the number of drops per minute that fall in the drip chamber.

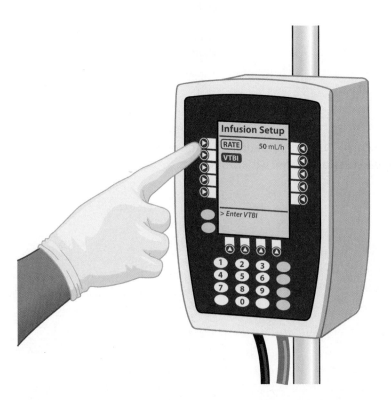

FIGURE 10-18   Most infusion devices can be programmed to deliver a set number of milliliters per hour.

WARNING!

Potential for Large Errors with Large-Volume Infusion Devices

Some large-volume infusion devices can deliver volumes as large as 999 mL per hour or more. However, these infusion devices also have the capability of delivering volumes as small as 0.1 mL per hour. Therefore, these pumps can be used to deliver fluids and medications to tiny premature infants or very large adults. Because of the wide range of infusion volumes with traditional infusion pumps, the potential for error is high: "errors of 10, 100, 1,000 or 10,000 times the intended dose can be set inadvertently, with no limits!" (Kaufman, 2009). Double-checking infusion rates and application of the Rights of Medication Administration will help prevent this type of error.

LEARNING ACTIVITY 10-2   Determine the device that should be used to deliver the prescribed intravenous infusion order.

1.   Ampicillin 200 mg in 10 mL NS to infuse over 15 minutes
2.   Morphine sulfate 1 mg as needed by patient
3.   Rehydration fluids, $D_5\frac{1}{2}$ NS @ 150 mL/h

Additional Monitoring Devices

Other devices are available to assist nurses with monitoring intravenous infusions, including:

- **Volume-control set**—This device, also called burette, Buretrol, or VOLU-trol, is a safety device with a maximum capacity of 150 mL that is inserted between the IV bag and the infusion pump (**Figure 10-19**). Used often in pediatric settings to limit the amount of fluid available to the pump, the volume-control set prevents accidental fluid overload due to programming error or pump malfunction.

- **Controller**—This device measures drops per minute to maintain a preset flow rate (**Figure 10-20**). When a controller is not available a hand held device that produces sound to correspond with drop rate, can help the nurse establish a flow rate (**Figure 10-21**).

WARNING!

Gravity Matters!

Follow manufactures directions for bag height, because gravity, not a mechanical pump, forces the fluid into the vein.

Access Devices

Intravenous fluids may be infused through a peripheral vein or a central vein. The most common sites for peripheral (venous therapy) lines are veins in the hands and forearm. Central (venous therapy) lines are inserted into large veins, usually in the neck (jugular vein) or chest (subclavian vein).

Peripheral IV Therapy

A peripheral line is used for short-term IV therapy. To access peripheral veins, a **peripheral venous catheter**, a small flexible **cannula** (tube), is inserted over a needle into the vein, after which the needle is withdrawn. The hub (end) of the catheter is then connected to extension tubing with an injection port on

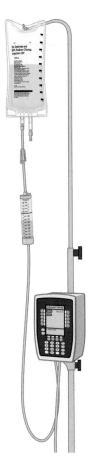

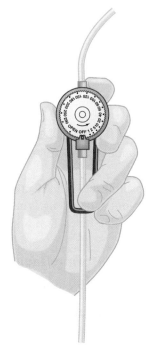

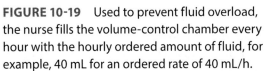

FIGURE 10-19 Used to prevent fluid overload, the nurse fills the volume-control chamber every hour with the hourly ordered amount of fluid, for example, 40 mL for an ordered rate of 40 mL/h.

FIGURE 10-20 To control the flow rate with this dial flow controller, the nurse turns the dial to the prescribed rate and the controller pinches the IV tubing to maintain a pre-set IV flow rate.

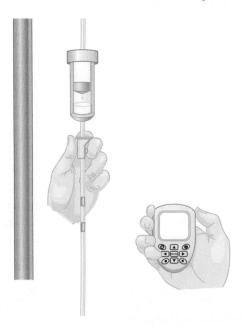

FIGURE 10-21 Enter the flow rate into this handheld device and it indicates, with sound, the appropriate drop rate tempo as the nurse adjusts the drop rate accordingly with the roller clamp.

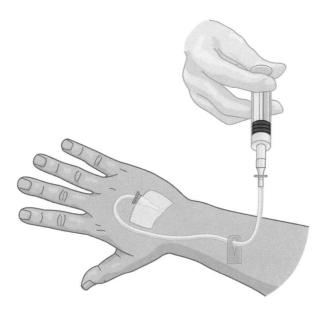

FIGURE 10-22   The nurse flushes this saline lock with a needless device.

the distal end that may serve as an access device for intermittent infusion/medication therapy or may be connected to primary tubing to administer a continuous infusion. Intermittent venous access devices are commonly called saline locks. **Saline locks** are devices that are periodically flushed with normal saline to maintain patency (**Figure 10-22**). Saline locks are accessed for intermittent infusion therapy with a needle or needleless access device. Intermittent IV medications may be given:

■ Via primary tubing into an intermittent access device

■ Through secondary tubing piggybacked to a primary line (IVPB medication)

■ Directly via IV push methods

An IV push (IV bolus) medication is injected directly into the venous access device over one to several minutes, while an IVPB medication is dripped into the vein from a mini-bag.

Central IV Therapy

A **central line** is used for long-term IV therapy and for infusion of very hypertonic solutions, such as highly concentrated electrolyte replacements, chemotherapy, and **total parenteral nutrition (TPN)**. These extremely hypertonic solutions are infused slowly through the thicker walled central veins (veins directly connected to the right atrium of the heart). By keeping the rate of infusion slow, the IV solution is diluted by the blood in these large vessels. IV chemotherapy refers to the infusion of drugs to destroy cancer cells. TPN is an IV solution that supplies all daily nutritional requirements. Various devices can be used for central IV therapy, including:

Clinical CLUE

A venous access device that is periodically flushed with heparin (a blood-thinning substance) is called a **heparin lock**. Before it was discovered that saline was sufficient to maintain patency of peripheral venous access devices, all devices were flushed with heparin and were referred to as "heparin locks." For this reason, some nurses use the terms *saline lock* and *heparin lock* interchangeably.

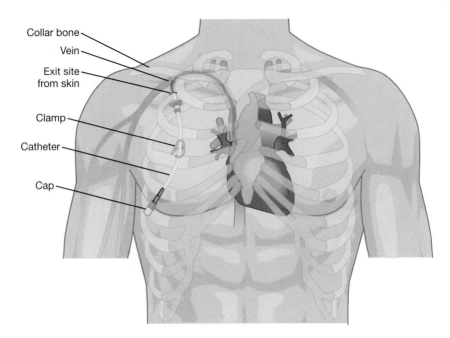

Collar bone

Vein

Exit site
from skin

Clamp

Catheter

Cap

FIGURE 10-23 This central line is inserted through the chest.

- Single-lumen lines (**Figure 10-23**)—Central venous catheters with one external **port** (entry to the intravenous catheter through which an IV infusion or syringe is attached) connected to a single **lumen** (channel through which fluids infuse)

- Triple-lumen lines (**Figure 10-24**)—Central venous catheters with three external ports, each attached to a separate lumen within the same intravenous catheter

- **Implantable subcutaneous infusion ports** (**Figure 10-25**) —Internal ports surgically placed below the clavicle with a catheter threaded through the subclavian vein

- **Peripherally inserted central catheter (PICC) lines**—Long central venous lines inserted into an arm vein (**Figure 10-26**) and threaded into a central vein

Clinical CLUE

The smaller, narrower, thinner walled peripheral veins cannot accommodate highly concentrated fluid. Ten percent (10%) dextrose in water is the maximal concentration of dextrose that can be administered as a continuous peripheral IV infusion. More concentrated solutions must be infused through a central vein.

Hypodermoclysis

Hypodermoclysis is the continuous subcutaneous infusion (CSI) of fluids. Subcutaneous tissue, for HDC, is accessed with a 21- or 23-gauge butterfly needle (**Figure 10-27**) to which tubing is attached through which fluids infuse. Because this infusion technique is considered easy and low risk, it can be administered at home by a nurse or family member. Once the needle is inserted into the fat tissue of the chest, abdomen, thigh, or upper arm, it is secured with an occlusive transparent dressing (**Figure 10-28**). The needle and site are changed every 1 to 2 days.

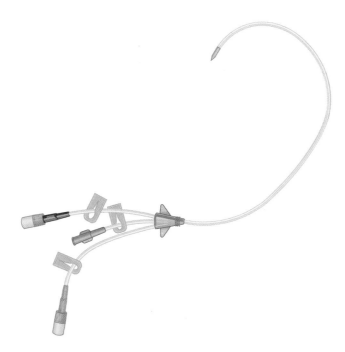

FIGURE 10-24   With a triple-lumen central line, three lines can be accessed simultaneously; for example, TPN can infuse continuously, while intermittent medications infuse into a second line and daily blood draws are done through a third line.

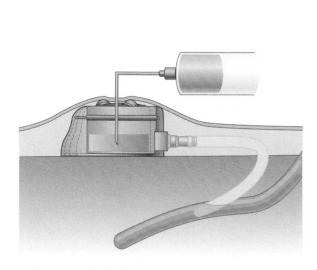

FIGURE 10-25   A port is accessed with a special needle and is a convenient method of intravenous access for patients that require long-term intravenous therapy.

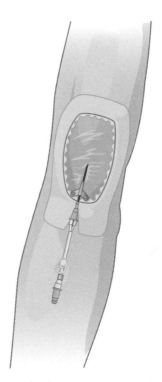

FIGURE 10-26   A peripherally inserted central catheter (PICC) line is usually inserted into the antecubital vein in the arm.

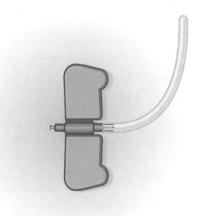

FIGURE 10-27 Hypodermoclysis requires a butterfly needle through which fluids are infused into subcutaneous tissue.

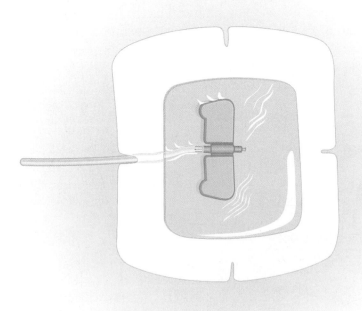

FIGURE 10-28 This occlusive dressing protects the needle used for HDC.

Clinical CLUE

HDC was widely practiced in the 1940s and 1950s until reports of shock caused by administration of hypertonic solutions led to abandonment of this practice by many providers. However, over the past two decades "clysis" has been regaining popularity. HDC, a safe alternative to IV therapy, is used in non-emergency situations. Moderately dehydrated elderly patients and hospice patients who are unable to take oral fluids or who have poor venous access are candidates for HDC (Mei and Auerhahn, 2009).

LEARNING ACTIVITY 10-3 Indicate whether the statement is true or false. Correct false statements.

1.   A volume-control set is used to prevent fluid volume overload.
2.   A PICC line is a peripheral line used for short-term venous access.
3.   TPN can be infused through a peripheral line.
4.   Hypodermoclysis is the subcutaneous infusion of fluids.

10-3   Infusion Flow Rate Calculations

To calculate infusion flow rate, the nurse needs to know the volume of fluid and the time frame for administration. Because most electronic devices regulate flow in mL/h, the nurse will need to calculate the numbers of milliliters per hour. When an electronic device is not used, the nurse will need to calculate the flow rate in gtt/min by counting the number of drops that fall in the drip chamber and manually adjusting the roller clamp to the appropriate number of drops per minute. Maintenance fluids and rehydration therapy usually require a continuous infusion, while an intermittent infusion is often used to administer medications and supplemental fluids. Continuous *medication* infusion rate calculations are covered in Chapter 14 (High-Alert Medications) and Chapter 15 (Critical Care Calculations).

Continuous Flow Rate Calculations

A typical continuous intravenous infusion order includes the IV solution and IV rate, for example $D_5\frac{1}{2}$ NS @ 125 mL/h. For most continuous IV infusion orders, the nurse will select a large IV bag (e.g., 1,000 mL or 500 mL). To implement the order in the previous example, the nurse will attach a primary line to a 1,000 mL bag of $D_5\frac{1}{2}$ NS, calculate the flow rate (if necessary), then establish the flow rate.

Electronically Regulated Flow Rates (mL/h)

Because most electronic infusion devices are programmed to deliver mL/h, many orders, such as the previous one, $D_5\frac{1}{2}$ NS @ 125 mL/h, require no flow rate calculation by the nurse. Once the primary tubing is attached to the solution, the tubing is threaded through the infusion device according to manufacturer instructions, and the device is programmed by the nurse with the ordered rate. If the IV infusion order does not include a rate, it should include the volume of solution and length of time over which the solution should infuse. To determine mL/h using ratio-proportion, $\frac{volume}{hours}$ is the (known) first ratio and the (unknown) second ratio is $\frac{x\,\text{mL}}{1\,\text{h}}$. Perhaps the formula method is the simplest way to determine mL/h (when no conversions are involved):

$$(\text{volume})\ \text{mL} \div (\text{time})\ \text{h} = x\ (\text{rate in mL/h}).$$

Example 1: Calculate the flow rate in mL/h for the IV infusion order.

Order: Infuse 1,000 mL D₅½ NS over 8 hours.

C: *Convert*—Because the volume is in mL and the time is in h, there are no conversions.

A: *Approximate*—Because 8 goes into 1,000 more than 100 times, the rate will be more than 100 mL/h.

S: *Solve*

Ratio-Proportion	Formula Method
$\dfrac{1,000 \text{ mL}}{8 \text{ h}} = \dfrac{x \text{ mL}}{1 \text{ h}}$ or $1,000 : 8 \text{ h} = x \text{ mL} : 1 \text{ h}$ $8x = 1,000$ $x = 125 \text{ mL/h}$	$1,000 \text{ mL} \div 8 \text{ h} = x \,(\text{mL/h})$ $1,000 \text{ mL} \div 8 \text{ h} = 125 \text{ mL/h}$

E: *Evaluate*

Ratio-Proportion	Formula Method
$\dfrac{1,000 \text{ mL}}{8 \text{ h}} = \dfrac{125 \text{ mL}}{1 \text{ h}}$ $8 \times 125 = 1,000 \times 1$ $1,000 = 1,000$	$1,000 \text{ mL} \div 8 \text{ h} = 125 \text{ mL/h}$ $125 \text{ mL/h} = 125 \text{ mL/h}$

Because the calculated amount accurately completes the equation and is consistent with the approximated rate, more than 100 mL/h, the answer is confirmed.

When conversions are required to determine mL/h, as in Example 2, dimensional analysis can be used. As stated in Chapter 7, dimensional analysis (DA) is the multiplication of a series of factors; therefore, to determine mL/h, the first factor starts with mL and the last factor ends with h. Factors must be inserted to allow all units of measurement to be cancelled except mL/h.

Example 2: Calculate the flow rate in mL/h for the IV infusion order.

Order: Infuse 3 L over 1 day.

C: *Convert*—Convert 3 L to 3,000 mL by moving the decimal to the right three places. Convert 1 day to 24 h. For DA, use the conversion factor $\frac{1,000 \text{ mL}}{1 \text{ L}}$ to cancel L (leaving mL in the numerator) and use the conversion factor $\frac{1 \text{ day}}{24 \text{ h}}$ to cancel day (leaving h in the denominator).

A: *Approximate*—Because 24 goes into 3,000 more than 100 times, the rate will be more than 100 mL/h.

S: *Solve*

Ratio-Proportion	Formula Method
$\dfrac{3,000 \text{ mL}}{24 \text{ h}} = \dfrac{x \text{ mL}}{1 \text{ h}}$ or $3,000 \text{ mL}: 24\text{h} = x \text{ mL}: 1\text{ h}$ $24x = 3,000$ $\dfrac{24x}{24} = \dfrac{3,000}{24}$ $x = 125 \text{ mL/h}$	$3,000 \text{ mL} \div 24 \text{ h} = x(\text{mL/h})$ $125 \text{ mL/h} = x$

Dimensional Analysis

$$x\left(\frac{\text{mL}}{\text{h}}\right) = \frac{1,000 \text{ mL}}{1 \text{ \sout{L}}} \times \frac{3 \text{ \sout{L}}}{1 \text{ \sout{day}}} \times \frac{1 \text{ \sout{day}}}{24 \text{ h}}$$

$$x = \frac{3,000 \text{ mL}}{24 \text{ h}}$$

$$x = 125 \text{ mL/h}$$

E: *Evaluate*

Ratio-Proportion	Formula Method
$\dfrac{3,000 \text{ mL}}{24 \text{ h}} = \dfrac{125 \text{ mL}}{1 \text{ h}}$ or $3,000 \text{ mL}: 24 \text{ h} = 125 \text{ mL}: 1\text{ h}$ $24 \times 125 = 3,000 \times 1$ $3,000 = 3,000$	$3,000 \text{ mL} \div 24 \text{ h} = 125 \text{ mL/h}$ $125 \text{ mL/h} = 125 \text{ mL/h}$

Dimensional Analysis

$$125\frac{\text{mL}}{\text{h}} = \frac{1,000 \text{ mL}}{1 \text{ \sout{L}}} \times \frac{3 \text{ \sout{L}}}{1 \text{ \sout{day}}} \times \frac{1 \text{ \sout{day}}}{24 \text{ h}}$$

$$125 \text{ mL/h} = \frac{3,000 \text{ mL}}{24 \text{ h}}$$

$$125 \text{ mL/h} = 125 \text{ mL/h}$$

Because the calculated amount accurately completes the equation and is consistent with the approximated rate, more than 100 mL/h, the answer is confirmed.

Electronic infusion devices are calibrated to whole numbers or to tenths, therefore IV rates are rounded to whole numbers or tenths. The decision for rounding depends on the calibration of the equipment. Because most infusion pumps are calibrated to the whole number, the nurse will most often round IV rates (in mL/h) to the whole number. However, in specialty areas such as critical care and pediatrics, the infusion devices used may be calibrated to tenths, in which case the IV rate should be rounded to tenths.

Rounding RULES!

- If the infusion pump is calibrated to the whole number, the IV rate should be rounded to the whole number.
- If the infusion pump is calibrated to tenths, the IV rate should be rounded to tenths.

LEARNING ACTIVITY 10-4   Use ratio-proportion, the formula method, or dimensional analysis to calculate the infusion rate in mL/h for each IV order, rounding to the whole number if necessary.

1.   **Order:** Infuse 1,000 mL D$_5$LR over 4 h.
2.   **Order:** Infuse 1.5 L over 15 h.
3.   **Order:** Infuse 1.25 L over 1 day.

Manually Regulated Flow Rates (gtt/min)

When no infusion pump is available, the nurse must calculate the flow rate in gtt/min. In order to determine a flow rate in gtt/min, the nurse must know the IV tubing **drop factor** (also called drip factor), a number based on the size or calibration of the drop that falls in the drip chamber. The drop factor, literally the number of drops in 1 milliliter, is found on the IV tubing package. IV tubing with macrodrop (large drop) calibration is available in three sizes: 10 gtt/mL, 15 gtt/mL, and 20 gtt/mL. **Figure 10-29** shows two different drop sizes. IV tubing with a microdrop (small drop) calibration is available in one size, 60 gtt/mL (**Figure 10-30**). Microdrop tubing is also called pedi-drip tubing, because low rates used for children can be manually regulated with this tubing.

Because the rate must be multiplied by the drop factor in order to calculate gtt/min, ratio-proportion is impractical to use. However, both the formula method and dimensional analysis can readily be used to calculate manually regulated IV flow rates. The formula for calculating IV flow rate in gtt/min is:

$$\frac{(\text{volume})\,\cancel{\text{mL}}}{(\text{time})\,\min} \times (\text{drop factor})\,\text{gtt}/\cancel{\text{mL}} = x\,(\text{rate in gtt/min})$$

When the unit of measurement, mL, is cancelled out in this equation, the flow rate is determined in gtt/min. This formula may be more easily remembered by using letters to denote each quantity in the equation: V for volume, T for time, C for drop factor calibration, and R for rate. The formula is:

$$\frac{V}{T} \times C = R$$

When using dimensional analysis for manually regulated flow rates to determine gtt/min:

- The first factor starts with gtt and is the drop factor, $\frac{\text{gtt}}{\text{mL}}$.
- The last factor ends with min, $\frac{1\,\text{h}}{60\,\min}$:

$$x\left(\frac{\text{gtt}}{\min}\right) = \frac{\text{gtt}}{\cancel{\text{mL}}} \times \frac{\cancel{\text{mL}}}{\min}$$

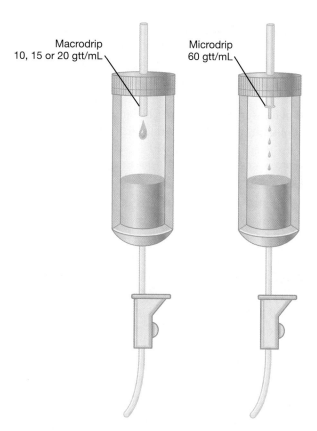

FIGURE 10-29   IV tubing with macrodrop calibration is available in three sizes (10, 15, or 20 gtt/mL), while microdrop is available in only one size (60 gtt/mL).

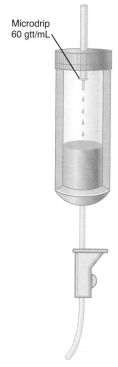

FIGURE 10-30   Tubing with a drop factor of 60 (60 gtt/mL) is also called microdrop (or microdrip) tubing.

■ A middle factor is needed if the time is given in hours, $\frac{mL}{h}$:

$$x \left(\frac{gtt}{min} \right) = \frac{gtt}{mL} \times \frac{mL}{h} \times \frac{1\,h}{60\,min}$$

When the terms (units of measurement) are cancelled in dimensional analysis equations for manually regulated flow rate calculations, gtt/min is left. The rate, in gtt/min, is then rounded to the whole number.

Rounding RULE!

■ Because only whole drops can be counted, manually regulated IV flow rate calculations are rounded to the whole number: 0.5 gtt or more is rounded up, and 0.4 gtt or less is rounded down.

Clinical CLUE

Manually regulated IVs infuse by gravity, therefore infusion solutions must be 2 to 3 feet above the level of the heart to provide adequate gravity flow. IV bags hung higher than this will infuse too quickly, while IV bags hung lower than this will infuse too slowly. Once the IV bag is hung at the correct height, nurses count the number of drops that fall into the drip chamber to establish the flow rate in gtt/min (**Figure 10-31**). To increase the flow rate, the roller clamp is moved up; to decrease the rate, the tubing is tightened by moving the roller clamp down. Because the flow rate of a manually regulated IV can be affected by the patient changing position, it is important that the nurse regularly check/adjust the infusion rate.

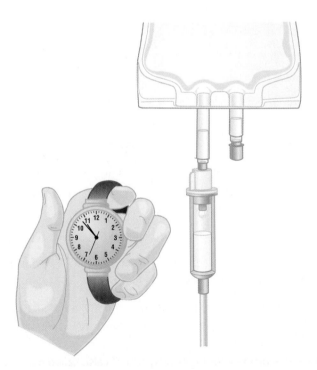

FIGURE 10-31   To establish the correct flow rate in gtt/min, count the number of drops for 1 full minute.

Example 1:   Calculate the flow rate for the following IV infusion order.

   Order: 1,000 mL LR at 100 mL/h, drop factor 15 gtt/mL

C: *Convert*—Convert 1 h to 60 min. For dimensional analysis, use the conversion factor 1 h/60 min.

A: *Approximate*—Because $\frac{100}{60}$ $\left(\frac{mL}{min}\right)$ is approximately 1.5, and 1.5 multiplied by the drop factor of 15 is slightly more than $20\,(1.5 \times 15)$, the drop rate will be slightly more than 20 gtt/min.

S: *Solve*—$V = 100$ mL, $T = 60$ min, $C = 15$ gtt/mL

Formula Method	Dimensional Analysis
$\dfrac{100\ \text{mL}}{60\ \text{min}} \times 15\ \text{gtt}/\text{mL} = x\ (\text{gtt}/\text{min})$ $\dfrac{1{,}500\ \text{gtt}}{60\ \text{min}} = x$ $25\ \text{gtt}/\text{min} = x$	$x(\text{gtt}/\text{min}) = \dfrac{15\ \text{gtt}}{1\ \text{mL}} \times \dfrac{100\ \text{mL}}{1\ \text{h}} \times \dfrac{1\ \text{h}}{60\ \text{min}}$ $x = \dfrac{1{,}500\ \text{gtt}}{60\ \text{min}}$ $x = 25\ \text{gtt}/\text{min}$

E: *Evaluate*

Formula Method	Dimensional Analysis
$\dfrac{100\ \text{mL}}{60\ \text{min}} \times 15\ \text{gtt}/\text{mL} = 25\ \text{gtt}/\text{min}$ $\dfrac{1{,}500\ \text{gtt}}{60\ \text{min}} = 25\ \text{gtt}/\text{min}$ $25\ \text{gtt}/\text{min} = 25\ \text{gtt}/\text{min}$	$25\ \text{gtt}/\text{min} = \dfrac{15\ \text{gtt}}{1\ \text{mL}} \times \dfrac{100\ \text{mL}}{1\ \text{h}} \times \dfrac{1\ \text{h}}{60\ \text{min}}$ $25\ \text{gtt}/\text{min} = \dfrac{1{,}500\ \text{gtt}}{60\ \text{min}}$ $25\ \text{gtt}/\text{min} = 25\ \text{gtt}/\text{min}$

Because the calculated amount completes the equation and is consistent with the approximated rate, slightly more than 20 gtt/min, the answer is confirmed.

It is important to note that the quantity of 1,000 mL in Example 1 is not needed to perform the calculation because the IV flow rate was already given in mL/h as is the case with most IV infusion orders. Because there are 60 minutes in 1 hour, for infusion orders given in mL/h, the quantity before minutes will always be 60. When infusion orders include a time frame greater than 1 hour, the nurse can compute the IV rate using the formula method in one of two ways:

- Using a two-step formula method, first convert the flow rate to mL/h and then calculate gtt/min using the formula $\frac{mL}{60\ min} \times \text{gtt}/\text{mL} = x$ (rate in gtt/min)

- Using a one-step formula method, convert the number of hours to minutes by multiplying the number of hours by 60 min/h and insert the calculated number of minutes into the formula $\frac{mL}{min} \times \text{gtt}/\text{mL} = x$ (rate in gtt/min)

The following order is solved using the one-step formula method, two-step formula method, and dimensional analysis.

Example 2: Calculate the infusion rate in gtt/min for the following order.

Order: Infuse 3,000 mL over 24 h using tubing with a drop factor of 10.

C: *Convert*—For the one-step formula method, convert 24 h to min: $24 \text{ h} \times 60 \text{ min/h} = 1,440 \text{ min}$; for the two-step formula method, convert 1 h to 60 min; and for dimensional analysis, use the conversion factors $\frac{10 \text{ gtt}}{1 \text{ mL}}$ (drop factor) and $\frac{1 \text{ h}}{60 \text{ min}}$.

A: *Approximate*—Because $\frac{3,000}{1,440}\left(\frac{\text{mL}}{\text{min}}\right)$ or $\frac{125}{60}\left(\frac{\text{mL}}{\text{min}}\right)$ is approximately 2, and 2 multiplied by the drop factor of 10 (2×10) is approximately 20, the drop rate will be about 20 gtt/min.

S: *Solve*

One-step formula method: $V = 3,000 \text{ mL}, \ T = 1,440 \text{ min}, \ C = 10 \text{ gtt/mL}$

Two-step formula method: $V = 125 \text{ mL}, \ T = 60 \text{ min}, \ C = 10 \text{ gtt/mL}$

One-Step Formula Method	Two-Step Formula Method
$\dfrac{3,000 \text{ mL}}{1,440 \text{ min}} \times 10 \text{ gtt/mL} = x \text{ (gtt/min)}$	Step 1: $3,000 \text{ mL} \div 24 \text{ h} = 125 \text{ mL/h}$
$\dfrac{30,000 \text{ gtt}}{1,440 \text{ min}} = x$	Step 2:
$20.8 \text{ gtt/min} = x$	$\dfrac{125 \text{ mL}}{60 \text{ min}} \times 10 \text{ gtt/mL} = x \text{ (gtt/min)}$
Rate is rounded to 21 gtt/min.	$\dfrac{1,250 \text{ gtt}}{60 \text{ min}} = x$
	$20.8 \text{ gtt/min} = x$
	Rate is rounded to 21 gtt/min.

Dimensional Analysis

$$x\left(\frac{\text{gtt}}{\text{min}}\right) = \frac{10 \text{ gtt}}{1 \text{ mL}} \times \frac{3,000 \text{ mL}}{24 \text{ h}} \times \frac{1 \text{ h}}{60 \text{ min}}$$

$$x = \frac{30,000 \text{ gtt}}{1,440 \text{ min}}$$

$$x = 20.8 \text{ gtt/min}$$

Rate is rounded to 21 gtt/min.

E: *Evaluate*

One-Step Formula Method	Two-Step Formula Method
$\dfrac{3,000 \text{ mL}}{1,440 \text{ min}} \times 10 \text{ gtt/mL} = 20.8 \text{ gtt/min}$	Step 1: 3,000 mL ÷ 24h = 125 mL/h
	Step 2:
$\dfrac{30,000 \text{ gtt}}{1,440 \text{ min}} = 20.8 \text{ gtt/min}$	$\dfrac{125 \text{ mL}}{60 \text{ min}} \times 10 \text{ gtt/mL} = 20.8 \text{ gtt/min}$
20.8 gtt/min = 20.8 gtt/min	$\dfrac{1,250 \text{ gtt}}{60 \text{ min}} = 20.8 \text{ gtt/min}$
	20.8 gtt/min = 20.8 gtt/min

Dimensional Analysis

$$20.8 \text{ gtt/min} = \frac{10 \text{ gtt}}{1 \text{ mL}} \times \frac{3,000 \text{ mL}}{24 \text{ h}} \times \frac{1 \text{ h}}{60 \text{ min}}$$

$$20.8 \text{ gtt/min} = \frac{30,000 \text{ gtt}}{1,440 \text{ min}}$$

$$20.8 \text{ gtt/min} = 20.8 \text{ gtt/min}$$

Because the calculated amount accurately completes the equation and the calculated rate is consistent with the approximated rate, roughly 20 gtt/min, the answer is confirmed.

LEARNING ACTIVITY 10-5   Using the formula method or dimensional analysis, calculate the infusion rate in gtt/min for each IV order, rounding to the whole number, if necessary.

1.   **Order:** Infuse 100 mL/h; drop factor 20.
2.   **Order:** Infuse 75 mL/h; drop factor 10.
3.   **Order:** Infuse 1,000 mL D$_5$LR over 4 h; drop factor 15.

Intermittent Flow Rate Calculations

Intermittent infusions are used to administer scheduled or prn intravenous medications and/or supplemental fluids. Intermittent infusions can be administered using secondary IV tubing piggybacked to a primary IV (IVPB) or via primary tubing inserted into a saline lock. Intermittent medications can also be delivered directly via the IV push or IV bolus method.

IV Piggyback Medications

Medications given via the IVPB method are usually infused through mini-bags in the sizes of 25, 50, 100, and 250 mL. Medications given in smaller volumes can be infused through a syringe pump or volume-control set (Such calculations are covered in Chapter 12, Dosage Calculations for Special Patient Populations). Infusion volume and time may or may not be included with intravenous medication orders. If not ordered, the nurse will seek this information from a drug reference. The infusion time for intermittent intravenous medications is often less than 1 hour; therefore, if using an electronic infusion device, the nurse will need to convert the rate to mL/h. Because there are 60 minutes in 1 hour, mL/h can be determined from minutes using:

- Ratio proportion, with first ratio as the ordered $\frac{\text{mL}}{\text{min}}$ and the second ratio $\frac{x \text{ mL}}{60 \text{ min}}$

- The formula method: $\frac{\text{mL}}{\cancel{\text{min}}} \times 60 \ \cancel{\text{min}}/\text{h} = x$ (rate in mL/h)

- Dimensional analysis using an equation similar to the formula method with the first factor, $\frac{\text{mL}}{\text{min}}$, and the second factor, $\frac{60 \text{ min}}{1 \text{ h}}$:

$$x \ (\text{mL/h}) = \frac{\text{mL}}{\cancel{\text{min}}} \times \frac{60 \ \cancel{\text{min}}}{1 \text{ h}}$$

Example 1:   Infuse 500 mg of ampicillin in 100 mL D$_5$W over 30 minutes.

> **NOTE:** To carry out this order, the nurse or pharmacist first reconstitutes 500 mg of ampicillin and then adds it to a 100 mL mini-bag of D$_5$W. The only information that is needed to calculate a basic infusion rate is the volume and the time (the quantity, 500 mg, is not used).

C: *Convert*—Because the volume is in mL, there is no conversion for ratio-proportion (R-P) or the formula method (FM). For dimensional analysis, the first factor is $\frac{100 \text{ mL}}{30 \text{ min}}$ and the last factor is $\frac{60 \text{ min}}{1 \text{ h}}$.

A: *Approximate*—Because 100 mL will infuse in 1 hour, at the rate of 100 mL/h, 100 mL will infuse in a half hour (twice as fast), at twice the rate (200 mL/h).

S: *Solve*

Ratio-Proportion	Formula Method
$\dfrac{100 \text{ mL}}{30 \text{ min}} = \dfrac{x \text{ mL}}{60 \text{ min}}$ or	$\dfrac{100 \text{ mL}}{30 \ \cancel{\text{min}}} \times 60 \ \cancel{\text{min}}/\text{h} = x \ (\text{mL/h})$
$100 \text{ mL}: 30 \text{ min} = x \text{ mL}: 60 \text{ min}$	$\dfrac{6{,}000 \text{ mL/h}}{30} = x$
$30x = 6{,}000$	$200 \text{ mL/h} = x$
$\dfrac{30x}{30} = \dfrac{6{,}000}{30}$	
$x = 200 \text{ mL per 60 min or } 200 \text{ mL/h}$	

Dimensional Analysis
$x \ (\text{mL/h}) = \dfrac{100 \text{ mL}}{30 \ \cancel{\text{min}}} \times \dfrac{60 \ \cancel{\text{min}}}{1 \text{ h}}$
$x = \dfrac{6{,}000 \text{ mL}}{30 \text{ h}}$
$x = 200 \text{ mL/h}$

E: *Evaluate*

Ratio-Proportion	Formula Method
$\dfrac{100\ mL}{30\ min} = \dfrac{200\ mL}{60\ min}$ or	$\dfrac{100\ mL}{30\ \cancel{min}} \times 60\ \cancel{min}/h = 200\ mL/h$
100 mL: 30 min = 200 mL: 60 min	$\dfrac{6{,}000\ mL/h}{30} = 200\ mL/h$
$30 \times 200 = 6{,}000$	$200\ mL/h = 200\ mL/h$
$6{,}000 = 6{,}000$	

Dimensional Analysis

$$200\ mL/h = \frac{100\ mL}{30\ \cancel{min}} \times \frac{60\ \cancel{min}}{1\ h}$$

$$200\ mL/h = \frac{6{,}000\ mL}{30\ h}$$

$$200\ mL/h = 200\ mL/h$$

Because the calculated amount accurately completes the equation and the calculated rate is consistent with the approximated rate, 200 mL/h, the answer is confirmed.

To calculate a manually regulated IV flow rate, the nurse can use the formula method or dimensional analysis, as shown in Example 2.

Example 2:   Infuse ampicillin 250 mg in 50 mL D_5W over 45 minutes; drop factor 20.

Recall, the only information needed to perform this (basic) IV flow rate calculation is the volume (mL), time (min), and drop factor (gtt/mL).

C: *Convert*—Because the time is needed in minutes and given in minutes, no conversion is needed.

A: *Approximate*—Because $\frac{50}{45}\left(\frac{mL}{min}\right)$ is approximately 1, and 1 multiplied by the drop factor of 20 (1×20) is approximately 20, the drop rate will be slightly more than 20 gtt/min.

S: *Solve*— $V = 50\ mL,\ T = 45\ min,\ C = 20\ gtt/mL$

Formula Method	Dimensional Analysis
$\dfrac{50\ \cancel{mL}}{45\ min} \times 20\ gtt/\cancel{mL} = x\ (gtt/min)$	$x\ (gtt/min) = \dfrac{20\ gtt}{1\ \cancel{mL}} \times \dfrac{50\ \cancel{mL}}{45\ min}$
$\dfrac{1{,}000\ gtt}{45\ min} = x$	$x = \dfrac{1{,}000\ gtt}{45\ min}$
$22.2 = x$	$x = 22.2\ gtt/min$
Rate is rounded to 22 gtt/min.	Rate is rounded to 22 gtt/min.

E: *Evaluate*

Formula Method	Dimensional Analysis
$\dfrac{50 \text{ mL}}{45 \text{ min}} \times 20 \text{ gtt/mL} = 22.2 \text{ gtt/min}$	$22.2 \text{ gtt/min} = \dfrac{20 \text{ gtt}}{1 \text{ mL}} \times \dfrac{50 \text{ mL}}{45 \text{ min}}$
$\dfrac{1{,}000 \text{ gtt}}{45 \text{ min}} = 22.2 \text{ gtt/min}$	$22.2 \text{ gtt/min} = \dfrac{1{,}000 \text{ gtt}}{45 \text{ mL}}$
$22.2 \text{ gtt/min} = 22.2 \text{ gtt/min}$	$22.2 \text{ gtt/min} = 22.2 \text{ gtt/min}$

Because the calculated amount accurately completes the equation and the calculated rate is consistent with the approximated rate, slightly more than 20 gtt/min, the answer is confirmed.

LEARNING ACTIVITY 10-6 Using the formula method or dimensional analysis, calculate the infusion rate for each intermittent IV medication order, rounding to the whole number if necessary.

1.   **Order:** Infuse cefazolin in 100 mL NS over 40 minutes via infusion pump.
2.   **Order:** Infuse cefazolin in 100 mL NS over 40 minutes; drop factor 10.

IV Bolus (Push) Medications

To administer medications using the IV bolus (also called "IV push") method, the nurse will draw up the needed dose and, with a syringe, administer the medication directly into an IV injection port (**Figure 10-32**). The nurse will need to determine, from a drug reference, the length of time over which

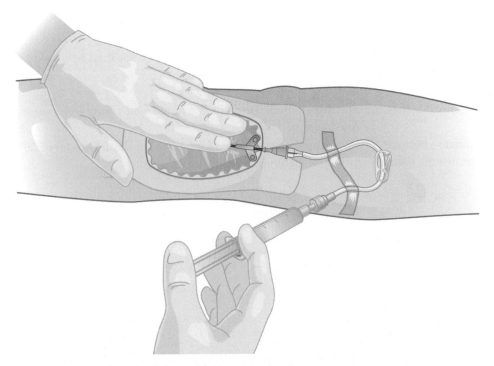

FIGURE 10-32   For IV bolus medications, the nurse will typically administer the medication through the IV tubing injection port closest to the patient.

a medication can be delivered and then, with rare exceptions, calculate the amount to inject at 15-second intervals. By administering small increments and waiting 15 seconds, the medication is diluted by the bloodstream and flush solutions. Most IV bolus medications are delivered over 1 to 5 minutes. Because there are four 15-second intervals in 1 minute, the number of intervals over which the medication should be administered is determined by multiplying the number of minutes (over which a medication should be pushed) by 4 intervals/minute (see **TABLE 10-2**).

WARNING!

Rapid IV Administration May Result in Toxicity

If IV medications are administered too rapidly, they may not be adequately diluted by the bloodstream. Too rapid administration may result in the patient experiencing the toxic effect of an otherwise safe dose.

After determining the number of bolus intervals, the nurse will calculate the volume of medication to administer in each interval by dividing the total volume of medication (plus diluent, if needed) by the number of bolus intervals.

Example 1:   Determine amount to draw up from supply and the volume of medication to be administered every 15 seconds.

Order: ketorolac 30 mg IV bolus q6h

Supply: ketorolac 30 mg/mL

Drug reference: "Administer undiluted 30 mg/min."

C: *Convert*—Because the order and supply are in mg, no conversion is needed.

A: *Approximate*—Because the order is the same as the supply, 1 mL will be needed. The time over which the medication is to be administered is 1 minute (60 seconds). There are four 15-second intervals in 60 seconds, therefore 0.25 mL will be administered every 15 seconds.

TABLE 10-2   Number of IV Medication Bolus Intervals per Length of Time Over Which Medication Is Administered

Length of Time Over Which Medication Is Delivered (in Minutes)	Number of 15-Second Bolus Intervals
1	4
2	8
3	12
4	16
5	20

S: *Solve*—First, determine the amount of ketorolac to draw up.

Ratio-Proportion	Formula Method
$\dfrac{30 \text{ mg}}{1 \text{ mL}} = \dfrac{30 \text{ mg}}{x \text{ mL}}$ or $30 \text{ mg} : 1 \text{ mL} = 30 \text{ mg} : x \text{ mL}$ $30x = 30$ $\dfrac{30x}{30} = \dfrac{30}{30}$ $x = 1 \text{ mL}$	$\dfrac{30 \text{ mg}}{30 \text{ mg}} \times 1 \text{ mL} = x \text{ (mL)}$ $\dfrac{30 \text{ mL}}{30} = x$ $1 \text{ mL} = x$

Dimensional Analysis
$x \text{ (mL)} = \dfrac{1 \text{ mL}}{30 \text{ mg}} \times \dfrac{30 \text{ mg}}{1}$ $x = \dfrac{30 \text{ mL}}{30}$ $x = 1 \text{ mL}$

E: *Evaluate*

Ratio-Proportion	Formula Method
$\dfrac{30 \text{ mg}}{1 \text{ mL}} = \dfrac{30 \text{ mg}}{1 \text{ mL}}$ $30 \times 1 = 1 \times 30$ $30 = 30$	$\dfrac{30 \text{ mg}}{30 \text{ mg}} \times 1 \text{ mL} = 1 \text{ mL}$ $\dfrac{30 \text{ mL}}{30} = 1 \text{ mL}$ $1 \text{ mL} = 1 \text{ mL}$

Dimensional Analysis
$1 \text{ mL} = \dfrac{1 \text{ mL}}{30 \text{ mg}} \times \dfrac{30 \text{ mg}}{1}$ $1 \text{ mL} = \dfrac{30 \text{ mL}}{30}$ $1 \text{ mL} = 1 \text{ mL}$

Because the calculated volume accurately completes the equation and is consistent with the approximated volume, 1 mL, the answer is confirmed.

Next, use Table 10-2 to determine or calculate the number of bolus intervals in 1 minute:

$$1 \text{ min} \times 4 \text{ intervals/min} = 4 \text{ intervals}$$

Next, calculate volume of medication to administer with each interval by dividing the total volume of medication by the number of intervals in 1 minute (4):

$$1 \text{ mL} \div 4 \text{ intervals} = 0.25 \text{ mL/interval}$$

To administer 1 mL of ketorolac IV push over 1 minute, the nurse will administer 0.25 mL per interval.

Some intravenous bolus medications must be further diluted before administration, in which case the nurse will determine the volume of medication to be administered per interval based on the amount of medication, plus diluent, as done in Example 2.

Example 2:   Determine amount to draw up from supply and the volume of medication to be administered every 15 seconds.

Order: hydromorphone 1.5 mg IV bolus q4h prn pain

Supply: hydromorphone 1 mg/mL

Drug reference: "Dilute in SW (sterile water) or NS (normal saline) a total of 5 mL (medication + diluent) and administer over 4 min."

C: *Convert*—Because the order and supply are in mg, no conversion is needed.

A: *Approximate*—Because the order is 1.5 times the supply of 1 mL (1.5 × 1), 1.5 mL will be needed. Per Table 10-2, there are sixteen 15-second intervals in 4 minutes. 5 mL (medication + diluent) divided by 16 intervals will be less than 0.5 mL administered per interval.

S: *Solve*—First, determine the amount of hydromorphone to draw up.

Ratio-Proportion	Formula Method
$\dfrac{1 \text{ mg}}{1 \text{ mL}} = \dfrac{1.5 \text{ mg}}{x \text{ mL}}$ or $1 \text{ mL} : 1 \text{ mL} = 1.5 \text{ mg} : x \text{ mL}$ $1x = 1.5$ $\dfrac{1x}{1} = \dfrac{1.5}{1}$ $x = 1.5 \text{ mL}$	$\dfrac{1.5 \text{ mg}}{1 \text{ mg}} \times 1 \text{ mL} = x \text{ (mL)}$ $\dfrac{1.5 \text{ mL}}{1} = x$ $1.5 \text{ mL} = x$

Dimensional Analysis

$$x \text{ (mL)} = \dfrac{1 \text{ mL}}{1 \text{ mg}} \times \dfrac{1.5 \text{ mg}}{1}$$

$$x = \dfrac{1.5 \text{ mL}}{1}$$

$$x = 1.5 \text{ mL}$$

E: *Evaluate*

Ratio-Proportion	Formula Method
$\dfrac{1\,mg}{1\,mL} = \dfrac{1.5\,mg}{1.5\,mL}$ $1 \times 1.5 = 1 \times 1.5$ $1.5 = 1.5$	$\dfrac{1.5\,\cancel{mg}}{1\,\cancel{mg}} \times 1\,mL = 1.5\,mL$ $\dfrac{1.5\,mL}{1} = 1.5\,mL$ $1.5\,mL = 1.5\,mL$

Dimensional Analysis

$$1.5\,mL = \dfrac{1\,mL}{1\,\cancel{mg}} \times \dfrac{1.5\,\cancel{mg}}{1}$$

$$1.5\,mL = \dfrac{1.5\,mL}{1}$$

$$1.5\,mL = 1.5\,mL$$

Because the calculated amount accurately completes the equation and is consistent with the approximated volume, 1.5 mL, the answer is confirmed.

The nurse will draw up 1.5 mL of hydromorphone. Because the hydromorphone must be diluted to a total of 5 mL, the nurse will add 3.5 mL of NS or SW to 1.5 mL of medication for a total volume of 5 mL.

Next, use Table 10-2 to determine or calculate the number of bolus intervals in 4 minutes:

$$4 \ \cancel{min} \times 4 \ intervals/\cancel{min} = 16 \ intervals$$

Next, calculate the volume of medication to administer with each interval by dividing the total volume of medication by the number of intervals (16):

$$5 \ mL \div 16 \ intervals = 0.3 \ mL/interval$$

To administer 5 mL of hydromorphone IV bolus over 4 minutes, the nurse will administer 0.3 mL/interval.

LEARNING ACTIVITY 10-7 Answer the following questions for each IV bolus medication order:

a.   What volume of medication will be administered?
b.   How many bolus intervals are needed?
c.   What volume of medication will be administered each interval?
1.   **Order:** Valium® 6 mg IV bolus stat
       Supply: Valium 5 mg/mL
       Reference: Administer undiluted over 1 minute.
2.   **Order:** diphenhydramine 75 mg IV q6h
       Supply: diphenhydramine 50 mg/mL
       Reference: Dilute with NS to a concentration of 25 mg/mL; administer over 3 minutes.

WARNING!

Patients Need Patience with IV Bolus Medications!

The Institute for Safe Medication Practices (ISMP) reported an incident in which an emergency room patient died after receiving a bolus dose of labetalol over a matter of seconds instead of over 2 minutes as indicated by the drug reference (Grissinger, 2007; ISMP, 2003). At least one study regarding medication errors reports that *95% of IV bolus drugs are administered too quickly* (Grissinger, 2007). It is imperative that nurses follow protocol (proper dilution and length of time over which medication should be delivered) for administration of IV bolus (push) medications.

10-4   Additional Intravenous Calculations

In addition to IV flow rate calculations, the nurse should be able to calculate how long an infusion should last or how much volume will infuse over a certain period of time.

Time Calculations

To anticipate when an infusion will be finished or when the next bag of IV solution is to be hung, a two-step process is used. The nurse calculates the duration of the volume to be infused (infusion time) and then adds that amount to the current time of day (start time). Infusion time can be calculated with all three methods of calculation, using the IV rate in mL/h and the total volume of IV solution, referred to as "total mL." The "total mL" is the total amount in the solution container or the amount left in the solution container.

Step 1: Calculate the infusion time:

- Ratio-proportion: Set up the proportion with the IV rate, $\frac{mL}{h}$, as the first ratio and $\frac{total\ mL}{x\ h}$ as the second ratio.

- Formula method: Use this formula: volume(mL) ÷ rate (mL/h) = time (h)

- Dimensional analysis: Because the time in hours is the unknown quantity, the first factor will be the rate, $\frac{h}{mL}$, and the second factor will be $\frac{total\ mL}{1}$.

Step 2: Add the infusion time to the start time.

To add international (also called "military") time:

- Convert the infusion time to hours and minutes.

- Separate the start time into hours and minutes.

- Add the hours; add the minutes.

- When minutes exceed 60, subtract 60 minutes and convert it to 1 hour, and add to the hour(s). For example, when the start time is 1235 and the infusion time is 5 h 35 min, to determine the end time:

  - Convert 1235 to 12 h 35 min.

$$\begin{array}{r} 12\ h\ 35\ min \\ +\ 05\ h\ 35\ min \\ \hline 17\ h\ 70\ min \end{array}$$

  - Add the hours; add the minutes: (as above)

  - Convert 70 min to 1 h 10 min and add to 17 h: $\begin{array}{r} 17\ h\ 00\ min \\ +01\ h\ 10\ min \\ \hline 18\ h\ 10\ min \end{array}$, therefore the infusion will end at 1810, or 6:10 p.m.

- When the added infusion time exceeds 2400, subtract 24 h 00 min from the total (because the day ends at 2400) to determine completion time on the next day. For example, when the start time is 2100 and the infusion time is 8 h, to determine the end time:

  - Convert 2100 to 21 h 00 min and 8 h to 08 h 00 min.

  $$21 \text{ h } 00 \text{ min}$$

  - Add the hours; add the minutes: $\underline{+08 \text{ h } 00 \text{ min}}$.

  $$29 \text{ h } 00 \text{ min}$$
  $$29 \text{ h } 00 \text{ min}$$

  - Subtract 24 h 00 min from the total: $\underline{-24 \text{ h } 00 \text{ min}}$, therefore the infusion will end at 0500, or 5:00 a.m.

  $$05 \text{ h } 00 \text{ min}$$

Example 1:   Determine the time the following order will be completed.

Order: 1,000 mL D_5½ NS @ 100 mL/h to start at 0730.

C: *Convert*—Because the volume is in mL and the time is in h, there are no conversions.

A: *Approximate*—Because 100 goes into 1,000 ten times, the infusion will last about 10 hours. If the infusion should run for 10 hours and is started at 7:30 a.m., and 7:30 p.m. is 12 hours later, the infusion should end 2 hours earlier at 5:30 p.m.

S: *Solve*

Step 1: Calculate the infusion time.

Ratio-Proportion	**Formula Method**
$\dfrac{100 \text{ mL}}{1 \text{ h}} = \dfrac{1,000 \text{ mL}}{x \text{ h}}$ or $100 \text{ mL} : 1 \text{ h} = 1,000 \text{ mL} : x \text{ h}$ $100x = 1,000$ $x = 10 \text{ } h$	$1,000 \text{ mL} \div 100 \text{ mL/h} = x \text{ (h)}$ $10 \text{ h} = x$

Dimensional Analysis

$$x \text{ (h)} = \frac{1 \text{ h}}{100 \text{ mL}} \times \frac{1,000 \text{ mL}}{1}$$

$$x = \frac{1,000 \text{ h}}{100}$$

$$x = 10 \text{ h}$$

E: *Evaluate*

Ratio-Proportion	Formula Method
$$\frac{100 \text{ mL}}{1 \text{ h}} = \frac{1,000 \text{ mL}}{10 \text{ h}}$$ 100 mL : 1 h = 1,000 mL : 10 h $100 \times 10 = 1 \times 1,000$ $1,000 = 1,000$	$1,000 \text{ mL} \div 100 \text{ mL/h} = 10 \text{ h}$ $10 \text{ h} = 10 \text{ h}$

Dimensional Analysis

$$10 \text{ h} = \frac{1 \text{ h}}{100 \text{ mL}} \times \frac{1,000 \text{ mL}}{1}$$

$$10 \text{ h} = \frac{1,000 \text{ h}}{100}$$

$$10 \text{ h} = 10 \text{ h}$$

Step 2: Add the infusion time to the start time.

$$
\begin{array}{r}
07 \text{ h } 30 \text{ min} \\
+10 \text{ h } 00 \text{ min} \\
\hline
17 \text{ h } 30 \text{ min}
\end{array}
$$

The infusion will finish at 1730, or 5:30 p.m.

Because the calculated amount accurately completes the equation and the calculated time is consistent with the approximated time, 5:30 p.m., the answer is confirmed.

When the infusion time calculation yields a decimal number, convert the decimal number to minutes by multiplying it by 60 min/h. For example, to convert 0.6 h to minutes, the equation is: $0.6 \text{ h} \times 60 \text{ min/h} = 36 \text{ min}$.

Example 2:   From the following order, determine the time the next bag of IV solution will be hung.

   Order: 1,000 mL D$_5$½ NS @ 150 mL/h; started at 1030

C: *Convert*—Because the volume is in mL and the time is in h, there are no conversions.

A: *Approximate*—Because 150 goes into 1,000 more than 6 times, but less than 7, the infusion will last more than 6, but less than 7, hours. If the infusion starts at 10:30 a.m. and 6 hours later is 4:30 p.m., the infusion will end (before 5:30 p.m.) at approximately 5:00 p.m.

S: *Solve*

Step 1: Calculate the infusion time.

Ratio-Proportion	Formula Method
$\dfrac{150 \text{ mL}}{1 \text{ h}} = \dfrac{1{,}000 \text{ mL}}{x \text{ h}}$ or $150 \text{ mL} : 1 \text{ h} = 1{,}000 \text{ mL} : x \text{ h}$ $150x = 1{,}000$ $x = 6.67 \text{ h}$	$1{,}000 \text{ mL} \div 150 \text{ mL}/\text{h} = x \text{ (h)}$ $6.67 \text{ h} = x$

Dimensional Analysis
$x \text{ (h)} = \dfrac{1 \text{ h}}{150 \text{ mL}} \times \dfrac{1{,}000 \text{ mL}}{1}$ $x = \dfrac{1{,}000 \text{ h}}{150}$ $x = 6.67 \text{ h}$

To convert 0.67 h to minutes, set up the equation:

$$0.67 \text{ h} \times 60 \text{ min}/\text{h} = 40.2 \text{ min (round to 40 min)}$$

E: *Evaluate*

Ratio-Proportion	Formula Method
$\dfrac{150 \text{ mL}}{1 \text{ h}} = \dfrac{1{,}000 \text{ mL}}{6.7 \text{ h}}$ or $150 \text{ mL} : 1 \text{ h} = 1{,}000 \text{ mL} : 6.67 \text{ h}$ $150 \times 6.67 = 1 \times 1{,}000$ $1{,}000.5 \cong 1{,}000$	$1{,}000 \text{ mL} \div 150 \text{ mL}/\text{h} = 6.67 \text{ (h)}$ $6.67 \text{ h} = 6.67 \text{ h}$

Dimensional Analysis
$6.67 \text{ h} = \dfrac{1 \text{ h}}{150 \text{ mL}} \times \dfrac{1{,}000 \text{ mL}}{1}$ $6.67 \text{ h} = \dfrac{1{,}000 \text{ h}}{150}$ $6.67 = 6.67 \text{ h}$

Step 2: Add the infusion time to the start time:

$$\begin{array}{r} 10 \text{ h } 30 \text{ min} \\ +\,06 \text{ h } 40 \text{ min} \\ \hline 16 \text{ h } 70 \text{ min} \end{array}$$

Convert 70 min to 1 h 10 min and add to 16 h:

$$16 \text{ h } 00 \text{ min}$$
$$+01 \text{ h } 10 \text{ min}$$
$$\overline{17 \text{ h } 10 \text{ min}}$$

The infusion will end at 1710, or 5:10 p.m.

Because the calculated amount accurately completes the equation and the calculated time is consistent with the approximated time, 5:00 p.m., the answer is confirmed.

Example 3:   From the following order, determine the time the next bag of IV solution will be hung.

Order: 1,000 mL D$_5$LR at 125 mL/h; the nurse notes 600 mL left prior to the end of the shift at 2215.

C: *Convert*—Because the volume is in mL and the time is in h, there are no conversions.

A: *Approximate*—Because 125 goes into 600 almost five times, the infusion will last almost 5 hours. Five hours after 10:15 p.m. is 3:15 a.m., therefore the infusion will end at approximately 3:00 a.m.

S: *Solve*

Step 1: Calculate the infusion time.

Ratio-Proportion	Formula Method
$\dfrac{125 \text{ mL}}{1 \text{ h}} = \dfrac{600 \text{ mL}}{x \text{ h}}$ or	$600 \text{ mL} \div 125 \text{ mL/h} = x \text{ (h)}$
125 mL: 1 h = 600 mL: x h	$4.8 \text{ h} = x$
$125x = 600$	
$x = 4.8 \text{ h}$	

Dimensional Analysis

$$x \text{ (h)} = \frac{1 \text{ h}}{125 \text{ mL}} \times \frac{600 \text{ mL}}{1}$$

$$x = \frac{600 \text{ h}}{125}$$

$$x = 4.8 \text{ h}$$

Note that the size of the bag (1,000 mL) used in this example is not needed to perform this calculation because the equation is based on the volume left in the bag, not the volume of solution at the start of the infusion.

To convert 0.8 h to minutes, set up the equation:

$$0.8 \text{ h} \times 60 \text{ min/h} = 48 \text{ min}$$

E: *Evaluate*

Ratio-Proportion	Formula Method
$$\frac{125 \text{ mL}}{1 \text{ h}} = \frac{600 \text{ mL}}{4.8 \text{ h}} \quad \text{or}$$ $$125 \text{ mL}: 1 \text{ h} = 600 \text{ mL}: 4.8 \text{ h}$$ $$125 \times 4.8 = 1 \times 600$$ $$600 = 600$$	$$600 \text{ mL} \div 125 \text{ mL/h} = 4.8 \text{ h}$$ $$4.8 \text{ h} = 4.8 \text{ h}$$

Dimensional Analysis
$$4.8 \text{ h} = \frac{1 \text{ h}}{125 \text{ mL}} \times \frac{600 \text{ mL}}{1}$$ $$4.8 \text{ h} = \frac{600 \text{ h}}{125}$$ $$4.8 \text{ h} = 4.8 \text{ h}$$

Step 2: Add the infusion time to the start time (current time noted by nurse):

$$
\begin{array}{r}
22 \text{ h } 15 \text{ min} \\
+04 \text{ h } 48 \text{ min} \\
\hline
26 \text{ h } 63 \text{ min}
\end{array}
$$

Convert 63 min to 1 h 03 min and add to 26 h:

$$
\begin{array}{r}
26 \text{ h } 00 \text{ min} \\
+01 \text{ h } 03 \text{ min} \\
\hline
27 \text{ h } 03 \text{ min}
\end{array}
$$

Because there are only 24 hours in a day, when the time exceeds 24 h, subtract 24 h 00 min:

$$
\begin{array}{r}
27 \text{ h } 03 \text{ min} \\
-24 \text{ h } 00 \text{ min} \\
\hline
03 \text{ h } 03 \text{ min}
\end{array}
$$

The infusion will end at 0303, or 3:03 a.m.

Because the calculated amount accurately completes the equations and the calculated time is consistent with the approximated time, 3:00 a.m., the answer is confirmed.

LEARNING ACTIVITY 10-8 Answer the following questions for each infusion order:

a. How much time is left until the next bag of solution is to be hung?
b. At what time should the nurse anticipate hanging the next bag of IV solution?
1. **Order:** 1,000 mL LR @ 75 mL/h; the nurse notes 700 mL left at the end of the shift at 2310
2. **Order:** 500 mL D$_5$½ NS @ 50 mL/h started at 0630
3. **Order:** 1,000 mL ½ NS @ 85 mL/h started at 0800; at 1400 the infusion pump reads 510 mL infused

Volume Calculations

To determine the total infusion intake, or to anticipate future infusion intake when monitoring a patient's fluid balance, the nurse performs volume calculations. Because most infusion devices track volume infused, nurses are most likely to calculate infusion volume for the purpose of anticipating or projecting fluid intake. Similar to time calculations, a two-step process is used:

Step 1: Calculate the infusion time.

Step 2: Calculate the infusion volume.

Infusion volume can be calculated with all three methods of calculation, using the IV rate in mL/h and the total time, referred to as "total h." The "total h" is the number of hours for which the nurse is determining the volume (to be) infused (infusion time).

Step 1: Calculate the infusion time by subtracting the start time from the end time.

To subtract international (or military) time:

- Separate the start time and the end time to hours and minutes.

- Subtract the start time from the end time:

  - Subtract the hours.

  - Subtract the minutes.

- When start time minutes are greater than end time minutes, borrow (subtract) 1 hour from the end time and convert it to 60 minutes and add to the end time minutes. For example, to determine the amount of time that has passed between a start time of 0815 and an end time of 1200:

  - First set up the equation: 12 h 00 min − 08 h 15 min

  - Because 15 min cannot be subtracted from 00 min, borrow 60 min (1 h) from 12 h and convert 12 h 00 min to 11 h 60 min:

$$
\begin{array}{r}
11\ \text{h}\ 60\ \text{min} \\
-\,08\ \text{h}\ 15\ \text{min} \\
\hline
03\ \text{h}\ 45\ \text{min}
\end{array}
$$

- If the end time is after midnight and the start time is before midnight, add 24 h 00 min to the end time before subtracting the start time. For example, if the start time is 2330 (23 h 30 min) and the end time is 0130 (01 h 30 min):

  - Add 24 h 00 min to the end time:
$$
\begin{array}{r}
24\ \text{h}\ 00\ \text{min} \\
+\,01\ \text{h}\ 30\ \text{min} \\
\hline
25\ \text{h}\ 30\ \text{min}
\end{array}
$$

  - Then, subtract the start time from the end time:

$$
\begin{array}{r}
25\ \text{h}\ 30\ \text{min} \\
-\,23\ \text{h}\ 30\ \text{min} \\
\hline
02\ \text{h}\ 00\ \text{min}
\end{array}
$$

Step 2: Calculate the infusion volume.

- Ratio-proportion: Set up the proportion with the IV rate, $\frac{\text{mL}}{\text{h}}$, as the first ratio and $\frac{x\ \text{mL}}{\text{total h}}$ as the second ratio.

- Formula method: Use the formula, $\text{time}(\cancel{h}) \times \text{rate}\ (\text{mL}/\cancel{h}) = \text{volume}\ (\text{mL})$

- Dimensional analysis: To calculate the volume in mL, the first factor is the rate, $\frac{\text{mL}}{h}$, and the next factor is $\frac{\text{total}\ \cancel{h}}{1}$.

Example 1: Calculate the infusion volume for the following order.

Order: 1,000 mL ½ NS @ 85 mL/h. If the infusion was started at 0630, how much will infuse before the end of the shift at 1430?

C: *Convert*—Because the volume is in mL and the time is in h, there are no conversions.

A: *Approximate*—From 6:30 a.m. to 2:30 p.m., 8 hours will pass. If the IV infuses at 85 mL/h for 8 hours, more than 640 mL ($8 \times 80 = 640$) will infuse.

S: *Solve*

Step 1: Determine the infusion time by subtracting the start time from the end time:

$$14\ h\ 30\ min$$
$$-06\ h\ 30\ min$$
$$\overline{08\ h\ 00\ min\ \text{or}\ 8\ h}$$

Step 2: Calculate the infusion volume.

Ratio-Proportion	Formula Method
$\dfrac{85\ \text{mL}}{1\ h} = \dfrac{x\ \text{mL}}{8\ h}$ or $85\ \text{mL}:1\ h = x\ \text{mL}:8\ h$ $85 \times 8 = x$ $680\ \text{mL} = x$	$8\ \cancel{h} \times 85\ \text{mL}/\cancel{h} = x\ (\text{mL})$ $680\ \text{mL} = x$

Dimensional Analysis
$x\ (\text{mL}) = \dfrac{85\ \text{mL}}{1\ \cancel{h}} \times \dfrac{8\ \cancel{h}}{1}$ $x = \dfrac{680\ \text{mL}}{1}$ $x = 680\ \text{mL}$

E: Evaluate

Ratio-Proportion	Formula Method
$\dfrac{85\ mL}{1\ h} = \dfrac{680\ mL}{8\ h}$ or 85 mL : 1 h = 680 mL : 8 h $85 \times 8 = 1 \times 680$ $680 = 680$	$8\ \cancel{h} \times 85\ mL/\cancel{h} = 680\ mL$ $680\ mL = 680\ mL$

Dimensional Analysis
$680\ mL = \dfrac{85\ mL}{1\ \cancel{h}} \times \dfrac{8\ \cancel{h}}{1}$ $680\ mL = \dfrac{680\ mL}{1}$ $680\ mL = 680\ mL$

Because the calculated amount accurately completes the equation and the calculated volume is consistent with the approximated volume, ~640 mL, the answer is confirmed.

When length of infusion time includes minutes, convert minutes to hours, by dividing minutes by 60 min/h; for example, to convert 20 minutes to hours, the equation is:

$$20\ \cancel{min} \div 60\ \cancel{min}/h = 0.33\ h$$

Example 2:   Calculate the infusion volume for the following order.

Order: 500 mL D5¼ NS @ 45 mL/h. If the infusion started at 1230, how much will infuse by the end of the shift at 1800?

C: *Convert*—Because the volume is in mL and the time is in h, there are no conversions.

A: *Approximate*—Between 12:30 p.m. and 6:00 p.m., 5 hours and 30 minutes, or 5.5 hours, will pass. By rounding 45 mL/h to 50 and rounding 5.5 hours to 5, approximately 250 mL (50 × 5) will infuse.

S: *Solve*

Step 1: Calculate the infusion time by subtracting the start time from the end time.

Because the start time minutes are greater than the end time minutes, borrow from the hour and convert 18 h 00 min to 17 h 60 min:

$$
\begin{array}{r}
17\ h\ 60\ min \\
-12\ h\ 30\ min \\
\hline
05\ h\ 30\ min
\end{array}
$$

Convert 30 min to hours:

$$30\ \cancel{min} \div 60\ \cancel{min}/h = 0.5\ h, \qquad \text{therefore 05 h 30 min is 5.5 h}$$

Step 2: Calculate the infusion volume.

Ratio-Proportion	Formula Method
$\dfrac{45\ mL}{1\ h} = \dfrac{x\ mL}{5.5\ h}$ or $45\ mL:1\ h = x\ mL:5.5\ h$ $45 \times 5.5 = x$ $247.5\ mL = x$ Round to 248 mL.	$5.5\ \cancel{h} \times 45\ mL/\cancel{h} = x\ (mL)$ $247.5\ mL = x$ Round to 248 mL.

Dimensional Analysis
$x\ (mL) = \dfrac{45\ mL}{1\ \cancel{h}} \times \dfrac{5.5\ \cancel{h}}{1}$ $x = \dfrac{247.5\ mL}{1}$ $x = 247.5\ mL$ Round to 248 mL.

E: Evaluate

Ratio-Proportion	Formula Method
$\dfrac{45\ mL}{1\ h} = \dfrac{247.5\ mL}{5.5\ h}$ or $45\ mL:1\ h = 247.5\ mL:5.5\ h$ $45 \times 5.5 = 247.5$ $247.5\ mL = 247.5$	$5.5\ \cancel{h} \times 45\ mL/\cancel{h} = 247.5\ mL$ $247.5\ mL = 247.5\ mL$

Dimensional Analysis
$247.5\ mL = \dfrac{45\ mL}{1\ \cancel{h}} \times \dfrac{5.5\ \cancel{h}}{1}$ $247.5\ mL = \dfrac{247.5\ mL}{1}$ $247.5\ mL = 247.5\ mL$

Because the calculated amount accurately completes the equation and the calculated volume is consistent with the approximated volume, ~250 mL, the answer is confirmed.

Note that the size of the bag in Example 1 (1,000 mL) and in Example 2 (500 mL) is not needed to calculate the infusion volume.

Example 3:   Calculate the infusion volume for the following order:

Order: $D_5\frac{1}{2}$ NS @ 110 mL/h. If the infusion started at 2230, how much will infuse before the end of the night shift at 0630?

C: *Convert*—Because the volume is in mL and the time is in h, there are no conversions.

A: *Approximate*—There are 8 hours between 10:30 p.m. and 6:30 a.m., therefore an IV running at 110 mL/h should infuse almost 900 mL in 8 hours.

S: *Solve*

Step 1: Calculate the infusion time by subtracting the start time from the end time.

Because the end time is after midnight and the start time is before midnight, add 24 h 00 min to the end time:

$$\begin{array}{r} 06 \text{ h } 30 \text{ min} \\ + 24 \text{ h } 00 \text{ min} \\ \hline 30 \text{ h } 30 \text{ min} \end{array}$$

Then, convert the start time to 22 h 30 min and subtract the start time from the end time:

$$\begin{array}{r} 30 \text{ h } 30 \text{ min} \\ - 22 \text{ h } 30 \text{ min} \\ \hline 08 \text{ h } 00 \text{ min} \end{array}$$

Step 2: Calculate the infusion volume.

Ratio-Proportion	Formula Method
$\dfrac{110 \text{ mL}}{1 \text{ h}} = \dfrac{x \text{ mL}}{8 \text{ h}}$ or $110 \text{ mL} : 1 \text{ h} = x \text{ mL} : 8 \text{ h}$ $110 \times 8 = x$ $880 \text{ mL} = x$	$8 \text{ h} \times 110 \text{ mL/h} = x \text{ (mL)}$ $880 \text{ mL} = x$

Dimensional Analysis

$$x \text{ (mL)} = \frac{110 \text{ mL}}{1 \text{ h}} \times \frac{8 \text{ h}}{1}$$

$$x = \frac{880 \text{ mL}}{1}$$

$$x = 880 \text{ mL}$$

E: *Evaluate*

Ratio-Proportion	**Formula Method**
$\dfrac{110 \text{ mL}}{1 \text{ h}} = \dfrac{880 \text{ mL}}{8 \text{ h}}$ or 110 mL : 1 h = 880 mL : 8 h $\quad\quad 110 \times 8 = 880$ $\quad\quad\quad 880 = 880$	$8\ \cancel{\text{h}} \times 110 \text{ mL}/\cancel{\text{h}} = 880 \text{ mL}$ $880 \text{ mL} = 880 \text{ mL}$

Dimensional Analysis

$$880 \text{ mL} = \frac{110 \text{ mL}}{1\ \cancel{\text{h}}} \times \frac{8\ \cancel{\text{h}}}{1}$$

$$880 \text{ mL} = \frac{880 \text{ mL}}{1}$$

$$880 \text{ mL} = 880 \text{ mL}$$

Because the calculated amount accurately completes the equation and the calculated volume is consistent with the approximated volume, ~900 mL, the answer is confirmed.

LEARNING ACTIVITY 10-9   Answer the following questions for each infusion order:

a.   What is the infusion time?
b.   What is the infusion volume?
1.   **Order:** 1,000 mL LR @ 75 mL/h. The infusion was started at 0630; project the volume intake prior to the end of the shift at 1800.
2.   **Order:** 500 mL D$_5$½ NS @ 50 mL/h started at 1830; project the volume intake by the end of the shift at 2300.
3.   **Order:** 1,000 mL D$_5$½ + 20 mEq KCl at 125 mL/h started at 1400; project the volume to be infused by 1900.

10-5   Monitoring IV Infusion Therapy

The nurse is responsible for ensuring the correct intravenous solution infuses at the prescribed rate. Additionally, the nurse monitors the patient during IV therapy to determine if the therapy produces the intended effect and observes for side effects or complications of IV infusion therapy.

Initial and Ongoing IV Checks

When initiating intravenous therapy and throughout the therapy, the nurse must apply the Rights of Medication Administration. The right patient must receive the right intravenous solution/medication, in the right amount, via the right route (IV), at the right time, for the right reason, followed by the right documentation. When initiating care for a patient with an IV infusion already in progress, the nurse checks the IV system from top (IV bag) to bottom (insertion site) to perform the "three checks" of IV therapy:

1. Check the container that the solution is correct.

2. Check the drip chamber or the infusion pump screen that the rate is correct.

3. Check the insertion site that the catheter is intact and the site is not compromised (red, swollen, cool and pale, or draining).

After the initial "three checks," the nurse continues to monitor IV therapy at regular intervals (see Clinical Clue), checking the site and rate each time. If a manually regulated IV is infusing too slow or too fast, the nurse adjusts the gtt/min according to the prescribed rate and drop factor. For example, if the nurse observes an infusion rate of 21 gtt/min, but the prescribed order indicates the rate should be 25 gtt/min, the nurse increases the rate to 25 gtt/min. When checking the rate, the nurse assesses if the correct volume has infused. If the correct volume has not infused, the nurse calculates the discrepancy between the actual volume infused and the prescribed volume that should have infused. If there is a significant difference between the actual and prescribed infusion volumes, the nurse notifies the provider. Applying a time tape to an IV allows the nurse to determine at a glance whether an IV is infusing at the correct rate. A **time tape** is a strip of tape attached to an IV container on which the nurse marks the:

- Start time at the top (container number, e.g., #1, #2, #3, may also be included).

- Fluid intervals—For example, for a 1,000 mL IV bag prescribed at 125 mL/h, the fluid intervals would be marked every 125 mL at 125 mL, 250 mL, 375, mL, 500 mL, 625, mL, 750 mL, 875 mL and 1,000 mL.

- End time written on the bottom (see **Figure 10-33**).

Time taping is routinely practiced by nurses working with manually regulated infusions, but can also be used for electronically regulated infusions. Using time tape for IVs infusing through electronic devices aids the nurse in determining that the device is working properly and delivering the correct volume at the appropriate rate.

Complications of IV Therapy

As with any intervention, the nurse monitors the patient for the intended effect and any adverse effect(s). If an infusion is delivered too quickly or too much solution is infused, a patient may experience circulatory

---

Clinical CLUE

The frequency of IV site assessment depends on a variety of factors, including:

- Age and condition of patient
- Type of infusion
- IV catheter location
- Healthcare setting

Many hospitals require hourly IV site assessment for specialty populations (e.g., neonates and the elderly) and q2h assessment for the general patient populations. Administration of certain chemotherapeutic medications requires IV site assessment every 5–60 minutes, depending on the medication. IV sites receiving **vesicant** solutions must be checked every 5–10 minutes. A vesicant is a chemical that causes blistering or tissue necrosis with **extravasation**, leakage into the surrounding tissue. Nurses must learn their agency's requirements for IV site assessment. The Infusion Nurses Society (2012) recommends site assessment at the following intervals:

- q4h for alert patients receiving nonirritant, nonvesicant solutions who are able to report complications
- q1–2h for critically ill patients with cognitive deficits
- q1h for neonatal and pediatric patients
- q5–10 min for patients receiving vesicant medications

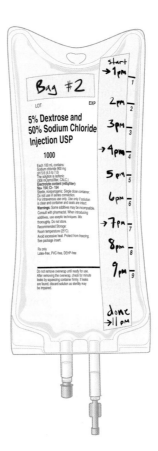

FIGURE 10-33 This time tape, marked at 100 mL intervals for a prescribed rate of 100 mL/h, provides the nurse with the ability to quickly check that the IV is infusing on time.

overload, manifested by an increase in heart rate and blood pressure, and other serious symptoms. If this occurs, the nurse decreases the IV rate and contacts the provider. A very slow rate used to maintain an IV is called a "keep open" or a **KVO** (keep vein open) or **TKO** (to keep open) rate. Keep open rates vary by institution but are generally 15–30 mL/h for adults and 5–10 mL/h for children.

Nurses also monitor patients receiving IV infusion therapy for site complications. The two most common IV site complications include:

- **Phlebitis**—inflammation of the vein caused by the IV fluids and/or additives, producing redness, swelling, and warmth surrounding the insertion site

- **Infiltration**—swelling at the insertion site that occurs when the IV cannula slips out of or pierces the vein, causing fluid to infuse into the surrounding tissue

LEARNING ACTIVITY 10-10 Answer the questions that relate to the following order.

Order: 1,000 mL D$_5$LR @ 150 mL/h to start at 0800 (via infusion pump into a left hand IV site)

1. Determine the fluid intervals with corresponding times (using traditional time) at which the nurse will time tape this solution.
2. At what time will this infusion be complete?
3. What will the nurse include in the "three checks" of IV therapy?
4. What will the nurse include in the ongoing IV checks?

Intravenous Incident ... Case Closure

Because the majority of patients have electronically regulated intravenous infusions, nurses (and nursing students) sometimes forget how to calculate manually regulated flow rates. Had the nursing student remembered the formula for determining manual flow in gtt/min, $\frac{mL}{min} \times \frac{(drop\ factor)gtt}{mL} = \frac{gtt}{min}$, or remembered the concepts of dimensional analysis for determining rate, this error could have been avoided. Many factors affect manually regulated flow rates, one of the most common of which is placement and position of the intravenous catheter in relation to the patient's heart and to the IV bag. As the patient moves, the IV rate can change. Thus, it is important to check the IV rate regularly to ensure that it is infusing on time.

Chapter Summary

Learning Outcomes	Points to Remember
10-1 Differentiate solutions used for infusion therapy.	• Isotonic—same osmolality as plasma/expands volume (NS, LR, D$_5$W, D$_5$¼ NS) • Hypotonic—fewer particles than plasma/moves fluid into cells (½ NS, D$_5$W [after glucose metabolizes]) • Hypertonic—more particles than plasma/moves fluid into bloodstream (D$_5$NS, D$_5$½ NS, D$_5$LR)

10-2 Identify equipment used for infusion therapy.	• Containers—1,000 mL, 500 mL, 250 mL, and mini-bags (100 mL, 50 mL)
	 • Tubing—primary (long) for continuous infusion and secondary (short) for intermittent (medication) infusion
	 • Monitoring equipment—infusion pumps, syringe pumps, smart (computerized) pumps, controllers, volume-control sets
	 • Access devices:
	   ○ Peripheral devices—inserted into a vein in the periphery (hand or arm) for short-term therapy (e.g., saline lock, heparin lock)
	   ○ Central devices—inserted into a central vein (subclavian or jugular) for long-term therapy (e.g., triple-lumen lines, ports, PICC lines)

10-3 Calculate infusion therapy flow rates.	• Electronic flow rates (mL/h): Example (time in hours): 3 L over 1 day Convert 3 L to 3,000 mL and 1 day to 24 h or use conversion factors $\frac{1,000\ mL}{1\ L}$ and $\frac{1\ day}{24\ h}$ <table><tr><td>**RP**</td><td>**FM**</td></tr><tr><td>$\frac{3,000\ mL}{24\ h} = \frac{x\ mL}{1\ h}$ $x = 125\ mL\ /\ h$</td><td>3,000 mL ÷ 24 h = 125 mL/h</td></tr></table>

DA

$$x \left(mL/h \right) = \frac{1{,}000 \ mL}{1 \ \text{L}} \times \frac{3 \ \text{L}}{1 \ \text{day}} \times \frac{1 \ \text{day}}{24 \ h}$$

- Manual flow rates (gtt/min): Use FM or DA.

Example: 125 mL/h with drop factor calibration 15 gtt/mL

Formula Method	Dimensional Analysis
$\dfrac{mL}{min} \times gtt/\text{mL} = x \ (gtt/min)$ or $$\dfrac{V}{T} \times C = R$$ $\dfrac{125 \ mL}{60 \ min} \times 15 \ gtt/mL = 31.25 \ gtt/min$ Round to 31 gtt/min.	$x \left(\dfrac{gtt}{min} \right) = \dfrac{15 \ gtt}{1 \ \text{mL}} \times \dfrac{125 \ \text{mL}}{1 \ \text{h}}$ $\times \dfrac{1 \ \text{h}}{60 \ min}$ $x = \dfrac{1{,}875 \ gtt}{60 \ min} = 31.25 \ gtt/min$

- IV push:
  - Calculate the volume of medication to draw up
  - Calculate the number of 15-second intervals in the length of time of administration (4 intervals/min)
  - Calculate the volume to push in each 15 sec interval
    mL of med (+ diluent) ÷ number of intervals

10-4 Calculate infusion time and volume.	Time calculations: • volume $\left(\text{mL} \right)$ ÷ rate (mL/h) = time (h) • To convert h to min: h × 60 min/h Volume calculations: • time $\left(\text{h} \right)$ × rate (mL/h) = volume (mL) • To convert min to h: min ÷ 60 min /h

10-5 Cite important observations to be made during infusion therapy.	• To initiate IV therapy, observe "Rights of Medication Administration."
	• Initial "three checks" of IV therapy:
	  1. Correct solution
	  2. Correct rate
	  3. Functional site
	• Ongoing checks at regular intervals (e.g., hourly)—check rate and site
	• Complications:
	  ○ Fluid volume overload—too much solution infused or delivered too quickly
	  ○ Infiltration—swelling due to IV fluid infusing into tissue surrounding IV site
	  ○ Phlebitis—inflammation of the vein

Homework

For exercises 1–5, match the IV solution name with the solution description. (LO 10-1)

1. D₅W

2. LR

3. D₅½ NS

4. D₅¼ NS

5. ½ NS

a. hypotonic fluid replacement solution for clients who do not need glucose

b. hypertonic in the bag, hypotonic in the body; typical maintenance fluid

c. isotonic solution that becomes hypotonic after glucose is metabolized

d. isotonic solution containing electrolytes

e. recommended maintenance fluid for children < 30 kg

For exercises 6–10, match the IV label with the solution descriptions a–e. (LO 10-1)

a. a combination of fluid and electrolytes

b. 0.9% sodium chloride

c. 5% dextrose in 0.225% sodium chloride

d. 5% dextrose in 0.45% sodium chloride with 20 mEq of potassium chloride

e. 5% dextrose in a Lactated Ringer's solution

6.

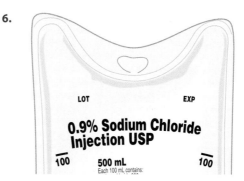

7.

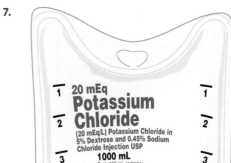

8.

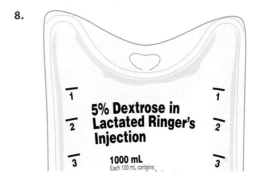

9.

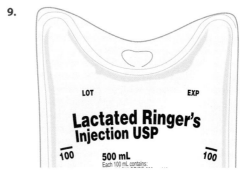

10.

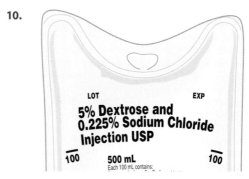

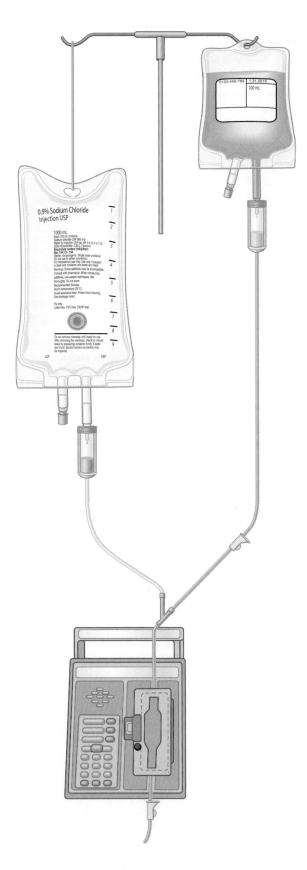

For exercises 11–16, label and describe the intravenous therapy equipment. (LO 10-2)

11. Primary tubing

12. Secondary tubing

13. Primary drip chamber

14. Primary roller clamp

15. Infusion pump

16. Injection port (to add medication to IV solutions)

For exercises 17–20, match the infusion device to the description. (LO 10-2)

17. Smart pump

a. a burette that is inserted between the IV bag and pump

18. PCA pump

b. a small-volume infusion device used for infants

19. Syringe pump

c. a computerized pump containing error prevention software

20. Volume-control set

d. delivers pain medicine when the patient presses a button

For exercises 21–26, calculate the electronically regulated IV flow rate in mL/h, rounding the rate to the whole number. (LO 10-3)

21. **Order:** Infuse 1,000 mL NS over 10 h.
22. **Order:** Infuse 1.3 L $D_5\frac{1}{2}$ NS over 8 h.
23. **Order:** Infuse 500 mL D_5W over 10 h.
24. **Order:** Infuse 1,000 mL LR over 6.5 h.
25. **Order:** Infuse 1,000 mL ½ NS over 12 h.
26. **Order:** Infuse 2 L $D_5\frac{1}{2}$ NS over 1 day.

For exercises 27–30, calculate the manually regulated IV flow rate in gtt/min for each drop factor. Manually regulated IV rates should be rounded to the whole number. (LO 10-3)

27. **Order:** Infuse 1,000 mL D_5W at 125 mL/h; drop factors 10, 15, 20, 60.
28. **Order:** Infuse 500 mL NS at 50 mL/h; drop factors 10, 15, 20, 60.
29. **Order:** Infuse 2 L $D_5\frac{1}{2}$ NS over 12 h; drop factors 10, 15, 20, 60.
30. **Order:** Infuse 1.5 L ½ NS over 10 h; drop factors 10, 15, 20, 60.

For exercises 31–36, calculate the IV flow rate in mL/h or gtt/min as indicated for each IVPB medication order. Round IV rates to the whole number. (LO 10-3)

31. **Order:** Infuse Zosyn® 3.375 g in 100 mL D_5W over 30 min q6h via infusion pump.
32. **Order:** Infuse Zosyn 3.375 g in 100 mL D_5W over 30 min q6h; drop factor 15.
33. **Order:** Infuse Dilantin® 250 mg in 50 mL NS over 45 min q8h via infusion pump.
34. **Order:** Infuse Dilantin 250 mg in 50 mL NS over 45 min q8h; drop factor 10.
35. **Order:** Infuse dexamethasone 4 mg in 50 mL D_5W over 15 min q12h.
36. **Order:** Infuse dexamethasone 4 mg in 50 mL D_5W over 15 min q12h; drop factor 60.

For exercises 37–40, for each IV bolus medication order, calculate the following (LO 10-3):
- Volume of medication to withdraw from the supply
- Amount of diluent to add to the medication
- Number of 15-second bolus intervals
- Volume of medication to administer for each interval

37. **Order:** lorazepam 2 mg IV bolus 30 min prior to chemotherapy
Supply: lorazepam 2 mg/mL
Reference: Dilute with an equal amount of SW (sterile water); administer over 2 minutes.
38. **Order:** diphenhydramine 100 mg IV bolus stat
Supply: diphenhydramine 50 mg/mL
Reference: Dilute with NS (normal saline) to a concentration of 25 mg/mL; administer over 4 minutes.
39. **Order:** famotidine 20 mg IV q12h
Supply: famotidine 10 mg/mL
Reference: Dilute with NS so each 4 mg is in 1 mL solution; administer each 10 mg over 1 minute.
40. **Order:** furosemide 40 mg q12h
Supply: furosemide 10 mg/mL
Reference: Administer undiluted over 2 minutes.

For exercises 41–43, calculate the infusion time and indicate the completion time for each order. (LO 10-4)

41. **Order:** 250 mL D_5W @ 50 mL/h to start at 2330
42. **Order:** 500 mL NS @ 75 mL/h to start at 1120
43. **Order:** 1,000 mL $D_5\frac{1}{2}$ NS @ 120 mL/h; 650 mL left at 0615

For exercises 44–46, calculate the infusion volume for each order. (LO 10-4)

44. **Order:** NS @ 100 mL/h for 2 h 30 min
45. **Order:** 1,000 mL D_5W @ 150 mL/h started at 1930; how much will infuse by 2200?
46. **Order:** 500 mL D5¼ NS @ 60 mL/h, started at 0015; how much will infuse by 0730?

For exercises 47–50, answer the questions that relate to the following order. (LO 10-5)

Order: 500 mL ½ NS @ 75 mL/h to start at 1615 via infusion pump into a right arm IV site

47. Determine the fluid intervals with corresponding times (using traditional time) at which the nurse will time tape this solution.
48. At what time will this infusion be complete?
49. What will the nurse include in the "three checks" of IV therapy?
50. What will the nurse include in the ongoing IV checks?

NCLEX-Style Review Questions

For questions 1–4, select the best response.

1. To infuse 3 L over 24 hours using tubing with a drop factor of 15, the nurse should establish a flow rate of:
   a. 31 gtt/min
   b. 125 gtt/min
   c. 188 mL/h
   d. 1,875 mL/h

2. To infuse ampicillin 500 mg in 50 mL D_5W over 30 minutes, the nurse should:
   a. Set the infusion pump to 10 mL/h.
   b. Establish the flow rate of 17 gtt/min.
   c. Establish the flow rate of 25 gtt/min.
   d. Set the secondary IV infusion rate on the pump to 100 mL/h.
   e. Not enough data to answer the question.

3. The nurse initiates the order for continuous intravenous infusion, $D_5\frac{1}{2}$ NS @ 150 mL/h, with a 1-liter bag of solution at 0900 and anticipates that the next liter bag should be ready to hang at:
   a. 1500
   b. 1540
   c. 1600
   d. 1607

4. The home care nurse is preparing to visit a patient ordered to receive long-term intravenous antibiotic therapy. The nurse expects that the patient will have which access device?
   a. Saline lock
   b. Heparin lock
   c. PICC line
   d. Large-volume infusion pump

For questions 5–6, select all that apply.

5. To administer an intermittent infusion of Zosyn 3.375 g in 100 mL D_5W IVPB over 30 minutes via infusion pump, the nurse should:
   a. Flush the saline lock prior to injecting the medication.
   b. Prime the secondary tubing.
   c. Set the IV infusion pump to 100 mL/h.
   d. Swab the injection port closest to the IV bag with alcohol.
   e. Establish a flow rate of 200 gtt/min.
   f. Calculate the flow rate in mL/h.
   g. Verify compatibility of the medication with the secondary IV solution.

6. Nursing responsibilities regarding intravenous therapy include:
   a. Checking the IV site at regular intervals, according to institutional policy
   b. Calculating the IV flow rate in mL/h
   c. Hanging the primary solution above the secondary solution
   d. Counting the flow rate in gtt/min
   e. Ordering the correct IV solution
   f. Observing the patient for complications
   g. Programming the infusion pump

REFERENCES

Centers for Disease Control and Prevention. (2011). 2011 guidelines for the prevention of intravascular catheter-related infections. Retrieved from http://www.cdc.gov/hicpac/BSI/07-bsi-background-info-2011.htmles-2011.html

Crawford, A., & Harris, H. (2011, May). IV fluids: What nurses need to know. *Nursing 2011, 41*(5), 30–38.

David, K. (October 2007). IV fluids: Do you know what's hanging and why? *Modern Medicine.* Retrieved from http://www.modernmedicine.com/modernmedicine/article/articleDetail.jsp?id=463604

Grissinger, M. (2007). How fast is too fast for delivering IV push medications? *Pharmacy & Therapeutics, 32*(3). Retrieved from http://www.ptcommunity.com/system/files/PTJ3203124.pdf

Infusion Nurses Society. (2012). Recommendations for frequency of assessment of the short peripheral catheter site. Retrieved from http://www.ins1.org/i4a/pages/index.cfm?pageid=3412

Institute of Safe Medication Practices. (2003, May 15). Medication safety alert: How fast is too fast for IV push medications? Retrieved from http://www.ismp.org/newsletters/acutecare/articles/20030515.asp

Kaufman, M. B. (2009, July 20). New IV smart pump technologies prevent medication errors, ADRs. *Formulary ENews.* Retrieved from http://formularyjournal.modernmedicine.com/formulary/Technology+News/New-IV-smart-pump-technologies-prevent-medication-/ArticleStandard/Article/detail/611706

Kee, J. L., Paulanka, B. J., & Polek, C. (2010). *Handbook of fluid, electrolyte, and acid-base imbalances* (3rd ed.). Clifton Park, NY: Cengage.

Mei, A., & Auerhahn, C. (2009, May 8). Hypodermoclysis: maintaining hydration in the frail older adult. *Annals of Long-Term Care*, *17*(5), 28–30.

Metheny, N. M. (2012). *Fluid and electrolyte balance: Nursing considerations* (5th ed.). Sudbury, MA: Jones & Bartlett Learning.

Chapter 10   ANSWER KEY

Learning Activity 10-1

1. Isotonic—tonicity (osmolarity) similar to plasma; examples include NS, LR
2. Hypotonic—lower osmolarity than plasma causing fluid to move from circulatory system to cells (tissue); for example, ½ NS
3. Hypertonic—higher osmolarity than plasma, causing fluid to move from the cells (tissue) into the circulatory system; examples include D_5NS, D_5LR, D_5½ NS (Note: These solutions are hypertonic in the IV container. When glucose is metabolized in the body, the tonicity is altered.)

Learning Activity 10-2

1. Syringe pump
2. PCA pump
3. Large-volume infusion pump

Learning Activity 10-3

1. True
2. False. A PICC line is a peripherally inserted central line used for long-term IV access.
3. False. TPN can be infused through a PICC line or other central line.
4. True

Learning Activity 10-4

1. 250 mL/h
2. 100 mL/h
3. 52 mL/h

Learning Activity 10-5

1. 33 gtt/min
2. 13 gtt/min
3. 63 gtt/min

Learning Activity 10-6

1. 150 mL/h
2. 25 gtt/min

Learning Activity 10-7

1. a. 1.2 mL, b. 4 intervals, c. 0.3 mL
2. a. 1.5 mL, b. 12 intervals, c. 0.25 mL

Learning Activity 10-8

1. a. 9.33 h or 9 h 20 min, b. 0830 or 8:30 a.m.
2. a. 10 h, b. 1630 or 4:30 p.m.
3. a. 5.76 h or 5 h 46 min, b. 1946 or 7:46 p.m.

Learning Activity 10-9

1. a. 11 h 30 min or 11.5 h, b. 862.5 or 863 mL
2. a. 4 h 30 min or 4.5 h, b. 225 mL
3. a. 5 h, b. 625 mL

Learning Activity 10-10

1. Start time 8:00 a.m. @ 0 mL, 150 mL @ 9:00 a.m., 300 mL @ 10:00 a.m., 450 mL @ 11:00 a.m., 600 mL @ 12:00 p.m., 750 mL @ 1:00 p.m., 900 mL@ 2:00 p.m., end time @ 2:40 p.m.
2. 1440 or 2:40 p.m.
3. Check that solution is D_5LR; check that pump is set to 150 mL/h, check left-hand insertion site for presence or absence of complications.
4. At regular intervals, check the site and rate, noting whether the volume is decreasing in the solution container according to the time tape. NOTE: Regular intervals are typically every 1–2 hours, but may be more frequent depending on variables such as age, condition of patient, or type of solution/medication infusion.

Homework

1. c
2. d
3. b
4. e
5. a
6. b
7. d
8. e
9. a
10. c

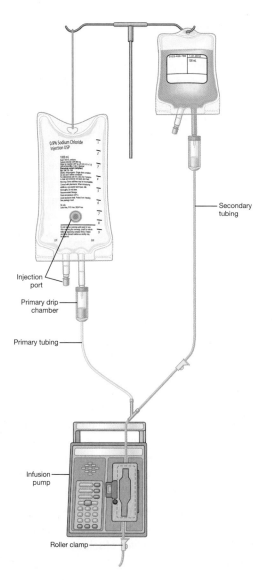

Secondary tubing

Injection port

Primary drip chamber

Primary tubing

Infusion pump

Roller clamp

11. Long IV tubing (which goes from the primary solution to the patient's IV insertion site) with injection ports and a one-way valve

12. Secondary tubing—short IV tubing (which goes from the secondary solution to the distal injection port of the primary line) used for intermittent medication administration

13. Primary drip chamber—site where drops fall and are counted per minute (when infusion is manually regulated)

14. Primary roller clamp—device on tubing used to adjust the gtt/min falling into the drip chamber for manually regulated IVs

15. Infusion pump—Electronic device used to regulate the IV flow rate in mL/h

16. Injection port—Site on IV bag where medication can be inserted

17. c
18. d
19. b
20. a
21. 100 mL/h
22. 163 mL/h
23. 50 mL/h
24. 154 mL/h
25. 83 mL/h
26. 83 mL/h
27. 21 gtt/min, 31 gtt/min, 42 gtt/min, 125 gtt/min
28. 8 gtt/min, 13 gtt/min, 17 gtt/min, 50 gtt/min
29. 28 gtt/min, 42 gtt/min, 56 gtt/min, 167 gtt/min
30. 25 gtt/min, 38 gtt/min, 50 gtt/min, 150 gtt/min
31. 200 mL/h
32. 50 gtt/min
33. 67 mL/h
34. 11 gtt/min
35. 200 mL/h
36. 200 gtt/min
37. Draw up 1 mL of medication; add 1 mL diluent for a total of 2 mL; 8 intervals; administer 0.25 mL/interval.
38. Draw up 2 mL of medication; add 2 mL diluent for a total of 4 mL; 16 intervals; administer 0.25 mL/interval.
39. Draw up 2 mL of medication; add 3 mL diluent for a total of 5 mL; 8 intervals; administer 0.63 mL/interval.
40. Draw up 4 mL of medication; add no diluent; 8 intervals; administer 0.5 mL/interval.
41. 5 h; 0430 or 4:30 a.m.
42. 6.67 h or 6 h 40 min; 1800 or 6:00 p.m.
43. 5.42 h or 5 h 25 min; 1140 or 11:40 a.m.
44. 250 mL
45. 375 mL
46. 435 mL
47. Start time 4:15 p.m. @ 0 mL, 5:15 p.m. @ 75 mL, 6:15 p.m. @ 150 mL, 7:15 p.m. @ 225 mL, 8:15 p.m. at 300 mL, 9:15 p.m. @ 375 mL, 10:15 p.m. @ 450 mL, end time @ 10:55 p.m.
48. 2255 or 10:55 p.m.
49. Check that solution is ½ NS; check that pump is set to 75 mL/h, check right-hand insertion site.
50. At regular intervals, check the site and rate, noting whether the volume is decreasing in the solution container according to the time tape. NOTE: Regular intervals are typically every 1–2 hours, but may be more frequent depending on variables such as age, condition of patient, or type of solution/medication infusion.

NCLEX-Style Review Questions

1. a

   Rationale: 3 L (3,000 mL) over 24 h = 125 mL/h; because a drop factor is given and no infusion pump is indicated, the rate will be in gtt/min. Because 125 mL is infusing every 60 minutes with a drop factor of 15, the rate will be 31 gtt/min.

2. d

   Rationale: Because no drop factor is given, the rate will be in mL/h. To infuse 50 mL over 30 minutes, the rate must be set to 100 mL/h.

3. b

   Rationale: 1,000 mL (1 L) running at 150 mL/h will last 6.67 h or 6 h 40 min. Because the IV started at 0900 (9:00 a.m.), it should finish 6 h 40 min later—at 1540, or 3:40 p.m.

4. c

   Rationale: For long-term infusion therapy, the patient will need a PICC line. Saline and heparin locks are used for short-term access devices. An infusion pump is an infusion device, not an access device.

5. b, d, f, g

   Rationale: To administer an intermittent infusion via IVPB, the nurse will first confirm the compatibility of the medication and the primary solution (g), then calculate the flow rate in mL/h (f) because the medication is being delivered via infusion pump. Then, the nurse will attach the 100 mL mini-bag to secondary tubing and prime it (b) and attach the secondary tubing to the primary tubing to the proximal port after swabbing it with alcohol (d). Finally, the nurse will program the infusion pump to deliver 200 mL/h. Because the medication is being given via IVPB, it will be connected to a primary solution; therefore, flushing the saline lock will not be necessary.

6. a, b, d, f, g

   Rationale: Nursing responsibilities regarding intravenous therapy include checking the IV site at regular intervals according to institutional policy (a), calculating the flow rate in mL/h (or gtt/min) (b) or counting the flow rate in gtt/min (or mL/h) (d), observing the patient for complications (f), and programming the infusion pump to deliver the solution at the correct rate (g). When hanging a secondary infusion (IVPB), the secondary medication will be hung higher than the primary bag so that gravity will cause the higher solution to infuse first. Although the nurse is responsible for checking that the correct solution is infusing, ordering the solution is the responsibility of the provider (licensed independent prescriber).

© Forfunlife/Shutterstock

Chapter 11

Solution Calculations

CHAPTER OUTLINE

11-1 Solution Concentration Calculations

11-2 Additional Solute and Solvent Calculations
    A.   Enteral Feeding Solutions
    B.   Topical Solutions

LEARNING OUTCOMES

Upon completion of the chapter, the student will be able to:

11-1 Calculate solution components based on percentages.

11-2 Calculate solute and solvent volumes based on solution strength.

KEY TERMS

diluent

full strength

hang time

solute

solvent

universal solvent

Case Consideration ... Formula Fiasco

A mother brings her newborn to the emergency room because the infant was vomiting large amounts of formula. The mother explained to the nurse that she had been feeding the infant 2–3 ounces of formula concentrate every 4 hours.

1. What went wrong?

2. How could this situation been avoided?

■ INTRODUCTION

Solution concentration is an important concept for nurses to understand. Nurses may be required to alter a solution strength to make it more or less concentrated, as desired by the licensed prescriber. Medical notation used to indicate solution strength includes percentages, ratios, and fractions.

11-1   Solution Concentration Calculations

Solution concentration expressed as a percentage, as noted in Chapter 9, specifies the number of grams per hundred milliliters. Recall from Chapter 10 that D_5W is dextrose 5% in water; therefore, this solution contains 5 grams of dextrose in every 100 mL of water. To calculate the amount of dextrose in a specific quantity of 5% dextrose solution, the nurse uses one of the three methods of calculation:

■ Ratio-proportion: The supply ratio is the first ratio, the total volume is the denominator of the second ratio, and the equation is set up as: $\frac{5\text{ g}}{100\text{ mL}} = \frac{x\text{ g}}{\text{total mL}}$

■ Formula method: $\frac{\text{total mL}}{\text{supply mL}} \times \text{g} = x \text{ (g)}$, applied to a calculation with 5% dextrose is:

$$\frac{\text{total } \cancel{\text{mL}}}{100 \ \cancel{\text{mL}}} \times 5 \text{ g} = x \text{ (g)}$$

■ Dimensional analysis: To solve for grams (g), the first factor is the supply, $\frac{\text{g}}{100\text{ mL}}$, and the next factor is the total volume as $\frac{\text{total mL}}{1}$. (Additional factors are inserted in the equation, as needed.) A calculation using 5% dextrose is set up as:

$$x \text{ (g)} = \frac{5 \text{ g}}{100 \ \cancel{\text{mL}}} \times \frac{\text{total } \cancel{\text{mL}}}{1}$$

Example 1:   Calculate the amount of dextrose in the ordered intravenous (IV) solution.

   Order: 500 mL D_5W

C: *Convert*—D_5W indicates the supply of dextrose is 5 g/100 mL. Because the quantity ordered is in mL and the supply is in mL, there is no conversion.

A: *Approximate*—Because the ordered quantity, 500 mL, is five times the 100 mL supply, the ordered amount of dextrose will be five times the 5 g supply of dextrose, which is 25 g.

S: *Solve*

Ratio-Proportion	Formula Method
$\dfrac{5\,g}{100\,mL} = \dfrac{x\,g}{500\,mL}$ or $5\,g : 100\,mL = x\,g : 500\,mL$ $100x = 2{,}500$ $x = 25\,g$	$\dfrac{500\,\cancel{mL}}{100\,\cancel{mL}} \times 5\,g = x\,(g)$ $\dfrac{2{,}500\,g}{100} = x$ $25\,g = x$

Dimensional Analysis
$x\,(g) = \dfrac{5\,g}{100\,\cancel{mL}} \times \dfrac{500\,\cancel{mL}}{1}$ $x = \dfrac{2{,}500\,g}{100}$ $x = 25\,g$

E: *Evaluate*

Ratio-Proportion	Formula Method
$\dfrac{5\,g}{100\,mL} = \dfrac{25\,g}{500\,mL}$ or $5\,g : 100\,mL = 25\,g : 500\,mL$ $100 \times 25 = 5 \times 500$ $2{,}500 = 2{,}500$	$\dfrac{500\,\cancel{mL}}{100\,\cancel{mL}} \times 5\,g = 25\,g$ $\dfrac{2{,}500\,g}{100} = 25\,g$ $25\,g = 25\,g$

Dimensional Analysis
$25\,g = \dfrac{5\,g}{100\,\cancel{mL}} \times \dfrac{500\,\cancel{mL}}{1}$ $25\,g = \dfrac{2{,}500\,g}{100}$ $25\,g = 25\,g$

Because the calculated amount accurately completes the equation and is consistent with the approximated amount, 25g, the answer is confirmed.

For solutions containing both dextrose and sodium chloride (NaCl), the amount of dextrose and NaCl will be calculated separately. Recall from Chapter 10 that normal saline (NS) is 0.9% sodium chloride, therefore it contains 0.9 g of NaCl per 100 mL solution.

Example 2:   Calculate the amount of dextrose and NaCl in the ordered IV solution.

Order: $1{,}000$ mL D_5NS

C: *Convert*—D_5NS indicates the supply of dextrose is 5 g/100 mL and the supply of NaCl is 0.9g/100 mL. Because the quantity ordered is in mL and the supply is in mL, there is no conversion.

A: *Approximate*—Because the ordered quantity, 1,000 mL, is 10 times the 100 mL supply:

- The ordered amount of dextrose will be 10 times the 5 g supply of dextrose, which is 50 g.
- The ordered amount of NaCl will be 10 times the 0.9 g supply of NaCL, which is 9 g.

S: *Solve*

Ratio-Proportion	Formula Method
Dextrose Calculation $$\frac{5\ g}{100\ mL} = \frac{x\ g}{1{,}000\ mL} \text{ or}$$ $$5\ g : 100\ mL = x\ g : 1{,}000\ mL$$ $$100x = 5{,}000$$ $$x = 50\ g$$	**Dextrose Calculation** $$\frac{1{,}000\ \cancel{mL}}{100\ \cancel{mL}} \times 5\ g = x\ (g)$$ $$\frac{5{,}000\ g}{100} = x$$ $$50\ g = x$$

Dimensional Analysis

Dextrose Calculation

$$x\ (g) = \frac{5\ g}{100\ \cancel{mL}} \times \frac{1{,}000\ \cancel{mL}}{1}$$
$$x = \frac{5{,}000\ g}{100}$$
$$x = 50\ g$$

Ratio-Proportion	Formula Method
NaCl Calculation $$\frac{0.9\ g}{100\ mL} = \frac{x\ g}{1{,}000\ mL} \text{ or}$$ $$0.9\ g : 100\ mL = x\ g : 1{,}000\ mL$$ $$100x = 900$$ $$x = 9\ g$$	**NaCl Calculation** $$\frac{1{,}000\ \cancel{mL}}{100\ \cancel{mL}} \times 0.9\ g = x\ (g)$$ $$\frac{900\ g}{100} = x$$ $$9\ g = x$$

Dimensional Analysis

NaCl Calculation

$$x\ (g) = \frac{0.9\ g}{100\ \cancel{mL}} \times \frac{1{,}000\ \cancel{mL}}{1}$$
$$x = \frac{900\ g}{100}$$
$$x = 9\ g$$

E: *Evaluate*

Ratio-Proportion

Dextrose Calculation

$$\frac{5\ g}{100\ mL} = \frac{50\ g}{1,000\ mL} \quad or$$

$5\ g : 100\ mL = 50\ g : 1,000\ mL$

$100 \times 50 = 5 \times 1,000$

$5,000 = 5,000$

Formula Method

Dextrose Calculation

$$\frac{1,000\ \cancel{mL}}{100\ \cancel{mL}} \times 5\ g = 50\ g$$

$$\frac{5,000\ g}{100} = 50\ g$$

$$50\ g = 50\ g$$

Dimensional Analysis

Dextrose Calculation

$$50\ g = \frac{5\ g}{100\ \cancel{mL}} \times \frac{1,000\ \cancel{mL}}{1}$$

$$50\ g = \frac{5,000\ g}{100}$$

$$50\ g = 50\ g$$

Ratio-Proportion

NaCl Calculation

$$\frac{0.9\ g}{100\ mL} = \frac{9\ g}{1,000\ mL} \quad or$$

$0.9\ g : 100\ mL = 9\ g : 1,000\ mL$

$100 \times 9 = 0.9 \times 1,000$

$900 = 900$

Formula Method

NaCl Calculation

$$\frac{1,000\ \cancel{mL}}{100\ \cancel{mL}} \times 0.9\ g = 9\ g$$

$$\frac{900\ g}{100} = 9\ g$$

$$9\ g = 9\ g$$

Dimensional Analysis

NaCl Calculation

$$9\ g = \frac{0.9\ g}{100\ \cancel{mL}} \times \frac{1,000\ \cancel{mL}}{1}$$

$$9\ g = \frac{900\ g}{100}$$

$$9\ g = 9\ g$$

Because the calculated amount accurately completes the equation and is consistent with the approximated quantities of dextrose, 50 g, and NaCl, 9 g, the answers are confirmed.

Recall from Chapter 10 that NaCl is present in IV solutions in concentrations other than 0.9% (NS), including:

- 0.45% NaCl, also called ½ NS

- 0.3% NaCl, also called ⅓ NS

- 0.225% NaCl, also called ¼ NS

$$\frac{0.225g}{100ml} \times 2.5$$

Example 3:   Calculate the amount of dextrose and NaCl that a patient will receive in 24 hours.

Order: 250 mL D_5 ¼ NS IV q6h

C: *Convert*—D_5¼ NS indicates the supply of dextrose is 5 g/100 mL and the supply of NaCl is 0.225 g/100 mL. Because q6h occurs 4 times per day, convert q6h to 4 doses/day.

A: *Approximate*—Because q6h occurs four times per day, 250 mL of IV solution will be administered four times for an approximate total of 1,000 mL. Because this total volume is 10 times the supply volume of 100 mL:

- The ordered amount of dextrose will be 10 times the supply amount of 5 g, which is 50 g.

- The ordered amount of NaCl will be 10 times the supply amount of 0.225 g, which is 2.25 g.

S: *Solve*

For ratio-proportion and the formula method, perform two steps:

Step 1: Calculate the total (24 h) volume of IV solution to be administered in 24 h based on 4 doses per day, because q6h occurs four times in 24 h.

Step 2: Calculate the number of grams of dextrose and NaCl in the 24 h volume.

Ratio-Proportion	**Formula Method**
Dextrose Calculation	Dextrose Calculation
Step 1:	Step 1:
$\dfrac{250\ mL}{1\ dose} = \dfrac{x\ mL/day}{4\ doses/day}$ or 250 mL: 1 dose = x mL/day: 4 doses/day $\quad x = 1,000\ mL/day$	250 mL/~~dose~~ × 4 ~~doses~~/day = x (mL/day) 1,000 mL/day = x
Step 2:	Step 2:
$\dfrac{5\ g}{100\ mL} = \dfrac{x\ g/day}{1,000\ mL/day}$ or $\quad$ 5 g: 100 mL = x g: 1,000 mL $\quad\quad 100x = 5,000$ $\quad\quad\quad x = 50\ g/day$	$\dfrac{1,000\ \cancel{mL}/day}{100\ \cancel{mL}} \times 5\ g = x(g/day)$ $\dfrac{5,000\ g/day}{100} = x$ $\quad$ 50 g/day = x

Dimensional Analysis

Dextrose Calculation

$$x\left(\frac{g}{day}\right) = \frac{5\ g}{100\ \cancel{mL}} \times \frac{250\ \cancel{mL}}{1\ \cancel{dose}} \times \frac{4\ \cancel{doses}}{1\ day}$$

$$x = \frac{5{,}000\ g}{100}$$

$$x = 50\ g/day$$

Ratio-Proportion

NaCl Calculation

$$\frac{0.225\ g}{100\ mL} = \frac{x\ g/day}{1{,}000\ mL/day}\quad \text{or}$$

$$0.225\ g : 100\ mL = x\ g : 1{,}000\ mL$$

$$100 = 225$$

$$x = 2.25\ g/day$$

Formula Method

NaCl Calculation

$$\frac{1{,}000\ \cancel{mL}/day}{100\ \cancel{mL}} \times 0.225\ g = x\ (g/day)$$

$$\frac{225\ g/day}{100} = x$$

$$2.25\ g/day = x$$

Dimensional Analysis

NaCl Calculation

$$x\left(\frac{g}{day}\right) = \frac{0.225\ g}{100\ \cancel{mL}} \times \frac{250\ \cancel{mL}}{1\ \cancel{dose}} \times \frac{4\ \cancel{doses}}{1\ day}$$

$$x = \frac{225\ g}{100\ day}$$

$$x = 2.25\ g/day$$

E: *Evaluate*

Ratio-Proportion

Dextrose Calculation

$$\frac{5\ g}{100\ mL} = \frac{50\ g}{1{,}000\ mL}\quad \text{or}$$

$$5\ g : 100\ mL = 50\ g : 1{,}000\ mL$$

$$100 \times 50 = 5 \times 1{,}000$$

$$5{,}000 = 5{,}000$$

Formula Method

Dextrose Calculation

$$\frac{1{,}000\ \cancel{mL}/day}{100\ \cancel{mL}} \times 5\ g = 50\ g/day$$

$$\frac{5{,}000\ g/day}{100} = 50\ g/day$$

$$50\ g/day = 50\ g/day$$

Dimensional Analysis

Dextrose Calculation

$$50\frac{g}{day} = \frac{5\ g}{100\ \cancel{mL}} \times \frac{250\ \cancel{mL}}{1\ \cancel{dose}} \times \frac{4\ \cancel{doses}}{1\ day}$$

$$50\ g/day = \frac{5,000\ g}{100\ day}$$

$$50\ g/day = 50\ g/day$$

Ratio-Proportion

NaCl Calculation

$$\frac{0.225\ g}{100\ mL} = \frac{2.25\ g/day}{1,000\ mL/day} \quad \text{or}$$

$$0.225\ g : 100\ mL = 2.25\ g : 1,000\ mL$$

$$100 \times (2.25) = 225$$

$$225 = 225$$

Formula Method

NaCl Calculation

$$\frac{1,000\ \cancel{mL}/day}{100\ \cancel{mL}} \times 0.225\ g = 2.25\ g/day$$

$$\frac{225\ g/day}{100} = x$$

$$2.25\ g/day = x$$

Dimensional Analysis

NaCl Calculation

$$2.25\frac{g}{day} = \frac{0.225\ g}{100\ \cancel{mL}} \times \frac{250\ \cancel{mL}}{1\ \cancel{dose}} \times \frac{4\ \cancel{doses}}{1\ day}$$

$$2.25\ g/day = \frac{225\ g}{100\ day}$$

$$2.25\ g/day = 2.25\ g/day$$

Because the calculated amount accurately completes the equation and is consistent with the approximate amounts of dextrose, 50 g, and NaCl, 2.25 g, the answers are confirmed.

LEARNING ACTIVITY 11-1 Calculate the IV solution components, as requested.

1. **Order:** 500 mL NS
2. **Order:** 0.5 L D_5W
3. **Order:** 1,000 mL $D_5\frac{1}{2}$ NS; calculate the amount of dextrose and NaCl in this solution.
4. **Order:** 1.5 L $D_{10}W$ q12h; calculate the amount of dextrose to be administered daily.

11-2 Additional Solute and Solvent Calculations

Sometimes nurses are required to prepare solutions to be used for feeding or for wound care. A solution may be prepared by mixing a concentrated substance or formula with one that is less concentrated. In this case, the more concentrated formula or solution is referred to as the **solute**. The less concentrated solution is typically referred to as the **solvent**. The solvent is also known as the solution that dilutes or dissolves, as described in the reconstitution section of Chapter 9. Also in Chapter 9, the solvent, referred to as the **diluent**, is the solution used to dissolve a powdered medication (a dry solute). Because water is the most commonly used solvent to dilute solutions, it is called the **universal solvent** (Helmenstine, 2012). Another common solvent is normal saline.

Enteral Feeding Solutions

Nutritional products are available in various forms:

- Ready-to-feed containers (**Figure 11-1**)

- Concentrated formulas (**Figure 11-2**)

- Powdered mixtures (**Figure 11-3**)

Ready-to-feed solutions are considered **full strength**, the typical concentration used to meet normal nutrient needs. Concentrated formulas and powdered mixtures, once mixed with water according to the manufacturer instructions, are considered full strength. Partial-strength formulas are created from full-strength formulas by adding water, the universal solvent. Partial-strength nutritional formulas are sometimes ordered for pediatric patients recovering from a gastrointestinal illness or surgery.

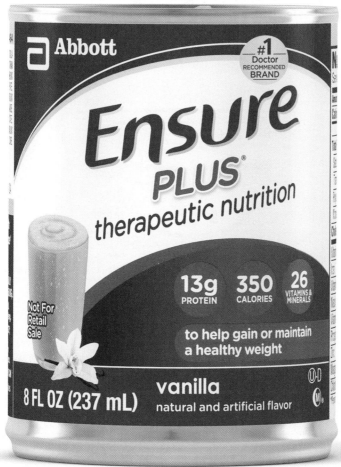

FIGURE 11-1   Ready-to-feed nutritional formulas do not require dilution with water, unless a partial-strength formula is ordered.

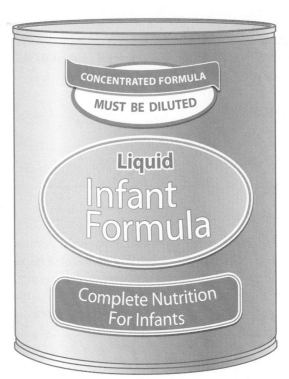

FIGURE 11-2 Concentrated formulas must be diluted (reconstituted) with water according to manufacturer instructions prior to feeding.

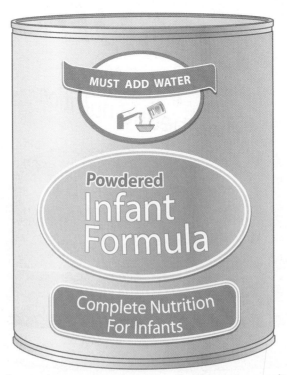

FIGURE 11-3 Formula powder must be reconstituted with water according to manufacturer instructions prior to feeding.

For partial-strength formulas, fractions are used to indicate solution strength, for example, ¼-strength Similac® 360 mL. This order indicates that ¼ of 360 mL should be solute (Similac), which means that the remaining volume, ¾ of 360 mL, should be solvent (water). To determine the amount of Similac (solute) and water (solvent) needed to create 360 mL of ¼-strength solution, calculations are done using one of the three methods:

- Ratio-proportion: The first ratio (fraction) is the solution strength and the second ratio is $\frac{\text{mL solute}}{\text{mL total solution}}$, thus the equation is: $\frac{1}{4} = \frac{x \text{ mL (solute)}}{360 \text{ mL}}$.

- Formula method: solution strength × total mL = x (mL solute). Mathematically, the word *of* acts like a multiplication sign; therefore, to determine the volume of solute (Similac), the equation is: $\frac{1}{4} \times 360 \text{ mL} = x \text{ (mL)}$.

- Dimensional analysis: The first factor is the total volume $\frac{\text{total mL}}{1}$ and the last factor is the solution strength. (Additional factors are inserted, when necessary.) To determine the volume of solute (Similac), the equation is: $x \text{ (mL)} = \frac{360 \text{ mL}}{1} \times \frac{1}{4}$.

To determine the amount of solvent, subtract the solute from the solution total:

$$360 \text{ mL (total solution)} - 90 \text{ mL (solute, Similac)} = 270 \text{ mL (solvent, water)}$$

As a time-saving measure, nurses often prepare enough nutritional solution for multiple feedings as indicated in the examples that follow.

Example 1:   Determine the amount of solute and solvent needed to prepare a 24-hour supply of the following nutritional order.

Order: ⅔-strength Isomil® 90 mL PO q3h

C: *Convert*—Because q3h occurs 8 times per day, convert q3h to 8 feedings/day.

A: *Approximate*—If one-third of 90 mL is 30 mL, then two-thirds of 90 mL is 60 mL, therefore 60 mL of Isomil, mixed with 30 mL of water, will be needed every 3 hours. Because q3h occurs eight times in 24 h, the quantities of solute, solvent, and solution are approximated as follows:

- Solute—Isomil: 60 mL × 8 is approximately 500 mL

- Solvent—Water: 30 mL × 8 is approximately 250 mL

- Solution—approximately 750 mL

S: *Solve*

For ratio-proportion and the formula method, perform two steps:

Step 1: Calculate the total (24 h) volume of solution based on eight feedings per day, because q3h occurs eight times in 24 h.

Step 2: Calculate the volume of solute (Isomil):

Ratio-Proportion	Formula Method
Step 1: $\dfrac{90 \text{ mL}}{1 \text{ feeding}} = \dfrac{x \text{ mL/day}}{8 \text{ feedings/day}}$ $x = 720 \text{ mL/day}$ Step 2: $\dfrac{2}{3} = \dfrac{x \text{ mL/day}}{720 \text{ mL/day}}$ or $2:3 = x \text{ mL}: 720 \text{ mL}$ $3x = 1,440$ $x = 480 \text{ mL/day}$	Step 1: $90 \dfrac{\text{mL}}{\text{fdg}} \times 8 \text{ fdg/day} = x \text{ (mL/day)}$ $720 \text{ mL/day} = x$ Step 2: $\dfrac{2}{3} \times 720 \text{ mL/day} = x \text{ (mL/day)}$ $\dfrac{1,440 \text{ mL/day}}{3} = x$ $480 \text{ mL/day} = x$

Dimensional Analysis

$$x \text{ (mL/day)} = \frac{90 \text{ mL}}{1 \text{ feeding}} \times \frac{8 \text{ feedings}}{1 \text{ day}} \times \frac{2}{3}$$

$$x = \frac{1,440 \text{ mL}}{3 \text{ day}}$$

$$x = 480 \text{ mL/day}$$

E: *Evaluate*

Ratio-Proportion	Formula Method
$\dfrac{2}{3} = \dfrac{480}{720}$ or $2:3 = 480:720$ $3 \times 480 = 2 \times 720$ $1,440 = 1,440$	$\dfrac{2}{3} \times 720 \text{ mL} = 480 \text{ mL}$ $\dfrac{1,440 \text{ mL}}{3} = 480 \text{ mL}$ $480 \text{ mL} = 480 \text{ mL}$

Dimensional Analysis

$$480 \frac{\text{mL}}{\text{day}} = \frac{90 \text{ mL}}{1 \text{ feeding}} \times \frac{8 \text{ feedings}}{1 \text{ day}} \times \frac{2}{3}$$

$$480 \text{ mL/day} = \frac{1,440 \text{ mL}}{3 \text{ day}}$$

$$480 \text{ mL/day} = 480 \text{ mL/day}$$

Finally, calculate the volume of water (solvent) to add to the Isomil to obtain the necessary volume of total solution:

$$720 \text{ mL (total solution)} - 480 \text{ mL Isomil (solute)} = 240 \text{ mL water (solvent)}$$

Because the calculated volumes of solute are consistent with the approximated volumes, 500 mL, solvent, 250 mL, and solution, 750 mL, the answers are confirmed.

To implement 'the order in Example 1, the nurse will feed orally 90 mL of reconstituted formula every 3 hours. Enteral feeding solutions are sometimes delivered via electronic feeding pump. Like IV pumps, feeding pumps are calibrated in mL/h. Therefore, feeding infusion rate calculations are done in the same way as electronic IV infusion rate calculations:

- $(\text{volume}) \text{ mL} \div (\text{time}) \text{ h} = x \ (\text{rate in mL/h})$
- $\dfrac{\text{mL}}{\text{min}} \times 60 \text{ min/h} = x \ (\text{rate in mL/h})$

If the route in the Example 1 order is changed to nasogastric tube (NGT) and an infusion time of 30 minutes is added, the new order will read: ⅔-strength Isomil 90 mL via NGT q3h; infuse over 30 min.

The nurse will calculate the infusion rate:

$$\frac{90 \text{ mL}}{30 \ \cancel{\text{min}}} \times 60 \ \cancel{\text{min}}/\text{h} = 180 \text{ mL/h}$$

To implement this order, the nurse will:

1. Fill a solution container (**Figure 11-4**) with 90 mL of reconstituted solution (per Example 1).

2. Set the feeding pump (Figure 11-4) to 180 mL/h.

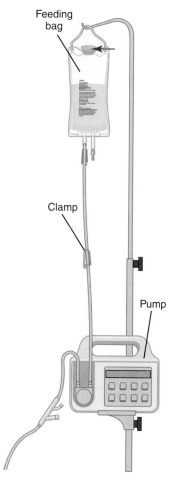

Feeding bag

Clamp

Pump

FIGURE 11-4   If the hang time for a nutritional formula is 4 hours, the nurse will add only enough solution for 4 hours to the solution container.

When a hospitalized child continues consuming partial-strength nutritional formula at home after discharge, the nurse provides the quantity of formula, water, and total solution in ounces instead of milliliters. To convert ounces to mL, use the conversion factor 1 oz/30 mL.

Example 2:   Determine the amount of solution, solute, and solvent *in oz* needed to prepare the following feeding order that the nurse will give to the parents of an infant recovering from a gastric illness.

Order: ¾-strength Prosobee® 180 mL via NGT q4h; infuse over 1 hour

C: *Convert*—For ratio-proportion and the formula method, convert 180 mL to 6 oz. For dimensional analysis, use the conversion factor 1 oz/30 mL.

A: *Approximate*—Six oz of Prosobee is needed every 4 hours. Half of 6 oz is 3 oz. Because ¾ is more than ½, then more than 3 oz but less than 6 oz, or approximately 5 oz of Prosobee, will be mixed with approximately 1 oz of water every 4 hours.

S: *Solve*

Calculate the volume of solute:

Ratio-Proportion	Formula Method
Step 1: $$\frac{30 \text{ mL}}{1 \text{ oz}} = \frac{x \text{ mL}}{6 \text{ oz}}$$ $$x = 180 \text{ mL}$$ **Step 2:** $$\frac{3}{4} = \frac{x \text{ oz}}{6 \text{ oz}} \text{ or}$$ $$3 : 4 = x \text{ oz} : 6 \text{ oz}$$ $$4x = 18$$ $$x = 4.5 \text{ oz}$$	**Step 1:** $$6 \text{ oz} \times 30 \text{ mL}/1 \text{ oz} = x \text{ (mL)}$$ $$180 \text{ mL} = x$$ **Step 2:** $$\frac{3}{4} \times 6 \text{ oz} = x \text{ (oz)}$$ $$\frac{18 \text{ oz}}{4} = x$$ $$4.5 \text{ oz} = x$$

Dimensional Analysis

$$x \text{ (oz)} = \frac{1 \text{ oz}}{30 \text{ mL}} \times \frac{180 \text{ mL}}{1} \times \frac{3}{4}$$

$$x = \frac{540 \text{ oz}}{120}$$

$$x = 4.5 \text{ oz}$$

E: *Evaluate*

Ratio-Proportion	Formula Method
$\dfrac{3}{4} = \dfrac{4.5}{6}$ or $3 : 4 = 4.5 : 6$ $4 \times 4.5 = 3 \times 6$ $18 = 18$	$\dfrac{3}{4} \times 6\text{ oz} = 4.5\text{ oz}$ $\dfrac{18\text{ oz}}{4} = 4.5\text{ oz}$ $4.5\text{ oz} = 4.5\text{ oz}$

Dimensional Analysis

$$4.5\text{ oz} = \frac{1\text{ oz}}{30\text{ mL}} \times \frac{180\text{ mL}}{1} \times \frac{3}{4}$$

$$4.5\text{ oz} = \frac{540\text{ oz}}{120}$$

$$4.5\text{ oz} = 4.5\text{ oz}$$

Calculate the volume of water (solvent) to add to the Prosobee to obtain the necessary volume of total solution:

$$6\text{ oz (total solution)} - 4.5\text{ oz Prosobee}^{\circledR}\text{ (solute)} = 1.5\text{ oz water (solvent)}$$

Because the calculated volumes are consistent with the approximated volumes of solute, 5 oz, and solvent, 1 oz, the answers are confirmed.

To implement the order in Example 2, every 4 hours the nurse will fill a solution container with 180 mL of reconstituted solution and set the feeding pump to 180 mL/h.

Clinical CLUE

Prior to administration of feeding via NGT, the nurse should check tube placement as described in Step 3 of "Clinical Clue ... Procedure for Administration of Medications via Enteral Tube" in Chapter 8.

Example 3:   Determine the amount of solute and solvent needed to prepare the tube feeding solution for a 12-hour shift.

Order: ½-strength Similac 35 mL/h via GT (**Figure 11-5**)

C: *Convert*—For Ratio-Proportion and the Formula Method, convert 35 mL/h to 420 mL total over 12 h; for dimensional analysis, use the conversion factor 12 h/1.

A: *Approximate*—Similac at 35 mL/h for 12 hours can be approximated by rounding 35 mL up to 40 and rounding 12 h down to 10, then multiplying 40×10 to obtain a solution total of approximately 400 mL. Because half of the solution will be solute, the other half will be solvent; therefore, approximately 200 mL Similac with 200 mL of water is needed.

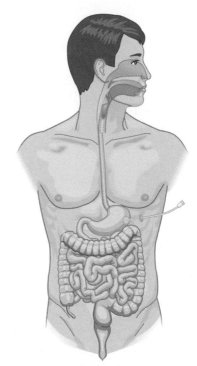

FIGURE 11-5   Enteral formulas can be administered orally or directly into the stomach through a tube, such as a gastrostomy tube (GT).

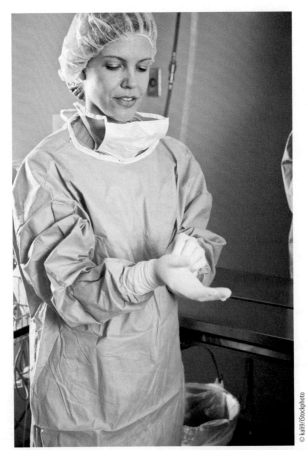

FIGURE 11-6   In some facilities, it is required that nurses wear masks, gowns, and gloves when preparing to administer enteral nutrition to reduce the spread of airborne bacteria.

S: *Solve*

For ratio-proportion and the formula method, perform two steps:

Step 1: Calculate the total volume of solution to be administered in 12 h.

Step 2: Calculate the volume of solute (Similac):

Ratio-Proportion	Formula Method
Step 1: $\dfrac{35 \text{ mL}}{1 \text{ h}} = \dfrac{x \text{ mL}}{12 \text{ h}}$ $x = 420 \text{ mL}$ Step 2: $\dfrac{1}{2} = \dfrac{x \text{ mL}}{420 \text{ mL}}$ or $1 : 2 = x \text{ mL} : 420 \text{ mL}$ $2x = 420$ $x = 210 \text{ mL}$	Step 1: $35 \text{ mL}/\cancel{h} \times 12 \cancel{h} = x \text{ (mL)}$ $420 \text{ mL} = x$ Step 2: $\dfrac{1}{2} \times 420 \text{ mL} = x \text{ (mL)}$ $\dfrac{420 \text{ mL}}{2} = x$ $210 \text{ mL} = x$

Dimensional Analysis

$$x \text{ (mL)} = \frac{35 \text{ mL}}{1 \cancel{h}} \times \frac{12 \cancel{h}}{1} \times \frac{1}{2}$$

$$x = \frac{420 \text{ mL}}{2}$$

$$x = 210 \text{ mL}$$

Finally, calculate the amount of water (solvent) to add to the Similac to obtain the necessary volume of total solution:

$$420 \text{ mL (total solution)} - 210 \text{ mL Similac (solute)} = 210 \text{ mL water (solvent)}$$

E: *Evaluate*

Ratio-Proportion	Formula Method
$\dfrac{1}{2} = \dfrac{210}{420}$ or $1 : 2 = 210 : 420$ $2 \times 210 = 1 \times 420$ $420 = 420$	$\dfrac{1}{2} \times 420 \text{ mL} = 210 \text{ mL}$ $\dfrac{420 \text{ mL}}{2} = 210 \text{ mL}$ $210 \text{ mL} = 210 \text{ mL}$

Dimensional Analysis

$$210 \text{ mL} = \frac{35 \text{ mL}}{1 \cancel{h}} \times \frac{12 \cancel{h}}{1} \times \frac{1}{2}$$

$$210 \text{ mL} = \frac{420 \text{ mL}}{2}$$

$$210 \text{ mL} = 210 \text{ mL}$$

Because the calculated volumes are consistent with the approximated volumes of solute, 200 mL; solvent, 200 mL; and solution, 400 mL, the answers are confirmed.

Clinical CLUE

Hang time is the time an enteral nutrition formula is considered safe for delivery to the patient at room temperature, beginning from the time when the formula was reconstituted, or decanted, or from the time when the original package seal was broken (Yantis & Velander, 2011). Because hang time for most pediatric nutritional formulas is 4 hours, only enough solution for 4 hours should be hung at one time. In the previous Example 3, once the total solution of 420 mL is prepared, one-third of it, 140 mL (35 mL/h × 4 h = 140 mL), will be added to the solution container (Figure 11-5) every 4 hours, while the remaining reconstituted solution should be refrigerated. The feeding pump will be set to 35 mL/h as ordered.

WARNING!

Be Certain the (Universal) Solvent Is Safe

Water, used to mix and dilute formulas in home care settings, can be tepid (room temperature) tap water, as long as it has been determined by the local or state health departments as safe to drink. To err on the side of caution, water can be sterilized by boiling it for 1 minute before mixing with formula. After boiling for 1 minute, the water should be cooled to room temperature. The water should sit at room temperature for no longer than 30 minutes. Once prepared, the formula is ready to feed without additional refrigeration or warming. Water used to mix and dilute formulas in healthcare settings should be sterile water (Yantis & Velander, 2011).

WARNING!

Be Certain the Solute and Solution Are Safe

The contamination of tube-feeding formulas can occur during the preparation process. When reconstituting powdered formulas, sterile technique should be used to avoid introducing pathogens. The hang time for most pediatric and reconstituted formulas is 4 hours, while some ready-to-hang containers may be hung for 24 hours or more. Nurses should follow healthcare agency policy and procedures for administration of enteral nutrition.

Topical Solutions

In addition to preparing feeding solutions, nurses may need to prepare topical solutions to be used as wound irrigants or cleansing solutions. For example, nurses may dilute stock solutions, such as hydrogen peroxide (H_2O_2) with a less concentrated liquid, such as normal saline (NS). As with nutritional formulas, fractions are often used to designate solution strength for topical solutions. In the next example the nurse will dilute H_2O_2, the solute, with NS, the solvent.

Example: Using normal saline as the solvent, calculate the amount of solute and solvent needed to prepare a daily supply of the following order.

Order: Clean the wound with ¼-strength hydrogen peroxide 2 oz q6h.

C: *Convert*—Because q6h occurs 4 times per day, convert q6h to 4 cleanings/day.

A: *Approximate*—Because q6h occurs four times per day, 2 oz of solution will be needed four times for an approximate total of 8 oz. One-fourth of 8 oz is 2 oz, therefore 2 oz of hydrogen peroxide, mixed with 6 oz of normal saline, will be needed for a daily supply of wound-cleaning solution.

S: *Solve*

For ratio-proportion and the formula method, perform two steps:

Step 1: Calculate the total volume of solution needed for a daily supply.

Step 2: Calculate the volume of solute (H_2O_2).

Ratio-Proportion	Formula Method
Step 1: $\dfrac{2 \text{ oz}}{1 \text{ cleaning}} = \dfrac{x \text{ oz/day}}{4 \text{ cleanings/day}}$ $x = 8 \text{ oz/day}$ Step 2: $\dfrac{1}{4} = \dfrac{x \text{ oz/day}}{8 \text{ oz/day}}$ or $1 : 4 = x \text{ oz} : 8 \text{ oz}$ $4x = 8$ $x = 2 \text{ oz/day}$	Step 1: $2\dfrac{\text{oz}}{\cancel{\text{cleaning}}} \times 4 \cancel{\text{ cleanings}}/\text{day} = x(\text{oz/day})$ $8 \text{ oz/day} = x$ Step 2: $\dfrac{1}{4} \times 8 \text{ oz/day} = x \text{ (oz/day)}$ $\dfrac{8 \text{ oz/day}}{4} = x$ $2 \text{ oz/day} = x$

Dimensional Analysis

$$x(\text{oz/day}) = \frac{2 \text{ oz}}{1 \cancel{\text{cleaning}}} \times \frac{4 \cancel{\text{ cleanings}}}{1 \text{ day}} \times \frac{1}{4}$$

$$x = \frac{8 \text{ oz}}{4 \text{ day}}$$

$$x = 2 \text{ oz/day}$$

E: *Evaluate*

Ratio-Proportion	Formula Method
$\dfrac{1}{4} = \dfrac{2}{8}$ or $1 : 4 = 2 : 8$ $4 \times 2 = 1 \times 8$ $8 = 8$	$\dfrac{1}{4} \times 8 \text{ oz/day} = 2 \text{ oz/day}$ $\dfrac{8 \text{ oz/day}}{4} = 2 \text{ oz/day}$ $2 \text{ oz/day} = 2 \text{ oz/day}$

Dimensional Analysis

$$2 \text{ oz/day} = \frac{2 \text{ oz}}{1 \cancel{\text{cleaning}}} \times \frac{4 \cancel{\text{ cleanings}}}{1 \text{ day}} \times \frac{1}{4}$$

$$2 \text{ oz/day} = \frac{8 \text{ oz}}{4 \text{ day}}$$

$$2 \text{ oz/day} = 2 \text{ oz/day}$$

Finally, calculate the amount of NS (solvent) to add to the H_2O_2, to obtain the necessary volume of total solution:

$$8 \text{ oz } (\text{total solution}) - 2 \text{ oz } H_2O_2 \text{ (solute)} = 6 \text{ oz NS (solvent)}$$

Because the calculated volumes are consistent with the approximated volumes of solute, 2 oz; solvent, 6 oz; and solution, 8 oz, the answers are confirmed.

Community health nurses may use household measures to carry out orders as reflected with the use of fluid ounces in the previous example. If a patient with the previous order were transferred to an inpatient setting, the provider would convert ounces to milliliters when placing the wound-cleansing order onto the patient's medical record. Because 1 oz = 30 mL, to create the cleansing solution needed in the previous example, the nurse would prepare 240 mL (8 oz) of total solution by mixing 60 mL (2 oz) of H_2O_2 with 180 mL (6 oz) of NS.

LEARNING ACTIVITY 11-2 Calculate in mL the amount of total solution, solute, and solvent for each order. For feeding orders, calculate the infusion rate in mL/h.

1. **Order:** ¾-strength Isomil 5 oz qid to infuse over 1 h; using water as the solvent, the nurse will prepare enough solution for 1 day.
2. **Order:** ½-strength Similac 1 oz per hour for 8 hours; prepare enough solution for 4 hours.
3. **Order:** ⅓-strength H_2O_2 1 oz q8h; using NS as the solvent, the nurse will prepare enough solution for 1 week.

Formula Fiasco ... Case Closure

1. Formula concentrate is a solute and needs to be diluted with a solvent (water) before feeding, according to manufacturer instructions (which is usually equal parts of solute and solvent).

2. Formula feeding instructions must be given to new parents prior to discharge from the hospital and should include information about the three types of formula preparations:

   • Ready-to-feed formula solution

   • Liquid concentrate, which needs to be diluted with water prior to feeding

   • Powdered formula, which needs to be mixed with water prior to feeding

Chapter Summary

Learning Outcomes	Points to Remember
11-1 Calculate solution components based on percentages.	Percent solutions indicate the number of g/100 mL of solution components. • D_5W contains 5 g dextrose/100 mL; $D_{10}W$ contains 10g dextrose/100 mL. Recall from Chapter 10: • NS, 0.9% NaCl, contains 0.9 g NaCl/100 mL. • ½ NS contains 0.45 g NaCl/100 mL. • ⅓ NS contains 0.3 g NaCl/100 mL. • ¼ NS contains 0.225 g NaCl/100 mL.

To calculate the amount of dextrose and NaCl in 250 mL $D_5\frac{1}{2}$ NS, the ratio-proportion (RP), formula method (FM), and dimensional analysis (DA) calculations are:

RP—Dextrose	RP—NaCl
$\dfrac{5\ g}{100\ mL} = \dfrac{x\ g}{250\ mL}$ $100x = 1{,}250$ $x = 12.5\ g$	$\dfrac{0.45\ g}{100\ mL} = \dfrac{x\ g}{250\ mL}$ $100x = 112.5$ $x = 1.125\ g$
FM—Dextrose	**FM—NaCl**
$\dfrac{250\ \cancel{mL}}{100\ \cancel{mL}} \times 5\ g = x\ (g)$ $\dfrac{1{,}250\ g}{100} = x$ $12.5\ g = x$	$\dfrac{250\ \cancel{mL}}{100\ \cancel{mL}} \times 0.45\ g = x\ (g)$ $\dfrac{112.5\ g}{100} = x$ $1.125\ g = x$
DA—Dextrose	**DA—NaCl**
$x\ (g) = \dfrac{5\ g}{100\ \cancel{mL}} \times \dfrac{250\ \cancel{mL}}{1}$ $x = \dfrac{1{,}250\ g}{100}$ $x = 12.5\ g$	$x\ (g) = \dfrac{0.45\ g}{100\ \cancel{mL}} \times \dfrac{250\ \cancel{mL}}{1}$ $x = \dfrac{112.5\ g}{100}$ $x = 1.125\ g$

11-2 Calculate solute and solvent based on solution strength.

For partial-strength solutions, fractions are used to designate solution strength. When using ratio-proportion or the formula method to calculate the volume of solute (concentrated solution) and solvent (product used to dilute), first calculate the total volume of solution that is needed, if necessary.

To calculate solute volume:

- RP: Use the solution strength fraction as the first ratio and the second ratio is $\frac{mL\ solute}{mL\ total\ solution}$.
- FM: Multiply the fraction by the total solution volume.
- DA: The first factor is the total volume ($\frac{total\ mL}{1}$) and the last factor is solution strength and additional factors are inserted as needed.

To calculate solvent volume: Subtract the solute from the solution total.

Example: Calculate the solute and solvent needed to prepare ¼-strength Enfamil® 240 mL q6h × 1 day.

For ratio-proportion and the formula method, perform two steps:

Step 1: Calculate the solution total based on four feedings per day, because q6h happens four times per day. For DA, insert the conversion factor 4 fdg/day in the equation.

Step 2: Calculate the solute (Enfamil) total.

RP	Step 1: $\dfrac{240 \text{ mL}}{1 \text{ fdg}} = \dfrac{x \text{ mL/day}}{4 \text{ fdg/day}}$ $x = 960 \text{ mL/day}$
	Step 2: $\dfrac{1}{4} = \dfrac{x \text{ mL/day}}{960 \text{ mL/day}}$ $x = 240 \text{ mL}$
FM	Step 1: $240 \text{ mL/}\cancel{\text{fdg}} \times 4 \cancel{\text{fdg}}\text{/day} = x \text{ (mL/day)}$ $\qquad\qquad 960 \text{ mL/day} = x$
	Step 2: $\dfrac{1}{4} \times 960 \text{ mL} = x$ $\qquad\qquad 240 \text{ mL} = x$
DA	$x \text{ (mL/day)} = \dfrac{1}{4} \times \dfrac{4 \cancel{\text{fdg}}}{1 \text{ day}} \times \dfrac{240 \text{ mL}}{1 \cancel{\text{fdg}}}$
	$x = \dfrac{960 \text{ mL}}{4 \text{ day}} = 240 \text{ mL/day}$

Solution total: 960 mL
Solute (Enfamil®) total: −240 mL
Solvent (water) total: 720 mL

Homework

For exercises 1–6, refer to the IV solution, $D_5\frac{1}{2}$ NS, to answer each question. (LO 11-1)

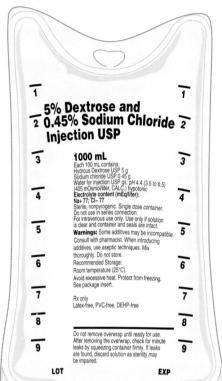

For exercises 7–10, refer to the IV solution, $D_{10}W$, to answer each question. (LO 11-1)

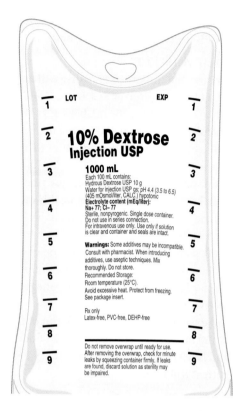

1. Calculate the amount of dextrose in the IV bag.
2. Calculate the amount of NaCl in the IV bag.
3. Calculate the amount of dextrose the patient will receive in 1 day with an IV infusing at 125 mL/h.
4. Calculate the amount of NaCl the patient will receive in 1 day with an IV infusing at 125 mL/h.
5. Calculate the amount of dextrose the patient will receive in 1 day with an IV infusing at 75 mL/h.
6. Calculate the amount of NaCl the patient will receive in 1 day with an IV infusing at 75 mL/h.

7. Calculate the amount of dextrose in the IV bag.
8. Calculate the amount of NaCl in the IV bag.
9. Calculate the amount of dextrose the patient will receive in 1 day with an IV infusing at 100 mL/h.
10. Calculate the amount of dextrose the patient will receive in 1 day with an IV infusing at 150 mL/h.

For exercises 11–15, refer to the following order:

Order: 500 mL $D_5\frac{1}{3}$ NS + 10 mEq KCl at 50 mL/h

11. Calculate the amount of dextrose in this IV solution.
12. Calculate the amount of NaCl in this IV solution.
13. If the nurse starts this infusion at 1130, how much should infuse by 1500?

14. If the nurse starts this infusion at 1130, how much dextrose will have infused by 1500?

15. If the nurse starts this infusion at 1130, how much NaCl will have infused by 1500?

For exercises 16–20, refer to the following order:

Order: 100 mL D_5W + 10 mEq KCl × 3 doses; infuse each via IVPB (secondary line) over 1 hour.

Supply: 10 mL vial of KCl 2 mEq/mL

16. To carry out this order, the nurse will need a total of _____ mL of KCl and will add _____ mL to each of three 100 mL bags of D_5W.

17. Calculate the amount of dextrose the patient will receive when the three doses of KCl are infused.

18. If this order is initiated at 1545, use traditional time to indicate what time this order will be completed if it is carried out without interruption.

19. If the patient has a primary infusion of $D_5\frac{1}{2}$ NS at 100 mL/h, calculate the volume of fluid (via primary and secondary IVs) the patient will receive in 1 day.

20. If the patient has a primary infusion of $D_5\frac{1}{2}$ NS at 100 mL/h, calculate the amount of dextrose and NaCl (via primary and secondary IVs) the patient will receive in 1 day.

For exercises 21–25, refer to the Isomil order. (LO 11-2)

Order: ¾-strength Isomil 3.5 oz q2h

21. Calculate the total solution for 24 hours.
22. Calculate the solute volume in ounces.
23. Calculate the solute volume in milliliters.
24. Calculate the solvent volume in ounces.
25. Calculate the solvent volume in milliliters.

For exercises 26–30, refer to the Similac order. (LO 11-2)

Order: ⅔-strength Similac 25 mL/h via GT

26. Calculate the total solution needed for 1 day.
27. Calculate the solute volume.
28. Calculate the solvent volume.
29. The hang time for Similac is 4 hours. How much Similac should the nurse add to the solution container every 4 hours?
30. If the patient is also receiving IV fluid $D_5\frac{1}{3}$ NS at 20 mL/h, calculate the patient's total fluid intake during a 12-hour shift.

For exercises 31–41, refer to the Enfamil order. (LO 11-2)

Order: At 0900 start GT feedings with Enfamil, increasing the strength and volume as follows:

Day 1
- ¼-strength Enfamil 60 mL q3h × 12 h, then advance to
- ½-strength Enfamil 80 mL q4h × 12 h, then advance to

Day 2
- ¾-strength Enfamil 120 mL q6h × 12 h, then advance to
- Full-strength Enfamil one 8 oz can q12h

31. Calculate the total solution to be administered from 0900 to 2100 on Day 1.

32. Calculate the amount of solute and solvent needed to prepare the solution needed from 0900 to 2100 on Day 1.

33. Calculate the total solution to be administered from 2100 to 0900 on Day 1.

34. Calculate the amount of solute and solvent needed to prepare the solution needed from 2100 to 0900 on Day 1.

35. Calculate the total solution to be administered from 0900 to 2100 on Day 2.

36. Calculate the amount of solute and solvent needed to prepare the solution needed from 0900 to 2100 on Day 2.

37. Calculate the total solution in mL to be administered from 2100 to 0900 on Day 2.

38. Calculate the amount of solute and solvent needed to prepare the solution needed from 2100 to 0900 on Day 2.

39. Calculate the total volume of solution the patient will receive in 48 hours.

40. Calculate the number of 8 oz cans of Enfamil the nurse will need to prepare enough solution for 2 days.

41. Calculate the number of cups of water the nurse will need to prepare enough solution for 2 days.

For exercises 42–44, refer to the povidone-iodine order. (LO 11-2)

Order: Use NS as a solvent and cleanse wound with 3 oz of ⅓-strength povidone-iodine q3h.

42. Calculate the total volume in mL of solution needed for 1 day.

43. Calculate the volume in mL of povidone-iodine needed for 1 day.

44. Calculate the volume in mL of NS needed for 1 day.

For exercises 45–47, refer to the following order. (LO 11-2)

Order: Cleanse wound with 2 oz of ½-strength H_2O_2 qid

45. Calculate the total volume in mL of solution needed for 2 days.
46. Calculate the volume in mL of H_2O_2 needed for 2 days.
47. Calculate the volume in mL of NS needed for 2 days.

For exercises 42–44, refer to the following order. (LO 11-2)

Ordetr: Provide skeletal pin care with 1 oz of ⅓-strength H_2O_2 tid.

48. Calculate the total volume in mL of solution needed for 1 week.
49. Calculate the total volume in mL of H_2O_2 needed for 1 week.
50. Calculate the total volume in mL of NS needed for 1 week.

NCLEX-Style Review Questions

For questions 1–4, select the best response.

1. The licensed prescriber orders 24 oz of a pre-packaged nutritional formula, with a hang time of 24 hours, to be delivered via feeding pump over 12 hours. The nurse will set the pump to deliver _____ mL/h.
   a. 2
   b. 10
   c. 60
   d. Not enough information provided to answer the question

2. To prepare a ⅔-strength solution of Similac 0.3 L to run over 4 hours, the nurse will need _____ mL Similac®, _____ mL water, and will set the feeding pump to _____ mL/h. (LO 11-2)
   a. 200, 100, 50
   b. 100, 200, 75
   c. 100, 200, 50
   d. 200, 100, 75

3. To create a partial-strength nutritional formula, the nurse will use: (LO 11-2)
   a. Water, the universal solvent
   b. Water, the universal solute
   c. Saline, the universal solute
   d. Saline, the universal solvent

4. The nurse recognizes that ½ NS IV solution is: (LO 11-1)
   a. 0.5% sodium chloride, 0.5 g per 100 mL of solution
   b. 0.45% sodium chloride, 0.45 g per 100 mL of solution
   c. 0.5% sodium chloride, 0.5 g per liter of solution
   d. 0.45% sodium chloride, 0.45 g per mL

For question 5–6, select all that apply.

5. The provider orders ¾-strength Enfamil infant formula 1 oz to be given q2h. To prepare enough solution for 1 day, the nurse will need: (LO 11-2)
   a. 90 mL solute
   b. 90 mL solvent
   c. 270 mL solute
   d. 270 mL solvent
   e. 3 oz Enfamil
   f. 3 oz water
   g. 12 oz Enfamil
   h. 12 oz total solution

6. The patient has an IV 1,000 mL of D_5NS infusing. Concerned about the patient's history of diabetes, a family member asked the nurse to explain the components of the IV solution. The nurse correctly explains that the IV solution includes: (LO 11-1)
   a. 5 grams of dextrose
   b. 50 grams of dextrose
   c. 1,000 grams of dextrose
   d. 0.9 grams of sodium chloride
   e. 9 grams of sodium chloride
   f. 90 grams of sodium chloride
   g. 1,000 grams of sodium chloride

REFERENCES

Helmenstine, A. M. (2012). *Why is water the universal solvent?* Retrieved from http://chemistry.about.com /od/waterchemistry/f/Why-Is-Water-The -Universal-Solvent.htm

Yantis, M. A., & Velander, R. (2011, September). Untangling enteral nutrition guidelines. *Nursing 2011, 41*(9), 32–38.

Chapter 11   ANSWER KEY

Learning Activity 11-1
1. 4.5 g NaCl
2. 25 g dextrose
3. 50 g dextrose, 4.5 g NaCl
4. 300 g dextrose, 150, g q12h

Learning Activity 11-2

1. Total solution: 600 mL/day
   Solute: 450 mL Isomil
   Solvent: 150 mL water
   Infusion rate: 150 mL/h
2. Total solution: 120 mL for 4 h
   Solute: 60 mL Similac
   Solvent: 60 mL water
   Infusion rate: 30 mL/h
3. Total solution: 90 mL/day; 630 mL for 1 week
   Solute: 210 mL H_2O_2
   Solvent: 420 mL NS

Homework

1. 50 g dextrose
2. 4.5 g NaCl
3. 150 g dextrose
4. 13.5 g NaCl
5. 90 g dextrose
6. 8.1 g NaCl
7. 100 g dextrose
8. N/A: There is no NaCl in this IV solution.
9. 240 g dextrose
10. 360 g dextrose
11. 25 g dextrose
12. 1.5 g NaCl
13. 175 mL
14. 8.75 g dextrose
15. 0.525 g NaCl
16. 15 mL, 5 mL
17. 15 g dextrose (5 g dextrose per 100 mL D_5W)
18. 6:45 p.m.
19. 2,415 mL (2,100 mL via primary infusion, 315 mL via secondary infusion)
20. 120 g dextrose (105 g via primary infusion, 15 g via secondary infusion), 9.45 g NaCl (via primary infusion)
21. 42 oz (1,260 mL) total solution
22. 31.5 oz Isomil
23. 945 mL Isomil
24. 10.5 oz water
25. 315 mL water
26. 600 mL
27. 400 mL Similac
28. 200 mL water
29. 100 mL
30. 540 mL total fluid intake (240 mL IV fluid + 300 mL Similac)
31. 240 mL
32. Solute (Enfamil)—60 mL; solvent (water)—180 mL
33. 240 mL
34. Solute (Enfamil)—2120 mL; solvent (water)—120 mL
35. 240 mL
36. Solute (Enfamil)—180 mL; solvent (water)—60 mL
37. 240 mL
38. N/A: The patient will be receiving full-strength formula from 2100 to 0900 on Day 2.
39. 960 mL
40. three 8-oz cans Enfamil
41. 1½ cups water
42. 720 mL total solution
43. 240 mL povidone-iodine
44. 480 mL NS
45. 480 mL total solution
46. 240 mL H_2O_2
47. 240 mL NS
48. 630 mL total solution
49. 210 mL H_2O_2
50. 420 mL NS

NCLEX-Style Review Questions

1. c
   Rationale: 24 oz = 720 mL; 720 mL divided by 12 h = 60 mL/h
2. d
   Rationale: The nurse will need 300 mL of solution of which $^2/_3$ (200 mL) is Similac⁻ and the balance, 100 mL, is water. To run 300 mL over 4 hours, the nurse will set the feeding pump to 75 mL/h.
3. a
   Rationale: Partial-strength formulas are created from full-strength formulas by adding water, the universal solvent.
4. b
   Rationale: Because NS is 0.9% sodium chloride, ½ NS is 0.45% sodium chloride, because 0.45 is half of 0.9. Percent, by definition, means what part of 100 something is, and percent solution concentrations indicate the number of grams per 100 mL. Therefore, 0.45% sodium chloride (½ NS) refers to 0.45 g/100 mL of solution.
5. b, c, f, h
   Rationale: The nurse will need 12 oz total solution (h); ¾ of the 12 oz—that is, 9 oz or 270 mL should be Enfamil/solute(c) and the balance (3 oz or 90 mL) should be water/solvent (b, f).
6. b, e
   Rationale: The IV solution, D_5NS, contains 5 g dextrose/100 mL and 0.9 g NaCl/100 mL; therefore, a 1,000 mL IV bag will contain 50 g dextrose and 9 g NaCl.

© Forfunlife/Shutterstock

Chapter 12

Dosage Calculations for Special Patient Populations

CHAPTER OUTLINE

LEARNING OUTCOMES

Upon completion of the chapter, the student will be able to:

12-1 Identify factors that impact drug dosing in special populations.

12-2 Perform weight-based safe dose calculations.

12-3 Perform safe dose calculations based on body surface area.

12-4 Determine minimum dilution volumes for intravenous medication administration.

KEY TERMS
absorption
body surface area (BSA)
BSA-based dosing
creatinine clearance
distribution
elimination
fixed dosing
geriatric
IV flush
IV syringe pumps
metabolism
pediatric
pharmacokinetics
polypharmacy
safe dose range (SDR)
volume-control set
weight-based dosing

Case Consideration ... Conversion Confusion

The nursing student, privileged to witness a birth and assist with newborn care, weighed the infant and recorded a weight of 2,500 grams. After converting 2,500 g to 2.5 kg, the student calculated the weight in pounds to be 5.5 lb. After swaddling the infant and placing him in his mother's arms, the student joyfully exclaimed, "The baby weighs 5 lb 5 oz!"

1. What went wrong?

2. How could this situation been avoided?

■ INTRODUCTION

Before administration of medication, the nurse must know that the dose ordered is safe. Safe dose information, determined by the drug manufacturer, is listed on the drug label or on the package insert. This information can also be found in a drug reference. Drug doses are generally determined by one of three approaches: fixed dosing, weight-based dosing, or body surface area–based dosing. **Body surface area (BSA)**, the total surface area of the body, is a more sensitive indicator of body size than body weight as it takes into account both height and weight.

Fixed dosing is dosing applied to homogeneous populations, such as average-sized adults. Dosing based on body weight or BSA assumes that drug dose parameters increase in proportion with increasing body size. **Weight-based dosing** is drug dosing that varies according to body weight, while **BSA-based dosing** varies according to BSA. Doses based on body weight and BSA are applied to medications used for special patient populations that require extra care and consideration regarding medication administration.

12-1   Factors That Impact Drug Dosing in Special Patient Populations

There are several special patient populations, but two populations that are routinely served by nurses in both inpatient and outpatient settings include the **geriatric** (age 65 or older) and **pediatric** (birth through age 18) patient populations. How drugs are used by the body differs greatly in these two populations.

Pharmacokinetics

Pharmacokinetics is the study of how drugs move through the body or the study of these four processes, which can easily be remembered using the acronym ADME:

- **Absorption**—The movement of a drug into the bloodstream

- **Distribution**—The movement of a medication into body tissues and fluids

- **Metabolism**—The transformation of a drug into chemicals used by the body

- **Elimination**—The movement of a medication out of the body

The pharmacokinetics of acetaminophen (Tylenol®), as noted on the package insert, indicate that this medication is:

- Absorbed mainly in the small intestine

- Distributed throughout most body fluids, except fat

- Metabolized (converted to and/or combined with other chemicals) in the liver

- Eliminated in several hours through the urine

This example demonstrates that adequately functioning body systems are needed for movement of medications throughout the body. Because the function of body systems vary throughout an individual's life, and the impact of medications is affected by the function of body systems, medication dosing may need to be altered during the ages and stages of life when body function is minimized.

Pediatric Patients

Multiple factors impact medication dosing for pediatric patients, making children more susceptible to the effects and adverse effects of drugs. Such factors include:

- Decreased stomach acid production

- Immature liver and kidney function

- Decreased circulation to muscles

- Variable weights and BSA

- Increased metabolism

- Higher percentage of water composing body weight

To maximize drug effect while minimizing adverse effects, safe doses of pediatric medications must be carefully determined. Pediatric doses may be ordered according to body weight or BSA. A major focus of this chapter is safe dose calculation for the pediatric population.

Geriatric Patients

As with children, age-related factors, such as decreased liver and kidney function, poor circulation, and decreased stomach acid production, impact medication dosing for older adults. Additional factors that affect medication dosing in the geriatric population include:

- **Polypharmacy**—Referring to multiple medications taken by one patient, polypharmacy (**Figure 12-1**) increases the chances of drugs interacting or interfering with one another, which may minimize the intended effect of a drug while increasing its side effects. From 2002 to 2012, the percentage of people over 60 who take five or more medications jumped from 22% to 37% (LaPook, 2012).

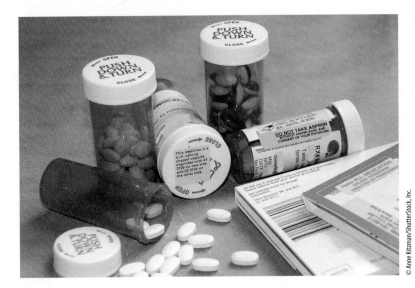

FIGURE 12-1 When observing patients after medication administration, nurses should consider the possible effects of polypharmacy.

- **Creatinine clearance**—The rate at which creatinine, a byproduct of muscle metabolism, is cleared or filtered by the kidneys and is thereby decreased as a normal part of the aging process. Many drug package inserts provide information about safe dosages based on creatinine clearance.

In addition to consideration of the multiple factors that impact medication dosing in the geriatric population, some medication doses for elderly patients are ordered based on body weight or BSA. Although most calculations in this chapter are based on the pediatric population, the same calculations are used for adult weight-based or BSA calculations.

LEARNING ACTIVITY 12-1 Match the terms with the appropriate descriptive phrase.

1.	Process by which a medication enters the bloodstream	a.	Polypharmacy
2.	Causes drug–drug interactions	b.	Absorption
3.	Used to determine safe medication doses	c.	Distribution
		d.	Body surface area

12-2 Weight-Based Calculations

Prior to administration of medications, nurses must ensure that an ordered dose is safe by checking a drug reference to determine recommended weight-based dosages. Because children metabolize medications more rapidly than adults, they typically need more medication per kilogram of body weight than adults. For this reason, nurses should use a pediatric-specific drug reference when checking pediatric drug doses.

Most weight-based medications are based on body weight in kilograms, therefore the nurse needs to convert pounds and ounces, and grams to kilograms, by recalling these equivalencies or conversion factors:

- 1 lb = 16 oz

- 1 kg = 2.2 lb

- 1 kg = 1,000 g

The nurse obtains weight-based dosing information from a drug reference to calculate the safe dose (also called recommended dose) or safe dose range. The drug reference indicates the amount of drug per kilogram of body weight (e.g., 5 mg/kg). This quantity is placed in a ratio-proportion against the patient's weight in kilograms or is multiplied by the patient's weight in kilograms for the formula method and dimensional analysis:

- Ratio-proportion: $\frac{5 \text{ mg}}{1 \text{ kg}} = \frac{x \text{ mg}}{\text{pt's wt in kg}}$

- The formula method: $5 \text{ mg/kg} \times \text{pt wt in kg} = x \text{ (mg)}$

- Dimensional analysis: $x \text{ (mg)} = \frac{5 \text{ mg}}{1 \text{ \cancel{kg}}} \times \frac{\text{pt wt in \cancel{kg}}}{1}$

In each of these equations x will be the recommended or safe dose of medication in milligrams. Safe medication doses are given in the unit of measurement in which the drug is supplied, such as g/kg, mcg/kg, units/kg, mEq/kg, and so on. Therefore, safe dose calculations yield the safe amount of medication in the same unit of measurement as the supply.

When calculating a safe dose, the nurse takes into account whether the weight-based dosing information pertains to a single dose, a single dose range, a daily dose, or a daily dose range.

Calculating a Safe Single Dose (SSD)

The safe dose information for a drug that is given one time or on an as-needed basis is based on a single dose and may be indicated "per dose" or "/dose" in the drug reference manual. For example, the safe dose of ibuprofen may be listed as "10 mg/kg" or "10 mg/kg/dose." The distinction "/dose" should be used with RP and FM while the factor "1/1 dose" should be included in the DA equation. This becomes important when the nurse compares the calculated safe dose to the ordered dose.

Example: Calculate the safe single dose of ibuprofen for a child who weighs 33 lb. The drug reference states, "The recommended dose of ibuprofen is 10 mg/kg/dose."

Ratio-Proportion	Formula Method
Step 1: Convert lb to kg:	Step 1: Convert lb to kg:
$\dfrac{2.2 \text{ lb}}{1 \text{ kg}} = \dfrac{33 \text{ lb}}{x \text{ kg}}$	$\dfrac{1 \text{ kg}}{2.2 \text{ \cancel{lb}}} \times 33 \text{ \cancel{lb}} = x \text{ (kg)}$
$15 \text{kg} = x$	$x = 15 \text{ kg}$
Step 2: Calculate SSD:	Step 2: Calculate SSD:
$\dfrac{10 \text{ mg/dose}}{1 \text{ kg}} = \dfrac{x \text{ mg/dose}}{15 \text{ kg}}$	$10 \text{ mg/\cancel{kg}/dose} \times 15 \text{ \cancel{kg}} = x \text{ (mg/dose)}$
or	$150 \text{ mg/dose} = x$
$10 \text{ mg/dose} : 1 \text{ kg} = x \text{ mg/dose} : 15 \text{kg}$	
$1 \times x = 10 \times 15$	
$x = 150 \text{ mg/dose}$	

Dimensional Analysis

Convert lb to kg using conversion factor 1 kg/2.2 lb:

$$x \, (\text{mg/dose}) = \frac{10 \text{ mg}}{1 \text{ kg}} \times \frac{1 \text{ kg}}{2.2 \text{ lb}} \times \frac{33 \text{ lb}}{1} \times \frac{1}{1 \text{ dose}}$$

$$x = \frac{330 \text{ mg}}{2.2 \text{ dose}}$$

$$x = 150 \text{ mg/dose}$$

The safe dose of acetaminophen for a 15 kg (33 lb) child is 150 mg per dose.

Calculating a Safe Single Dose Range

Some medication safe doses are determined within a range. To determine a **safe dose range (SDR)**, the nurse must calculate the minimum safe dose and the maximum safe dose, and the amount between these two quantities is considered the safe dose range of medication. For example, the minimum and maximum safe doses of a medication with a recommended safe dose range of 5 to 10 mg/kg/dose are calculated as follows:

- 5 mg/kg/dose × kg = x (mg/dose) (minimum safe dose)

- 10 mg/kg/dose × kg = x (mg/dose) (maximum safe dose)

The safe dose range falls within (and includes) these two values.

Example: Calculate the safe dose range of codeine for an 8.8 lb infant. The drug reference indicates, "The safe dose range for codeine is 0.25–0.5 mg/kg/dose."

Ratio-Proportion	Formula Method
Step 1: Convert lb to kg: $$\frac{2.2 \text{ lb}}{1 \text{ kg}} = \frac{8.8 \text{ lb}}{x \text{ kg}}$$ $$x = 4 \text{ kg}$$ Step 2: Calculate minimum safe dose $$\frac{0.25 \text{ mg/dose}}{1 \text{ kg}} = \frac{x \text{ mg/dose}}{4 \text{ kg}}$$ or 0.25 mg/dose : 1 kg = x mg/dose : 4 kg $$1 \times x = 0.25 \times 4$$ $$x = 1 \text{ mg/dose}$$	Step 1: Convert lb to kg: $$\frac{1 \text{ kg}}{2.2 \text{ lb}} \times 8.8 \text{ lb} = x \, (\text{kg})$$ $$4 \text{ kg} = x$$ Step 2: Calculate minimum safe dose: 0.25 mg/kg/dose × 4 kg = x (mg/dose) 1 mg/dose = x Step 3: Calculate maximum safe dose: 0.5 mg/kg/dose × 4 kg = x (mg/dose) 2 mg/dose = x

Step 3: Calculate maximum safe dose:

$$\frac{0.5\ \text{mg/dose}}{1\ \text{kg}} = \frac{x\ \text{mg/dose}}{4\ \text{kg}}$$

or

$$0.5\ \text{mg/dose}:1\ \text{kg} = x\ \text{mg/dose}:4\ \text{kg}$$

$$1 \times x = 0.5 \times 4$$

$$x = 2\ \text{mg/dose}$$

Dimensional Analysis

Step 1: Calculate minimum safe dose; use conversion factor 1 kg/2.2 lb:

$$x\ (\text{mg/dose}) = \frac{0.25\ \text{mg}}{1\ \cancel{\text{kg}}} \times \frac{1\ \cancel{\text{kg}}}{2.2\ \cancel{\text{lb}}} \times \frac{8.8\ \cancel{\text{lb}}}{1} \times \frac{1}{1\ \text{dose}}$$

$$x = \frac{2.2\ \text{mg}}{2.2/\text{dose}}$$

$$x = 1\ \text{mg/dose}$$

Step 2: Calculate maximum safe dose; use conversion factor 1 kg/2.2 lb:

$$x\ (\text{mg/dose}) = \frac{0.5\ \text{mg}}{1\ \cancel{\text{kg}}} \times \frac{1\ \cancel{\text{kg}}}{2.2\ \cancel{\text{lb}}} \times \frac{8.8\ \cancel{\text{lb}}}{1} \times \frac{1}{1\ \text{dose}}$$

$$x = \frac{4.4\ \text{mg}}{2.2/\text{dose}}$$

$$x = 2\ \text{mg/dose}$$

- The minimum safe dose of codeine for a 4 kg (8.8 lb) infant is 1 mg per dose.

- The maximum safe dose of codeine for a 4 kg (8.8 lb) infant is 2 mg per dose.

- The safe dose range of codeine for a 4 kg (8.8 lb) infant is 1–2 mg per dose.

Clinical CLUE

Certain categories of medications are typically ordered on an as needed (prn) basis; therefore, safe doses of such drugs are usually determined per dose or per dose range:

- Antipyretics (fever-reducing medications), for example, acetaminophen: 15 mg/kg/dose

- Analgesics (pain-relieving medications), for example, morphine: 0.2–0.5 mg/kg/dose

LEARNING ACTIVITY 12-2 Determine the safe dose or safe dose range of each medication for a newborn who weighs 3,575 grams and for an infant who weighs 10 lb 8 oz. Round kilogram weights to the tenths.

1. Acetaminophen—15 mg/kg/dose
2. Potassium chloride—0.5 to 1 mEq/kg/dose

> ### Rounding RULE
>
> Convert ounces to pounds before converting pounds to kilograms. Do not round the resulting weight in pounds prior to converting to kilograms. As a final step, once converted to kilograms, the weight should be rounded to the tenths.
>
> **Example:**   Convert 5 lb 6 oz to kilograms.
>
> - Convert 6 oz to lb: $\frac{1\text{ lb}}{16\text{ oz}} \times 6 \text{ oz} = 0.375$ lb.
>
> - Combine partial pounds with whole pounds: $5\text{ lb} + 0.375\text{ lb} = 5.375$ lb.
>
> - Convert 5.375 lb to kg: $\frac{1\text{ kg}}{2.2\text{ lb}} \times 5.375 \text{ lb} = 2.443$ kg.
>
> - Round 2.443 to 2.4 kg.

Calculating a Safe Daily Dose (SDD)

Safe doses for medications that are ordered on a scheduled basis rather than a prn basis are usually based on a daily dose, indicated "per day" or "/day" in the drug reference. For example, the safe dose of clarithromycin is 15 mg/kg/day. The distinction "/day" should be used with RP and FM while the factor "1/1 day" should be included in the DA equation. Proper labeling, when calculating, will eliminate confusion by prompting the nurse to compare a safe daily dose to an ordered daily dose rather than comparing a safe daily dose to an ordered single dose.

Example: Calculate the safe daily dose and the safe single dose of clarithromycin for a child who weighs 66 lb. Regarding clarithromycin, the drug reference states, "The recommended dose is 15 mg/kg/day divided q12h."

Ratio-Proportion	Formula Method
Step 1: Convert lb to kg: $$\frac{2.2\text{ lb}}{1\text{ kg}} = \frac{66\text{ lb}}{x\text{ kg}}$$ $$x = 30\text{ kg}$$ Step 2: Calculate the SDD: $$\frac{15\text{ mg/day}}{1\text{ kg}} = \frac{x\text{ mg/day}}{30\text{ kg}}$$ or $$15\text{ mg/day}:1\text{ kg} = x\text{ mg/day}:30\text{ kg}$$ $$1 \times x = 15 \times 30$$ $$x = 450\text{ mg/day}$$	Step 1: Convert lb to kg: $$\frac{1\text{ kg}}{2.2\text{ lb}} \times 66\text{ lb} = x\,(\text{kg})$$ $$30\text{ kg} = x$$ Step 2: Calculate the SDD: $$15\text{ mg/kg/day} \times 30\text{ kg} = x\,(\text{mg/day})$$ $$450\text{ mg/day} = x$$

Dimensional Analysis

Calculate the SDD; use the conversion factor 1 kg/2.2 lb:

$$x\,(\text{mg/day}) = \frac{15\text{ mg}}{1\text{ kg}} \times \frac{1\text{ kg}}{2.2\text{ lb}} \times \frac{66\text{ lb}}{1} \times \frac{1}{1\text{ day}}$$

$$x = \frac{990\text{ mg}}{2.2/\text{day}}$$

$$x = 450\text{ mg/day}$$

The safe dose of clarithromycin for a 30 kg (66 lb) child is 450 mg per day.

To determine the safe single dose using ratio-proportion or the formula method, divide the daily dose by the number of doses per day. Because q12h occurs two times per day, the safe single dose of clarithromycin is calculated as follows:

$$450 \text{ mg/day} \div 2 \text{ doses/day} = 225 \text{ mg/dose}$$

Therefore, the safe dose of clarithromycin for a 30 kg (66 lb) child is 225 mg per dose.

When using dimensional analysis, multiply by the frequency factor, 12 h/1 dose, and the conversion factor, 1 day/24 h:

$$x \text{ (mg/dose)} = \frac{15 \text{ mg}}{1 \text{ kg}} \times \frac{30 \text{ kg}}{1} \times \frac{1}{1 \text{ day}} \times \frac{1 \text{ day}}{24 \text{ h}} \times \frac{12 \text{ h}}{1 \text{ dose}}$$

$$x \text{ (mg/dose)} = \frac{5,400 \text{ mg}}{24 \text{ dose}} = 225 \text{ mg/dose}$$

Therefore, the safe dose of clarithromycin for a 30 kg child is 225 mg per dose.

Calculating a Safe Daily Dose Range

Some daily medication safe doses are determined within a range, such as 10 to 20 mg/kg/day. In this case, the nurse will perform two calculations, the first to obtain the minimum safe dose and the second to obtain the maximum safe dose. After determining the safe daily dose range, if desired, the nurse may determine the minimum and maximum safe single doses by dividing both the minimum and maximum safe daily doses by the number of doses per day. Or, if using dimensional analysis, multiply by the frequency factor and the conversion factor 1 day/24 h.

Example:　Calculate the safe daily dose range and the safe single dose range of ampicillin for a 10 kg child. Regarding ampicillin, the drug reference recommends "50–100 mg/kg/day in divided doses q6h." For ratio-proportion and the formula method, the safe single dose range is calculated after determining the number of doses per day. Because q6h occurs 4 times per day, there are 4 doses per day.

Ratio-Proportion	Formula Method
Minimum daily dose:	Minimum daily dose:
$\dfrac{50 \text{ mg/day}}{1 \text{ kg}} = \dfrac{x \text{ mg/day}}{10 \text{ kg}}$　or	$50 \text{ mg/kg/day} \times 10 \text{ kg} = x \text{ (mg/day)}$
$50 \text{ mg/day} : 1 \text{ kg} = x \text{ mg/day} : 10 \text{ kg}$	$500 \text{ mg/day} = x$
$1 \times x = 50 \times 10$	Minimum single dose:
$x = 500 \text{ mg/day}$	$500 \text{ mg/day} \div 4 \text{ doses/day} = \text{(mg/dose)}$
Minimum single dose:	$125 \text{ mg/dose} = x$
$\dfrac{500 \text{ mg}}{4 \text{ doses}} = \dfrac{x \text{ mg}}{1 \text{ dose}}$　or	
$500 \text{ mg} : 4 \text{ doses} = x \text{ mg} : 1 \text{ dose}$	
$4x = 500$	
$x = 125 \text{ mg/dose}$	

Maximum daily dose:

$$\frac{100 \text{ mg/day}}{1 \text{ kg}} = \frac{x \text{ mg/day}}{10 \text{ kg}} \text{ or}$$

$$100 \text{ mg/day} : 1 \text{ kg} = x \text{ mg/day} : 10 \text{ kg}$$

$$1 \times x = 100 \times 10$$

$$x = 1,000 \text{ mg/day}$$

Maximum single dose:

$$\frac{1,000 \text{ mg}}{4 \text{ doses}} = \frac{x \text{ mg}}{1 \text{ dose}} \text{ or}$$

$$1,000 \text{ mg} : 4 \text{ doses} = x \text{ mg} : 1 \text{ dose}$$

$$4x = 1,000$$

$$x = 250 \text{ mg/dose}$$

Maximum daily dose:

$$100 \text{ mg/} \cancel{\text{kg}} \text{/day} \times 10 \ \cancel{\text{kg}} = x \ (\text{mg/day})$$

$$1,000 \text{ mg/day} = x$$

Maximum single dose:

$$1,000 \text{ mg/} \cancel{\text{day}} \div 4 \text{ doses/} \cancel{\text{day}} = (\text{mg/dose})$$

$$250 \text{ mg/dose} = x$$

Dimensional Analysis

Minimum daily dose:

$$x \ (\text{mg/day}) = \frac{50 \text{ mg}}{1 \ \cancel{\text{kg}}} \times \frac{10 \ \cancel{\text{kg}}}{1} \times \frac{1}{1 \text{ day}}$$

$$x = \frac{500 \text{ mg}}{1 \text{ day}}$$

$$x = 500 \text{ mg/day}$$

Minimum single dose:

$$x \ (\text{mg/dose}) = \frac{500 \text{ mg}}{1 \ \cancel{\text{day}}} \times \frac{1 \ \cancel{\text{day}}}{24 \ \cancel{\text{h}}} \times \frac{6 \ \cancel{\text{h}}}{1 \text{ dose}}$$

$$x = \frac{3,000 \text{ mg}}{24 \text{ dose}} = 125 \text{ mg/dose}$$

Maximum daily dose:

$$x \ (\text{mg/day}) = \frac{100 \text{ mg}}{1 \ \cancel{\text{kg}}} \times \frac{10 \ \cancel{\text{kg}}}{1} \times \frac{1}{1 \text{ day}}$$

$$x = \frac{1,000 \text{ mg}}{1 \text{ day}}$$

$$x = 1,000 \text{ mg/day}$$

Maximum single dose:

$$x \ (\text{mg/dose}) = \frac{1,000 \text{ mg}}{1 \ \cancel{\text{day}}} \times \frac{1 \ \cancel{\text{day}}}{24 \ \cancel{\text{h}}} \times \frac{6 \ \cancel{\text{h}}}{1 \text{ dose}}$$

$$x = \frac{6,000 \text{ mg}}{24 \text{ dose}} = 250 \text{ mg/dose}$$

- The minimum daily dose of ampicillin for a 10 kg child is 500 mg per day.

- The maximum daily dose of ampicillin for a 10 kg child is 1,000 mg per day.

- The safe daily dose range of ampicillin for a 10 kg child is 500 to 1,000 mg per day.

- The minimum single dose of ampicillin for a 10 kg child is 125 mg per dose.

- The maximum single dose of ampicillin for a 10 kg child is 250 mg per dose.

- The safe single dose range of ampicillin for a 10 kg child is 125 to 250 mg per dose.

Clinical CLUE

The safe dose and safe dose range of medications that are typically ordered on a scheduled basis are usually determined per day rather than per dose. For example, because antibiotics and cardiac medications are scheduled around the clock, drug references usually provide information regarding the safe daily dose/dose range of these drugs. From this information, the nurse will calculate the safe daily dose/dose range and:

- Compare it to the ordered daily dose or

- Determine the single dose/dose range and compare the ordered (single) dose

LEARNING ACTIVITY 12-3 The recommended dose of amoxicillin is 20 to 40 mg/kg/day in divided doses q12h. For a 12 lb, 4 oz infant, calculate the:

1. Minimum daily dose
2. Maximum daily dose
3. Minimum single dose
4. Maximum single dose

Comparing a Safe Dose to an Ordered Dose

After calculating a safe dose, the nurse compares the ordered dose to the calculated safe dose. If the ordered dose matches the safe dose or falls within the safe dose range, the nurse can proceed with medication administration. If the ordered dose does not match the safe (recommended) dose or does not fall within the (recommended) SDR, the nurse should not administer the medication, but should contact the authorized prescriber right away.

Example 1:   Determine if the order is safe, and, if safe, calculate the amount, in mL, to administer.

   Order: acetaminophen 140 mg PO q4h prn fever greater than 38.5°C for a 20 lb 6 oz child

Reference: Recommended dose of acetaminophen is 15 mg/kg per dose.

  Supply: Acetaminophen 80 mg/ 1/2 teaspoon (see **Figure 12-3**).

Step 1: Convert weight to kg using the conversion factors $\frac{1 \text{ kg}}{2.2 \text{ lb}}$ and $\frac{1 \text{ lb}}{16 \text{ oz}}$.

Step 2: Calculate the safe dose.

© Francois Etienne du Plessis/ShutterStock, Inc.

Clinical CLUE

Weight-based medications require accurate weights to be recorded in charts. In the interest of time, a prescriber may order medications based on a reported weight instead of an actual weight. This may cause a discrepancy in the safe dose calculation obtained by the nurse and the prescriber. Consider the following scenario:

- A parent reports to the physician their child's weight as 23 pounds. The physician converts this weight to 10.5 kg (23 lb × 1 kg/2.2 lb = 10.45 or 10.5 kg).

- Because the recommended dose of acetaminophen is 15 mg/kg/dose, the prescriber orders 158 mg to be given, based on this recommended (safe) dose calculation:

$$\frac{15 \text{ mg}}{1 \text{ kg}} \times \frac{10.5 \text{ kg}}{1} \times \frac{1}{1 \text{ dose}} = 157.5 \text{ or } 158 \text{ mg/dose}.$$

- The nurse obtains the child's actual weight of 22 pounds and converts it to 10 kg:

$$22 \text{ lb} \times \frac{1 \text{ kg}}{2.2 \text{ lb}} = 10 \text{ kg}$$

- The nurse calculates the safe dose using the actual weight of 10 kg:

$$\frac{15 \text{ mg}}{\text{kg}} \times \frac{10 \text{ kg}}{1} \times \frac{1}{1 \text{ dose}} = 150 \text{ mg/dose}$$

Because of the discrepancy between the dose ordered and the safe dose calculation, the nurse questions the order. This discrepancy can be avoided if patient weights are promptly obtained and recorded. (**Figure 12-2**)

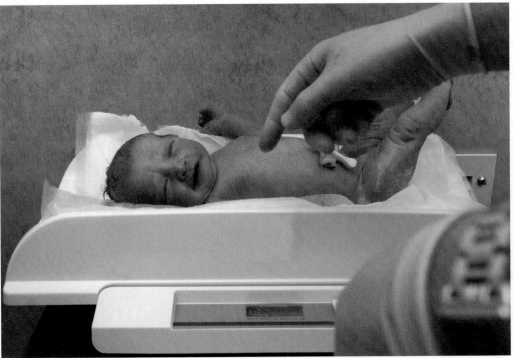

FIGURE 12-2   Accurate weights are needed for weight-based medication doses.

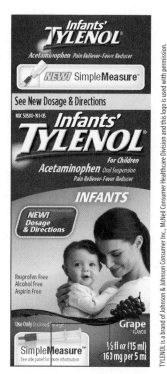

FIGURE 12-3 Acetaminophen label showing supply of 160 mg/5 mL which is equivalent to 80 mg/1/2 tsp.

Step 3: Determine whether the ordered dose is safe by comparing it to the safe dose.

Step 4: Calculate the amount to administer or contact the prescriber if the ordered dose is not safe.

Ratio-Proportion	Formula Method
Step 1a: Convert oz to lb:	Step 1a: Convert oz to lb:
$$\frac{1\,lb}{16\,oz} = \frac{x\,lb}{6\,oz}\ \text{ or}$$	$$\frac{1\,lb}{16\,\cancel{oz}} \times 6\ \cancel{oz} = x\ (lb)$$
$$1\,lb : 16\,oz = x\,lb : 6\,oz$$	$$0.375\,lb = x$$
$$16x = 6$$	Step 1b: Combine partial pounds with whole pounds.
$$x = 0.375\,lb$$	$$x = 20\,lb + 0.375\,lb$$
Step 1b: Combine partial pounds with whole pounds:	$$x = 20.375\,lb$$
$$x = 20\,lb + 0.375\,lb$$	Step 1c: Convert 20.375 lb to kg.
$$x = 20.375\,lb$$	$$\frac{1\,kg}{2.2\,\cancel{lb}} \times 20.375\ \cancel{lb} = x\ (kg)$$
	$$9.26136\,kg = x$$
	round to 9.3 kg

Step 1c: Convert 20.375 lb to kg:

$$\frac{1\,kg}{2.2\,lb} = \frac{x\,kg}{20.375\,lb} \quad or$$

$$1\,kg : 2.2\,lb = x\,kg : 20.375\,lb$$

$$2.2x = 20.375\,lb$$

$$x = 9.26\ or\ 9.3\,kg$$

Step 2: Calculate SSD:

$$\frac{15\,mg/dose}{1\,kg} = \frac{x\,mg/dose}{9.3\,kg} \quad or$$

$$15\,mg/dose : 1\,kg = x\,mg/dose : 9.3\,kg$$

$$1 \times x = 15 \times 9.3$$

$$x = 139.5\,mg/dose$$

Step 2: Calculate SSD:

$$15\,mg/\cancel{kg}/dose \times 9.3\,\cancel{kg} = x$$

$$139.5\,mg/dose = x$$

Dimensional Analysis

Steps 1a, 1b, 1c, and 2 are combined:

$$x\,(mg/dose) = \frac{15\,mg}{1\,\cancel{kg}} \times \frac{1\,\cancel{kg}}{2.2\,lb} \times \left[\frac{20\,lb}{1} + \left(\frac{6\,\cancel{oz}}{1} \times \frac{1\,lb}{16\,\cancel{oz}} \right) \right] \times \frac{1}{1\,dose}$$

$$x = \frac{15\,mg}{2.2\,\cancel{lb}} \times \frac{20.375\,\cancel{lb}}{1\,dose}$$

$$x = \frac{305.625\,mg}{2.2\,dose}$$

$$x = 138.92\,mg/dose$$

Step 3: Compare the ordered dose to the recommended dose.

Because the ordered dose is 140 mg and the calculated recommended doses are 139.5 mg and 138.92 mg, the dose is considered safe. Note that with the dimensional analysis approach, because there is no internal rounding, the answer is more exact and slightly lower than the amount calculated using ratio-proportion and the formula method. When there is only a slight difference between the ordered dose and calculated safe dose, it is usually acceptable to proceed with medication administration; however, to err on the side of caution, the nurse should contact the prescriber if there is any question when comparing the ordered dose to the safe calculated dose.

Step 4: Because the ordered dose is safe, the nurse can now use the CASE approach to determine the amount to administer.

C: *Convert*—Because the order and supply are in mg, there is no conversion needed for the amount. Because the supply volume is given in teaspoons (tsp) and the answer requested is mL, convert ½ tsp to 2.5 mL; for dimensional analysis, use the conversion factor 1 tsp/5 mL.

A: *Approximate*—The ordered dose, 140 mg, is almost two times the supply amount of 80 mg, therefore almost two times the supply volume of ½ tsp (i.e., almost 1 tsp [5 mL]) will be needed to administer the ordered dose.

S: *Solve*

Ratio-Proportion	Formula Method
$$\frac{80 \text{ mg}}{2.5 \text{ mL}} = \frac{140 \text{ mg}}{x \text{ mL}} \text{ or}$$	$$\frac{140 \text{ mg}}{80 \text{ mg}} \times 2.5 \text{ mL} = x \text{ (mL)}$$
$80 \text{ mg}:2.5 \text{ mL} = 140 \text{ mg}:x \text{ mL}$	$$\frac{350 \text{ mL}}{80} = x$$
$80x = 350$	$4.375 \text{ mL} = x$
$$\frac{80x}{80} = \frac{350}{80}$$	Round to tenths; $x = 4.4 \text{ mL}$
$x = 4.375 \text{ mL}$	
Round to tenths; $x = 4.4 \text{ mL}$	

Dimensional Analysis

$$x \text{ (mL)} = \frac{\frac{1}{2} \text{ tsp}}{80 \text{ mg}} \times \frac{5 \text{ mL}}{1 \text{ tsp}} \times \frac{140 \text{ mg}}{1}$$

$$x = \frac{350 \text{ mL}}{80}$$

$$x = 4.375 \text{ mL}$$

Round to tenths; $x \text{ mL} = 4.4 \text{ mL}$

E: *Evaluate*

Ratio-Proportion	Formula Method
$$\frac{80 \text{ mg}}{2.5 \text{ mL}} = \frac{140 \text{ mg}}{4.375 \text{ mL}} \text{ or}$$	$$\frac{140 \text{ mg}}{80 \text{ mg}} \times 2.5 \text{ mL} = 4.375 \text{ mL}$$
$80 \text{ mg}:2.5 \text{ mL}$	$$\frac{350 \text{ mL}}{80} = 4.375 \text{ ml}$$
$= 140 \text{ mg}:4.375 \text{ mL}$	$4.375 \text{ mL} = 4.375 \text{ mL}$
$80 \times 4.375 = 2.5 \times 140$	
$350 = 350$	

Dimensional Analysis

$$4.375 \text{ mL} = \frac{\frac{1}{2} \text{ tsp}}{80 \text{ mg}} \times \frac{5 \text{ mL}}{1 \text{ tsp}} \times \frac{140 \text{ mg}}{1}$$

$$4.375 \text{ mL} = \frac{350 \text{ mL}}{80}$$

$$4.375 \text{ mL} = 4.375 \text{ mL}$$

Because the calculated volume accurately completes the equation and is consistent with the approximated volume, the answer, 4.4 mL, is confirmed.

WARNING!

Compare Apples to Apples: Safe Single Dose to Ordered Single Dose ... Safe Daily Dose to Ordered Daily Dose!

When calculating safe doses, it is important to distinguish safe single dose calculations from safe daily dose calculations. Convert daily doses to single doses or single doses to daily doses for comparison. For example, the safe dose of gentamicin may be referenced as "2.5 mg/kg (q8h)," which refers to the safe single dose. Because there are three single doses in 1 day (24 h), the safe daily dose is 7.5 mg/kg/day. If the drug reference gives the safe daily dose, 7.5 mg/kg/day, to determine if 75 mg q8h of gentamicin is safe for a 30 kg child, the nurse has two options:

1. Calculate both the safe daily dose and the ordered daily dose; then compare the ordered daily dose to the safe daily dose.

   Safe daily dose:

   $$\frac{7.5 \text{ mg}}{1 \text{ kg}} \times \frac{30 \text{ kg}}{1} \times \frac{1}{1 \text{ day}} = 225 \text{ mg/day}$$

   Ordered daily dose:

   $$\frac{75 \text{ mg}}{\text{dose}} \times \frac{3 \text{ doses}}{1 \text{ day}} = 225 \text{ mg/day}$$

   Safe daily dose (225 mg) = ordered daily dose (225 mg), therefore the ordered dose is safe.

2. Calculate the safe daily dose, determine the safe single dose, then compare the safe single dose to the ordered single dose.

   Safe daily dose:

   $$\frac{7.5 \text{ mg}}{1 \text{ kg}} \times \frac{30 \text{ kg}}{1} \times \frac{1}{1 \text{ day}} = 225 \text{ mg/day}$$

   Safe single dose:

   $$225 \text{ mg/day} \div 3 \text{ doses/day} = 75 \text{ mg/dose}$$

   Safe single dose $\left(75 \text{ mg}\right)$ = ordered $\left(\text{single}\right)$ dose $\left(75 \text{ mg}\right)$, therefore the ordered dose is safe.

Always compare safe *daily* doses to ordered *daily* doses and compare safe *single* doses to ordered *single* doses.

Example 2:   Determine if the order is safe, and, if safe, calculate the amount, in mL, to administer.

Order: erythromycin lactobionate 250 mg IV q6h for an adult weighing 185 lb

Reference: Recommended daily dosage of erythromycin lactobionate for adult patients is 15–20 mg/kg/day to be administered in 4 divided doses.

Supply: See **Figure 12-4**.

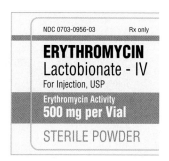

FIGURE 12-4

Ratio-Proportion	Formula Method
Step 1: Convert lb to kg:	Step 1: Convert lb to kg:
$$\frac{1\,kg}{2.2\,lb} = \frac{x\,kg}{185\,lb}$$	$$\frac{1\,kg}{2.2\,lb} \times 185\,\cancel{lb} = x\,(kg)$$
$$2.2x = 185\,lb$$	$$x = 84.09\,kg$$
$$x = 84.09\,kg$$	Round to 84.1 kg
Round to 84.1 kg	Step 2a: Calculate minimum daily dose:
Step 2a: Calculate minimum daily dose:	$$15\,mg/\cancel{kg}/day \times 84.1\,\cancel{kg} = x\,(mg/day)$$
$$\frac{15\,mg/day}{1\,kg} = \frac{x\,mg/day}{84.1\,kg}\ \ or$$	$$1,261.5\,mg/day = x$$
$$15\,mg/day:1\,kg = x\,mg/day:84.1\,kg$$	
$$x = 1,261.5\,mg/day$$	
Step 2b: Calculate maximum daily dose:	Step 2b: Calculate maximum daily dose:
$$\frac{20\,mg/day}{1\,kg} = \frac{x\,mg/day}{84.1\,kg}\ \ or$$	$$20\,mg/\cancel{kg}/day \times 84.1\,\cancel{kg} = x\,(mg/day)$$
$$20\,mg/day:1\,kg = x\,mg/day:84.1\,kg$$	$$1,682\,mg/day = x$$
$$x = 1,682\,mg/day$$	

Dimensional Analysis

Steps 1 and 2 are combined.

Calculate minimum daily dose; use conversion factor $\frac{1\,kg}{2.2\,lb}$:

$$x\,(mg/day) = \frac{15\,mg}{1\,\cancel{kg}} \times \frac{1\,\cancel{kg}}{2.2\,\cancel{lb}} \times \frac{185\,\cancel{lb}}{1} \times \frac{1}{1\,day}$$

$$x = \frac{2,775\,mg}{2.2\,day}$$

$$x = 1,261.3636$$

$$x = 1,261.4\,mg/day$$

Calculate maximum daily dose; use conversion factor $\frac{1\,kg}{2.2\,lb}$:

$$x\ (mg/day) = \frac{20\ mg}{1\ \cancel{kg}} \times \frac{1\ \cancel{kg}}{2.2\ lb} \times \frac{185\ lb}{1} \times \frac{1}{1\ day}$$

$$x = \frac{3{,}700\ mg}{2.2\ day}$$

$$x = 1{,}681.8181$$

$$x = 1{,}681.8\ mg/day$$

- The minimum daily dose of erythromycin for a 185 lb adult is 1,261.5 or 1,261.4 mg per day.

- The maximum daily dose of erythromycin for a 185 lb adult is 1,682 or 1,681.8 mg per day.

- The safe daily dose range of erythromycin for a 185 lb adult is 1,261–1,682 mg per day.

Step 3: Compare the ordered dose to the safe dose.

Because the ordered dose, 250 mg, is to be given four times daily (q6h), the daily dose $(4 \times 250\ mg)$ would be 1 g or 1,000 mg. Because 1,000 mg per day is outside the safe daily dose range of 1,261 to 1,682 mg, the order is not safe.

Step 4: Because the order is not safe, the nurse will not carry out this drug order but instead will contact the prescriber for a new order.

If desired with Example 2, the nurse could calculate the safe single dose of erythromycin and then compare it to the single dose of erythromycin ordered. To determine the safe single dose of erythromycin, the nurse should divide the daily dose by the number of doses per day. Recall that the drug reference states that erythromycin should be given "in 4 divided doses." Therefore, the conversion factor 1 day/4 doses is inserted into the above DA equation or the recommended daily dose will be divided by 4 to determine the safe single dose:

$$1{,}261\ mg/\cancel{day} \div 4\ doses/\cancel{day} = 315.25\ or\ 315\ mg/dose$$

$$1{,}682\ mg\ mg/\cancel{day} \div 4\ doses/\cancel{day} = 420.5\ or\ 421\ mg/dose,\ therefore:$$

- The minimum single dose of erythromycin for a 185 lb adult is 315 mg per dose.

- The maximum single dose of erythromycin for a 185 lb adult is 421 mg per dose.

- The safe single dose range of erythromycin for a 185 lb adult is 315 to 421 mg per dose.

Because the dose ordered, 250 mg, is outside the safe dose range, the nurse should contact the prescriber for a new order right away.

LEARNING ACTIVITY 12-4 Apply the following orders to a 15 kg child and:

a. Calculate the safe daily dose/dose range.
b. Compare the ordered daily dose to the safe daily dose/dose range.
c. Determine whether the nurse should calculate the amount to administer (for a single dose) or contact the prescriber.

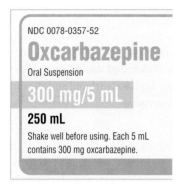

FIGURE 12-5

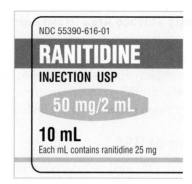

FIGURE 12-6

1.   **Order:** Oxcarbazepine 75 mg PO bid
      Reference: Safe dose of oxycarbazepine is 8–10 mg/kg/day in divided doses q12h.
      Supply: See **Figure 12-5**.
2.   **Order:** Zantac® 15 mg IV q8h
      Reference: Recommended dose of ranitidine is 2–4 mg/kg/day in divided doses q6–8h.
      Supply: See **Figure 12-6**.
3.   **Order:** albuterol sulfate 2 mg PO tid
      Reference: Recommended pediatric dosage of albuterol sulfate is 0.3 mg/kg/day in three divided
      doses, not to exceed 2 mg tid.
      Supply: See **Figure 12-7**.

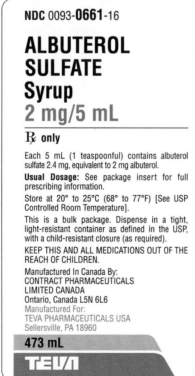

FIGURE 12-7

12-3   Body Surface Area (BSA) Calculations

Body surface area is used to calculate safe dosages of highly potent drugs and drugs given to vulnerable populations. Examples of types of medications that may require BSA-based dosing include pediatric medications, chemotherapy drugs, and medications given to patients who have suffered serious burn injuries, are receiving radiation treatment, or are undergoing open heart surgery.

Calculation of BSA

Body surface area is the total surface area of the body expressed in square meters (m^2). BSA is calculated using metric or household measurements of height and weight. Common formulas for calculating BSA include:

- BSA metric formula $m^2 = \sqrt{\dfrac{ht(cm) \times wt(kg)}{3,600}}$
- BSA household formula $m^2 = \sqrt{\dfrac{ht(in) \times wt(lb)}{3,131}}$

Clinical CLUE

The constants 3,600 in the metric formula and 3,131 in the household formula were derived, through research, by measuring the BSA for a large sample of people and comparing it with the formula height $\times$ weight. On average, it was found that height $\times$ weight needs to be divided by 3,600 when using metric units and 3,131 when using household units to get the BSA.

Rounding RULE

When calculating BSA, round quantities less than 1 to hundredths and quantities greater than 1 to tenths.

Example 1:   Calculate the BSA for a 4 ft 3 in tall 7-year-old child who weighs 55 pounds.

Convert 4 feet, 3 inches to inches:

$$12 \text{ in}/\cancel{ft} \times 4 \ \cancel{ft} = 48 \text{ in}$$

$$48 \text{ in} + 3 \text{ in} = 51 \text{ in}$$

Choose the BSA household formula:

$$m^2 = \sqrt{\frac{51 \text{ in } \times 55 \text{ lb}}{3,131}} = \sqrt{\frac{2,805}{3,131}} = \sqrt{0.896} = 0.95$$

Example 2:   Calculate the BSA for an infant who weighs 7,540 g and is 65 cm long.

Convert 7,540 g to 7.54 kg.

Choose the BSA metric formula:

$$m^2 = \sqrt{\frac{65 \text{ cm } \times 7.54 \text{ kg}}{3,600}} = \sqrt{\frac{490.1}{3,600}} = \sqrt{0.136} = 0.37$$

Example 3:   Calculate the BSA for a 5 ft 5 in adult who weighs 155 lb.

Convert 5 feet, 5 inches to inches: $12 \text{ in}/\text{ft} \times 5 \text{ ft} = 60 \text{ in}$

$$60 \text{ in} + 5 \text{ in} = 65 \text{ in}$$

Choose the BSA household formula:

$$m^2 = \sqrt{\frac{65 \text{ in} \times 155 \text{ lb}}{3,131}} = \sqrt{\frac{10,075}{3,131}} = \sqrt{3.218} = 1.8$$

LEARNING ACTIVITY 12-5 For the given measurements, calculate the BSA using the household formula or the metric formula.

1.   25 in, 16 lb
2.   175 cm, 75.5 kg
3.   4 ft 6 in, 95 lb
4.   51 cm, 3,636 g

Using a Nomogram to Determine Body Surface Area

The West Nomogram is a graph used to estimate BSA (**Figure 12-8**). This graph includes height (in inches and centimeters) on the left, weight (in pounds and kilograms) on the right, and BSA (in square meters) in the center. To determine BSA using the West Nomogram, a straight line connecting

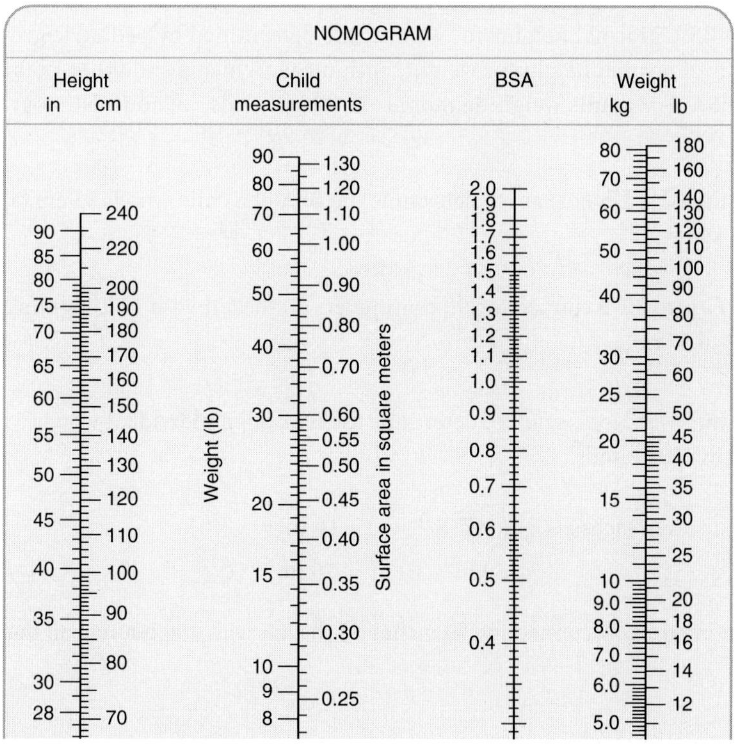

FIGURE 12-8   The West Nomogram is used for estimation of body surface area (BSA).

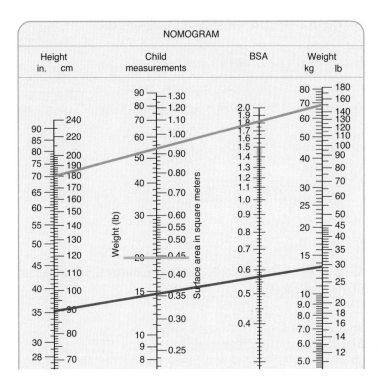

FIGURE 12-9 Using the West Nomogram, the nurse can determine that the BSA of a 90 cm, 13 kg child is 0.57 m² (red line); the BSA of a 5 ft 10 in, 150 lb individual is 1.8 m² (blue line); the BSA of a 9.1 kg infant of normal height and weight is 0.44 m² (green line).

height and weight is made and the point at which this line intersects the BSA column indicates the estimated BSA in square meters. The West Nomogram also includes an insert that can be used to identify BSA for children of normal height for weight by locating the weight on the graph and reading the corresponding BSA. Normal heights for weights are determined by pediatric growth charts. When not sure if a child is of normal height for weight, both measurements should be obtained and used to determine the BSA. For adults weighing more than 180 pounds, an adult Nomogram is available (see Appendix F).

Example 1: Use the West Nomogram to determine the BSA of a child who is 85 cm tall and weighs 13.5 kg.

See the red line on **Figure 12-9** connecting 90 centimeters on the left with 13 kilograms on the right, revealing the BSA = 0.57 m².

Example 2: Use the West Nomogram to determine the BSA of an individual who is 5 ft 10 in tall and weighs 150 pounds.

Convert 5 feet, 10 inches to inches: $\left(\frac{12 \text{ in}}{1 \text{ ft}} \times 5 \text{ ft} \right) + 10 \text{ in} = x \text{ (in)}$

$60 \text{ in} + 10 \text{ in} = 70 \text{ in}$

See the blue line on Figure 12-9 connecting 70 inches on the left with 150 pounds on the right, revealing the BSA = 1.8 m².

Example 3: Use the West Nomogram to determine the BSA of an infant of normal height and weight who weighs 9.1 kg.

Convert 9.1 kg to pounds: $\frac{2.2 \text{ lb}}{1 \text{ kg}} \times 9.1 \text{ kg} = 20 \text{ lb}$

See the green line on Figure 12-9 identifying the BSA of a 20-pound infant as 0.44 m².

LEARNING ACTIVITY 12-6 For the given measurements, determine the BSA using the West Nomogram.

1.   ht = 35 in; wt = 35 lb
2.   ht = 70 cm; wt = 9.4 kg
3.   ht = 4 ft 4 in; wt = 75 lb
4.   normal ht for wt; wt = 40 kg

Calculation of BSA-Based Doses

When the drug reference indicates that a safe medication dose is BSA based, the nurse will first determine the BSA. The nurse will then calculate the safe dose/safe dose range in the same way that a weight-based dose is calculated. The safe dose per square meters (e.g., 2.5 mg/m²) will be placed in a ratio-proportion against the patient's BSA in square meters or will be multiplied by the patient's BSA in square meters for the formula method and dimensional analysis:

- Ratio-proportion: $\frac{\text{safe dose [2.5 mg]}}{1 \text{ m}^2} = \frac{x \text{ mg}}{\text{pt BSA in m}^2}$

- The formula method: safe dose $\frac{[2.5 \text{ mg}]}{\text{m}^2} \times$ pt BSA in $\text{m}^2 = x \text{ (mg)}$

- Dimensional analysis: $x \text{ (mg)} = \frac{\text{safe dose [2.5 mg]}}{1 \text{ m}^2} \times \frac{\text{pt wt in m}^2}{1}$

In each of these equations, x will be the recommended or safe dose of medication in milligrams. Safe medication doses are given in the unit of measurement in which the drug is supplied, such as g/m², mcg/m², units/m², or mEq/m². Therefore, safe dose calculations should yield the safe amount of medication in the same unit of measurement in which the drug is supplied.

As with weight-based calculations, the nurse must take into account whether the BSA-based dosing information pertains to a single dose, a single dose range, a daily dose, or a daily dose range.

Example 1: Determine if the order is safe and, if safe, calculate the amount, in mL, to administer.

Order: vinblastine 2 mg IV q Monday for a child who weighs 45 lb 8 oz and is 45 inches tall

Reference: Recommended dose of vinblastine is 2.5 mg/m² in a single dose weekly.

Supply: vinblastine solution 1 mg/mL

Step 1: Calculate the BSA:

- Convert 45 lb 8 oz to lb:

$$x \text{ (lb)} = \left(\frac{1 \text{ lb}}{16 \text{ oz}} \times \frac{8 \text{ oz}}{1} \right) + 45 \text{ lb} = 45\frac{1}{2} \text{ lb} = 45.5 \text{ lb}$$

- Choose the BSA household formula:

$$m^2 = \sqrt{\frac{45 \text{ in} \times 45.5 \text{ lb}}{3,131}} = \sqrt{\frac{2,047.5}{3,131}} = \sqrt{0.654} = 0.81$$

Step 2: Calculate the safe dose:

Ratio-Proportion	Formula Method
$$\frac{2.5 \text{ mg/dose}}{1 \text{ m}^2} = \frac{x \text{ mg/dose}}{0.81 \text{ m}^2}$$ or $2.5 \text{ mg/dose}: 1 \text{ m}^2 = x \text{ mg/dose}: 0.81 \text{ m}^2$ $1 \times x = 2.5 \times 0.81$ $x = 2.025; \text{round to 2 mg/dose}$	$2.5 \text{ mg/}\cancel{\text{m}^2}\text{/dose} \times 0.81 \cancel{\text{m}^2} = x \,(\text{mg/dose})$ $2.025 \text{ mg/dose} = x$ round to 2 mg/dose

Dimensional Analysis
$$x \,(\text{mg/dose}) = \frac{2.5 \text{ mg}}{1 \cancel{\text{m}^2}} \times \frac{0.81 \cancel{\text{m}^2}}{1} \times \frac{1}{1 \text{ dose}}$$ $$x = \frac{2.025 \text{ mg}}{1 \text{ dose}}$$ round to 2 mg/dose

Step 3: Determine whether the dose ordered is safe. Because 2 mg is ordered and 2 mg is the calculated safe dose, the dose ordered is safe.

Step 4: Calculate the amount to administer:

C: *Convert*—Because the order and supply are in mg, there is no conversion.

A: *Approximate*—The ordered dose, 2 mg, is two times the supply amount of 1 mg, therefore two times the supply volume of 1 mL (i.e., 2 mL) will be needed to administer the ordered dose.

S: *Solve*

Ratio-Proportion	Formula Method
$$\frac{1 \text{ mg}}{1 \text{ mL}} = \frac{2 \text{ mg}}{x \text{ mL}} \quad \text{or}$$ $1 \text{ mg}: 1 \text{ mL} = 2 \text{ mg}: x \text{ mL}$ $1 \times x = 1 \times 2$ $x = 2$ $x = 2 \text{ mL}$	$$\frac{2 \cancel{\text{mg}}}{1 \cancel{\text{mg}}} \times 1 \text{ mL} = x \,(\text{mL})$$ $$\frac{2 \text{ mL}}{1} = x$$ $2 \text{ mL} = x$

Dimensional Analysis

$$x\,(\text{mL}) = \frac{1\,\text{mL}}{1\,\cancel{\text{mg}}} \times \frac{2\,\cancel{\text{mg}}}{1}$$

$$x = \frac{2\,\text{mL}}{1}$$

$$x = 2\,\text{mL}$$

E: *Evaluate*

Ratio-Proportion	**Formula Method**
$\dfrac{1\,\text{mg}}{1\,\text{mL}} = \dfrac{2\,\text{mg}}{2\,\text{mL}}$ or $1\,\text{mg} : 1\,\text{mL} = 2\,\text{mg} : 2\,\text{mL}$ $1 \times 2 = 1 \times 2$ $2 = 2$	$\dfrac{2\,\cancel{\text{mg}}}{1\,\cancel{\text{mg}}} \times 1\,\text{mL} = 2\,\text{mL}$ $\dfrac{2\,\text{mL}}{1} = 2\,\text{mL}$ $2\,\text{mL} = 2\,\text{mL}$
Dimensional Analysis	
$2\,\text{mL} = \dfrac{1\,\text{mL}}{1\,\cancel{\text{mg}}} \times \dfrac{2\,\cancel{\text{mg}}}{1}$ $2\,\text{mL} = \dfrac{2\,\text{mL}}{1}$ $2\,\text{mL} = 2\,\text{mL}$	

Because the calculated volume accurately completes the equation and is consistent with the approximated volume, the answer, 2 mL, is confirmed.

Example 2:   Determine if the order is safe, and, if safe, calculate the amount, in mL, to administer.

   Order: vincristine 4 mg IV q Friday for a child who weighs 45 kg and is 155 cm tall

Reference: Recommended dose of vincristine is 1.5 to 2 mg/m² in a single dose weekly.

   Supply: vincristine solution 1 mg/mL

Step 1: Calculate the BSA with the metric formula:

$$m^2 = \sqrt{\frac{45\ \text{kg}\ \times\ 155\ \text{cm}}{3,600}} = \sqrt{\frac{6,975}{3,600}} = \sqrt{1.94} = 1.4$$

Step 2: Calculate the safe dose range:

Ratio-Proportion	Formula Method
Step 2a: Minimum single dose: $\dfrac{1.5 \text{ mg/dose}}{1 \text{ m}^2} = \dfrac{x \text{ mg/dose}}{1.4 \text{ m}^2}$ or $1.5 \text{ mg} : 1 \text{ m}^2 = x \text{ mg} : 1.4 \text{ m}^2$ $1 \times x = 1.5 \times 1.4$ $x = 2.1 \text{ mg/dose}$	Step 2a: Minimum single dose: $1.5 \text{ mg/} \cancel{\text{m}^2} \text{/dose} \times 1.4 \, \cancel{\text{m}^2} = x \text{ (mg/dose)}$ $2.1 \text{ mg/dose} = x$
Step 2b: Maximum single dose: $\dfrac{2 \text{ mg/dose}}{1 \text{ m}^2} = \dfrac{x \text{ mg/dose}}{1.4 \text{ m}^2}$ or $2 \text{ mg} : 1 \text{ m}^2 = x \text{ mg} : 1.4 \text{ m}^2$ $1 \times x = 2 \times 1.4$ $x = 2.8 \text{ mg/dose}$	Step 2b: Maximum single dose: $2 \text{ mg/} \cancel{\text{m}^2} \text{/dose} \times 1.4 \, \cancel{\text{m}^2} = x \text{ (mg/dose)}$ $2.8 \text{ mg/dose} = x$

Dimensional Analysis

Minimum single dose:

$$x \text{ (mg/dose)} = \frac{1.5 \text{ mg}}{1 \, \cancel{\text{m}^2}} \times \frac{1.4 \, \cancel{\text{m}^2}}{1} \times \frac{1}{1 \text{ dose}}$$

$$x = \frac{2.1 \text{ mg}}{1 \text{ dose}}$$

$$x = 2.1 \text{ mg/dose}$$

Maximum single dose:

$$x \text{ (mg/dose)} = \frac{2 \text{ mg}}{1 \, \cancel{\text{m}^2}} \times \frac{1.4 \, \cancel{\text{m}^2}}{1} \times \frac{1}{1 \text{ dose}}$$

$$x = \frac{2.8 \text{ mg}}{1 \text{ dose}}$$

$$x = 2.8 \text{ mg/dose}$$

Step 3: Determine whether the dose ordered is safe. The safe dose range of vincristine is 2.1 to 2.8 mg per (weekly) dose. Because the ordered dose, 4 mg, does not fall in the safe dose range, the dose is not safe.

Step 4: Because the dose is not safe, the nurse will contact the prescriber.

LEARNING ACTIVITY 12-7 Apply the following orders to a child who weighs 17.2 kg and is 100 cm tall.

a.   Calculate or use the West Nomogram to determine the BSA.
b.   Calculate the safe daily dose/dose range.

c.   Compare the ordered daily dose to the safe daily dose/dose range.

d.   Determine whether the nurse should calculate the amount to administer or contact the prescriber.

1.   **Order:** Interferon 2,070,000 units subcut at 8:00 a.m. on Monday, Wednesday, and Friday
        Supply: Interferon 5,000,000 units/mL
        Reference: Interferon 3 million units/m^2 three times weekly

2.   **Order:** Doxorubicin 20 mg IV daily on Monday, Tuesday, and Wednesday
        Supply: Doxorubicin 2 mg/mL
        Reference: Doxorubicin is administered to children 25 to 30 mg/m^2/day IV × 3 days every 4 weeks.

12-4   Minimum Drug Dilution Calculations

As detailed in Chapter 10, most intravenous (IV) medications are further diluted and administered intermittently via the IV bolus (push) method or via the IV piggyback (IVPB) method. Medications not approved for the IV push method are given via the IVPB method or as a continuous infusion unless a minimum dilution volume is required, as is the case with infants, small children, and fluid-restricted adults. IV medications should be given to infants, children, and fluid-restricted adults in the smallest volume possible in order to prevent fluid overload. Special equipment required to administer intravenous medications in minimal fluid volumes includes **volume-control sets (Figure 12-10)** and **IV syringe pumps (Figure 12-11)**. A volume-control set, IV tubing with a fluid chamber that is filled intermittently with fluid directly from the IV solution, prevents fluid overload as it delivers small volumes of fluid over a specified period of time.

As explained in Chapter 11, most IV medications are further diluted with normal saline (NS) or compatible IV fluid prior to administration. To determine the minimum fluid volume needed to further dilute an intravenous medication, the nurse should first consult a drug reference. This information is typically referenced under "IV Administration Guidelines" for each medication and includes phrases such as "concentration" or "concentration for administration." The drug reference indicates the amount of drug per milliliter of diluent; for example, the concentration for administration of ampicillin is

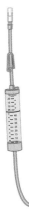

FIGURE 12-10   A volume-control set is used to regulate small hourly fluid volumes and to administer intermittent IV medications. Volume-control sets are microdrop sets and, therefore, have a drop factor of 60 gtt/mL.

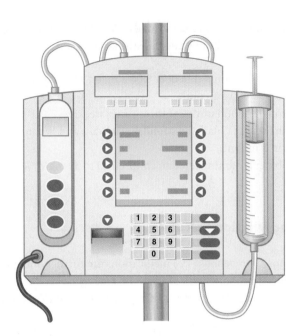

FIGURE 12-11 A syringe pump is also used to regulate small hourly fluid volumes and to administer intermittent IV medications.

30 mg/mL. The concentration for administration can be inserted into the calculation methods in the same manner as the supply volume:

- Ratio-proportion: $\frac{30\ mg}{1\ mL} = \frac{ordered\ dose\ in\ mg}{x\ mL}$

- The formula method: $\frac{ordered\ dose\ in\ \cancel{mg}}{30\ \cancel{mg}} \times 1\ mL = x\ (mL)$

- Dimensional analysis: $x\ (mL) = \frac{1\ mL}{30\ \cancel{mg}} \times \frac{ordered\ dose\ in\ \cancel{mg}}{1}$

In each of these equations, x is the recommended or safe volume of diluent in which to infuse the ordered dose of medication. Safe medication concentrations for administration are given in the unit of measurement in which the drug is supplied, such as g/mL, mcg/mL, units/mL, or mEq/mL. Therefore, minimum dilution calculations should yield, per milliliter, the safe amount of medication in the same unit of measurement in which the drug is supplied.

Clinical CLUE

Diluents, solutions used to dilute medications, include normal saline (NS), sterile water (SW), and compatible IV solutions. The nurse needs to consult a drug reference to determine appropriate diluents for medications.

Some medications allow for a dilution range, for example, the safe concentration for administration of Unasyn® is 3–45 mg/mL. In this example, 3 mg/mL is the minimum concentration and 45 mg/mL is the maximum concentration. When the dilution volume is calculated using the minimum concentration, the maximum dilution is determined. When the dilution volume is calculated using the maximum concentration, the minimum dilution is determined.

Example 1:   Calculate the dilution volume needed to administer 500 mg of ampicillin. The drug reference indicates the safe concentration for administration is 30 mg/mL.

Ratio-Proportion	Formula Method
Minimum dilution volume:	Minimum dilution volume:

$$\frac{30 \text{ mg}}{1 \text{ mL}} = \frac{500 \text{ mg}}{x \text{ mL}} \text{ or}$$

$$30 \text{ mg} : 1 \text{ mL} = 500 \text{ mg} : x \text{ mL}$$

$$30 \times x = 1 \times 500$$

$$30x = 500$$

$$x = 16.7 \text{ or } 17 \text{ mL}$$

Formula Method — Minimum dilution volume:

$$\frac{500 \text{ mg}}{30 \text{ mg}} \times 1 \text{ mL} = x \text{ (mL)}$$

$$16.7 \text{ or } 17 \text{ mL} = x$$

Dimensional Analysis

Minimum dilution volume:

$$x \text{ (mL)} = \frac{1 \text{ mL}}{30 \text{ mg}} \times \frac{500 \text{ mg}}{1}$$

$$x = \frac{500 \text{ mL}}{30}$$

$$x = 16.7 \text{ or } 17 \text{ mL}$$

This example indicates that the nurse will administer 500 mg of ampicillin in a minimum fluid volume of 16.7 or 17 mL.

Example 2:   Calculate the minimum and maximum dilution volumes needed to administer 240 mg of Unasyn. The drug reference indicates the safe concentration for administration is 3–45 mg/mL.

NOTE: When calculating using minimum concentration first, the first value yielded is maximum dilution volume.

Ratio-Proportion	Formula Method
Maximum dilution volume:	Maximum dilution volume:

$$\frac{3 \text{ mg}}{1 \text{ mL}} = \frac{240 \text{ mg}}{x \text{ mL}} \text{ or}$$

$$3 \text{ mg} : 1 \text{ mL} = 240 \text{ mg} : 1 \text{ mL}$$

$$3 \times x = 1 \times 240$$

$$3x = 240$$

$$x = 80 \text{ mL}$$

Formula Method — Maximum dilution volume:

$$\frac{240 \text{ mg}}{3 \text{ mg}} \times 1 \text{ mL} = x \text{ (mL)}$$

$$80 \text{ mL} = x$$

Minimum dilution volume:

$$\frac{45 \text{ mg}}{1 \text{ mL}} = \frac{240 \text{ mg}}{x \text{ mL}} \text{ or}$$

$$45 \text{ mg}: 1 \text{ mL} = 240 \text{ mg}: 1 \text{ mL}$$

$$45 \times x = 1 \times 240$$

$$45x = 240$$

$$x = 5.3 \text{ mL}$$

Minimum dilution volume:

$$\frac{240 \text{ mg}}{45 \text{ mg}} \times 1 \text{ mL} = x \text{ (mL)}$$

$$5.3 \text{ mL} = x$$

Dimensional Analysis

Maximum dilution volume:

$$x \text{ (mL)} = \frac{1 \text{ mL}}{3 \text{ mg}} \times \frac{240 \text{ mg}}{1}$$

$$x = \frac{240 \text{ mL}}{3}$$

$$x = 80 \text{ mL}$$

Minimum dilution volume:

$$x \text{ (mL)} = \frac{1 \text{ mL}}{45 \text{ mg}} \times \frac{240 \text{ mg}}{1}$$

$$x = \frac{240 \text{ mL}}{45}$$

$$x = 5.3 \text{ mL}$$

- The minimum volume of diluent needed to administer 240 mg of Unasyn, 5.3 mL, is yielded by the maximum concentration, 45 mg/mL.

- The maximum volume of diluent needed to administer 240 mg of Unasyn, 80 mL, is yielded by the minimum concentration, 3 mg/mL.

- After drawing up 240 mg of Unasyn, the nurse must further dilute it in 5.3 to 80 mL of solution.

Rounding RULE

Minimum and maximum dilution volumes can be rounded, if necessary:

- Minimum volumes can be rounded up but should not be rounded down, because the calculated volume is the minimum amount (less volume would make the solution too concentrated).

- Maximum volumes can be rounded down but should not be rounded up, because the calculated volume is the maximum amount (more volume would make the solution too dilute).

Example: A dilution range of 4.4 to 10.5 mL can be rounded to 5–10 mL.

LEARNING ACTIVITY 12-8 Calculate the minimum dilution volume needed for administration of each ordered medication. Round volumes to the whole number, if necessary.

1.   **Order:** 250 mg clindamycin IV q6h
      Reference: The concentration of clindamycin is not to exceed 18 mg/mL.
2.   **Order:** 400 mg vancomycin IV q8h
      Reference: Concentration for administration of vancomycin is 1–5 mg/mL.

Calculations for Medications Administered via Volume-Control Sets

A volume-control set is primary intravenous tubing with a 150 mL capacity chamber that connects to an IV solution. This device can be used to regulate IV fluid infusion or to administer intermittent IV medications. To regulate IV fluid infusion, the nurse fills the chamber with 1 to 2 hours' worth of IV fluid at a time for the purpose of preventing fluid overload, particularly with pediatric and geriatric patients. For intermittent medication administration, the nurse injects the medication through the injection port at the top of the chamber and fills the chamber with the appropriate amount of diluent. To complete the medication administration, an **IV flush** is administered immediately after the medication is infused. An IV flush is a small volume of IV fluid, 10–15 mL, needed to clear the medication from the IV tubing and deliver it completely into the patient's vein.

A volume-control set, which can be regulated manually or electronically, is most often manually regulated. Volume-control sets are microdrop sets; therefore, for manually regulated infusions, the nurse will use the drop factor of 60 gtt/mL to calculate the infusion rate (**Figure 12-12**). To calculate the infusion rate, the nurse must seek from a drug reference the amount of time, in minutes, over which to infuse the medication. Both the medication and the flush must infuse over the specified period of time. To calculate

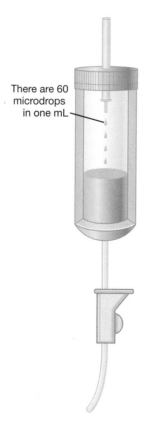

There are 60 microdrops in one mL

FIGURE 12-12 Volume-control sets have this drip chamber below with a drop factor of 60 gtt/mL.

a manually regulated IV flow rate, the nurse can use the formula method or dimensional analysis as detailed in Chapter 10:

- Formula method: $\frac{mL}{min} \times 60$ gtt/mL = x (gtt/min)

- Dimensional analysis: x (gtt/min) = $\frac{60 \text{ gtt}}{1 \text{ } mL} \times \frac{mL}{min}$

Example: Perform the following calculations needed to administer the ordered medication via volume-control set, followed by a 15 mL flush.

Step 1: Calculate the amount to administer (volume of medication to inject into the volume-control set).

Step 2: Calculate the dilution volume (volume of IV fluid in which the medication will be further diluted).

Step 3: Add the flush volume to the dilution volume and flush volume, then calculate the infusion rate in gtt/min.

Order: cimetidine 75 mg IV q6h

Supply: cimetidine 150 mg/mL

Reference: Administer cimetidine in a concentration of 5.8 mg/mL over 20 minutes.

Step 1: To calculate the amount to administer, refer to the order and supply.

C: *Convert*—Because the order is in milligrams and the supply is in milligrams, there is no conversion.

A: *Approximate*—The ordered dose, 75 mg, is half of the supply amount of 150 mg. Therefore, half of the supply volume, 0.5 mL, will be needed to administer the ordered dose.

S: *Solve*

Ratio-Proportion	Formula Method
$\frac{150 \text{ mg}}{1 \text{ mL}} = \frac{75 \text{ mg}}{x \text{ mL}}$ or	$\frac{75 \text{ mg}}{150 \text{ mg}} \times 1 \text{ mL} = x \text{ (mL)}$
150 mg : 1 mL = 75 mg : x mL	$0.5 \times 1 \text{ mL} = x$
$150 \times x = 1 \times 75$	$0.5 \text{ mL} = x$
$150x = 75$	
$x = 0.5 \text{ mL}$	

Dimensional Analysis

$$x \text{ (mL)} = \frac{1 \text{ mL}}{150 \text{ mg}} \times \frac{75 \text{ mg}}{1}$$

$$x = \frac{75 \text{ mL}}{150}$$

$$x = 0.5 \text{ mL}$$

E: *Evaluate*

Ratio-Proportion	Formula Method
$\dfrac{150 \text{ mg}}{1 \text{ mL}} = \dfrac{75 \text{ mg}}{0.5 \text{ mL}}$ or	$\dfrac{75 \text{ mg}}{150 \text{ mg}} \times 1 \text{ mL} = 0.5 \text{ mL}$
150 mg : 1 mL = 75 mg : 0.5 mL	$0.5 \times 1 \text{ mL} = 0.5 \text{ mL}$
$150 \times 0.5 = 1 \times 75$	$0.5 \text{ mL} = 0.5 \text{ mL}$
$75 = 75$	

Dimensional Analysis

$$0.5 \text{ mL} = \frac{1 \text{ mL}}{150 \text{ mg}} \times \frac{75 \text{ mg}}{1}$$

$$0.5 \text{ mL} = \frac{75 \text{ mL}}{150}$$

$$0.5 \text{ mL} = 0.5 \text{ mL}$$

Because the calculated volume accurately completes the equation and is consistent with the approximated volume, 0.5 mL, the answer is confirmed.

Step 2: To calculate the volume of IV fluid needed to further dilute the medication, refer to the concentration, 5.8 mg/mL, and calculate the minimum dilution:

Ratio-Proportion	Formula Method
Minimum dilution:	Minimum dilution:
$\dfrac{5.8 \text{ mg}}{1 \text{ mL}} = \dfrac{75 \text{ mg}}{x \text{ mL}}$ or	$\dfrac{75 \text{ mg}}{5.8 \text{ mg}} \times 1 \text{ mL} = x \text{ (mL)}$
5.8 mg : 1 mL = 75 mg : *x* mL	12.9 or 13 mL = *x*
$5.8 \times x = 1 \times 75$	
$5.8x = 75$	
$x = 12.9 \text{ or } 13 \text{ mL}$	

Dimensional Analysis

Minimum dilution:

$$x \text{ (mL)} = \frac{1 \text{ mL}}{5.8 \text{ mg}} \times \frac{75 \text{ mg}}{1}$$

$$x = \frac{75 \text{ mL}}{5.8}$$

$$x = 12.9 \text{ or } 13 \text{ mL}$$

The nurse will inject 0.5 mL of cimetidine into the volume-control set and fill the chamber with 12.5 mL of IV fluid to reach the 13 mL calibration.

Step 3: To calculate the infusion rate to administer this medication over 20 minutes, the nurse will add the diluted medication volume, 13 mL, and the flush volume, 15 mL, and then apply the formula method or dimensional analysis for manually regulated IV flow rates, using the drop factor for volume-control sets, 60 gtt/mL:

Formula Method	Dimensional Analysis
$$\frac{(13 \text{ mL} + 15 \text{ mL})}{20 \text{ min}} \times 60 \text{ gtt/mL} = x \,(\text{gtt/min})$$ $$\frac{28 \text{ mL}}{20 \text{ min}} \times 60 \text{ gtt/mL} = x$$ $$\frac{1,680 \text{ gtt}}{20 \text{ min}} = x$$ $$84 \text{ gtt/min} = x$$	$$x \,(\text{gtt/min}) = \frac{60 \text{ gtt}}{1 \text{ mL}} \times \frac{(13 \text{ mL} + 15 \text{ mL})}{20 \text{ min}}$$ $$x = \frac{60 \text{ gtt}}{1 \text{ mL}} \times \frac{28 \text{ mL}}{20 \text{ min}}$$ $$x = \frac{1,680 \text{ gtt}}{20 \text{ min}}$$ $$x = 84 \text{ gtt/min}$$

To infuse the medication and the IV flush over 20 minutes, the nurse will:

- Run the diluted medication, 13 mL, at a flow rate of 84 gtt/min, then

- Fill the volume-control chamber with the 15 mL and run at a flow rate of 84 gtt/min

Clinical CLUE

When using a manually-regulated volume-control set, the nurse will need to calculate the amount of time it will take for the medication to infuse in order to anticipate when to return to the patient to infuse the flush. For the previous example, the medication in 13 mL will infuse at 84 gtt/min. To calculate the amount of time this will take the nurse should recall the manually-regulated IV rate formula from Chapter 10: $\frac{\text{Vol (mL)}}{\text{T (minutes)}} \times \text{drop factor} = \text{rate}$. The infusion time calculation for this example is:

$$\frac{13 \text{ mL}}{x \text{ min}} \times 60 \text{ gtt/mL} = 84 \text{ gtt/min}$$

$$\frac{780}{x \text{ min}} = \frac{84}{1}$$

$$84 x = 780$$

$$x = 9.3 \text{ min}$$

Recall from the example that the medication + flush will infuse over 20 minutes. If the medication will take just over 9 minutes to infuse (as indicated by this equation), then the 15 mL flush will infuse in just under 11 minutes.

LEARNING ACTIVITY 12-9 Calculate the IV flow rate in gtt/min for each ordered medication to be given via volume-control set.

1. **Order:** furosemide 50 mg IV q8h diluted in 5 mL (10 mg/mL) IV solution, followed by a 15 mL flush; infuse over 1 hour

2. **Order:** tobramycin 40 mg IV q8h diluted in 8 mL (5 mg/mL) IV solution, followed by a 15 mL flush; infuse over 30 min

Calculations for Medications Administered via Syringe Pump

Like volume-control sets, syringe pumps are used to deliver small, precise volumes of fluid, with or without medication, over a specified period of time. While a volume-control set holds a maximum fluid volume of 150 mL, a syringe pump is used to infuse volumes of 1 to 60 mL using a correspondingly sized syringe. Medications infused through syringe pumps should be followed by normal saline flush of 10 to 15 mL. Calculations for medications administered through a syringe pump are similar to calculations for volume-control sets with the exception that the flow rate is determined in mL/h. To calculate the infusion rate, the nurse must seek from a drug reference the amount of time, in minutes, over which to infuse the medication. As with volume-control set calculations, both the medication and the flush must infuse over the specified period of time. To calculate the flow rate in mL/h, the nurse can use ratio-proportion, the formula method, or dimensional analysis as detailed in Chapter 10:

- Ratio-proportion: $\frac{mL}{min} = \frac{x\ mL}{60\ min}$

- The formula method: $\frac{mL}{min} \times 60\ \cancel{min}/h = x\ (mL/h)$

- Dimensional analysis: $x\ (mL/h) = \frac{mL}{min} \times \frac{60\ \cancel{min}}{1\ h}$

Example: Perform the following calculations needed to administer the ordered medication via syringe pump, followed by a 10 mL NS flush.

Step 1: Calculate the volume of medication to administer.

Step 2: Calculate the volume of diluent (NS or SW) needed to further dilute the medication.

Step 3: Add the dilution volume and flush volume, then calculate the infusion rate in mL/h for the total volume to be infused.

Order: dexamethasone 32 mg IV q6h

Supply: dexamethasone 10 mg/mL

Reference: Administer dexamethasone in a concentration of 4 mg/mL over 15 minutes.

Step 1: To calculate the volume of medication needed, refer to the order and supply and apply the CASE method:

C: *Convert*—Because the order is in milligrams and the supply is in milligrams, there is no conversion.

A: *Approximate*—The ordered dose, 32 mg, is more than three times the supply. Therefore, more than three times the supply volume of 1 mL, or more than 3 mL, will be needed to administer the ordered dose.

S: *Solve*

Ratio-Proportion	Formula Method
$\frac{10\ mg}{1\ mL} = \frac{32\ mg}{x\ mL}$ or	$\frac{32\ \cancel{mg}}{10\ \cancel{mg}} \times 1\ mL = x\ (mL)$
10 mg : 1 mL = 32 mg : x mL	$3.2 \times 1\ mL = x$
$10 \times x = 1 \times 32$	3.2 mL = x
$10x = 32$	
$x = 3.2\ mL$	

Dimensional Analysis

$$x \, (\text{mL}) = \frac{1 \, \text{mL}}{10 \, \cancel{\text{mg}}} \times \frac{32 \, \cancel{\text{mg}}}{1}$$

$$x = \frac{32 \, \text{mL}}{10}$$

$$x = 3.2 \, \text{mL}$$

E: *Evaluate*

Ratio-Proportion	**Formula Method**
$\dfrac{10 \, \text{mg}}{1 \, \text{mL}} = \dfrac{32 \, \text{mg}}{3.2 \, \text{mL}}$ or	$\dfrac{32 \, \cancel{\text{mg}}}{10 \, \cancel{\text{mg}}} \times 1 \, \text{mL} = 3.2 \, \text{mL}$
$10 \, \text{mg} : 1 \, \text{mL} = 32 \, \text{mg} : 3.2 \, \text{mL}$	$3.2 \times 1 \, \text{mL} = 3.2 \, \text{mL}$
$10 \times 3.2 = 1 \times 32$	$3.2 \, \text{mL} = 3.2 \, \text{mL}$
$32 = 32$	

Dimensional Analysis

$$3.2 \, \text{mL} = \frac{1 \, \text{mL}}{10 \, \cancel{\text{mg}}} \times \frac{32 \, \cancel{\text{mg}}}{1}$$

$$3.2 \, \text{mL} = \frac{32 \, \text{mL}}{10}$$

$$3.2 \, \text{mL} = 3.2 \, \text{mL}$$

Because the calculated volume accurately completes the equation and is consistent with the approximated volume, more than 3 mL, the answer is confirmed.

Step 2: To calculate the volume of fluid needed to further dilute the medication, refer to the concentration, 4 mg/mL, and calculate the minimum dilution:

Ratio-Proportion	**Formula Method**
$\dfrac{4 \, \text{mg}}{1 \, \text{mL}} = \dfrac{32 \, \text{mg}}{x \, \text{mL}}$ or	$\dfrac{32 \, \cancel{\text{mg}}}{4 \, \cancel{\text{mg}}} \times 1 \, \text{mL} = x \, (\text{mL})$
$4 \, \text{mg} : 1 \, \text{mL} = 32 \, \text{mg} : x \, \text{mL}$	$8 \, \text{mL} = x$
$4 \times x = 1 \times 32$	
$4x = 32$	
$x = 8 \, \text{mL}$	

Dimensional Analysis

$$x\,(\text{mL}) = \frac{1\,\text{mL}}{4\,\cancel{\text{mg}}} \times \frac{32\,\cancel{\text{mg}}}{1}$$

$$x = \frac{32\,\text{mL}}{4}$$

$$x = 8\,\text{mL}$$

With a 10 mL syringe, the nurse will draw up 3.2 mL of dexamethasone and then draw up an additional volume of normal saline or sterile water for a total volume of 8 mL.

Step 3: To calculate the infusion rate to administer this medication over 15 minutes, the nurse will add the diluted medication volume, 8 mL, and the flush volume, 10 mL, and then apply ratio-proportion, the formula method, or dimensional analysis for calculating IV flow rates in mL/h:

Ratio-Proportion

$$\frac{(8\,\text{mL} + 10\,\text{mL})}{15\,\text{min}} = \frac{x\,\text{mL}}{60\,\text{min}}$$

or

$$18\,\text{mL} : 15\,\text{min} = x\,\text{mL} : 60\,\text{min}$$

$$\frac{18\,\text{mL}}{15\,\text{min}} = \frac{x\,\text{mL}}{60\,\text{min}}$$

$$15x = 1{,}080$$

$$\frac{15x}{15} = \frac{1{,}080}{15}$$

$$x = 72\,\text{mL per } 60\,\text{min or } 72\,\text{mL/h}$$

Formula Method

$$\frac{(8\,\text{mL} + 10\,\text{mL})}{15\,\text{min}} \times 60\,\text{min/h} = x\,(\text{mL/h})$$

$$\frac{18\,\text{mL}}{15\,\cancel{\text{min}}} \times 60\,\cancel{\text{min}}/\text{h} = x$$

$$\frac{1{,}080\,\text{mL/h}}{15} = x$$

$$72\,\text{mL/h} = x$$

Dimensional Analysis

$$x\,(\text{mL/h}) = \frac{(8\,\text{mL} + 10\,\text{mL})}{15\,\text{min}} \times \frac{60\,\text{min}}{1\,\text{h}}$$

$$x = \frac{18\,\text{mL}}{15\,\cancel{\text{min}}} \times \frac{60\,\cancel{\text{min}}}{1\,\text{h}}$$

$$x = \frac{1{,}080\,\text{mL}}{15\,\text{h}}$$

$$x = 72\,\text{mL/h}$$

LEARNING ACTIVITY 12-10 Calculate the IV flow rate in mL/h for each ordered medication to be given via syringe pump.

1. **Order:** ondansetron 4 mg IV stat diluted in 4 mL (1 mg/mL) NS or SW, followed by a 10 mL NS flush; infuse over 15 min

2. **Order:** propanolol 10 mg IV q12h diluted in 5 mL (2 mg/mL) NS or SW, followed by a 10 mL NS flush; infuse over 10 min

Clinical CLUE

Although smart pumps have the capability of converting mL/min to mL/h after this infusion device has been programmed with the volume and time, it is important for nurses to perform flow rate calculations to verify that infusion devices function with accuracy! So-called smart pumps have been known to "outsmart" the operator when an internal setting has overridden the rate programmed by the nurse. This has resulted in the patient receiving the wrong dose of medication. Always do the math and observe the rate.

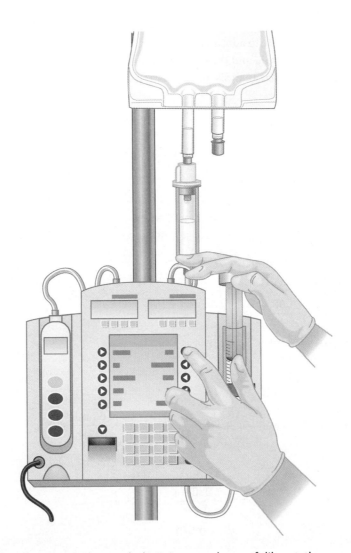

FIGURE 12-13   After drawing up the needed minimum volume of diluent, the nurse inserts the medication into the syringe, then attaches the syringe to the patient's existing IV tubing for infusion.

Conversion Confusion ... Case Closure

The nursing student correctly converted 2,500 grams to kilograms and 2.5 kg to 5.5 lbs. However, before reporting the weight in pound and ounces, the student should have converted the decimal fraction 0.5 pounds to ounces, using the conversion factor $\frac{16 \text{ oz}}{1 \text{ lb}}$:

$$x(\text{oz}) = \frac{16 \text{ oz}}{1 \text{ lb}} \times \frac{0.5 \text{ lb}}{1}$$

$$x = 8 \text{ oz}$$

After converting 0.5 lb to 8 ounces, the student can correctly report the newborn's weight as 5 lb 8 oz. Worse than providing new parents with misinformation, inaccurate weights can lead to drug dosing errors. To avoid this type of error, many institutions post weight conversion charts that can serve as a means of double-checking a calculated conversion. Nurses (and students) should get in the habit of double-checking weight conversions before reporting and recording this data.

Chapter Summary

Learning Outcomes	Points to Remember
12-1 Identify factors that impact drug dosing in special populations.	Factors include age, pharmacokinetics, weight, body weight, BSA, polypharmacy, and creatinine clearance: • Pharmacokinetics—the study of how drugs move throughout the body; includes absorption, distribution, metabolism, and elimination • Polypharmacy—multiple medications taken by one patient leads to drug interactions • Creatinine clearance—filtering of drugs through the kidneys decreases with age; many medication package inserts include safe dose information based on creatinine clearance
12-2 Perform weight-based safe dose calculations.	Four Steps 1. Convert weight to kg, if applicable. 2. Calculate safe dose or doses (minimum and maximum, if safe dose range is supplied). For example, the safe dose is 5 mg/kg: 　o Ratio-proportion: $\frac{5 \text{ mg}}{1 \text{ kg}} = \frac{x \text{ mg}}{\text{pt wt in kg}}$ 　o The formula method: 5 mg/kg × pt wt in kg = x (mg) 　o Dimensional analysis: $x(\text{mg}) = 5\frac{\text{mg}}{1\text{kg}} \times \frac{\text{pt wt in kg}}{1}$ NOTE: mg can be substituted for the unit of measurement in which a drug is supplied (e.g., mcg, g, mEq, units). 3. Compare the ordered dose to the safe dose calculation(s). NOTE: Be sure to compare a single safe dose calculation to a single dose ordered or a daily safe dose calculation to a daily dose ordered. 4. Calculate the amount to administer using the CASE approach or contact the prescriber if the dose is unsafe.

12-3 Perform safe dose calculations based on body surface area.	**Four Steps**
	1. Determine BSA:
	  o BSA metric formula $m^2 = \sqrt{\dfrac{ht(cm) \times wt(kg)}{3,600}}$
	  o BSA household formula $m^2 = \sqrt{\dfrac{ht(in) \times wt(lb)}{3,131}}$
	  o Use Nomogram: Connect height and weight, and the point at which the line intersects the BSA column is the estimated BSA.
	2. Calculate safe dose or doses (minimum and maximum, if safe dose range is supplied). For example, the safe dose is 2.5 mg/m²:
	  o Ratio-proportion: $\dfrac{2.5\ mg}{1\ m^2} = \dfrac{x\ mg}{pt\ BSA\ in\ m^2}$
	  o The formula method: $2.5\ mg/m^2 \times pt\ BSA\ in\ \cancel{m^2} = x\ (mg)$
	  o Dimensional analysis: $x\ (mg) = \dfrac{2.5\ mg}{1\ \cancel{m^2}} \times \dfrac{pt\ BSA\ in\ \cancel{m^2}}{1}$
	3. Compare the calculated safe dose to the ordered dose.
	4. Calculate the amount to administer using the CASE approach or contact the prescriber if the ordered dose is unsafe.

12-4 Determine minimum dilution volumes for intravenous medication administration.	Look up concentration for administration in drug reference—for example, 30 mg/mL, then calculate the dilution volume using: • Ratio-proportion: $\dfrac{30\ mg}{1\ mL} = \dfrac{ordered\ dose\ in\ mg}{x\ mL}$ • Formula method: $\dfrac{ordered\ dose\ in\ \cancel{mg}}{30\ \cancel{mg}} \times 1\ mL = x\ (mL)$ • Dimensional analysis: $x\ (mL) = \dfrac{1\ mL}{30\ \cancel{mg}} \times \dfrac{ordered\ dose\ in\ \cancel{mg}}{1}$ If a dilution concentration range is given—for example, 30–100 mg/mL, calculate the minimum dilution (maximum concentration) and maximum dilution (minimum concentration). Volume-Control Set Calculations Add medication volume + flush volume (10–15 mL); then perform manually regulated IV rate calculation using a drop factor of 60 gtt/mL: $$\dfrac{\cancel{mL}}{min} \times 60\ gtt/\cancel{mL} = x\ (gtt/min)$$ Syringe Pump Calculations Add medication volume + flush volume (10–15 mL); then perform electronically regulated IV rate calculation: $$\dfrac{vol\ (mL)}{h} = mL/h \quad or \quad \dfrac{mL}{\cancel{min}} \times 60\ \cancel{min}/h = x\ (mL/h)$$

Homework

For exercises 1–5, indicate whether the statement is true or false. Convert false statements to true statements. (LO 12-1)

1. Distribution refers to the movement of a medication into body tissues and fluids.

2. Drugs ordered according to body surface area take into account the patient's height and weight.

3. The process by which drugs are moved out of the body is called creatinine clearance.

4. Decreased stomach acid production in both geriatric and pediatric patients makes these patient populations more susceptible to adverse effects of drugs.

5. Polypharmacy refers to the transformation of drugs into chemicals used by the body.

For exercises 6–10, convert the weights to kilograms. Round quantities to the tenth, if necessary. (LO 12-2)

6. 6 lb 6 oz = _____ kg

7. 121 lb = _____ kg

8. 8 lb 12 oz _____ kg

9. 5,250 g _____ kg

10. 10 lb 10 oz _____ kg

For exercises 11–15, calculate the minimum safe single dose and maximum safe single dose. (LO 12-2)

11. Vancomycin 10 to 15 mg/kg/dose IV q12h for an infant who weighs 10 lb 8 oz

12. Diphenhydramine 1 to 1.5 mg/kg/dose PO 30 min ā bedtime for a 145 lb patient

13. Ceftazidime 33.3 to 50 mg/kg/dose q8h for an infant who weighs 25 lb

14. Digoxin 10 to 15 mcg/kg/dose once daily for a child who weighs 74 lb

15. Furosemide 0.5 to 2 mg/kg/dose q12h for a neonate who weighs 4,800 g

For exercises 16–18, refer to the following order, supply, and reference information. (LO 12-2)

> **Order:** ticarcillin disodium 1.5 g IV q6h
>
> **Supply:** 3 g vial; add 6 mL sterile water to yield a concentration of 385 mg/mL
>
> **Reference:** ticarcillin 200–300 mg/kg/day in four divided doses

16. Calculate the safe daily dose range for a 55 lb child.

17. Calculate the safe single dose range or the ordered daily dose and determine if the ordered dose is safe.

18. Determine the nurse's next action: Calculate the amount to administer or contact the authorized prescriber.

For exercises 19–20, refer to the following order, supply, and reference information. (LO 12-2)

> **Order:** acyclovir 30 mg IV q8h
>
> **Supply:** 0.25 g vial acyclovir; mix with 10 mL sterile water or 0.9% sodium chloride for a concentration of 25 mg/mL
>
> **Reference:** acyclovir 10 mg/kg q8h for children 3 months old to 12 years old; acyclovir 20 mg/kg q8h for infants 1–3 months of age; acyclovir 10 mg/kg q12h for neonates

19. Calculate the safe single dose for a 10 lb infant who is 2 months old.

20. Determine the nurse's next action: Calculate the amount to administer or contact the prescriber.

For exercises 21–23, refer to the following order, supply, and reference information. (LO 12-2)

> **Order:** amoxicillin 150 mg PO q8h
>
> **Supply/Reference:** Per label, "20-40 mg/kg/day in divided doses every eight hours"

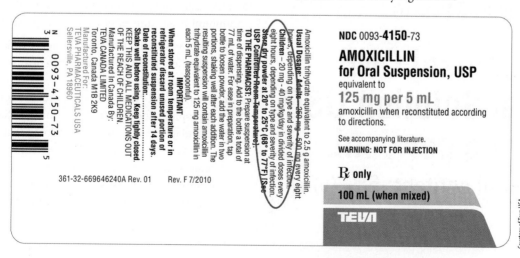

21. Calculate the safe daily dose range for a 44 lb child.
22. Calculate the safe single dose range or the ordered daily dose and determine if the ordered dose is safe.
23. Determine the nurse's next action: Calculate the amount to administer or contact the prescriber.

For exercises 24–27, refer to the following order, supply, and reference information. (LO 12-2)

> **Order:** valproic acid 0.5 g PO q12h
>
> **Supply:**

NDC 0093-**9633**-16

VALPROIC ACID
Oral Solution USP
250 mg/5 mL

Each 5 mL contains the equivalent of
250 mg valproic acid as the sodium salt.

℞ only

Courtesy of Teva USA

Reference: Initial oral dose for children is 15–45 mg/kg/day.

24. Is the ordered dose safe for a 23 kg child?
25. Is the ordered dose safe for a 33 kg child?
26. Is the ordered dose safe for a 43 kg child?
27. If the ordered dose is safe for a 23 kg, 33 kg, and 43 kg child, calculate the amount to administer. If the ordered dose is not safe, determine the nurse's next action.

For exercises 28–30, refer to the following order, supply, and reference information. (LO 12-2)

> **Order:** prednisolone 30 mg PO q12h
>
> **Supply:**

NDC 0093-**6118**-16

**PrednisoLONE
Oral Solution USP
15 mg per 5 mL**
alcohol content: 5% (v/v)

Courtesy of Teva USA

Reference: Recommended dose of prednisolone is 1–2 mg/kg/day in divided doses twice daily; maximum 60 mg/day.

28. Calculate the safe daily dose range for a 50 lb child.
29. Compare the ordered daily dose to the safe dose range and determine if the ordered dose is safe.
30. Determine the nurse's next action: Calculate the amount to administer or contact the prescriber.

For exercises 31–33, refer to the following order, supply, and reference information. (LO 12-2)

> **Order:** calcitriol 0.5 mcg PO daily
>
> **Supply:**

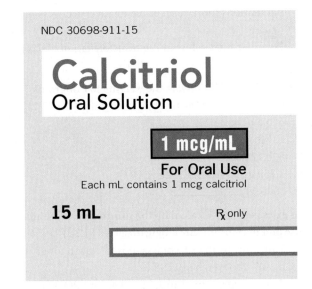

NDC 30698-911-15

Calcitriol
Oral Solution

1 mcg/mL

For Oral Use
Each mL contains 1 mcg calcitriol

15 mL   ℞ only

Reference: Recommended dose of calcitriol is 0.04–0.08 mcg/kg/day.

31. Calculate the safe dose range of calcitriol for a 9.5 kg infant.
32. Compare the ordered dose to the safe dose range and determine if the ordered dose is safe.
33. Determine the nurse's next action: Calculate the amount to administer or contact the prescriber.

For exercises 34–38, use the measurements, order, supply, and reference information given to answer questions a, b, c, and d. (LO 12-3)

> a. Use the West Nomogram (Figure 12-8) or the appropriate formula to determine the BSA.
> b. Calculate the safe dose or safe dose range.
> c. Compare the ordered daily dose to the safe dose range and determine if order is safe.
> d. Determine the nurse's next action: Calculate the amount to administer or contact the prescriber.

34. **Measurements:** 4 ft 2 in; 75 lb
    Order: cortisone 50 mg PO q6h
    Supply:

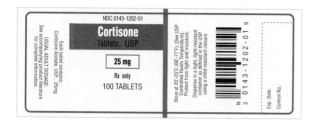

Reference: Recommended dose of oral cortisone is 75 to 300 mg/m²/day in divided doses q6–8h.

35. **Measurements:** 80 cm; 12 kg
    Order: triamcinolone 15 mg IM daily
    Supply:

$40\,mg = \dfrac{15\,g}{X}$

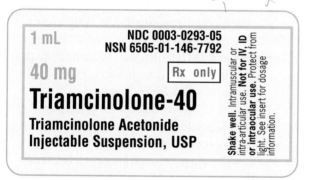

Reference: Recommended dose of triamcinolone is 3.2 to 48 mg/m² given every 1 to 7 days.

36. **Measurements:** 3 ft; 30 lb
    Order: methotrexate 7.5 mg PO q Monday and Thursday
    Supply: methotrexate 5 mg tablets
    Reference: Recommended dose for children is 10–30 mg/m² two times per week.

37. **Measurements:** 200 cm; 72.7 kg
    Order: cisplatin 0.15 g IV every 4 weeks
    Supply:

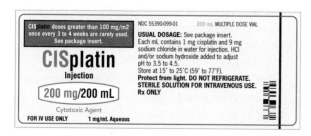

Reference: Safe dose of cisplatin is 75–100 mg/m² every 4 weeks.

38. **Measurements:** 150 cm; 40 kg
    Order: cyclophosphamide 0.1 g PO daily X 6 days
    Supply: cyclophosphamide 50 mg tablets
    Reference: Safe dose of cyclophosphamide is 60–250 mg/m²/day.

For exercises 39–40, use the information provided to calculate the weight-based safe daily dose range and safe single dose range. (LO 12-2)

39. Wt: 5 kg; SDR of amoxicillin: 25–50 mg/kg/day divided q8h
40. Wt: 50 lb; SDR of digoxin: 5–10 mcg/kg/day

For exercises 41–42, using the order and drug reference information, match the quantity, i–iv, with the terminology, a–d. (LO 12-4)

41. **Order:** kanamycin 115 mg IV q12h
    Reference: Concentration for administration of kanamycin is 2.5–5 mg/mL (23–46 mL).
    a. Minimum concentration   i. 46 mL
    b. Maximum concentration   ii. 5 mg/mL
    c. Minimum dilution volume   iii. 2.5 mg/mL
    d. Maximum dilution volume   iv. 23 mL

42. **Order:** cefotaxime 1.2 g IV q8h
    Reference: Concentration for administration of cefotaxime is 20–60 mg/mL.
    a. Minimum concentration   i. 60 mL
    b. Maximum concentration   ii. 20 mg/mL
    c. Minimum dilution volume   iii. 60 mg/mL
    d. Maximum dilution volume   iv. 20 mL

For exercises 43–45, using the order and drug reference information, calculate the minimum dilution volume rounded to the whole number. (LO 12-4)

43. **Order:** caspofungin acetate 50 mg IV daily
    Reference: Concentration for administration of caspofungin is 0.4–0.5 mg/mL.
44. **Order:** ceftazidime 0.5 g IV q8h
    Reference: Concentration for administration of ceftazidime is 40 mg/mL.
45. **Order:** Primaxin® 160 mg IV q6h
    Reference: Concentration for administration of Primaxin® is 2.5–5 mg/mL.

For exercises 46–47, use the order, supply, and drug reference information to perform calculations a–c needed to administer the ordered medication via volume-control set, *followed by a 15 mL flush.* (LO 12-4)

a. Calculate the volume of medication to inject into the volume-control set.
b. Calculate the volume of IV fluid in which the medication will be further diluted. Round volume to the whole number.

c. Calculate the infusion rate (of the medication and flush) in gtt/min. (Volume-control sets have a drop factor of 60 gtt/mL.)

46. **Order:** pantoprazole 40 mg IV daily
    Supply: pantoprazole 40 mg vial; reconstitute with 10 mL NS to a concentration of 4 mg/mL
    Reference: Further dilute with NS to a concentration of 0.8 mg/mL; administer over 15 min.

47. **Order:** valproate sodium 0.15 g IV q12h
    Supply: 5 mL vial containing valproate sodium 100 mg/mL
    Reference: Administer valproate sodium in a concentration of 2 mg/mL over 60 min.

For exercises 48–49, use the order, supply, and drug reference information to perform calculations a–c needed to administer the ordered medication via syringe pump, *followed by a 10 mL NS flush.* (LO 12-4)

   a. Calculate the volume of medication to draw up.
   b. Calculate the volume of diluent (NS) needed to further dilute the medication. Round volume to the whole number.
   c. Calculate the infusion rate (of the medication and flush) in mL/h.

48. **Order:** cimetidine 45 mg IV q6h
    Supply: cimetidine 150 mg/mL
    Reference: Administer cimetidine in a concentration of 15 mg/mL over 20 min.

49. **Order:** gentamicin 50 mg IV q8h
    Supply: gentamicin 80 mg/2 mL
    Reference: Administer gentamicin in a concentration of 2 mg/mL over 2 h.

For exercise 50, use the order, supply, and drug reference information to answer questions a–g. (LO 12-2, 12-4)

   a. Calculate the safe daily dose range.
   b. Calculate the safe single dose range.
   c. Determine if the ordered dose is safe.
   d. Calculate the volume of medication to draw up.
   e. Calculate the minimum dilution (rounded to the whole number, if necessary).
   f. Calculate the maximum dilution (rounded to the whole number, if necessary).
   g. Calculate the infusion rate of the medication to infuse the medication via volume-control set in the minimum fluid volume followed by a 15 mL flush.

50. **Order:** acyclovir 0.5 g IV q8h for a 77 lb child
    Supply: 20 mL vial containing acyclovir 25 mg/mL
    Reference: The recommended dose of acyclovir is 30–60 mg/kg/day in 3 divided doses. Acyclovir should be administered in a concentration of 7–10 mg/mL over 1 hour.

NCLEX-Style Review Questions

For questions 1–4, select the best response.

1. Clindamycin 60 mg PO q6h is ordered for an 8 kg infant. The safe dose range of clindamycin is 25–40 mg/kg/day in divided doses every 6–8 hours. The supply of clindamycin is 75 mg/5 mL. From this information, the nurse determines: (LO 12-2)
   a. The order is safe; administer 0.8 mL.
   b. The order is too low; administer the ordered dose and contact the authorized prescriber for an additional dose.
   c. The order is safe; administer 4 mL.
   d. The order is too high; contact the authorized prescriber for a new order.

2. Oncaspar® 1,200 International Units IM stat is ordered for a child with the following measurements: ht, 90 cm; wt, 16 kg; BSA, 0.63 m². The recommended dose of Oncaspar for children with a BSA more than 0.6 m² is 2,500 International Units/m² q 14 days. The supply of Oncaspar is 750 International Units/mL. From this information, the nurse determines: (LO 12-3)
   a. The dose is safe; administer 1.6 mL.
   b. The dose is too low; contact the prescriber.
   c. The dose is safe; administer 0.63 mL.
   d. The dose is too high; contact the prescriber.

3. The dosage strength of acetaminophen is 160 mg/tsp. The recommended dose of acetaminophen, 15 mg/kg/dose, is ordered for a 5 lb, 14 oz infant. The nurse determines: (LO 12-2)
   a. 194 mg is the recommended dose and measures 1.2 tsp in a calibrated medicine spoon
   b. 40 mg is the recommended dose and draws up 1.3 mL into an oral syringe
   c. 40 mg is the recommended dose and measures 4 mL in a medicine cup
   d. 35 mg is the recommended dose and measures 1.1 mL in a calibrated medicine spoon

4. Vancocin® 40 mg IV q6h is ordered. Vancocin should be further diluted to a concentration of 1–5 mg/mL. The nurse uses this information to calculate the: (LO 12-4)
   a. Minimum dilution 8 mL; maximum dilution 40 mL
   b. Minimum concentration 8 mL; maximum concentration 40 mL
   c. Minimum dilution 40 mL; maximum dilution 200 mL
   d. Minimum concentration 40 mL; maximum concentration 200 mL

For questions 5–6 select all that apply.

5. Gentamicin 50 mg IV q8h is ordered. The supply is gentamicin 80 mg/2 mL. The drug reference states that gentamicin should be further diluted to a concentration of 2 mg/mL and infused over 1 hour. The nurse should: (LO 12-4)

   a. Inject 0.63 mL of gentamicin into the volume-control set.

   b. Inject 0.63 mL of gentamicin into a 100 mL mini-bag of NS.

   c. Inject 1.3 mL of gentamicin into a 100 mL mini-bag of NS.

   d. Inject 1.3 mL of gentamicin into the volume-control set.

   e. Inject 2.6 mL of gentamicin into a volume-control set.

   f. Inject 2.6 mL of gentamicin into a 100 mL mini-bag of NS.

   g. Fill the volume-control set with IV fluid to the 25 mL calibration.

   h. Infuse the gentamicin via IVPB at 100 mL/h.

   i. Infuse the gentamicin followed by a 15 mL flush at 40 gtt/min.

6. Nurses should know that children are more susceptible to adverse medication effects due to: (LO 12-1)

   a. Increased metabolism

   b. Polypharmacy

   c. Increased stomach acid production

   d. Immature liver and kidney function

   e. Lower percentage of water composing body weight

   f. Variable weights and body surface area

REFERENCES

Collopy, K. T. (2010). Medication considerations. *EMS World*. Retrieved from http://www.emsworld.com/article/10319449/medication-considerations?page=5

Deglin, J. H., Vallerand, A. H., & Sanoski, C. A. (2011). *Davis's drug guide for nurses* (12th ed.) Philadelphia, PA: F.A. Davis.

LaPook, J. (2012). Multiple medications: Growing polypharmacy problem. Retrieved from http://www.cbsnews.com/8301-18563_162-57402912/multiple-medications-growing-polypharmacy-problem/

Mosteller, R. D. (October 22, 1987). Simplified calculation of body-surface area. *New England Journal of Medicine, 317*(17), 1098. Retrieved from http://www.medcalc.com/body.html

U.S. National Library of Medicine. (2012). Drug dosing based on weight and body surface area: Mathematical assumptions and limitations in obese adults. *Pharmacotherapy, 32*(9), 856–868. Retrieved from http://www.ncbi.nlm.nih.gov/pubmed/22711238

Chapter 12   ANSWER KEY

Learning Activity 12-1

1. b
2. a
3. d

Learning Activity 12-2

1. 54 mg for 3.6 kg newborn; 72 mg for 4.8 kg infant
2. 1.8–3.6 mEq for 2.6 kg newborn; 2.4–4.8 mEq for 4.8 kg infant

Learning Activity 12-3

1. 112 mg
2. 224 mg
3. 56 mg
4. 112 mg

Learning Activity 12-4

1. a. 120–150 mg/day
   b. Ordered daily dose, 150 mg, falls in the 120–150 mg safe dose range, therefore, is safe.
   c. Administer 1.3 mL.
2. a. 30–60 mg/day
   b. Ordered daily dose, 45 mg, falls in the 30–60 mg safe dose range, therefore, is safe.
   c. Administer 0.6 mL.
3. a. 4.5 mg/day
   b. Ordered daily dose, 6 mg, exceeds the safe daily dose, 4.5 mg.
   c. Contact the provider.

Learning Activity 12-5

1. 0.36 m^2
2. 1.9 m^2
3. 1.3 m^2
4. 0.23 m^2

Learning Activity 12-6

1. 0.64 m^2
2. 0.43 m^2
3. 1.1 m^2
4. 1.3 m^2

Learning Activity 12-7

1. a. 0.69 m^2
    b. Safe dose is 2,070,000 three times weekly.
    c. Ordered dose is safe.
    d. Administer 0.41 mL.
2. a. 0.69 m^2
    b. SDR is 17.25–20.7 mg/day.
    c. Ordered dose is safe.
    d. Administer 10 mL.

Learning Activity 12-8

1. 14 mL
2. 80 mL

Learning Activity 12-9

1. 20 gtt/min
2. 46 gtt/min

Learning Activity 12-10

1. 56 mL/h
2. 90 mL/h

Homework

1. True
2. True
3. False. The process by which drugs are moved out of the body is called elimination. Creatinine clearance is the rate at which creatinine is cleared by the kidneys.
4. True
5. False. Metabolism refers to the transformation of drugs into chemicals used by the body. Polypharmacy refers to multiple medications taken by one patient.
6. 2.9
7. 55
8. 4
9. 5.3
10. 4.8
11. Minimum dose 48 mg; maximum dose 72 mg
12. Minimum dose 66 mg; maximum dose 99 mg
13. Minimum dose 380 mg; maximum dose 570 mg
14. Minimum dose 336 mcg; maximum dose 504 mcg
15. Minimum dose 2.4 mg; maximum dose 9.6 mg
16. Safe daily dose range is 5,000–7,500 mg/day.
17. SSD range = 1,250–1,875 mg/day vs. dose ordered = 1,500 mg (daily dose ordered = 6,000 mg); dose ordered is safe.
18. Draw up 3.9 mL of reconstituted ticarcillin.
19. 90 mg q8h
20. Dose is too low; contact the provider.
21. 400–800 mg/day
22. SDR is 133–267 mg/day or daily dose ordered is 450 mg/day.
23. Dose ordered, 150 mg, falls in the SDR, 133–267 mg/day. Daily dose ordered, 450 mg, falls in the daily dose range, 400–800 mg/day; therefore, the nurse should administer 6 mL.
24. Yes, 345–1,035 mg/day is safe; 1,000 mg/day is ordered.
25. Yes, 495–1,485 mg/day is safe; 1,000 mg/day is ordered.
26. Yes, 645–1,935 mg/day is safe; 1,000 mg/day is ordered.
27. For a 23 kg, 33 kg, or 43 kg child, administer 10 mL.
28. 23–45 mg/day
29. Ordered daily dose, 60 mg/day, is too high.
30. Contact the provider.
31. 0.38 to 0.76 mcg/day
32. 0.5 mcg, the ordered dose, falls in the SDR, 0.38–0.76 mcg.
33. Administer 0.5 mL.
34. a. 1.1 m^2
    b. 82.5 to 330 mg/day
    c. Dose is safe; 50 mg/dose falls in the dose range 20.6–82.5 mg; 200 mg/day falls in daily range 82.5–330 mg.
    d. Administer 2 tablets.
35. a. 0.52 m^2
    b. SDR is 1.7–25 mg/day.
    c. 15 mg is ordered and falls in SDR.
    d. Administer 0.38 mL.
36. a. 0.59 m^2
    b. SDR is 5.9 to 17.7 mg/dose.
    c. Ordered dose, 7.5 mg, falls in SDR, 5.9 to 17.7 mg/dose, therefore is safe.
    d. Administer 1½ tablets.
37. a. 2.0 m^2
    b. SDR is 150 to 200 mg q 4 wk.
    c. Ordered dose, 150 mg, falls in SDR, 150–200 mg, therefore is safe.
    d. Administer 150 mL.
38. a. 1.3 m^2
    b. SDR is 78 to 325 mg/day.
    c. Ordered dose, 100 mg, falls in SDR, 78–325 mg, therefore is safe.
    d. Administer 2 tab.
39. 125–250 mg/day; 42–83 mg/dose (q8h)
40. 114–227 mcg daily
41. a. iii
    b. ii
    c. iv
    d. i

42. a. ii
    b. iii
    c. iv
    d. i
43. 100 mL
44. 13 mL
45. 32 mL
46. a. 10 mL
    b. 50 mL
    c. 260 gtt/min
47. a. 1.5 mL
    b. 75 mL
    c. 90 gtt/min
48. a. 0.3 mL
    b. 2.7 mL
    c. 39 mL/h
49. a. 1.3 mL
    b. 23.7 mL
    c. 17.5 mL/h
50. a. 1,050–2,100 mg/day
    b. 350–700 mg/dose
    c. Yes
    d. 20 mL
    e. 50 mL
    f. 71 mL
    g. 65 gtt/min or 65 mL/h

NCLEX-Style Review Questions

1. c
   Rationale: The safe daily range is 200–320 mg/day. The safe dose range is 50–80 mg/dose; therefore, the ordered dose, 60 mg, is safe. Because the supply is 75 mg/5 mL, the nurse will draw up 4 mL.
2. b
   Rationale: The safe dose is 1,575 International Units. The ordered dose, 1,200 International Units, is too low. The nurse should contact the provider.

3. b
   Rationale: 5 lb 14 oz = 5.875 lb, which converts to 2.7 kg. The safe dose based on this weight is 40 mg. To administer 40 mg from a supply of 160 mg/5 mL (1 tsp), the nurse will measure 1.3 mL in an oral syringe.
4. a
   Rationale: 40 mg divided by the maximum concentration, 5 mg/mL, yields a minimum dilution volume of 8 mL. 40 mg divided by the minimum concentration, 1 mg/mL, yields a maximum dilution volume of 40 mL.
5. d, g, i
   Rationale: To obtain 50 mg from a supply of 80 mg/2 mL, the nurse will draw up 1.3 mL and inject it into a volume-control set (d) rather than a 100 mL mini-bag, which is too much volume for a pediatric patient. To determine the concentration for administration, the dose, 50 mg, is divided by the concentration 2 mg/mL to yield a dilution volume of 25 mL, thus the nurse will add 24 mL to the 1.3 mL of medication in the volume-control set (g). To calculate the infusion rate for the medication to infuse over 1 hour, the nurse will add the medication and flush (25 + 15 = 40 mL), and, using a microdrop (60 gtt/mL) volume-control set, the nurse will establish a flow rate of 40 gtt/min.
6. a, d, f
   Rationale: Factors that make children more susceptible to the effects and adverse effects of drugs include decreased stomach acid production, immature liver and kidney function (d), decreased circulation to muscles, variable weights and body surface area (f), increased metabolism (a), and higher percentage of water composing body weight.

© Forfunlife/Shutterstock

Chapter 13

Hydration and Nutrition Calculations

CHAPTER OUTLINE

LEARNING OUTCOMES

Upon completion of the chapter, the student will be able to:

13-1   Calculate daily pediatric fluid requirements.

13-2   Calculate daily pediatric caloric requirements.

13-3   Calculate major nutrient quantities.

13-4   Perform fluid resuscitation calculations using the Parkland Formula.

KEY TERMS

calorie requirement

caloric

carbohydrate

complex carbohydrate

daily fluid requirement (DFR)

fat

fluid resuscitation

hypovolemic shock

lipid

maintenance fluids

nutrient dense

percent daily value (%DV)

protein

simple carbohydrate

Case Consideration ... Fluid Fiasco

A pediatric patient weighing 14 kg is recovering from gastroenteritis. The physician decreases the intravenous fluid intake to 10 mL/h and explains to the parents that the child may be discharged when an adequate oral fluid intake is taken and tolerated. The parents ask the nursing student, "How much fluid intake is considered adequate?" The student encourages the parents to give the child as much fluid as possible. After 24 hours, the child's fluid intake is 240 mL via the intravenous route and 1.5 L given orally for a total of 1,740 mL over the course of the day.

1. What went wrong?

2. How could this situation have been avoided?

■ INTRODUCTION

Clinical nursing calculations include computations regarding nutrition and hydration. This chapter covers weight-based fluid and caloric requirement calculations and addresses analysis of intake and output. Because a child's body size varies greatly during the pediatric years (birth to 18 years old), pediatric nutrition and hydration requirements vary according to weight. Weight-based calculations determine 24-hour, or daily, requirements. Nurses must be able to analyze nutrient and hydration status to determine if and when patients' needs are met.

13-1   Pediatric Daily Fluid Requirement (DFR) Calculations

Fluid imbalances pose a greater threat to children than to adults because their bodies are composed of a greater percentage of water than adults. To prevent fluid overload or dehydration, nurses need to calculate and sustain a child's **maintenance fluids**, the amount of fluid a patient needs to maintain normal hydration as described in Chapter 10. Maintenance fluids, also called **daily fluid requirement (DFR)**, are based on body weight and are calculated using the formulas in **TABLE 13-1**.

Calculating DFR is accomplished in two steps:

Step 1: Convert weight to kilograms, if necessary.

Step 2: Select and apply the appropriate formula from Table 13-1.

TABLE 13-1 Formulas for Calculating Daily Fluid Requirements (DFR)/Maintenance Fluids	
Weight	**DFR Formulas**
0–10 kg	100 mL/kg/day
11–20 kg	1,000 mL/day (for 1st 10 kg) + 50 mL/kg/day (for each kg between 10 and 20 kg)
Over 20 kg	1,500 mL/day (for 1st 20 kg) + 20 mL/kg/day (for each kg over 20 kg)

Example 1:   Calculate the DFR for a newborn who weighs 3,300 grams.

Step 1: Convert 3,300 g to 3.3 kg.

Step 2: Apply the formula for 0–10 kg in Table 13-1.

$$100 \text{ mL/} \cancel{\text{kg}}\text{/day} \times 3.3 \text{ } \cancel{\text{kg}} = x$$
$$330 \text{ mL/day} = x$$

Example 2:   Calculate the DFR for a child who weighs 35 pounds.

Step 1: Convert 35 lb to kg:

$$\frac{1 \text{ kg}}{2.2 \text{ lb}} = \frac{x \text{ kg}}{35 \text{ lb}}, \quad x = 15.9 \text{ kg} \quad \text{or} \quad 35 \text{ } \cancel{\text{lb}} \times \frac{1 \text{ kg}}{2.2 \text{ } \cancel{\text{lb}}} = 15.9 \text{ kg}$$

Step 2: Apply the formula for 11–20 kg in Table 13-1. Note the weight between 10 and 20 kg is 5.9 kg.

$$1,000 \text{ mL/day} + (50 \text{ mL/} \cancel{\text{kg}}\text{/day} \times 5.9 \text{ } \cancel{\text{kg}}) = x$$
$$1,000 \text{ mL/day} + 295 \text{ mL/day} = 1,295 \text{ mL/day}$$

Example 3:   Calculate the DFR for a child who weighs 75 pounds.

Step 1: Convert 75 lb to kg:

$$\frac{1 \text{ kg}}{2.2 \text{ lb}} = \frac{x \text{ kg}}{75 \text{ lb}}, \quad x = 34.1 \text{ kg} \quad \text{or} \quad 75 \text{ } \cancel{\text{lb}} \times \frac{1 \text{ kg}}{2.2 \text{ } \cancel{\text{lb}}} = 34.1 \text{ kg}$$

Step 2: Apply the formula for 11–20 kg. Note the weight over 20 kg is 14.1 kg.

$$1,500 \text{ mL/day} + (20 \text{ mL/} \cancel{\text{kg}}\text{/day} \times 14.1 \text{ } \cancel{\text{kg}}) = x$$
$$1,500 \text{ mL/day} + 282 \text{ mL/day} = 1,782 \text{ mL/day}$$

WARNING!

Document Weights in Kilograms!

Accurate weights are important (**Figure 13-1**). Nurses weigh patients as soon as possible upon admission. Weights should be documented only in kilograms. A Pennsylvania Patient Safety Authority (2009) study that analyzed the significance of accurate weights reported that "more than 25% of the 479 reports mention breakdowns that occurred when the patient's weight, measured in pounds or kilograms, was erroneously documented as the patient's weight in kilograms or pounds, respectively."

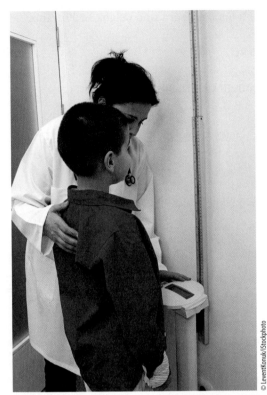

FIGURE 13-1 Actual weights should be used for fluid and nutrition weight-based calculations.

Clinical CLUE

If daily weights are prescribed for a nutritional problem, they should be done at the same time every day (usually before breakfast), with the same amount of clothing, preferably after voiding, using the same scale. This will minimize the number of variables affecting the weight and thus promote greater accuracy.

Information obtained from DFR calculations are used by:

■ The provider to determine the IV flow rate for a child who is taking minimal to no fluids by mouth

■ The nurse to determine if the child's fluid needs are being met by the oral and/or intravenous fluid intake

Assuming the children in the previous Examples 1–3 are taking in nothing by mouth, the provider calculates the hourly IV flow rate for each by dividing the daily maintenance fluids by 24 hours:

Example 1: 330 mL/~~day~~ ÷ 24 h/~~day~~ = 13.75 or 13.8 mL/h

Example 2: 1,295 mL/~~day~~ ÷ 24 h/~~day~~ = 53.95 or 54 mL/h

Example 3: 1,782 mL/~~day~~ ÷ 24 h/~~day~~ = 74.25 or 74.3 mL/h

Rounding RULE

Because rounding is done according to equipment, and intravenous infusion pumps in the pediatric setting are typically calibrated to tenths (of a milliliter), pediatric IV rates should be rounded to tenths. It is also worth noting that IV rates in critical care settings are often rounded to tenths.

LEARNING ACTIVITY 13-1 Calculate the DFR for each weight and then determine the hourly IV flow rate, assuming that there will be no oral intake.

1.   4,500 g
2.   33 lb
3.   27 kg

Assessing Intake

The nurse uses information obtained from DFR calculations to determine if patient intake is adequate by comparing actual (or expected) intake to the DFR. This is accomplished in three steps:

Step 1: Convert weight to kilograms (if necessary) and calculate the DFR.

Step 2: Convert the volume to milliliters (if necessary) and calculate the daily (24-hour) intake.

Step 3: Compare the actual daily intake to the DFR.

Example 1:   Determine if a 13½ lb infant is meeting his DFR if he consumes 3½ ounces of formula q4h.

Step 1: Convert 13.5 lb to kg and calculate the DFR for this weight:

$$\frac{1 \text{ kg}}{2.2 \text{ lb}} = \frac{x \text{ kg}}{13.5 \text{ lb}}, \quad x = 6.1 \text{ kg} \quad \text{or} \quad 13.5 \text{ lb} \times \frac{1 \text{ kg}}{2.2 \text{ lb}} = 6.1 \text{ kg}$$

$$100 \text{ mL/kg/day} \times 6.1 \text{ kg} = 610 \text{ mL/day}$$

Step 2a: Convert 3.5 ounces to mL:

$$\frac{1 \text{ oz}}{30 \text{ mL}} = \frac{3.5 \text{ oz}}{x \text{ mL}}, \quad x = 105 \text{ mL} \quad \text{or} \quad 3.5 \text{ oz} \times \frac{30 \text{ mL}}{1 \text{ oz}} = 105 \text{ mL}$$

Step 2b: Calculate the expected mL/day intake:

Because q4h occurs 6 times per day, 105 mL × 6/day = 630 mL/day.

Step 3: Compare the expected daily intake, 630 mL/day, to the DFR, 610 mL/day, and determine that this infant's daily consumption will slightly exceed his DFR, thus his daily fluid needs will be met.

Clinical CLUE

DFR is a minimum amount of fluid needed to meet fluid needs. Often, actual oral intake will exceed the DFR. To determine appropriateness of intake, it should always be evaluated along with output (See "Measuring Output," next section). When the nurse is in doubt of whether or not fluid intake is excessive, the provider should be contacted.

Example 2:   Determine if a newborn who weighs 6 lb 6 oz and consumes ½ oz q2h will meet her DFR.

Step 1a: Convert 6 oz to lb: $\frac{1 \text{ lb}}{16 \text{ oz}} = \frac{x \text{ lb}}{6 \text{ oz}}, x = 0.375$ lb or $6 \text{ oz} \times \frac{1 \text{ lb}}{16 \text{ oz}} = 0.375$ lb, therefore 6 lb 6 oz = 6.375 lb.

Step 1b: Convert 6.375 lb to kg:

$$\frac{1\ \text{kg}}{2.2\ \text{lb}} = \frac{x\ \text{kg}}{6.375\ \text{lb}}, \quad x = 2.9\ \text{kg} \quad \text{or} \quad 6.375\ \cancel{\text{lb}} \times \frac{1\ \text{kg}}{2.2\ \cancel{\text{lb}}} = 2.9\ \text{kg}$$

Step 1c: Calculate DFR:

$$100\ \text{mL/}\cancel{\text{kg}}\text{/day} \times 2.9\ \cancel{\text{kg}} = 290\ \text{mL/day}$$

Step 2a: Convert ½ oz to 15 mL:

$$\frac{1}{2}\ \cancel{\text{oz}} \times \frac{30\ \text{mL}}{1\ \cancel{\text{oz}}} = 15\ \text{mL}$$

Step 2b: Calculate the expected mL/day intake:

Because q2h occurs 12 times per day, determine the mL/day intake by multiplying 15 mL by 12:

$$15\ \text{mL} \times 12\text{/day} = 180\ \text{mL/day}$$

Step 3: Compare the DFR to the expected intake. Because the infant requires 290 mL/day but is expected to consume only 180 mL, the nurse determines that this child's fluid needs will not be met. The nurse will consult the provider and possibly obtain an order for IV fluids for this child.

Example 3:   Determine if an infant who weighs 17 kg is meeting his DFR by consuming 8 oz of formula q3h.

Step 1: Because the weight is already in kilograms, no weight conversion is needed. Note the formula for 11–20 kg is needed, and the weight between 11 and 20 kg is 7 kg. The DFR is calculated as follows:

$$1,000\ \text{mL/day} + (50\ \text{mL/}\cancel{\text{kg}}\text{/day} \times 7\ \cancel{\text{kg}})$$
$$= 1,000\ \text{mL/day} + 350\ \text{mL/day} = 1,350\ \text{mL/day}$$

Step 2a: Convert 8 oz to 240 mL:

$$8\ \cancel{\text{oz}} \times \frac{30\ \text{mL}}{1\ \cancel{\text{oz}}} = 240\ \text{mL}$$

Step 2b: Calculate the expected mL/day intake:

Because q3h occurs 8 times per day, calculate mL/day by multiplying this intake by 8:

$$240\ \text{mL} \times 8\text{/day} = 1,920\ \text{mL/day}$$

Step 3: The nurse should note that the infant's intake, 1,920 mL/day, will greatly exceed the DFR:

$$1,920\ \text{mL/day [actual intake]} - 1,350\ \text{mL/day [DFR]} = 570\ \text{mL excess fluid intake}$$

Excessive fluid can lead to electrolyte imbalance, respiratory distress, and other health concerns. The nurse should contact the provider and report this information immediately so appropriate measures can be taken to avoid or manage the effects of fluid overload.

LEARNING ACTIVITY 13-2 Determine if hydration requirements will be met in each situation.

1.   A 66 lb child is NPO after surgery and is receiving IV fluids at 71 mL/h.
2.   An 18.7 kg infant is recovering from gastroenteritis and consuming 6 oz of fluid q6h and receiving IV fluids at 30 mL/h.

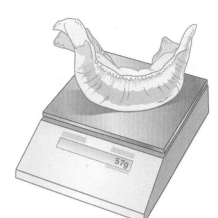

FIGURE 13-2 To determine urine output, the nurse weighs the wet diaper and subtracts the dry diaper weight.

Measuring Output

Fluid intake is usually assessed in conjunction with output. Expected urine output for pediatric clients is 1–2 mL/kg/h. With the knowledge that 1 mL of liquid weighs 1 gram, nurses measure infant output by weighing diapers and subtracting the dry diaper weight (**Figure 13-2**). For example, if the dry diaper weight is 30 g, urine output contained in a wet diaper weighing 150 g is 120 mL. In addition to monitoring intake, the nurse also monitors output to evaluate hydration status of patients. Evaluation of pediatric output is a three-step process:

Step 1: Calculate the total urine output for the shift.

Step 2: Calculate the expected output by converting the weight to kilograms or determining the conversion factor for dimensional analysis (if necessary) and applying the formula for expected urine output, 1–2 mL/kg/h.

> **NOTE:** If actual output exceeds expected output, the nurse should compare actual output to intake. In general output should be 50–100% of intake.

Step 3: Compare expected output to actual output.

Example: During a 12-h shift, a 15-lb infant has 3 wet diapers weighing 50 g, 85 g, and 60 g. The dry diaper weight is 25 g. Calculate the output and compare it to the expected urine output.

Step 1: Calculate the output by subtracting 25 g from each wet diaper and add the weights:

$$(50 \text{ g} - 25 \text{ g}) + (85 \text{ g} - 25 \text{ g}) + (60 \text{ g} - 25 \text{ g})$$
$$= 25 \text{ g} + 60 \text{ g} + 35 \text{ g} = 120 \text{ g}$$

Because 1 g (diaper weight) = 1 mL (urine output), 120 g = 120 mL.

Step 2: To determine the expected urine output with dimensional analysis, use the conversion factor 1 kg/2.2 lb, then calculate both the minimum (1 mL/kg/h) and maximum (2 mL/kg/h) output expected during the 12-h shift. To use the formula method, the weight in pounds must be converted to kg before calculating the minimum and maximum outputs.

Formula Method	Dimensional Analysis
Step 2a: $15 \ \cancel{lb} \times \dfrac{1 \ kg}{2.2 \ \cancel{lb}} = 6.81 \ \text{or} \ 6.8 \ kg$ Step 2b: $1 \ mL/\cancel{kg}/\cancel{h} \times 6.8 \ \cancel{kg} \times 12 \ \cancel{h} = x \ (mL)$ $\mathbf{82 \ mL \ (min)} = x$ $2 \ mL/\cancel{kg}/\cancel{h} \times 6.8 \ \cancel{kg} \times 12 \ \cancel{h} = x \ (mL)$ $\mathbf{163 \ mL \ (max)} = x$	$x \ (mL) = \dfrac{1 \ mL}{1 \ \cancel{kg}} \times \dfrac{1 \ \cancel{kg}}{2.2 \ \cancel{lb}} \times \dfrac{15 \ \cancel{lb}}{1 \ \cancel{h}} \times \dfrac{12 \ \cancel{h}}{1}$ $x = \dfrac{180 \ mL}{2.2} = \mathbf{82 \ mL \ (min)}$ $x \ (mL) = \dfrac{2 \ mL}{1 \ \cancel{kg}} \times \dfrac{1 \ \cancel{kg}}{2.2 \ \cancel{lb}} \times \dfrac{15 \ \cancel{lb}}{1 \ \cancel{h}} \times \dfrac{12 \ \cancel{h}}{1}$ $x = \dfrac{360 \ mL}{2.2} = \mathbf{164 \ mL \ (max)}$

Step 3: The actual urine output, 120 mL, falls in the expected urine output range, 82–164 mL. This information assists the nurse in determining that this patient is adequately hydrated.

Clinical CLUE

Normal adult urine output is 0.5 to 1 mL/kg/h. Minimum adult urine output is 30 mL/h.

LEARNING ACTIVITY 13-3 Calculate the actual urine output and expected urine output for each example.

1. During an 8 h shift, a 10 kg infant has two wet diapers weighing 95 g and 75 g. The dry diaper weight is 20 g.
2. During a 12 h shift, a 3,940 g infant has three wet diapers weighing 35 g, 25 g, and 44 g. The dry diaper weight is 15 g.

Clinical CLUE

Diaper weights are only necessary when strict intake and output measurement is needed. When strict output measurement is not required, wet diaper count, instead, is recorded. An output of 6–10 wet diapers per day reflects adequate (intake and) output.

13-2 Pediatric Daily Caloric Requirement Calculations

Just as fluid requirements vary with age and weight, caloric requirements also vary. A **calorie** is a unit of energy used to fuel the body, thus measuring calories is like measuring the amount of fuel needed (or

Age	Caloric Requirement
Birth to 6 months	120 cal/kg/day
6 months to 1 year	110 cal/kg/day
1–3 years old	100 cal/kg/day
3–6 years old	75–90 cal/kg/day
6–12 years old	60–75 cal/kg/day
12–18 years old	30–60 cal/kg/day

TABLE 13-2   These Caloric Requirements Are Geared Toward Average-Sized, Healthy Children in Each Age Group

consumed) by the body. **Caloric requirement**, the number of calories to meet energy needs and sustain growth, is based on weight. Energy needs per kilogram of body weight decrease with age, as reflected in **TABLE 13-2**.

To evaluate caloric intake, the nurse will:

Step 1: Convert the weight to kilograms or select the appropriate weight conversion factor(s) when using dimensional analysis (if necessary).

Step 2: Select and apply the appropriate caloric requirement from Table 13-2.

Step 3: Calculate the daily caloric intake and compare it to the daily caloric requirement. To calculate caloric intake, the nurse needs to know the caloric content of infant formulas. Most standard infant formulas contain 20 calories/ounce. This conversion factor is multiplied by the number of ounces consumed.

Clinical CLUE

Actual caloric intake will most likely not exactly match the expected caloric intake, but in general, is usually within 10% of the expected caloric intake.

Example: Calculate the caloric requirements of a 3-month-old infant who weighs 10 lb 6 oz and determine if needs are being met by consuming 5 oz standard formula (20 cal/oz) every 4 hours.

Step 1: For ratio-proportion and the formula method, convert 10 lb 6 oz to kg. For dimensional analysis, use the conversion factors 1 kg/2.2 lb and 1 lb/16 oz.

Step 2: Choose from Table 13-2 the caloric requirement for birth to 6 months old: 120 cal/kg/day.

Ratio-Proportion	Formula Method
Step 1: Convert 10 lb 6 oz to kg:	Step 1: Convert 10 lb 6 oz to kg:

Ratio-Proportion

Step 1: Convert 10 lb 6 oz to kg:

$$\frac{16\ oz}{1\ lb} = \frac{6\ oz}{x\ lb}$$
$$x = 0.375\ lb$$
so 10 lb 6 oz = 10.375 lb
$$\frac{1\ kg}{2.2\ lb} = \frac{x\ kg}{10.375\ lb}$$
$$x = 4.72\ kg$$

Step 2: Calculate calories:

$$\frac{120\ cal}{1\ kg} = \frac{x\ cal}{4.72\ kg}\ or$$
120 cal: 1 kg = x cal: 4.72 kg
$$1 \times x = 120 \times 4.72$$
$$x = \textbf{566 cal per day}$$

Formula Method

Step 1: Convert 10 lb 6 oz to kg:

$$6\ \cancel{oz} \times \frac{1\ lb}{16\ \cancel{oz}} = 0.375\ lb$$
so 10 lb 6 oz = 10.375 lb
$$10.375\ \cancel{lb} \times \frac{1\ kg}{2.2\ \cancel{lb}} = 4.72\ kg$$

Step 2: Calculate calories:

$$120\ cal/\cancel{kg}/day \times 4.72\ \cancel{kg} = x\ (cal/day)$$
$$\textbf{566 cal/day} = \textbf{\textit{x}}$$

Dimensional Analysis

$$x\ (cal/day) = \frac{120\ cal}{1\ \cancel{kg}} \times \frac{1\ \cancel{kg}}{2.2\ lb} \times \left[\frac{10\ lb}{1} + \left(\frac{6\ oz}{1} \times \frac{1\ lb}{16\ oz} \right) \times \frac{1}{1\ day} \right]$$
$$x = \frac{120\ cal}{2.2\ \cancel{lb}} \times \frac{10.375\ \cancel{lb}}{1\ day}$$
$$x = \frac{1,245\ cal}{2.2\ day}$$
$$x = \textbf{566 cal/day}$$

Step 3: Because q4h occurs 6 times in a day, the daily caloric intake is calculated as follows:

$$5\ oz/\cancel{feeding} \times 6\ \cancel{feeding}/day = 30\ oz/day$$
$$30\ \cancel{oz}/day \times 20\ cal/\cancel{oz} = 600\ cal/day$$

From this calculation, the nurse determines that the daily caloric intake of 600 cal/day meets the expected caloric intake of 566 cal/day.

Rounding RULE

For average-sized, healthy children, caloric requirements are approximate, therefore, calculations can be rounded to the whole number.

LEARNING ACTIVITY 13-4 For each example, calculate the daily caloric requirement and amount of standard (20 cal/oz) formula needed per day to meet this requirement.

1. 2-month-old that weighs 10 lb 8 oz
2. 4-month-old that weighs 14 lb

Clinical CLUE

Breastfeeding exclusively for the first 6 months of life is recommended by the American Academy of Pediatrics (2012). Formula is only used when a mother chooses not to breastfeed or if she has a medical condition contraindicating breastfeeding. Solid foods are added between the ages of 4 and 6 months. The addition of solid foods will decrease the amount of formula required.

13-3   Nutrient Calculations

The main nutrients that supply calories are called energy nutrients. There are three energy nutrients: carbohydrates, proteins, and fats. **Carbohydrates**, manufactured by plants, are a major source of fuel for the body. **Simple carbohydrates**, sometimes called sugars, are found in fruits, milk, and sweeteners, such as sugar, honey, and corn syrup. **Complex carbohydrates** include starches and are found in grains, cereals, pastas, vegetables, and fruits. In addition to providing energy, **proteins** are called the body's building blocks because they perform many functions in the body, including building and repairing tissue. Food sources of protein include meat, poultry, seafood, dairy, eggs, and many plant-based foods. **Fats**, also called **lipids**, provide energy to fuel the body when carbohydrates are not available. In addition to being a fuel source for the body, fats play a role in nutrient absorption, insulation, and maintaining body temperature.

Caloric Content of Energy Nutrients

Carbohydrates contain 4 calories per gram and should account for approximately 60% of the calories in a typical healthy diet. Protein also contains 4 calories per gram and supplies about 10% of the calories in a typical healthy diet. Fat has the highest caloric content, with 9 calories per gram and should compose no more than 30% of the calories in a healthy diet (U.S. Food and Drug Administration [FDA], 2013). To calculate the number of carbohydrate, protein, or fat calories in a serving of food, use the appropriate conversion factor (4 cal/g of carbohydrate, 4 cal/g of protein, 9 cal/g of fat) and set up the ratio-proportion, or use the formula method or dimensional analysis.

Example: Calculate the number of carbohydrate, protein, fat, and total calories in an egg omelet with the following nutrition facts:

- 0.42 g carbohydrate

- 6.48 g protein

- 7.33 g fat

Add the total calories and round to the whole number.

Ratio-Proportion	Formula Method
$\dfrac{4\ cal}{1\ g} = \dfrac{x\ cal}{0.42\ g}$ $x = $ **1.68 cal** (carbohydrate)	$4\,cal/g \times 0.42\ g = $ **1.68 cal** (carbohydrate)
$\dfrac{4\ cal}{1\ g} = \dfrac{x\ cal}{6.48\ g}$ $x = $ **25.92 cal** (protein)	$4\,cal/g \times 6.48\ g = $ **25.92 cal** (protein)

$$\frac{9\ cal}{1\ g} = \frac{x\ cal}{7.33\ g}$$

$x = $ **65.97 cal** (fat)

$9\ cal/\cancel{g} \times 7.33\ \cancel{g} = $ **65.97 cal**
(fat)

1.68 + 25.92 + 65.97
= **94 cal** (total)

1.68 + 25.92 + 65.97
= **94 cal** (total)

Dimensional Analysis

$$x\ cal = \left(\frac{4\ cal}{1\ \cancel{g}} \times \frac{0.42\ \cancel{g}}{1}\right) + \left(\frac{4\ cal}{1\ \cancel{g}} \times \frac{6.48\ \cancel{g}}{1}\right) + \left(\frac{9\ cal}{1\ \cancel{g}} \times \frac{7.33\ \cancel{g}}{1}\right)$$

$x\ cal = $ **1.68 cal** [carb] + **25.92 cal** [prot] + **65.97 cal** [fat]

$x\ cal = $ **93.57 or 94 cal** [total]

LEARNING ACTIVITY 13-5 Calculate the number of carbohydrate, protein, fat, and total calories for each food item. Round total calories to the whole number.

1.   1 slice ($\frac{1}{8}$ of a 12-inch diameter) of pizza: 26.1 g carbohydrate, 10.6 g protein, 10 g fat
2.   4 oz vanilla ice cream: 19 g carbohydrate, 2.5 g protein, 7 g fat

---

Clinical CLUE

Fiber is a complex carbohydrate that passes through the body without being digested and, therefore, does not supply the body with energy or nutrients. Its role is to provide dietary bulk to regulate the movement of food through the digestive system. To count net carbohydrates or "net carbs" for dieting purposes, some diets allow for subtraction of fiber grams from the total carbohydrate grams.

Calculating Percentage of Major Nutrients

The **percent daily value (%DV)** is the percentage in one serving of a particular product that contributes to the recommended daily intake of a nutrient. Percent daily value is included on nutrition labels and helps individuals assess nutrient content and make comparisons between products. Using nutrition labels, nurses and other healthcare professionals can help clients select **nutrient-dense** foods that are rich in nutrients but low in calories. Most %DVs on nutrition labels are based on a 2,000-calorie diet. **TABLE 13-3**, derived from the FDA's Food Labeling Guide, compares the %DV of carbohydrate, protein, and fat across three different diets.

To calculate the %DV of a food item:

Step 1: Examine the nutrition label to determine the number of grams per serving.

Step 2: Divide number of grams per serving by the diet-appropriate recommended grams/day (per Table 13-3) and convert this value to a percentage.

TABLE 13-3   Recommended Percent Daily Value for Energy Nutrients for Adults and Children 4 Years and Older

Nutrient (%DV)	2,200-Calorie Diet Recommended g/day	2,000-Calorie Diet Recommended g/day	1,800-Calorie Diet Recommended g/day
Carbohydrate (55–60%)	303–330 g	275–300 g	248–270 g
Protein (10–15%)	55–83 g	50–75 g	45–68 g
Fat (30%)	73 g	65 g	60 g

Example: Calculate the %DV of carbohydrate, protein, and fat per serving of cheese-flavored crackers (see **Figure 13-3**) for a 1,800-calorie diet.

Step 1: The nutrition label (Figure 13-3) indicates the number of grams per serving as 20 g carbohydrate, 4 g protein, and 4.5 g fat.

Step 2: Table 13-3 indicates that for a 1,800-calorie diet, the recommended grams per day for each energy nutrient are 248–270 g carbohydrate, 45–68 g protein, and 60 g fat. Therefore, the %DV for each nutrient is calculated as follow:

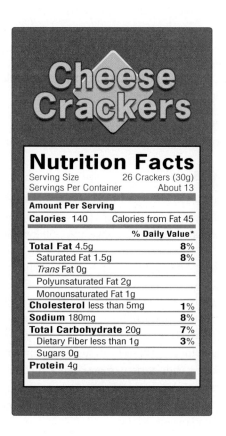

FIGURE 13-3   Nutrition label for cheese-flavored crackers.

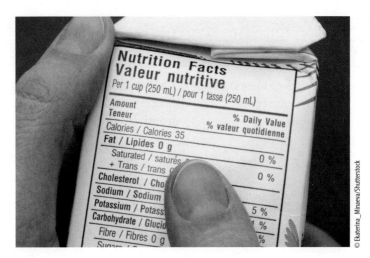

FIGURE 13-4 Nutrition labels enable healthcare consumers to determine how individual foods meet their nutritional needs.

- Carbohydrate: $\frac{20\text{ g}}{248\text{ g}} = 0.08 = 8\%$; $\frac{20\text{ g}}{270\text{ g}} = 0.07 = 7\%$. Therefore, the %DV is 7–8%.
- Protein: $\frac{4\text{ g}}{45\text{ g}} = 0.09 = 9\%$; $\frac{4\text{ g}}{68\text{ g}} = 0.06 = 6\%$. Therefore, the %DV is 6–9%
- Fat: $\frac{4.5\text{ g}}{60\text{ g}} = 0.08$. Therefore, the %DV is 8%.

From this information, an individual can determine that, while 130 calories per serving is not excessive, the amount of energy nutrients is low and, therefore, cheese-flavored crackers would not be considered a nutrient-dense snack.

LEARNING ACTIVITY 13-6 For the snack item listed, calculate the %DV of carbohydrate, protein, and fat based on the indicated diet.

1. 1 cup of peanuts containing 24 g carbohydrate, 38 g protein, 72 g fat; 2,000-calorie diet
2. 1 cup of sliced avocado containing 12 g carbohydrate, 3 g protein, 21 g fat; 2200-calorie diet

Nutrient-Restricted Diets

Nutrient-restricted diets are ordered when necessary for a particular health issue. For example, patients with kidney disease may be placed on a weight-based, protein-restricted diet of 0.7 g/kg/day. For a 150 lb individual, the protein restriction is calculated after converting 150 lb to 68.2 kg:

$$0.7 \text{ g/kg/day} \times 68.2 \text{ kg} = 47.74 \text{ or g/day}$$

An overweight patient or one patient with gallbladder disease may be placed on a fat restriction of 50 g/day. In these and many other instances, it will be important for the healthcare professional to teach patients to read and interpret nutrition labels.

When patients are unable to take food or fluids by mouth, nutrients may be delivered through tube feedings or via the intravenous route. A wide variety of nutritional formulas are available to provide proper nutrition to patients with diverse nutritional needs. Monitoring nutrient intake of individuals with altered nutrition may provide the nurse and other healthcare professionals with valuable information about a patient's condition and/or treatment plan.

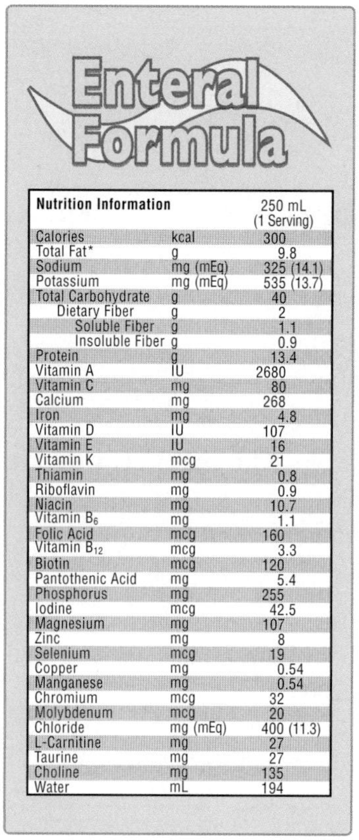

Nutrition Information		250 mL (1 Serving)
Calories	kcal	300
Total Fat*	g	9.8
Sodium	mg (mEq)	325 (14.1)
Potassium	mg (mEq)	535 (13.7)
Total Carbohydrate	g	40
Dietary Fiber	g	2
Soluble Fiber	g	1.1
Insoluble Fiber	g	0.9
Protein	g	13.4
Vitamin A	IU	2680
Vitamin C	mg	80
Calcium	mg	268
Iron	mg	4.8
Vitamin D	IU	107
Vitamin E	IU	16
Vitamin K	mcg	21
Thiamin	mg	0.8
Riboflavin	mg	0.9
Niacin	mg	10.7
Vitamin B_6	mg	1.1
Folic Acid	mcg	160
Vitamin B_{12}	mcg	3.3
Biotin	mcg	120
Pantothenic Acid	mg	5.4
Phosphorus	mg	255
Iodine	mcg	42.5
Magnesium	mg	107
Zinc	mg	8
Selenium	mcg	19
Copper	mg	0.54
Manganese	mg	0.54
Chromium	mcg	32
Molybdenum	mcg	20
Chloride	mg (mEq)	400 (11.3)
L-Carnitine	mg	27
Taurine	mg	27
Choline	mg	135
Water	mL	194

FIGURE 13-5 In addition to information regarding energy nutrients, nutrition labels provide vitamin and mineral content.

Example: A patient who is NPO is receiving nutritional formula via gastrostomy tube at 100 mL/h from 7:00 p.m. to 7:00 a.m. Refer to the nutrition label (**Figure 13-5**) to calculate daily intake of total calories, carbohydrate calories, protein calories, and fat calories.

Step 1: Determine total volume of nutritional formula to be infused in 1 day (24 h). Because the formula will infuse for only 12 out of 24 h (7:00 p.m.–7:00 a.m.), the total daily intake is calculated as follows:

$$100\ \text{mL}/\cancel{\text{h}} \times 12\ \cancel{\text{h}} = 1,200\ \text{mL}$$

Step 2: Determine the nutrient information per serving and use the appropriate conversion factor to calculate the caloric content of carbohydrate, protein, and fat. The label indicates that each 250 mL serving contains 40 g carbohydrate, 13.4 g protein, and 9.8 g fat. Calculate the number of carbohydrate, protein, fat, and total calories per serving.

Ratio-Proportion	Formula Method
$\frac{4\ \text{cal}}{1\ \text{g}} = \frac{x\ \text{cal}}{40\ \text{g}}$ $x =$ **160 cal** (carbohydrate)	$4\ \text{cal}/\cancel{\text{g}} \times 40\ \cancel{\text{g}} =$ **160 cal** (carbohydrate)
$\frac{4\ \text{cal}}{1\ \text{g}} = \frac{x\ \text{cal}}{13.4\ \text{g}}$ $x =$ **53.6 cal** (protein)	$4\ \text{cal}/\cancel{\text{g}} \times 13.4\ \cancel{\text{g}} =$ **53.6 cal** (protein)

$$\frac{9 \text{ cal}}{1 \text{ g}} = \frac{x \text{ cal}}{9.8 \text{ g}}$$

$$x = 88.2 \textbf{ cal } (\text{fat})$$

$$9 \text{ cal/} \cancel{\text{g}} \times 9.8 \cancel{\text{g}} = \textbf{88.2 cal}$$
(fat)

$160 + 54 + 88 = \textbf{302 cal (total)}$ | $160 + 54 + 88 = \textbf{302 cal (total)}$

Dimensional Analysis

$$x \text{ cal} = \left(\frac{4 \text{ cal}}{1 \cancel{\text{g}}} \times \frac{40 \cancel{\text{g}}}{1} \right) + \left(\frac{4 \text{ cal}}{1 \cancel{\text{g}}} \times \frac{13.4 \cancel{\text{g}}}{1} \right) + \left(\frac{9 \text{ cal}}{1 \cancel{\text{g}}} \times \frac{9.8 \cancel{\text{g}}}{1} \right)$$

$$x \text{ cal} = \textbf{160 cal } [\text{carb}] + \textbf{53.6 cal } [\text{prot}] + \textbf{88.2 cal } [\text{fat}]$$

$$x \text{ cal} = \textbf{301.8 or 302 cal } [\textbf{total}]$$

Step 2: Calculate the number of carbohydrate, protein, fat, and total calories to infuse in 1 day, using the total volume to be infused, 1,200 mL.

Ratio-Proportion

$$\frac{160 \text{ cal}}{250 \text{ mL}} = \frac{x \text{ cal}}{1,200 \text{ mL}}$$
$$x = \textbf{768 cal } (\text{carbohydrate})$$

$$\frac{54 \text{ cal}}{250 \text{ mL}} = \frac{x \text{ cal}}{1,200 \text{ mL}}$$
$$x = \textbf{259.2 cal } (\text{protein})$$

$$\frac{88 \text{ cal}}{250 \text{ mL}} = \frac{x \text{ cal}}{1,200 \text{ mL}}$$
$$x = \textbf{422.4 cal } (\text{fat})$$

$768 + 259.2 + 422.4 = 1,449.6$
   or **1,450 cal (total)**

Formula Method

$$\frac{1,200 \cancel{\text{mL}}}{250 \cancel{\text{mL}}} \times 160 \text{ cal} = \textbf{768 cal}$$
(carbohydrate)

$$\frac{1,200 \cancel{\text{mL}}}{250 \cancel{\text{mL}}} \times 54 \text{ cal} = \textbf{259.2 cal}$$
(protein)

$$\frac{1,200 \cancel{\text{mL}}}{250 \cancel{\text{mL}}} \times 88 \text{ cal} = \textbf{422.4 cal}$$
(fat)

$768 + 259.2 + 422.4$
   $= 1,449.6$ or **1,450 cal (total)**

Dimensional Analysis

$$x \text{ cal} = \left(\frac{160 \text{ cal}}{250 \cancel{\text{mL}}} \times \frac{1,200 \cancel{\text{mL}}}{1} \right) + \left(\frac{54 \text{ cal}}{250 \cancel{\text{mL}}} \times \frac{1,200 \cancel{\text{mL}}}{1} \right) + \left(\frac{88 \text{ cal}}{250 \cancel{\text{mL}}} \times \frac{1,200 \cancel{\text{mL}}}{1} \right)$$

$$x \text{ cal} = \textbf{768 cal } [\text{carb}] + \textbf{259.2 cal } [\text{prot}] + \textbf{422.4 cal } [\text{fat}]$$

$$x \text{ cal} = 1,449.6 \text{ or } \textbf{1,450 cal } [\textbf{total}]$$

Calculating total daily caloric intake will enable the nurse to determine if a patient's nutritional needs are being met.

13-4   Fluid Resuscitation

When a patient has a large fluid volume deficit resulting in a low blood pressure, **fluid resuscitation** is implemented. Fluid resuscitation is the administration of a large volume of intravenous fluid over a relatively short period of time (e.g., infusion of normal saline [NS] at 1,000 mL/h). Fluid resuscitation is one of the most important aspects in managing the care of patients experiencing **hypovolemic shock**. Hypovolemic shock is a life-threatening condition in which 20% or more of the body's blood or fluid supply is lost. With such severe loss of fluids, the heart is unable to pump sufficient blood throughout the body, which leads to organ failure. To evaluate the effect of fluid resuscitation, the nurse monitors vital signs and urine output frequently. For example, while infusing NS at 1,000 mL/h, the nurse may assess the blood pressure every 15–30 minutes and monitor the urine output on an hourly basis. Once the blood pressure stabilizes and the urine output is at least 30 mL/h, the nurse will contact the provider for a change in infusion rate.

Patients with extensive burns suffer a significant fluid loss that can lead to hypovolemic shock. Fluid resuscitation is used to correct this fluid loss. Estimating the extent of the burn injury is necessary to calculate fluid replacement needs. One method of estimating the percentage of total body surface area (%TBSA) burned is the "Rule of Nines" (**Figure 13-6**). The Rule of Nines indicates that each of these major body parts comprises 9% of total body surface area: the head, each arm, the front of each leg, the back of each leg. The chest and back are each approximately 18% (2 × 9%) of total body surface area. In the pediatric patient, the head comprises 18% of the body surface area, while the legs are each 14%.

The amount of fluid replacement ordered for burn-injured patients is determined using a standardized formula, such as Parkland's Burn Formula:

$$24 \text{ h fluid requirement in mL} = \%TBSA \times \text{wt in kg} \times 4 \text{ mL/kg}$$

- ½ of this total is administered over the first 8 h

- ½ of this total is administered over the next 16 h

Example: Using the Rule of Nines and Parkland's Burn Formula, calculate the hourly IV infusion rate for 24 hours for a 75 kg patient who sustained burns on the chest and both sides of the right arm. Round IV rates to whole numbers.

Step 1: Calculate the %TBSA using the Rule of Nines:

$$\%TBSA = 18\% \text{ (chest)} + 9\% \text{ (arm)} = 27\%$$

Step 2: Calculate the 24 h fluid requirements:

$$27 \times 75 \text{ kg} \times 4 \text{ mL/kg} = 8,100 \text{ mL}$$

Step 3: Calculate the rate for the first 8 h (½ of the total divided by 8 h):

$$\left(\frac{8,100 \text{ mL}}{2} \right) \div 8 \text{ h} = 506 \text{ mL/h}$$

Step 4: Calculate the rate for the next 16 h (½ of the total divided by 16 h):

$$\left(\frac{8,100 \text{ mL}}{2} \right) \div 16 \text{ h} = 253 \text{ mL/h}$$

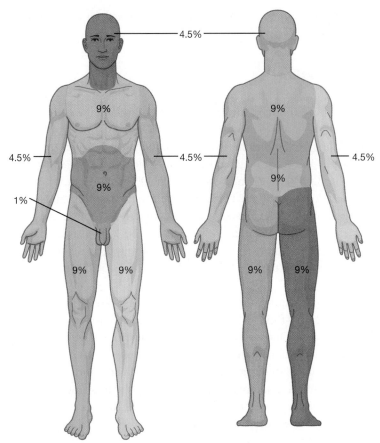

FIGURE 13-6 The Rule of Nines simplifies the process of determining %TBSA by using multiples of 9 to estimate the surface area burned. NOTE: In the pediatric patient, the head comprises 18% and the legs are each 14% of the TBSA.

LEARNING ACTIVITY 13-7 Using the Rule of Nines and Parkland's Burn Formula, calculate the hourly IV infusion rate for 24 hours for each patient.

1. 50 kg adult patient with burns on the front and back of both legs
2. 5 kg child with burns on the front and back of both legs

Fluid Fiasco … Case Closure

Based on the formula for calculating daily maintenance fluids (100 mL/kg/day for the first 10 kg, 50 mL/kg/day for the next 10 kg, 20 mL/kg/day for the remaining weight), the 24-hour fluid intake for a 14 kg child should be 1,200 mL (1,000 mL for the first 10 kg and 200 mL for the remaining 4 kg). By encouraging the parents to give their child as much fluid as possible, he received 540 mL more than necessary, almost 50% more than maintenance requirements. Fluid overloading a patient can lead to cardiovascular complications and electrolyte imbalances. This situation could have been avoided by explaining to the parents the appropriate weight-based fluid needs for their child. Furthermore, if the intake is calculated and analyzed each shift by the nurse, fluid overload would be minimized, as it would have been determined much sooner.

Chapter Summary

Learning Outcomes	Points to Remember
13-1 Calculate daily pediatric fluid requirements.	Formulas to Calculate Maintenance Fluids or Daily Fluid Requirements (DFR): • 0–10 kg: 100 mL/kg/day • 10–20 kg: 1,000 mL/day (for first 10 kg) + 50 mL/kg/day (for each kg between 10 and 20 kg) • Over 20 kg: 1,500 mL/day (for first 20 kg) + 20 mL/kg/day (for each kg over 20 kg) • Normal urine output: 1–2 mL/kg/h
13-2 Calculate daily pediatric caloric requirements.	Birth to 6 months old: 120 cal/kg/day 6 months to 1 year old: 110 cal/kg/day 1–3 years old: 100 cal/kg/day 3–6 years old: 75–90 cal/kg/day 6–12 years old: 60–75 cal/kg/day 12–18 years old: 30–60 cal/kg/day Standard infant formula contains 20 cal/oz.
13-3 Calculate major nutrient quantities.	Carbohydrate—4 cal/g Protein—4 cal/g Fat—9 cal/g
13-4 Perform fluid resuscitation calculations using the Parkland Formula.	The Rule of Nines: • The head, each arm, the front of each leg, and the back of each leg each comprise 9% of total body surface area (TBSA). • Chest and back are each approximately 18% TBSA. • In pediatric patients, the head comprises 18% TBSA, while the legs are each 14%. Parkland Formula: 24-hour fluid requirement in mL = %TBSA × pt wt in kg × 4 mL/kg • ½ of this total is administered over 8 h • ½ of this total is administered over 16 h

Homework

For exercises 1–5, calculate the DFR and determine the hourly IV rate needed to meet the DFR for each weight indicated, assuming there is no oral intake. Round IV rates to tenths. (LO 13-1)

1. 4,000 g
2. 25 lb
3. 8 lb 5 oz
4. 47 lb
5. 35 kg

For exercises 6–10, calculate the DFR, calculate the 24 h intake, and state whether the intake is sufficient, deficient, or excessive for each example, assuming a normal hydration status. (LO 13-1)

6. A 15 lb infant consumes 3 oz formula q4h.
7. A 2,500 g premie is NPO, receiving IV fluids at 10.4 mL/h.
8. A postoperative newborn weighing 7 lb, 10 oz is taking 1.5 oz q3h and receiving IV fluids at 15 mL/h.
9. A 33 kg child consumes 1 cup of fluid q6h and receives IV fluids at 20 mL/h.
10. A 10 lb 15 oz infant is NPO receiving IV fluids at 20.8 mL/h.

For exercises 11–15, calculate the expected 24 h urine output range (1–2 mL/kg/h) for the specified weight. (LO 13-1)

11. 18½ lb
12. 18.5 kg
13. 4,500 g
14. 8 lb 4 oz
15. 14.4 kg

For exercises 16–20, calculate the 8 h shift urine output based on a dry diaper weight of 20 g and determine if the output falls in the expected 8 h urine output range for the specified weight. (LO 13-1)

16. Infant weight: 3,335 g; diaper weights: 40 g, 50 g
17. Infant weight: 10 lb 6 oz; diaper weight: 95 g
18. Infant weight: 12.8 kg; diaper weights: 49 g, 75 g
19. Infant weight: 13 lb 8 oz; diaper weights: 66 g, 99 g
20. Infant weight: 4,550 g; diaper weight: 58 g

For exercises, 21–25, calculate the daily caloric requirements. (LO 13-2)

21. 1-month-old who weighs 9 lb 5 oz
22. 2-year-old who weighs 12.5 kg
23. 5-year-old who weighs 42 lb
24. 10-year-old who weighs 69 lb
25. 7-month-old who weighs 8 kg

For exercises 26–30, calculate the newborn caloric requirements and determine how many ounces of standard formula (20 cal/oz) per feeding are needed to meet the caloric requirements in each example. Round calories and ounces to the whole number. (LO 13-2)

26. A 1-month-old who weighs 8 lb 15 oz and is fed q3h
27. A 6½-month-old who weighs 7.5 kg and is fed 5 times per day
28. An 8-month-old who weighs 18 lb 11 oz and is fed q4h
29. A 5-month-old who weighs 6,075 g and is fed q2–3h
30. An 11-month-old who weighs 22 lb and is fed q3–4h

For exercises 31–35, calculate the carbohydrate, protein, fat, and total calories in one serving of each food item. Round total calories to the whole number. (LO 13-3)

31. 1 cereal bar: 20.64 g carbohydrate, 1.22 g protein, 2.15 g fat
32. 1 cup of 1% milk: 12.18 g carbohydrate, 8.22 g protein, 2.37 g fat
33. ⅔ cup of Greek-style yogurt: 5 g carbohydrate, 11 g protein, 8 g fat
34. ¼ cup of cashews: 9 g carbohydrate, 5 g protein, 14 g fat
35. ½ cup of granola: 40.18 g carbohydrate, 5.12 g protein, 6.12 g fat

For exercises 36–37, for the food item listed, using Table 13-3, calculate the %DV of carbohydrates, proteins, and fats based on a 2,000-calorie diet. Round percentages to the whole number. (LO 13-3)

36. 1 cup eggnog containing 20 g carbohydrate, 12 g protein, 11 g fat
37. 1 cup cooked oatmeal containing 27 g carbohydrate, 6 g protein, 3.2 g

For exercises 38–40, answer the questions by interpreting the following nutrition label for sliced almonds. (LO 13-3)

38. What is the serving size?
39. Calculate the total carbohydrate, protein, and fat calories in one serving.

40. The %DV on the label is based on a 2,000-calorie diet. Calculate the %DV of carbohydrate, fat, and protein for a 1,800-calorie diet comprising 30% fat, 55–60% carbohydrate, and 10–15% protein.

Nutrition Facts

Serving Size 1 cup, sliced 92 g (92 g)

Amount Per Serving

Calories 529

	% Daily Value*
Total Fat 45g	69%
Saturated Fat 3.4g	17%
Trans Fat 0g	
Cholesterol 0mg	0%
Sodium 1mg	0%
Total Carbohydrate 20g	6%
Dietary Fiber 11g	44%
Sugars 3.6g	
Protein 20g	

Vitamin A	0% •	Vitamin C	0%
Calcium	25% •	Iron	20%

*Percent Daily Values are based on a 2,000 calorie diet. Your daily values may be higher or lower depending on your calorie needs.

Data from the United States Department of Agriculture.

For exercises 41–43, refer to the following order to be administered to a patient who is unable to take oral food and fluids. (LO 13-3)

Order: Nutritional formula 1.5 cal/mL at 50 mL/h via GT; administer 8 oz water bid

41. Calculate the total number of calories to infuse daily.
42. Calculate the total fluid intake (in mL) to infuse daily.
43. A new daily feeding, started at 0630 is discontinued from 1330 to 1630 while the patient is off the unit for an MRI. The provider orders the nurse to reset the feeding and increase the rate to ensure that the initial prescribed amount infuses in 24 h. At what rate will the GT feeding be set?

For exercises 44–45, indicate whether the statement is true or false. Correct false statements. (LO 13-3)

44. Because protein and carbohydrate are both 4 calories/g, they compose the same %DV in a typical 2,000-calorie diet.
45. Nutrient-dense foods are high in caloric, carbohydrate, and protein content, but low in fat content.

For exercises, 46–48, answer the questions regarding a 132 lb adult who sustained burns on the chest and both sides of both arms. (LO 13-4)

46. Use the Rule of Nines to calculate the %TBSA burned.
47. Use the Parkland Formula to calculate the fluid resuscitation requirements for 1 day.
48. Calculate the IV rates to distribute half of the fluids over 8 hours and the other half of the fluids over 16 hours.

For exercises 49–50, answer the questions regarding a 44 lb child who sustained burns on both sides of the right arm and right leg.

49. Use the Rule of Nines to calculate the %TBSA burned.
50. Use the Parkland Formula to calculate the fluid resuscitation requirements for 1 day.

NCLEX-Style Review Questions

For questions 1–4, select the best response.

1. The daily fluid requirement (DFR) for a newborn weighing 8 lb 8 oz is: (LO 13-1)
   a. 16.1 mL/h
   b. 390 mL/day
   c. 400 mL/day
   d. 880 mL/day
   e. None of the above
2. Newborns generally lose 5–10% of their birth weight during the first few days of life but regain it by the 7th to 10th day. Parents of a newborn whose weight at 3 days old is 3,210 g and whose birth weight was 3,465 g should be told: (LO 13-2)
   a. "Your baby has lost a lot of weight. You should ensure that she consumes at least 120 cal/kg/day."
   b. "Your baby's weight loss is within normal limits. Normal caloric intake should be about 400 calories per day."

c. "Your baby has lost too much weight. It would be helpful to consult a nutritionist for advice."

d. "All babies lose weight in the first few days of life. You have nothing to worry about."

3. To treat a 15 lb, 6-month-old infant who has gastroenteritis and is unable to take oral fluids due to severe vomiting, the provider orders $D_5\frac{1}{4}$ NS with the following instructions: Double the maintenance fluids for 2 hours, then run the IV at a DFR rate. The nurse correctly sets the IV pump at: (LO 13-1)

a. 56.6 mL/h for 2 h, then 28.3 mL/h

b. 62.5 mL/h for 2 h, then 32.3 mL/h

c. 137.5 mL/h for 2 h, then 68.8 mL/h

d. None of the above

4. After keeping a 5-day food diary, a patient reports an average consumption of 300 g of carbohydrates per day. For a 2,200-calorie diet, the nurse determines this carbohydrate intake is: (LO 13-3)

a. 0.5% of the diet and suggests that this is appropriate for a typical diet

b. 9% of the diet and recommends a 40% increase

c. 13% of the diet and recommends a slight decrease

d. 55% of the diet and suggests that this is an appropriate amount

e. None of the above

For questions 5–6, select all that apply.

5. To interpret a nutrition label, the nurse knows: (LO 13-3)

a. Proteins contain 4 g/cal.

b. There are 9 cal/g of fat.

c. One serving contains the nutrients listed.

d. Proteins and carbohydrates contain the same number of calories per gram.

e. All of the above

6. A patient weighing 198 lb is placed on a protein restriction of 0.7 g/kg/day for renal disease. The patient, unable to take food or fluids by mouth, is receiving nutritional formula containing 42 g protein/L to deliver 62.5 mL/h via GT. (LO 13-3)

a. The patient's weight is 90 kg.

b. In 24 hours, the patient will receive 1,500 mL.

c. In 24 hours, the patient will receive 42 g protein.

d. The nurse should contact the provider, because the protein content is insufficient to meet the patient's needs.

e. The nurse should contact the provider, because the protein content exceeds the ordered protein restriction.

f. The nurse should maintain the tube-feeding rate as ordered.

REFERENCES

American Academy of Pediatrics. (2012). Breastfeeding and the use of human milk. *Pediatrics, 129*(3), e827–e841. Retrieved from http://pediatrics.aap publications.org/content/early/2012/02/22 /peds.2011-3552

Augustine, Jodi. (2012, February 24). Balancing carbs, protein, and fat. *Group Health*. Retrieved from http://www.ghc.org/healthAndWellness/?item=/ common/healthAndWellness/conditions/diabetes /foodBalancing.html

Beach, P., Revai, K., & Niebuhr, V. (2008). *Core concepts of pediatric[e-book]*. Retrieved from http://www .utmb.edu/pedi_ed/CORE/Nutrition/page_08.htm

Grodner, M., Long, S., & Walkingshaw, B. C. (2011). Life span health promotion: Pregnancy, lactation, and infancy. In *Foundations and clinical applications of nutrition: A nursing process approach* (5th ed.). St. Louis, MO: Elsevier.

Harvard School of Public Health. (2014). *The nutrition source: Protein*. Retrieved from http://www.hsph .harvard.edu/nutritionsource/what-should-you-eat /protein/

Kelley, J. W. (2013). How to calculate pediatric intake & output. Retrieved from http://www.livestrong.com /article/82974-calculate-pediatric-intake-output/

Khan, S. (2010). Average child weight by age. *Buzzle*. Retrieved from http://www.buzzle.com/articles /average-child-weight-by-age.html

Kirkpatrick, T., & Tobias, K. (2010). *Pediatric age-specific self-learning module for clinical staff*. UCLA Health System. Retrieved from http://download-pdfguide .rhcloud.com/ucla-health-system-pediatric-age -specific-self-learning-module/

Kurkchubasche, A. G (Ed.). (n.d.). *Hasbro Children's Hospital pediatric surgery handbook*. Retrieved from http://med.brown.edu/pedisurg/Brown /Handbook/Nutrition.html

Lewis, S. L., Dirksen, S. R., Heitkemper, M. M., & Bucher, L. (2014). *Medical-surgical nursing: Assessment and management of clinical problems* (9th ed., pp. 450–472). St. Louis, MO: Elsevier.

Mahan, L. K., Escott-Stump, S., & Raymond, J. L. (2012). Nutrition in infancy. In *Krause's food and the nutrition care process* (13th ed., pp. 375–383). St. Louis, MO: Elsevier.

Methodist Children's Hospital. (2012). *Pediatric reference guide*. Retrieved from www.methodistaircare.com

Pennsylvania Patient Safety Authority. (2009). Medication errors: Significance of accurate patient weights. *Pennsylvania Patient Safety Advisory*. Retrieved from http://www.patientsafetyauthority.org/ADVI SORIES/AdvisoryLibrary/2009/mar6(1)/Pages/10. aspx

U.S. Food and Drug Administration. (2013). *Guidance for industry: A food labeling guide*. Retrieved from http://www.fda.gov/Food/GuidanceRegulation /GuidanceDocumentsRegulatoryInformation /LabelingNutrition/ucm064928.htm

Chapter 13   ANSWER KEY

Learning Activity 13-1
1. DFR = 450 mL; IV rate = 18.8 mL/h
2. DFR = 1,250 mL; IV rate = 52.1 mL/h
3. DFR = 1,640 mL; IV rate = 68.3 mL/h

Learning Activity 13-2
1. Yes, the DFR for 30 kg = 1,700 mL/day; 71 mL/h × 24 h/ day = 1,704 mL/day
2. Yes, the DFR for 18.7 kg is 1,435 mL/day; the child consumes 720 mL/day and receives 720 mL/day of IV fluid for a total of 1,440 mL/day

Learning Activity 13-3
1. Actual output = 130 mL; expected output = 80 to 160 mL
2. Actual output = 59 mL; expected output = 47 to 95 mL

Learning Activity 13-4

(Note: Internal rounding [rounding before final answer is achieved], used with ratio-proportion and the formula method, may yield answers that slightly differ from answers achieved with dimensional analysis.)
1. 573 cal/day needed; 29 oz formula/day needed
2. 764 cal/day needed; 38 oz formula/day needed

Learning Activity 13-5
1. 104.4 carbohydrate cal, 42.4 protein cal, 90 fat cal, 237 total calories
2. 76 carbohydrate cal, 10 protein cal, 63 fat cal, 149 total calories

Learning Activity 13-6
1. 8–9% carbohydrate, 51–76% protein, 111% fat
2. 4% carbohydrate, 4–5% protein, 29% fat

Learning Activity 13-7
1. %TBSA = 36%; fluid resuscitation requirements = 7,200; IV rate = 450 mL/h × 8h followed by 225 mL/h × 16 h
2. %TBSA = 28%; fluid resuscitation requirements = 560 mL; IV rate = 35 mL/h × 8h followed by 17.5 mL/h × 16 h

Homework

(Note: Internal rounding [rounding before final answer is achieved], used with ratio-proportion and the formula method, may yield answers that slightly differ from answers achieved with dimensional analysis.)
1. 400 mL; 16.7 mL/h
2. 1,070 mL; 44.6 mL/h
3. 380 mL; 15.8 mL/h
4. 1,528 mL; 16.7 mL/h
5. 1,800 mL; 75 mL/h
6. DFR = 680 mL, intake 540 mL, deficient
7. DFR = 250 mL, intake 250 mL (rounded from 249.6), sufficient
8. DFR = 350 mL, intake = 720 mL (360 mL PO + 360 mL IV), excessive
9. DFR = 1,760 mL, intake 1,440 (960 mL PO + 480 mL IV), deficient
10. DFR = 500 mL, intake 499 mL, sufficient
11. 202 to 404 mL
12. 444 to 888 mL
13. 108 to 216 mL
14. 90 to 180 mL
15. 346 to 692 mL
16. Actual output: 50 mL, yes—expected output 27–53 mL
17. Actual output 75 mL, yes—expected output 38–76 mL
18. Actual output 84 mL, no, output low—expected output 102–205 mL
19. Actual output 125 mL, no, output is high—expected output 49–98 mL
20. Actual output 38 mL, yes—expected output 36–73 mL
21. 508 cal/day
22. 1,250 cal/day
23. 1,432 to 1,718 cal/day
24. 1,882 to 2,352 cal/day
25. 880 cal/day
26. 488 cal/day; 24.4 oz formula needed per day; 3 oz formula per feeding
27. 825 cal/day; 41 oz formula needed per day; 8 oz formula per feeding needed, may vary with solid food intake

28. 934 cal/day; 47 oz formula needed per day; 8 oz formula per feeding needed, may vary with solid food intake
29. 729 cal/day; 36 oz formula needed per day; 3–5 oz formula per feeding needed
30. 1,100 cal/day; 55 oz formula needed per day; 7–9 oz formula per feeding needed, may vary with solid food intake
31. Carbohydrate—82.56 cal; protein—4.88 cal; fat—19.35 cal; total calories—107
32. Carbohydrate—48.72 cal; protein—32.88 cal; fat—21.33 cal; total calories—103
33. Carbohydrate—20 cal; protein—44 cal; fat—72 cal; total calories—136
34. Carbohydrate—36 cal; protein 20 cal; fat—126 cal; total calories—182
35. Carbohydrate—106.72 cal; protein—20.48 cal; fat—55.08 cal; total calories—182
36. 7% DV carbohydrate, 16–24% DV protein, 17% DV fat
37. 9–10% DV carbohydrate, 8–12% DV protein, 5% DV fat
38. One cup
39. 80 carbohydrate calories, 80 protein calories, 405 fat calories
40. Per Table 13-3, a 1,800 cal diet should contain 248–270 g carbohydrate, 45–68 g protein, and 60 g fat. One serving of sliced almonds would provide 7–8% DV carbohydrate, 29–44% DV protein, 75% DV fat.
41. 1,800 calories
42. 1,200 mL formula + 480 mL water = 1,680 mL
43. The feeding will restart at 1630 and infuse at 61 mL/h from 1630 to 0630.
44. False—Protein and carbohydrate both contain 4 cal/g; however, they compose a different percentage of a typical 2,000 cal diet. Proteins should compose 10–15% of the daily calories and carbohydrates should compose 55–60% of the daily calories.
45. False—Nutrient-dense foods are high in nutrient content, but low in calories.
46. 36% TBSA
47. 8,640 mL
48. 540 mL/h × 8 h followed by 270 mL/h × 16 h
49. 23%
50. 1,840 mL

NCLEX-Style Review Questions

1. b
   Rationale: 8 oz is ½ lb, therefore 8 lb 8 oz = 8.5 lb; 8.5 ÷ 2.2 lb/kg = 3.86 or 3.9 kg; DFR is 100 mL/kg/day × 3.9 kg = 390 mL/day; 390 mL/day
2. b
   Rationale: 3,465 g (birth weight) – 3210 g (current weight) = 255 g, which represents a 7% weight loss (255 g/3,465 g = 0.07 = 7%); caloric intake for a newborn is 120 cal/kg/day × 3.2 kg = 384 cal/day. Therefore, the nurse should tell the parent, "Your baby's weight loss is within normal limits and intake should be approximately 400 cal/day."
3. a
   Rationale: 15 lb divided by 2.2 lb/kg = 6.8 kg; 6.8 kg × 100 mL/kg/day = 680 mL/day; the maintenance IV rate for a DFR of 680 is 28.3 mL/h (680 mL divided by 24 h/day); the instructions are to double the maintenance rate for 2 hours, so the nurse would increase the IV rate to 56.6 mL/h for 2 hours, then drop it to 28.3 mL/h.
4. d
   Rationale: Carbohydrate intake should compose 55–60% of daily intake for healthy individuals. 300 g of carbohydrate contains 1,200 calories (4 cal/g). This represents 55% of the diet (1,200 divided by 2,000 = 0.5454 = 55%).
5. b, c, d
   Rationale: There are 9 cal/g of fat. One serving contains the nutrients listed on a nutrition label. Proteins and carbohydrates contain the same number of calories per gram.
6. a, b, f
   Rationale: 198 lb × 1 kg/2.2 lb = 90 kg; 62.5 mL/h × 24 h = 1,500 mL/day; maintain tube-feeding rate as ordered; protein intake should be 0.7 g/kg/day × 90 kg = 63 g/day; 1,500 mL of nutritional formula containing 42 g/L will deliver 63 g of protein/day.

© Forfunlife/Shutterstock

Chapter 14

High-Alert Medications

CHAPTER OUTLINE

LEARNING OUTCOMES

Upon completion of the chapter, the student will be able to:

14-1 Determine appropriate insulin, amount, and device.

14-2 Perform calculations for intravenous and subcutaneous heparin administration.

KEY TERMS

activated partial thromboplastin time (aPTT)

anticoagulant

basal insulin

basal rate

blood glucose correction
factor

carbohydrate insulin dose

correction insulin

duration

fixed combination insulin

high-alert medications

hospitalist

insulin pumps

insulin sensitivity factor

insulin-to-carbohydrate ratio

loading dose

low molecular weight heparin
(LMWH)

mealtime insulin

onset

peak

total mealtime bolus dose

U-100

U-500

unfractionated heparin (UH)

weight-based heparin
protocol

Case Consideration ... What's in a Unit?

Humulin® R regular insulin 4 units subcut was ordered. The nurse, using the following insulin supply and syringe, drew up and administered the amount of insulin shown:

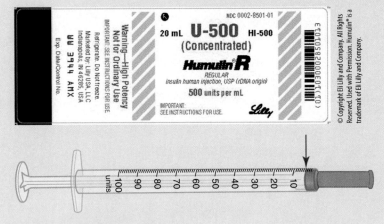

1. What went wrong?
2. How could this situation have been avoided?

■ INTRODUCTION

High-alert medications are medications that, if given erroneously, can result in serious harm and possibly death. Nurses, as well as other health professionals, need to be on "high alert" when ordering, transcribing, procuring, calculating dosage, and administering any medication on the Institute for Safe Medication Practices (ISMP, 2012b) "List of High-Alert Medications" (**Figure 14-1** and **Figure 14-2**). Deaths in several states have resulted from patients receiving insulin instead of heparin. In 2007, the ISMP identified two main causes: (1) product packaging, and (2) "mental slips"(ISMP, 2012a). This chapter focuses on two high-alert medications: insulin and heparin.

445

Classes/Categories of Medications
adrenergic agonists, IV (e.g., **EPINEPH**rine, phenylephrine, norepinephrine)
adrenergic antagonists, IV (e.g., propranolol, metoprolol, labetalol)
anesthetic agents, general, inhaled and IV (e.g., propofol, ketamine)
antiarrhythmics, IV (e.g., lidocaine, amiodarone)
antithrombotic agents, including: ■ anticoagulants (e.g., warfarin, low molecular weight heparin, IV unfractionated heparin) ■ Factor Xa inhibitors (e.g., fondaparinux, apixaban, rivaroxaban) ■ direct thrombin inhibitors (e.g., argatroban, bivalirudin, dabigatran etexilate) ■ thrombolytics (e.g., alteplase, reteplase, tenecteplase) ■ glycoprotein IIb/IIIa inhibitors (e.g., eptifibatide)
cardioplegic solutions
chemotherapeutic agents, parenteral and oral
dextrose, hypertonic, 20% or greater
dialysis solutions, peritoneal and hemodialysis
epidural or intrathecal medications
hypoglycemics, oral
inotropic medications, IV (e.g., digoxin, milrinone)
insulin, subcutaneous and IV
liposomal forms of drugs (e.g., liposomal amphotericin B) and conventional counterparts (e.g., amphotericin B desoxycholate)
moderate sedation agents, IV (e.g., dexmedetomidine, midazolam)
moderate sedation agents, oral, for children (e.g., chloral hydrate)
narcotics/opioids ■ IV ■ transdermal ■ oral (including liquid concentrates, immediate and sustained-release formulations)
neuromuscular blocking agents (e.g., succinylcholine, rocuronium, vecuronium)
parenteral nutrition preparations
radiocontrast agents, IV
sterile water for injection, inhalation, and irrigation (excluding pour bottles) in containers of 100 mL or more
sodium chloride for injection, hypertonic, greater than 0.9% concentration

Specific Medications
EPINEPHrine, subcutaneous
epoprostenol (Flolan), IV
insulin U-500 (special emphasis)*
magnesium sulfate injection
methotrexate, oral, non-oncologic use
opium tincture
oxytocin, IV
nitroprusside sodium for injection
potassium chloride for injection concentrate
potassium phosphates injection
promethazine, IV
vasopressin, IV or intraosseous

*All forms of insulin, subcutaneous and IV, are considered a class of high-alert medications. Insulin U-500 has been singled out for special emphasis to bring attention to the need for distinct strategies to prevent the types of errors that occur with this concentrated form of insulin.

Background
Based on error reports submitted to the ISMP National Medication Errors Reporting Program, reports of harmful errors in the literature, studies that identify the drugs most often involved in harmful errors, and input from practitioners and safety experts, ISMP created and periodically updates a list of potential high-alert medications. During May and June 2014, practitioners responded to an ISMP survey designed to identify which medications were most frequently considered high-alert drugs by individuals and organizations. Further, to assure relevance and completeness, the clinical staff at ISMP, members of the ISMP advisory board, and safety experts throughout the US were asked to review the potential list. This list of drugs and drug categories reflects the collective thinking of all who provided input.

Reproduced from the Institute for Safe Medication Practices (ISMP).

FIGURE 14-1 The ISMP refers to medications that are associated with harmful or fatal outcomes from medication administration errors as "high-alert medications." This is a list of high-alert medications administered in the acute care setting.

WARNING!

Insulin Is Implicated in Approximately One-Third of All Major Injurious Medication Errors!

"[Insulin] is in the top five 'high-risk' medications that account for about one third of all major drug-related, injurious medication errors. One analysis indicated the 33% of errors causing death within 48 hrs involved insulin therapy." (Jacobi et al., 2012)

Classes/Categories of Medications	Specific Medications
antiretroviral agents (e.g., efavirenz, lami**VUD**ine, raltegravir, ritonavir, combination antiretroviral products)	car**BAM**azepine
chemotherapeutic agents, oral (excluding hormonal agents) (e.g., cyclophosphamide, mercaptopurine, temozolomide)	chloral hydrate liquid, for sedation of children
hypoglycemic agents, oral	heparin, including unfractionated and low molecular weight heparin
immunosuppressant agents (e.g., aza**THIO**prine, cyclo**SPORINE**, tacrolimus)	met**FORMIN**
insulin, all formulations	methotrexate, non-oncologic use
opioids, all formulations	midazolam liquid, for sedation of children
pediatric liquid medications that require measurement	propylthiouracil
pregnancy category X drugs (e.g., bosentan, ISOtretinoin)	warfarin

Background
Based on error reports submitted to the ISMP Medication Errors Reporting Program (ISMP MERP), reports of harmful errors in the literature, and input from practitioners and safety experts, ISMP created a list of potential high-alert medications. During June-August 2006, 463 practitioners responded to an ISMP survey designed to identify which medications were most frequently considered high-alert drugs by individuals and organizations. In 2008, the preliminary list and survey data as well as data about preventable adverse drug events from the ISMP MERP, the Pennsylvania Patient Safety Reporting System, the FDA MedWatch database, databases from participating pharmacies, public litigation data, literature review, and a small focus group of ambulatory care pharmacists and medication safety experts were evaluated as part of a research study funded by an Agency for Healthcare Research and Quality (AHRQ) grant. This list of drugs and drug categories reflects the collective thinking of all who provided input. This list was created as part of the AHRQ funded project "Using risk models to identify and prioritize outpatient high-alert medications" (Grant # 1P20HS017107-01).

Reproduced from the Institute for Safe Medication Practices (ISMP).

FIGURE 14-2 The ISMP refers to medications that are associated with harmful or fatal outcomes from medication administration errors as "high-alert medications." This is a list of high-alert medications administered in the community and ambulatory care settings.

14-1 Insulin

Insulin is a hormone that facilitates blood glucose (BG) passage into the cell for nourishment, and into the liver for fat storage. Inadequate insulin results in high blood glucose levels and improper metabolism of carbohydrates and fats. Insulin is produced in the pancreas and is released into the bloodstream slowly and continuously as a "**basal rate**" to support normal cellular function. When blood glucose increases at mealtime or whenever food is ingested, a spurt of insulin is released by the pancreas to normalize the glucose level. Some individuals do not produce enough insulin or are resistant to the insulin produced. Both **basal insulin**, synthetic human insulin that provides long-term coverage, and **mealtime insulin**, synthetic human insulin that provides quick blood glucose control, are available for these individuals. Nursing errors associated with insulin administration are often related to administering the wrong type or amount of insulin.

Insulin Labels and Types

There are several different basal, mealtime, and **fixed combination** (combination of basal and mealtime) insulins available for patient use. Each type of insulin has an onset, peak, and duration. The **onset** is the length of time it takes for the insulin to start lowering blood glucose. The **peak** is the time at which the insulin has its maximum effect, and the **duration** is the length of time the insulin effects last. It is important to recognize the difference in labeling and action of insulins, especially because some labels and names are similar.

WARNING!

Do Not Substitute Brands or Types of Insulin Unless Ordered!

Onset of action, peak, and duration vary between brands and types of insulin, and may require a change of dose if substituted. Also, insulin concentration may vary from 100 units/mL to 200 units/mL, 300 units/mL or 500 units/mL. Therefore, any change in insulin requires an order.

Basal Insulin

Basal insulin is used to provide energy (in the form of glucose) to the cells for basic metabolic functioning of all the body systems. The dose of basal insulin targets the individual's basal metabolic rate, but does not meet the increased insulin demand associated with food intake. Therefore, (if dosed correctly) the basal insulin dose should not cause low blood glucose if the patient is restricted from eating (Magaji & Johnston, 2011). Basal insulin is either intermediate acting or long acting. Basal insulin is administered subcutaneously and cannot be administered intravenously. Intermediate-acting insulin, also called neutral protamine Hagedorn (NPH) insulin, is the only type of basal insulin that can be combined with mealtime insulin in the same syringe or vial. It is a white (cloudy) suspension that needs to be gently agitated to suspend the particles before preparing or administering the dose. Although NPH may have some effect up to 24 hours, its therapeutic effect generally lasts 12–18 hours. NPH is often prescribed twice a day. Humulin® N is NPH insulin (manufactured by Lilly) (**Figure 14-3**). It begins to take effect within 2–3 hours and has a maximal effect between 4 and 12 hours, with a pronounced or peak effect in 6 hours. Novolin® N is NPH insulin manufactured by Novo Nordisk (**Figure 14-4**). It is similar to Humulin N, but starts working within 1.5 hours, which is sooner than Humulin N.

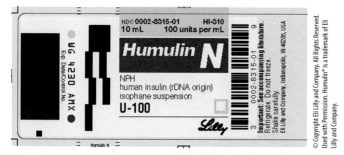

FIGURE 14-3   Humulin® N (Lilly Pharmaceutical) NPH insulin.

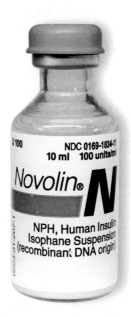

FIGURE 14-4   Novolin® N (Novo Nordisk Pharmaceutical) NPH insulin.

Neutral protamine Hagedorn is the name of the protein molecule in this type of insulin that makes the solution appear cloudy. This protein molecule decreases the absorption rate of insulin to give it a slower, more sustained effect than rapid-acting and short-acting insulins. NPH is classified as an intermediate-acting insulin as noted in **TABLE 14-1**.

TABLE 14-1	Insulin Categories, Types, Action Times			
Category	**Type**	**Onset**	**Peak**	**Duration**
Basal Insulin	**Intermediate Acting (NPH)**			
	Humulin® N	2–4 hours	4–12 hours	Up to 24 hours
	Novolin® N	1.5 hours	4–12 hours	
	Long Acting			
	Glargine (Lantus®)	1–1½ hours	No peak	20–24 hours
	Detemir (Levemir®)	1–2 hours	6–8 hours	Up to 24 hours
Mealtime Insulin	**Rapid Acting**			
	Lispro (Humalog®)	15–30 min	30–90 min	3–5 hours
	Aspart (NovoLog®)	10–20 min	40–50 min	3–5 hours
	Glulisine (Apidra®)	20–30 min	30–90 min	1–2½ hours
	Short Acting (Regular)			
	Humulin® R	10–75 min	3 hours	8 hours
	Novolin® R	30 min	2½–5 hours	8–12 hours
	Fixed Combination			
	Humalog® 75/25 Humalog® 50/50	15–30 min	30–90 min and again in 4–12 hours	Up to 24 hours
	NovoLog® 70/30 NovoLog® 50/50	10–20 min	40–50 min and again in 4–12 hours	
	Humulin® 70/30	10–75 min	3 hours and again in 4–12 hours	
	Novolin® 70/30	30 min	2.5–5 hours and again up to 12 hours	

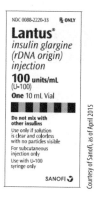

FIGURE 14-5   Lantus® (Sanofi Pharmaceutical) glargine insulin.

Long-acting acting basal insulins (glargine and detemir per Table 14-1) have a therapeutic effect for 24 hours and are, therefore, administered once a day. Long-acting insulin is not mixed with other insulin in the same syringe or vial. Glargine insulin is manufactured by Sanofi-Aventis as Lantus® insulin (**Figure 14-5**).

Lantus insulin has no peak, so it has a more consistent effect than detemir insulin, which peaks in 6–8 hours. Detemir is manufactured by Novo Nordisk as Levemir® (**Figure 14-6**).

Mealtime Insulin

Mealtime insulin is fast acting and is classified as either rapid-acting or short-acting. It is prescribed in *anticipation* of the amount of carbohydrates that are about to be consumed. A prescribed amount of insulin is ordered for a specific quantity of carbohydrates, usually for every 15 g of carbohydrate (refer to Chapter 13 to count carbohydrates). In general, mealtime insulin is not administered if the patient is NPO or if the premeal blood glucose is less than 70 mg/dL (Magaji & Johnston, 2011). This type of insulin is also utilized for **correction insulin**. A bolus dose of correction insulin is administered to correct *existing* high blood glucoses from food or other causes, such as (some) medications or illness. Short-acting insulin is also called regular insulin. It is difficult to use regular insulin as mealtime insulin in the hospital, because it should be administered 30 minutes before eating, and meal tray delivery times may vary. Rapid-acting insulin, having the fastest onset but shortest duration, is preferable for mealtime insulin in the hospital. Because rapid-acting insulin should be administered subcutaneously with the "first bite" of a meal or within 15 minutes after the first bite, it is easier to time with the arrival of food trays. When administered at the correct time, mealtime insulin peaks as the blood glucose level rises. Short-acting (regular insulin) and rapid-acting insulin (aspart and glulisine) can also be administered intravenously. There are three different types of rapid-acting insulin (**Figure 14-7**, **Figure 14-8**, and **Figure 14-9**):

- Lispro (Humalog®, manufactured by Lilly)

- Aspart (NovoLog®, manufactured by Novo Nordisk)

- Glulisine (Apidra®, manufactured by Sanofi-Aventis)

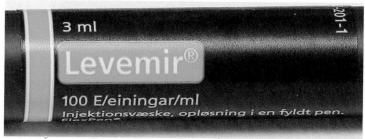

FIGURE 14-6   Levemir® (Novo Nordisk Pharmaceutical) detemir insulin.

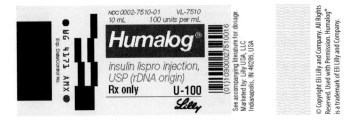

FIGURE 14-7 Humalog® (Lilly Pharmaceutical) lispro insulin.

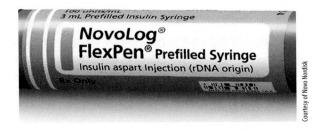

FIGURE 14-8 NovoLog® (Novo Nordisk Pharmaceutical) aspart insulin.

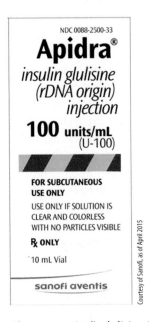

FIGURE 14-9 Apidra® (Sanofi Aventis Pharmaceutical) glulisine insulin.

WARNING!

U-100 and U-500 Insulin Are Not the Same Concentration!

U-100 insulin has a concentration of 100 units per 1 mL, while **U-500** insulin is five times stronger than U-100 insulin, with a concentration of 500 units per 1 mL. Regular insulin is the only type of insulin that is concentrated as U-100 and U-500. Only U-100 regular insulin can be administered intravenously; U-500 is too concentrated for IV administration.

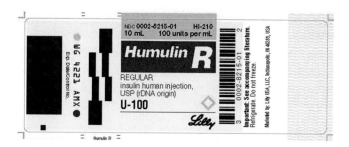

FIGURE 14-10   Humulin® R U-100 (Lilly Pharmaceutical) regular insulin contains 100 units per 1 mL.

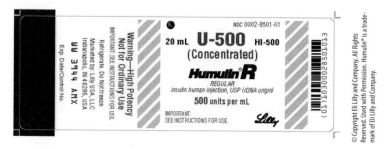

FIGURE 14-11   Humulin® R U-500 (Lilly Pharmaceutical) regular U-500 insulin contains 500 units per 1 mL.

Short-acting insulin, also called regular insulin, has a slower onset than rapid-acting insulin, but peaks the same as and lasts longer than rapid-acting insulin (**Figure 14-10**, **Figure 14-11**, and **Figure 14-12**). There are two brands of regular insulin manufactured for use in the United States. Only Humulin® R, manufactured by Lilly, is offered as U-100 (100 units per mL) and U-500 (500 units per mL) concentrations. Humulin R regular insulin U-100 may be administered through the intravenous (IV) or subcutaneous (subcut) routes. Humulin R regular insulin U-500 may only be administered through the subcutaneous route. Regular insulin concentrated to U-500 is used for patients with insulin resistance who require dosages greater than 200 units/day. Regular U-500 insulin, due to its high concentration, has mealtime and basal characteristics. Regular U-500 insulin peaks in 30 minutes and lasts up to 24 hours. Regular U-500 insulin should be drawn up in a 1 mL tuberculin syringe *not a U-100 insulin syringe*.

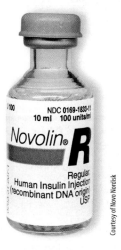

FIGURE 14-12   Novolin® (Novo Nordisk Pharmaceutical) regular insulin is U-100 concentration.

Clinical CLUE

Regular U-500 (concentrated) insulin is packaged by Lilly in a box marked with diagonal brown stripes. Regular U-500 (concentrated) insulin is supplied in a 20 mL vial with brown diagonal stripes on the label. This is to distinguish it from regular U-100 insulin, which is supplied in a 10 mL vial that is boxed and labeled with a yellow band instead of brown stripes. Always read the label, but if you are holding a 20 mL vial, read the label again.

Novolin R is regular insulin manufactured by Novo Nordisk®.

Fixed Concentration Mixed Insulin

Fixed concentration mixed insulin is a combination of NPH and rapid-acting or short-acting insulin (**Figure 14-13**, **Figure 14-14**, **Figure 14-15**, **Figure 14-16**, **Figure 14-17** and **Figure 14-18**). This combination can only be administered as a subcut injection given with a syringe or insulin pen. It cannot be given IV or via insulin pump. Mixed insulin lists the percentage of NPH insulin to the percentage of mealtime insulin; for example, Humalog® Mix 75/25 is 75% NPH and 25% Humalog insulin.

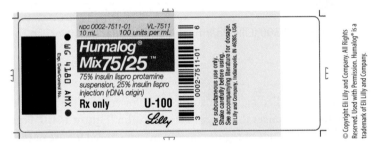

FIGURE 14-13   Humalog® Mix 75/25 is fixed concentration of 75% Humulin® N and 25% Humalog® U-100 insulins.

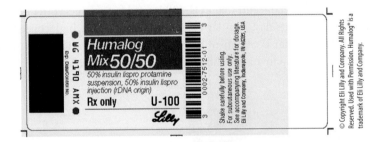

FIGURE 14-14   Humalog® Mix 50/50 is a fixed concentration of 50% Humulin® N and 50% Humalog® U-100 insulins.

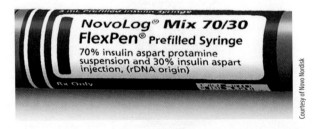

FIGURE 14-15   NovoLog® 70/30 is a fixed concentration of 70% Novolin® N and 30% NovoLog® U-100 insulins.

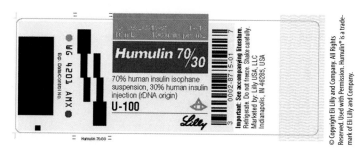

FIGURE 14-16   Humulin® Mix 70/30 is a fixed concentration of 70% Humulin® N and 30% Humulin® R U-100 insulins.

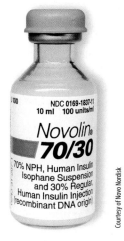

FIGURE 14-17   Novolin® 70/30 is a fixed concentration of Novolin® N and Novolin® R U-100 insulins.

LEARNING ACTIVITY 14-1   Refer to **Figures 14-18, 14-19,** and **14-20** to answer, the following questions.

1.   Which insulin is required to administer the following order?
       Order: Novolin® N insulin 30 units subcut
2.   Which is the rapid-acting insulin?

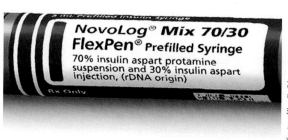

FIGURE 14-18

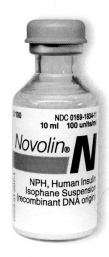

FIGURE 14-19

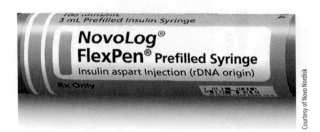

FIGURE 14-20

Insulin Administration by Syringe

Recall from Chapter 3 that insulin syringes are available in three sizes (100 unit 1 mL, 50 unit 0.5 mL, and 30 unit 0.3 mL), but are calibrated exclusively for U-100 insulin. U-100 insulin should be measured in U-100 insulin syringes and *not* in syringes calibrated in milliliters, such as a 1 mL tuberculin syringe. However, U-500 insulin should always be drawn up into a 1 mL syringe.

WARNING!

Do Not Use a U-100 Insulin Syringe for U-500 Insulin!

Insulin syringes are calibrated for U-100 insulin, so they should only be used for U-100 insulin. U-500 insulin should be drawn up into a 1 mL tuberculin syringe. To prevent dosage errors, The Joint Commission (TJC) and the ISMP recommend that a 1 mL syringe be used to administer U-500 insulin. They also recommend that the prescriber write both the number of units and the volume, in mL, of insulin required to administer the dose—for example, Humulin® R U-500 regular insulin 200 units (0.4 mL) subcut daily before breakfast (ISMP, 2011).

Single Dosage Insulin

Preparing U-100 insulin when only one dosage is ordered requires no calculation. To prepare, use a U-100 insulin syringe and draw up the ordered U-100 insulin to the unit calibration that corresponds to the ordered dose. Carefully select the correct insulin vial, and have another nurse verify the insulin and amount withdrawn matches the order. When administering U-500 insulin, calculate the volume in mL to be administered by using the dosage strength (supply), 500 units/1 mL. Although the prescriber orders the volume to be administered, for patient safety, the nurse should always calculate the volume to be administered.

Example 1: Determine the amount to administer for the following order:

    Order: Humulin R U-500 regular insulin 300 (0.6 mL) units subcut

    Supply: Humulin R U-500 regular insulin (500 units/1 mL) (**Figure 14-21**)

C: *Convert*—Because the order is in units and the supply is in units, there is no conversion.

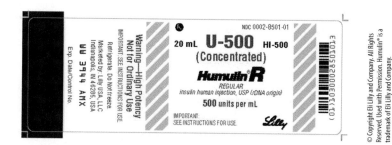

© Copyright Eli Lilly and Company. All Rights Reserved. Used with Permission. Humulin® is a trademark of Eli Lilly and Company.

FIGURE 14-21

A: *Approximate*—The ordered dose, 300 units, is slightly more than ½ the supply amount of 500 units; therefore, the amount to administer will be slightly more than ½ the supply volume of 1 mL, which is slightly more than 0.5 mL.

S: *Solve*

Ratio-Proportion

$$\frac{500 \text{ units}}{1 \text{ mL}} = \frac{300 \text{ units}}{x \text{ mL}} \quad \text{or}$$

500 units : 1 mL = 300 units : x mL

$$500x = 300$$

$$\frac{500x}{500} = \frac{300}{500}$$

$$x = 0.6 \text{ mL}$$

Formula Method

$$\frac{300 \text{ units}}{500 \text{ units}} \times 1 \text{ mL} = x \text{ (mL)}$$

$$\frac{300 \text{ mL}}{500} = x$$

$$0.6 \text{ mL} = x$$

Dimensional Analysis

$$x \text{ (mL)} = \frac{1 \text{ mL}}{500 \text{ units}} \times \frac{300 \text{ units}}{1}$$

$$x = \frac{300 \text{ mL}}{500}$$

$$x = 0.6$$

E: *Evaluate*

Ratio-Proportion

$$\frac{500 \text{ units}}{1 \text{ mL}} = \frac{300 \text{ units}}{0.6 \text{ mL}} \quad \text{or}$$

500 units : 1 mL = 300 units : 0.6 mL

$$500 \times 0.6 = 1 \times 300$$

$$300 = 300 \text{ mL}$$

Formula Method

$$\frac{300 \text{ units}}{500 \text{ units}} \times 1 \text{ mL} = 0.6 \text{ mL}$$

$$\frac{300 \text{ mL}}{500} = 0.6 \text{ mL}$$

$$0.6 \text{ mL} = 0.6 \text{ mL}$$

Dimensional Analysis

$$0.6 \text{ mL} = \frac{1 \text{ mL}}{500 \text{ units}} \times \frac{300 \text{ units}}{1}$$

$$0.6 \text{ mL} = \frac{300 \text{ mL}}{500}$$

$$0.6 \text{ mL} = 0.6 \text{ mL}$$

Because the calculated amount, 0.6 mL, accurately completes the equation and is consistent with the approximated volume, the answer is confirmed.

Example 2:   Determine the amount to administer for the following order:

Order: Humulin R U-500 regular insulin 225 (0.45 mL) units subcut

Supply: Humulin R U-500 regular insulin (500 units/1 mL) (Figure 14-21)

C: *Convert*—Because the order is in units and the supply is in units, there is no conversion.

A: *Approximate*—The ordered dose, 225 units, is slightly less than ½ the supply amount 500 units; therefore, the amount to administer will be slightly less than ½ the supply volume of 1 mL, or slightly less than 0.5 mL.

S: *Solve*

Ratio-Proportion

$$\frac{500 \text{ units}}{1 \text{ mL}} = \frac{225 \text{ units}}{x \text{ mL}} \quad \text{or}$$

500 units : 1 mL = 225 units : x mL

$$500x = 225$$

$$\frac{500x}{500} = \frac{225}{500}$$

$$x = 0.45 \text{ mL}$$

Formula Method

$$\frac{225 \text{ units}}{500 \text{ units}} \times 1 \text{ mL} = x \text{ (mL)}$$

$$\frac{225 \text{ mL}}{500} = x$$

$$0.45 \text{ mL} = x$$

Dimensional Analysis

$$x \text{ (mL)} = \frac{1 \text{ mL}}{500 \text{ units}} \times \frac{225 \text{ units}}{1}$$

$$x = \frac{225 \text{ mL}}{500}$$

$$x = 0.45$$

E: Evaluate

Ratio-Proportion	Formula Method
$\dfrac{500 \text{ units}}{1 \text{ mL}} = \dfrac{225 \text{ units}}{0.45 \text{ mL}}$ or 500 units : 1 mL = 225 units : 0.45 mL $500 \times 0.45 = 1 \times 225$ $225 = 225$	$\dfrac{225 \text{ units}}{500 \text{ units}} \times 1 \text{ mL} = 0.45 \text{ mL}$ $\dfrac{225 \text{ mL}}{500} = 0.45 \text{ mL}$ $0.45 \text{ mL} = 0.45 \text{ mL}$

Dimensional Analysis

$$0.45 \text{ mL} = \frac{1 \text{ mL}}{500 \text{ units}} \times \frac{225 \text{ units}}{1}$$

$$0.45 \text{ mL} = \frac{225 \text{ mL}}{500}$$

$$0.45 \text{ mL} = 0.45 \text{ mL}$$

Because the calculated amount, 0.45 mL, accurately completes the equation and is consistent with the approximated volume, the answer is confirmed.

LEARNING ACTIVITY 14-2 Refer to **Figures 14-22** through **14-36** and select the appropriate insulin and syringe to administer each ordered dose. Mark the correct calibration on the selected syringe.

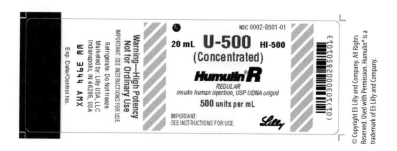

FIGURE 14-22

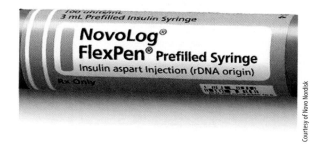

Courtesy of Novo Nordisk

FIGURE 14-23

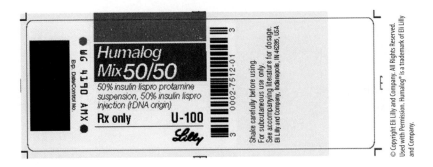

FIGURE 14-24

© Copyright Eli Lilly and Company. All Rights Reserved. Used with Permission. Humalog® is a trademark of Eli Lilly and Company.

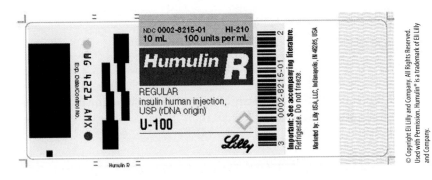

FIGURE 14-25

© Copyright Eli Lilly and Company. All Rights Reserved. Used with Permission. Humulin® is a trademark of Eli Lilly and Company.

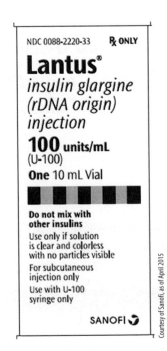

FIGURE 14-26

Courtesy of Sanofi, as of April 2015

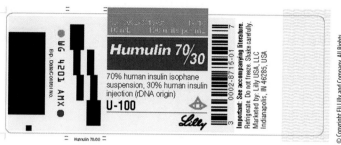

© Copyright Eli Lilly and Company. All Rights Reserved. Used with Permission. Humulin® is a trademark of Eli Lilly and Company.

FIGURE 14-27

1.   Lantus® insulin 42 units subcut daily before breakfast
        Figure _____

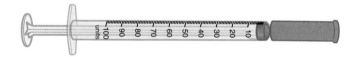

FIGURE 14-28

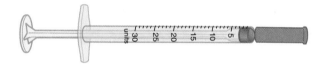

FIGURE 14-29

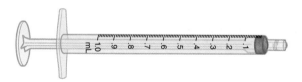

FIGURE 14-30

2.   Humulin R U-500 regular insulin 250 units (0.5 mL) subcut ac daily
        Figures _____

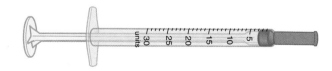

FIGURE 14-31

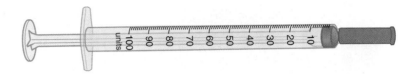

FIGURE 14-32

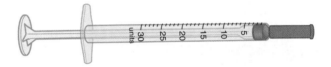

FIGURE 14-33

3. Humalog 50/50 insulin 20 units subcut bid before breakfast and dinner
    Figures _____

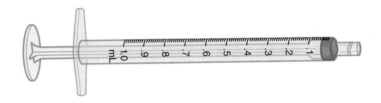

FIGURE 14-34

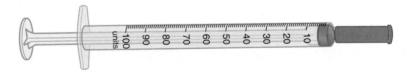

FIGURE 14-35

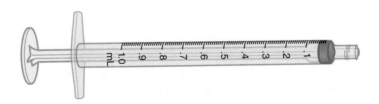

FIGURE 14-36

Correction Insulin (Sliding Scale Insulin Coverage)   When blood glucose levels (measured in mg/dL) are elevated, sliding scale insulin coverage is often ordered, as indicated in **TABLE 14-2**. Fast-acting or rapid-acting insulin is ordered in several dosages that each correspond to a blood glucose range on the sliding scale. The order for sliding scale insulin must include the type of insulin, as well as the frequency of

TABLE 14-2	Insulin Sliding Scale Example		
Humalog® Sliding Scale Subcutaneous Insulin Coverage			
Capillary Blood Glucose (mg/dL)	☐ **Low Dose**	☐ **Moderate Dose**	☐ **High Dose**
Less than 70	Institute hypoglycemic protocol	Institute hypoglycemic protocol	Institute hypoglycemic protocol
Less than 145	No coverage	No coverage	No coverage
145–185	1 unit	2 units	3 units
186–225	2 units	3 units	4 units
226–245	3 units	4 units	5 units
246–275	4 units	5 units	6 units
276–315	5 units	6 units	7 units
Greater than 315	6 units	7 units	8 units

blood glucose checks. Because the amount of insulin required to lower the glucose level is dependent on the patient's sensitivity to insulin, **hospitalists** (doctors who practice in hospitals) generally use low, moderate, and high correctional insulin scales. The prescriber determines the patient's sensitivity to insulin and then chooses a scale.

Example 1:   The patient's blood glucose (BG) before lunch is 232 mg/dL. Using Table 14-2, determine how much Humalog insulin should be administered.

   Order: Moderate-dose Humalog sliding scale insulin coverage subcut ac and at bedtime

   Supply: Humalog U-100 insulin

The BG 232 is between 226 and 245 mg/dL. The moderate dose scale indicates 4 units of Humalog® U-100 insulin should be administered subcutaneously.

Example 2:   The patient's BG before lunch is 110 mg/dL. Using Table 14-2, determine how much Humalog insulin should be administered.

   Order: Low-dose Humalog sliding scale insulin coverage subcut ac and at bedtime

   Supply: Humalog U-100 insulin

The BG 110 is less than 145 mg/dL, therefore, *no* Humalog U-100 insulin should be administered.

LEARNING ACTIVITY 14-3 Refer to the high-dose scale in Table 14-2 to determine the amount of insulin to be administered.

1.   The patient's BG before breakfast is 310 mg/dL.
      Administer _____ units
2.   The patient's BG before dinner is 240 mg/dL.
      Administer _____ units
3.   The patient's BG before bedtime is 160 mg/dL.
      Administer _____ units

Combining Mealtime Insulin and NPH Insulin

Mealtime and NPH insulin can be combined in the same syringe. This reduces the number of injections the patient requires. The only basal insulin that can be combined in the same syringe with mealtime insulin is NPH insulin. The sequence of combining insulins is important. Always fill the syringe with the prescribed mealtime insulin before adding the NPH insulin. Two phrases used to remember this sequence are, "fast first" and "clear before cloudy." Mealtime insulin is clear and faster acting than NPH insulin, which is a white, cloudy suspension.

Clinical CLUE

When combining insulins in the same syringe, follow the steps listed here and add the mealtime insulin to the syringe before the NPH:

1. Wipe the tops of both vials with alcohol.

2. Inject air into the NPH insulin vial.

3. Inject air into the mealtime insulin vial.

4. While the needle is still in the mealtime vial, invert the vial and withdraw the mealtime insulin dose.

5. Rotate the NPH vial to suspend the cloudy insulin.

6. Insert the needle into the NPH vial, invert and withdraw the NPH insulin dose.

7. Rock the syringe back and forth several times to mix the insulins.

Example: Indicate the calibration marks on the syringe where the plunger will be drawn for the basal insulin dose and the mealtime insulin dose (**Figure 14-37**).

10 units Humulin R insulin plus 22 units Humulin N insulin

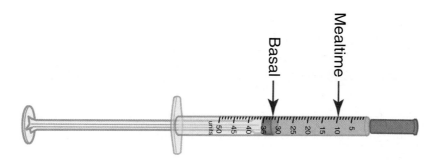

FIGURE 14-37   The nurse draws up 10 units of Humulin R then 22 units of Humulin N, for a total of 32 units in the syringe.

LEARNING ACTIVITY 14-4 For the following insulin dosages, indicate the calibration marks where the plunger must be drawn for the basal insulin dose and the mealtime insulin dose.

1.   8 units Humulin R insulin plus 12 units Humulin N insulin

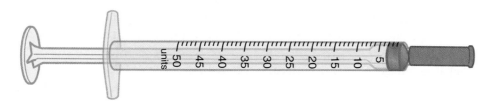

FIGURE 14-38

2.   30 units Humulin N insulin plus 10 units Humalog insulin

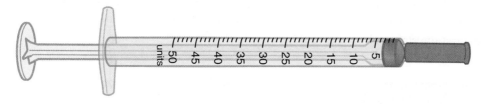

FIGURE 14-39

3.   27 units Novolin N insulin plus 12 units NovoLog insulin

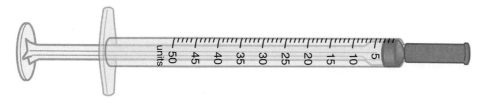

FIGURE 14-40

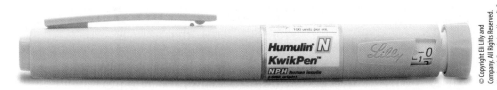

© Copyright Eli Lilly and Company. All Rights Reserved. Used with Permission. Humulin® is a trademark of Eli Lilly and Company.

FIGURE 14-41   Insulin pens are manufactured for different types and concentrations of insulin. Always read the manufacturer's instructions for priming the pen, because different pens may require a different priming volume.

Insulin Pens

Many patients prefer disposable prefilled insulin pens over using a vial and syringe (Davis, Foral, Dull, and Smith, 2013). Insulin pens look like a pen or marker and are used instead of syringes to administer subcutaneous insulin. They are supplied as prefilled disposable pens or reusable pens with prefilled insulin cartridges (Gebel, 2012) (**Figure 14-41**). After proper priming and needle application, the insulin dose is dialed on the pen, and a plunger or button is depressed to administer the dose. All pens are for single patient use and cannot be shared with other patients, even if a new needle is attached. Although insulin pens were designed for patient self-administration, many hospital pharmacies are supplying insulin pens for nurses to administer insulin (ISMP, 2015).

Clinical CLUE

Some pens have a digital dose display that can be misinterpreted if read upside down (e.g., 25 units looks like 52 units on the digital display if read upside down). People who use the pen with their left hand are more prone to read the display upside down. Teach all patients how to read the display.

Clinical calculations for ordering the correct number insulin pens are required, because the volume contained in the pen and the number of days the insulin can be stored once opened vary (TABLE 14-3). The community-based nurse may need to calculate the number of pens a patient requires while on vacation or away from home.

To determine the number of pens and pen packs required, refer to Table 14-3 and:

1. Determine the total number of doses to be administered by multiplying the number of doses ordered per day by the number of days.

2. Calculate the number of full doses in the pen. Because each device in Table 14-3 contains 3 mL of U-100 insulin, each device contains 300 units of insulin. To calculate the number of full doses per pen, divide the total number of units in each pen, 300 units, by the number of units per dose. Round any remainder down to the whole number.

3. Calculate the number of pens needed to deliver the total number of doses by dividing total doses by the number of full doses per pen.

4. Calculate the number of pen packs required by dividing the number of pens required by 5, the number of pens in each package.

TABLE 14-3	Insulin Pen/Cartridges with Storage Instructions	
Insulin Pens or Cartridge (3 mL Devices, 5 per Pack)	**Storage (Unopened)**	**Storage (After Opening)**
Humulin N Original Prefilled Pen	Until expiration date Refrigerated	14 days, room temperature, below 86°F (30°C) *Do not refrigerate.*
Humulin 70/30 Original Prefilled Pen	Until expiration date Refrigerated	10 days, room temperature, below 86°F (30°C) *Do not refrigerate.*
Humalog Mix 75/25™ KwikPen®	10 days, room temperature, below 86°F (30°C) Until expiration date, refrigerated	10 days, room temperature, below 86°F (30°C) *Do not refrigerate.*
Humalog Mix 50/50™ KwikPen®	10 days, room temperature, below 86°F (30°C) Until expiration date, refrigerated	10 days, room temperature, below 86°F (30°C) *Do not refrigerate.*
Humalog KwikPen®	28 days, room temperature, below 86°F (30°C) Until expiration date, refrigerated	28 days, room temperature, below 86°F (30°C) *Do not refrigerate.*
Humalog Cartridge	28 days, room temperature, below 86°F (30°C) Until expiration date, refrigerated	28 days, room temperature, below 86°F (30°C) *Do not refrigerate.*
Levemir® FlexPen®	Until expiration date, refrigerated	42 days, room temperature, below 86°F (30°C) *Do not refrigerate.*

Example: Determine the number of insulin pens required to administer the following order over a 3-week period.

Order: Humalog Mix 50/50 KwikPen insulin 47 units subcut bid before breakfast and dinner.

1.   Determine the number of doses to be administered:

$$x = \frac{2 \text{ doses}}{1 \text{ day}} \times \frac{7 \text{ days}}{1 \text{ week}} \times \frac{3 \text{ weeks}}{1}$$

$$x = \frac{42 \text{ doses}}{1}$$

42 doses will be administered over 3 weeks.

2. Calculate the number of full doses in the pen:

$$\frac{300 \text{ units}}{1 \text{ pen}} \div \frac{47 \text{ units}}{1 \text{ dose}} =$$

$$\frac{300 \text{ units}}{1 \text{ pen}} \times \frac{1 \text{ dose}}{47 \text{ units}} = 6.38 \text{ doses/pen}$$

There are 6 full doses per pen.

3. Calculate the number of pens needed to deliver the total number of doses.

$$\frac{42 \text{ total doses}}{6 \text{ (full) doses per pen}} = 7 \text{ pens}$$

4. Calculate the number of pen boxes required:

$$\frac{7 \text{ pens}}{5 \text{ pens per pack}} = 1.4 \text{ packs, which rounds up to 2 whole packs}$$

2 pen packs will be needed for a 3-week timeframe. As indicated in Table 14-3, unopened pens should be refrigerated.

NOTE: The nurse should check expiration date and storage instructions as noted in Table 14-3. If a pen is expected to expire prior to ability to use all doses, extra pens should be ordered, as needed.

Nurses comfortable with DA, can combine all steps into one equation:

$$x(\text{packs}) = \frac{1 \text{ pack}}{5 \text{ pens}} \times \frac{1 \text{ pen}}{300 \text{ units}} \times \frac{47 \text{ units}}{1 \text{ dose}} \times \frac{2 \text{ doses}}{1 \text{ day}} \times \frac{7 \text{ days}}{1 \text{ week}} \times \frac{3 \text{ weeks}}{1}$$

$$x = \frac{1,974 \text{ packs}}{1,500}$$

$$x = 1.316 \text{ packs; round to 2 packs}$$

LEARNING ACTIVITY 14-5 Determine the number of insulin pens and packages for each order and duration.

1. **Order:** Humulin 70/30 Original Prefilled Pen 30 units subcut bid before breakfast and dinner
   Duration: 1 week

2. **Order:** Humalog KwikPen insulin 6 units subcut tid before meals
   Duration: 4 weeks

Insulin Pumps

Insulin pumps are small, portable continuous subcutaneous infusion devices that are attached to the patient, under the skin, and designed to infuse insulin 24 hours a day (**Figure 14-42**). The pump infuses a continuous basal rate of rapid-acting insulin and can also be programmed to administer additional bolus doses. Some insulin pumps have programs that adjust the basal rate at different times of day to more closely mimic the basal rate of insulin released naturally by the pancreas.

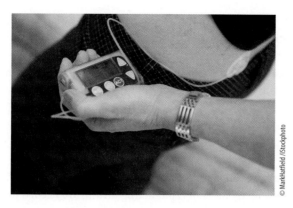

FIGURE 14-42   Patients can easily deliver extra doses of insulin as needed from an insulin pump that is secured to a site on the body. Flexible tubing delivers the insulin through a small cannula implanted under the skin.

Bolus Dose Calculation

Insulin bolus doses are based on the number of carbohydrates (CHO) about to be consumed at a meal. Bolus doses may also be given to correct elevated blood glucose levels from infection or other sources.

High Blood Glucose Correction

Dosage calculation for correcting high blood glucose is based on the current blood glucose, the target blood glucose, and **blood glucose correction factor**. The blood glucose correction factor, also called the **insulin sensitivity factor**, is the dose of insulin required to decrease the blood glucose by 50 mg/dL and is determined by the prescriber. To correct a high blood glucose:

- Subtract the target blood glucose from the current blood glucose.

- Divide the difference by 50 mg/dL.

- Multiply the quotient by the blood glucose correction factor:

$$\frac{\text{current blood glucose (mg/dL)} - \text{target blood glucose (mg/dL)}}{50 \text{ (mg/dL)}}$$
$$\times \text{ blood glucose correction factor (units)}$$
$$= \text{High blood glucose correction dose (units)}$$

Example 1A: The patient's blood glucose is 270 mg/dL. The target blood glucose is 120 mg/dL. The blood glucose correction factor is 1. How much rapid-acting insulin is required to lower the patient's blood glucose to the target range?

$$\frac{270 \text{ mg/dL} - 120 \text{ mg/dL}}{50 \text{ mg/dL}} \times 1 \text{ unit} = x \text{ (units)}$$

$$\frac{150 \ \cancel{\text{mg/dL}}}{50 \ \cancel{\text{mg/dL}}} \times 1 \text{ unit} = x$$

$$3 \times 1 \text{ unit} = x$$

$$3 \text{ units} = x$$

The high blood glucose correction dose is 3 units of rapid-acting insulin.

Total Mealtime Insulin Dose Calculation

To calculate the total mealtime insulin dose, add the high blood glucose correction dose to the **carbohydrate insulin dose**. The carbohydrate insulin dose is the amount of insulin required to dispose of the total number of carbohydrates (in grams) in the meal. To calculate the carbohydrate insulin dose, the pre-scriber must determine a patient's **insulin-to-carbohydrate ratio**, which is the amount of carbohydrate disposed of by 1 unit of insulin. The average insulin-to-carbohydrate ratio is 12–15 g CHO disposed by 1 unit of regular insulin. The carbohydrate insulin dose is calculated by multiplying the total meal carbohy-drate in grams (g) by the insulin to carbohydrate ratio (unit/g):

total carbohydrate (g) × insulin-to-carbohydrate ratio (unit/g) = carbohydrate insulin dose (units)

Example 1B: The same patient is about to eat 60 g of carbohydrates; the insulin to carbohydrate ratio is 15 g/unit. How many units of rapid-acting insulin are needed to dispose of this carbohy-drate load?

$$60 \cancel{g} \times 1 \text{ unit}/15 \cancel{g} = 4 \text{ units}$$

The carbohydrate insulin dose is 4 units of rapid-acting insulin.

To determine the **total mealtime bolus dose**, the total number of units to administer as the bolus dose, add the carbohydrate insulin dose to the high blood glucose correction dose:

carbohydrate insulin dose (units) + high blood sugar correction dose (units)

= total mealtime bolus dose (units)

Example 1C: Based on the high blood glucose correction dose calculated in Example 1A and the carbo-hydrate insulin dose calculated in Example 1B, determine the total mealtime bolus dose:

4 units + 3 units = 7 units

The patient should administer 7 units of insulin as a bolus dose via insulin pump just prior to eating.

Calculations for determining bolus doses administered via insulin pump can also be used to determine the bolus doses for insulin administered with a pen or syringe.

Rounding RULE!

To prevent hypoglycemia:

- Do not round high blood glucose correction dose or carbohydrate insulin dose.
- After both doses are combined, round total mealtime bolus dose down to the whole unit, if fraction exists.

For example, high blood glucose correction dose: 2.6 units, carbohydrate insulin dose 3.2 units:

2.6 + 3.2 = 5.8   total mealtime bolus dose is 5 units

- Rounding fractional units down will prevent insulin overdose.

LEARNING ACTIVITY 14-6 Determine the high blood glucose correction dose, carbohydrate insulin dose, and total mealtime bolus dose for the following patients.

1. The patient is going to eat 60 g of carbohydrates and has a blood glucose of 180 mg/dL. The patient's target blood glucose is 120 mg/dL, the blood glucose correction factor is 2 units, and the insulin to carbohydrate ratio is 1 unit/7.5 g.
   High blood glucose correction dose _____
   Carbohydrate insulin dose _____
   Total mealtime bolus dose _____
2. The patient is going to eat 90 g of carbohydrates and has a blood glucose of 110 mg/dL. The patient's target blood glucose is 120 mg/dL, the blood glucose correction factor is 1 unit, and the insulin to carbohydrate ratio is 1 unit/10 g.
   High blood glucose correction dose _____
   Carbohydrate insulin dose _____
   Total mealtime bolus dose _____

Clinical CLUE

Subcutaneous insulin administration is not always appropriate in critically ill patients. These patients receive rapid-acting or short-acting insulin as a continuous IV infusion ordered in units/h. Frequent (i.e., every 1 to 2 hours) BG testing is performed. The dose/rate of the infusion is adjusted according to the BG and a correctional, sliding scale (intravenous) insulin order set (Jacobi et al., 2012).

14-2   Heparin

Heparin is an **anticoagulant**, a medication that decreases blood clot formation. There are two types of heparin: **unfractionated heparin (UH)**, which has large molecules, and **low molecular weight heparin (LMWH)**, which has small molecules. Unless specified as LMWH, heparin is assumed to be UH. UH can be administered IV or subcutaneously, but may not be administered intramuscularly (IM) due to the risk of hematoma, while LMWH is only administered subcutaneously. A platelet count should be performed prior to administering the first dose of any heparin and repeated during heparin therapy. All heparin is supplied in United States Pharmacopeia (USP) units and is administered with syringe calibrated in milliliters. Recall from Chapter 2 that a USP unit, similar to the International Unit, is a standard unit of measurement that determines the potency of a drug. The units on a U-100 insulin syringe are *not* the same as USP units of heparin. Only a syringe that is calibrated in milliliters should be used to measure a heparin dose. Heparin comes in different concentrations and containers. Careful reading of the label is critical to prevent lethal dosage errors.

Determining the Concentration for Subcutaneous Heparin

Recall from Chapter 9 that 1 mL is the maximal injection volume for a subcutaneous injection. This requires the nurse to select a concentration of heparin that will yield a 1 mL injection volume or less. Calculation for subcutaneous heparin is a basic dosage calculation as demonstrated in Chapter 9.

Example 1:   Determine the amount to administer for the following order and supply.

   Order: heparin 7,000 USP units subcut bid

   Supply: Select the appropriate concentration of UH from **Figures 14-43, 14-44** and **14-45**.

C: *Convert*—Because the order and supply are both in units, there is no conversion.

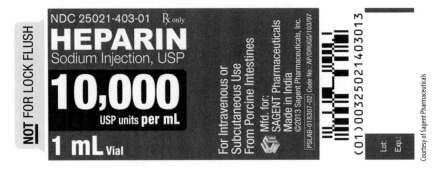

FIGURE 14-43

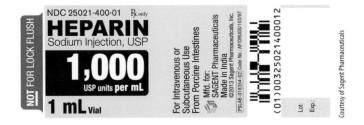

FIGURE 14-44

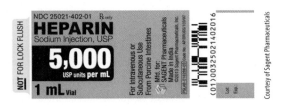

FIGURE 14-45

A: *Approximate*—The ordered dose, 7,000 units, needs to be contained in 1 mL or less. 7,000 units is more than 1,000 and 5,000, but less than 10,000, so heparin 10,000 units/mL will be used. Because 7,000 units is more than half of the supply of 10,000 units, more than half of the supply volume of 1 mL, that is, more than 0.5 mL of heparin 10,000 units per mL (Figure 14-43), will be administered.

S: *Solve*

Ratio-Proportion	Formula Method
$\dfrac{10,000\ \text{units}}{1\ \text{mL}} = \dfrac{7,000\ \text{units}}{x\ \text{mL}}$ or $10,000\ \text{units}:1\ \text{mL} = 7,000\ \text{units}:x\ \text{mL}$ $10,000x = 7,000$ $\dfrac{\cancel{10,000}x}{\cancel{10,000}} = \dfrac{7,000}{10,000}$ $x = 0.7\ \text{mL}$	$\dfrac{7,000\ \cancel{\text{units}}}{10,000\ \cancel{\text{units}}} \times 1\ \text{mL} = x\ (\text{mL})$ $\dfrac{7,000\ \text{mL}}{10,000} = x$ $0.7\ \text{mL} = x$

Dimensional Analysis

$$x \text{ (mL)} = \frac{1 \text{ mL}}{10,000 \text{ units}} \times \frac{7,000 \text{ units}}{1}$$

$$x = \frac{7,000 \text{ mL}}{10,000}$$

$$x = 0.7 \text{ mL}$$

E: *Evaluate*

Ratio-Proportion

$$\frac{10,000 \text{ units}}{1 \text{ mL}} = \frac{7,000 \text{ units}}{0.7 \text{ mL}} \text{ or}$$

$$10,000 \text{ units}: 1 \text{ mL} = 7,000 \text{ units}: 0.7 \text{ mL}$$

$$10,000 \times 0.7 = 7,000$$

$$7,000 = 7,000$$

Formula Method

$$\frac{7,000 \text{ units}}{10,000 \text{ units}} \times 1 \text{ mL} = 0.7 \text{ mL}$$

$$\frac{7,000 \text{ mL}}{10,000} = 0.7 \text{ mL}$$

$$0.7 \text{ mL} = 0.7 \text{ mL}$$

Dimensional Analysis

$$0.7 \text{ mL} = \frac{1 \text{ mL}}{10,000 \text{ units}} \times \frac{7,000 \text{ units}}{1}$$

$$0.7 \text{ mL} = \frac{7,000 \text{ mL}}{10,000}$$

$$0.7 \text{ mL} = 0.7 \text{ mL}$$

Because the calculated amount, 0.7 mL, accurately completes the equation and is consistent with the approximated volume, the answer is confirmed.

LEARNING ACTIVITY 14-7 Determine the amount to administer for the following orders and UH supplies.

1.   **Order:** heparin 5,000 units subcut bid
      Supply: Select the appropriate concentration of heparin from **Figures 14-46, 14-47,** and **14-48.**
2.   **Order:** heparin 8,000 units subcut tid
      Supply: Select the appropriate concentration of heparin from Figures 14-46, 14-47, and 14-48.

Clinical CLUE

Intermittent IV heparin, not ordered by weight, is calculated in the same way as subcutaneous heparin.

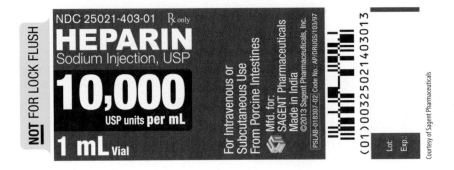

FIGURE 14-46

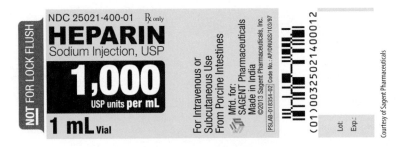

FIGURE 14-47

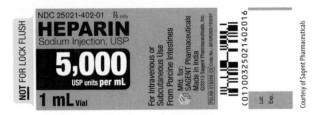

FIGURE 14-48

Intravenous Heparin Calculations

Heparin is often administered as a continuous IV infusion with intermittent IV push (IVP) or bolus doses ordered as needed, according to results of an intermittent lab test called **activated partial thromboplastin time (aPTT)**. This blood test, measured in seconds, indicates the how long it takes for blood to clot. The IV infusion rate is calculated separately from the IV bolus volume. Also, the IV infusion rate will be based on the concentration of the IV solution, while the IV bolus volume will be based on the dosage strength in the vial provided.

Clinical CLUE

Partial thromboplastin time (PTT) and aPTT are used to measure anticoagulation. An activator is added to the PTT to speed up clotting time (aPTT), which results in a narrower control range (Hammami, 2013). In the 1970s appropriate anticoagulation was determined to be 1.5 to 2.5 times the PTT control range (Lehman & Frank, 2009). Heparin is dosed according to the aPTT. In general, the goal is 1.5 to 2.5 times the aPTT control range, depending upon the patient's diagnosis.

Rounding RULE!

For weight-based heparin calculations, rounding is done according to equipment:

- Round weights to the tenth as most digital scales are calibrated to the tenth.

- Round IV rates in mL/h to the tenth or whole number, depending on the calibration of the infusion pump.

Weight-Based Bolus Doses

A weight-based heparin order will provide the number of units of heparin per 1 kg of body weight. This is a two-step process:

Step 1: Determine the number of units for the patient's weight in kg.

Step 2: Calculate the volume of heparin that contains the patient's dose.

Example: Use the following order and supply to calculate the amount in mL of heparin to administer to a 70 kg patient.

Order: heparin 60 units/kg IV bolus now

Supply: Heparin 1,000 units/mL

C: *Convert*—Because the order and supply are both in units, there is no conversion.

A: *Approximate*

Step 1: The ordered dose is 60 units per kg and the patient will need 70 times that amount (4,200 units) because the patient weighs 70 kg.

Step 2: Because there are 1,000 units of heparin per 1 mL, the volume to administer will be slightly more than 4 mL.

S: *Solve*

Ratio-Proportion	Formula Method
Step 1: Calculate the bolus dose in units: $$\frac{60 \text{ units}}{1 \text{ kg}} = \frac{x \text{ units}}{70 \text{ kg}}$$ or $$60 \text{ units} : 1 \text{ kg} = x \text{ units} : 70 \text{ kg}$$ $$x = 60 \times 70$$ $$x = 4,200 \text{ units}$$ The patient's bolus dose is 4,200 units.	Step 1: Calculate the bolus dose in units: $$\frac{60 \text{ units}}{1 \text{ kg}} \times 70 \text{ kg} = x \text{ (units)}$$ $$60 \text{ units} \times 70 = x$$ $$4,200 \text{ units} = x$$ The patient's bolus dose is 4,200 units.

Step 2: Calculate the volume to administer:

$$\frac{1,000 \text{ units}}{1 \text{ mL}} = \frac{4,200 \text{ units}}{x \text{ mL}} \text{ or}$$

$$1,000 \text{ units} : 1 \text{ mL} = 4,200 \text{ units} : x \text{ mL}$$

$$1,000x = 4,200$$

$$\frac{\cancel{1,000}x}{\cancel{1,000}} = \frac{4,200}{1,000}$$

$$x = 4.2 \text{ mL}$$

The volume to administer is 4.2 mL.

Step 2: Calculate the volume to administer:

$$\frac{4,200 \cancel{\text{ units}}}{1,000 \cancel{\text{ units}}} \times 1 \text{ mL} = x \text{ (mL)}$$

$$\frac{4,200 \text{ mL}}{1,000} = x$$

$$4.2 \text{ mL} = x$$

The volume to administer is 4.2 mL.

Dimensional Analysis

Step 1 and step 2 are combined:

$$x \text{ (mL)} = \frac{1 \text{ mL}}{1,000 \cancel{\text{ units}}} \times \frac{60 \cancel{\text{ units}}}{1 \cancel{\text{ kg}}} \times \frac{70 \cancel{\text{ kg}}}{1}$$

$$x = \frac{4,200 \text{ mL}}{1,000}$$

$$x = 4.2 \text{ mL}$$

The volume to administer is 4.2 mL.

E: *Evaluate*

Ratio-Proportion

Step 1: Calculate the bolus dose in units:

$$\frac{60 \text{ units}}{1 \text{ kg}} = \frac{4,200 \text{ units}}{70 \text{ kg}} \text{ or}$$

$$60 \text{ units} : 1 \text{ kg} = 4,200 \text{ units} : 70 \text{ kg}$$

$$60 \times 70 = 4,200$$

$$4,200 = 4,200$$

Step 2: Calculate the volume to administer:

$$\frac{1,000 \text{ units}}{1 \text{ mL}} = \frac{4,200 \text{ units}}{4.2 \text{ mL}} \text{ or}$$

$$1,000 \text{ units} : 1 \text{ mL} = 4,200 \text{ units} : 4.2 \text{ mL}$$

$$1,000 \times 4.2 = 4,200$$

$$4,200 = 4,200$$

Formula Method

Step 1: Calculate the bolus dose in units:

$$\frac{60 \text{ units}}{1 \cancel{\text{ kg}}} \times 70 \cancel{\text{ kg}} = 4,200 \text{ units}$$

$$60 \text{ units} \times 70 = 4,200 \text{ units}$$

$$4,200 \text{ units} = 4,200 \text{ units}$$

Step 2: Calculate the volume to administer:

$$\frac{4,200 \cancel{\text{ units}}}{1,000 \cancel{\text{ units}}} \times 1 \text{ mL} = 4.2 \text{ mL}$$

$$\frac{4,200 \text{ mL}}{1,000} = 4.2 \text{ mL}$$

$$4.2 \text{ mL} = 4.2 \text{ mL}$$

Dimensional Analysis

Step 1 and step 2 are combined:

$$4.2 \text{ mL} = \frac{1 \text{ mL}}{1,000 \text{ units}} \times \frac{60 \text{ units}}{1 \text{ kg}} \times \frac{70 \text{ kg}}{1}$$

$$4.2 \text{ mL} = \frac{4,200 \text{ mL}}{1,000}$$

$$4.2 \text{ mL} = 4.2 \text{ mL}$$

Because the calculated dose, 4,200 units, accurately completes the (Step 1) equation and is consistent with the approximated dose, the answer is confirmed. Because the calculated volume, 4.2 mL, accurately completes the (Step 2) equation and is consistent with the approximated volume, the answer is confirmed.

LEARNING ACTIVITY 14-8 Use the following orders and supplies to calculate the heparin dose in units and the heparin amount to administer in mL.

1.   **Order:** heparin 40 units/kg IV bolus now for a patient who weighs 60 kg
      Supply: Heparin 1,000 units/1 mL
2.   **Order:** heparin 35 units/kg IV bolus now; maximum dose 3,500 units for a patient who weighs
           120 kg
      Supply: Heparin 1,000 units/1 mL

Weight-Based Continuous IV Heparin Infusion

A weight-based heparin infusion order will provide the number of units of heparin per 1 kg of body weight per hour. Calculating the rate is a two-step process:

Step 1: Determine the number of units/h based on the patient's weight in kg.

Step 2: Calculate the IV rate in mL/h that delivers the patient's hourly dose of heparin.

Example: Use the following order and supply to calculate the rate of heparin in mL/h for a 70 kg patient.

   Order: heparin 16 units/kg/h IV infusion

   Supply: Heparin 25,000 units in 500 mL D_5W (50 units/mL)

C: *Convert*—Because the order and supply are both in units, there is no conversion.

A: *Approximate*

Step 1: The ordered dose is 16 units/kg/h, so the patient will need more than 700 units/h (10 units/h × 70 kg) but less than 1,400 units/h (20 units/h × 70 kg).

Step 2: Because there are 50 units of heparin per 1 mL, the infusion will be between 14 mL/h and 28 mL/h (i.e. 700 units/h divided by 50 units/mL = 14 mL/h; 1400 units/h divided by 50 units/mL = 28 mL/h).

S: *Solve*

Ratio-Proportion

Step 1: Calculate the dose in units/h:

$$\frac{16 \text{ units/h}}{1 \text{ kg}} = \frac{x \text{ units/h}}{70 \text{ kg}}$$

or

$$16 \text{ units/h} : 1 \text{ kg} = x \text{ units/h} : 70 \text{ kg}$$
$$x = 16 \times 70$$
$$x = 1{,}120 \text{ units/h}$$

The patient's dose is 1,120 units/h.

Step 2: Calculate the volume to administer 1,120 units:

$$\frac{50 \text{ units}}{1 \text{ mL}} = \frac{1{,}120 \text{ units}}{x \text{ mL}} \quad \text{or}$$
$$50 \text{ units/h} : 1 \text{ mL} = 1{,}120 \text{ units} : x \text{ mL}$$
$$50x = 1{,}120$$
$$\frac{50x}{50} = \frac{1{,}120}{50}$$
$$x = 22.4 \text{ mL}$$

To deliver 1,120 units/h, set the rate to 22.4 mL/h.

Formula Method

Step 1: Calculate the rate in units/h:

$$16 \text{ units/kg/h} \times 70 \text{ kg} = x \text{ (units/h)}$$
$$1{,}120 \text{ units/h} = x$$

The patient's dose is 1,120 units/h.

Step 2: Calculate the rate in mL/h

$$\frac{1{,}120 \text{ units/h}}{50 \text{ units}} \times 1 \text{ mL} = x \text{ (mL/h)}$$
$$22.4 \text{ mL/h} = x$$

The infusion rate is 22.4 mL/h.

Dimensional Analysis

Step 1 and step 2 are combined:

$$x \text{ (mL/h)} = \frac{1 \text{ mL}}{50 \text{ units}} \times \frac{16 \text{ units}}{1 \text{ kg}} \times \frac{70 \text{ kg}}{1} \times \frac{1}{1 \text{ h}}$$
$$x = \frac{1{,}120 \text{ mL}}{50 \text{ h}}$$
$$x = 22.4 \text{ mL/h}$$

The infusion rate is 22.4 mL/h.

E: *Evaluate*

Ratio-Proportion

Step 1: Calculate the dose in units/h:

$$\frac{16 \text{ units/h}}{1 \text{ kg}} = \frac{1{,}120 \text{ units/h}}{70 \text{ kg}} \quad \text{or}$$
$$16 \text{ units/h} : 1 \text{ kg} = 1{,}120 \text{ units/h} : 70 \text{ kg}$$
$$16 \times 70 = 1{,}120$$
$$1{,}120 = 1{,}120$$

Formula Method

Step 1: Calculate the dose in units/h:

$$16 \text{ units/kg/h} \times 70 \text{ kg} = 1{,}120 \text{ units/h}$$
$$1{,}120 \text{ units/h} = 1{,}120 \text{ units/h}$$

Step 2: Calculate the volume to administer 1,120 units:

$$\frac{50 \text{ units}}{1 \text{ mL}} = \frac{1,120 \text{ units}}{22.4 \text{ mL}} \text{ or}$$

50 units : 1 mL = 1,120 units : 22.4 mL

$50 \times 22.4 = 1,120$

$1,120 = 1,120$

Step 2: Calculate the rate in mL/h:

$$\frac{1,120 \text{ units/h}}{50 \text{ units}} \times 1 \text{ mL} = 22.4 \text{ mL/h}$$

22.4 mL/h = 22.4 mL/h

Dimensional Analysis

Step 1 and step 2 are combined:

$$22.4 \text{ mL/h} = \frac{1 \text{ mL}}{50 \text{ units}} \times \frac{16 \text{ units}}{1 \text{ kg}} \times \frac{70 \text{ kg}}{1} \times \frac{1}{1 \text{ h}}$$

$$22.4 \text{ mL/h} = \frac{1,120 \text{ mL}}{50 \text{ h}}$$

$22.4 \text{ mL/h} = 22.4 \text{ mL/h}$

Because the calculated dose, 1,120 unit/h, accurately completes the (Step 1) equation and is consistent with the approximated dose, the answer is confirmed. Because the calculated rate, 22.4 mL/h, accurately completes the (Step 2) equation and is consistent with the approximated rate, the answer is confirmed.

Clinical CLUE

Increased accuracy is not the only advantage of using dimensional analysis to solve advanced clinical calculations. Another advantage is the ability to incorporate multiple conversion factors into one equation rather than performing multi-step calculations. When using ratio-proportion or the formula method, weight-based heparin protocol calculations for weights given in pounds and ounces will require one or more conversion calculations in addition to the two-step process to determine bolus volumes or IV infusion rates. However, with dimensional analysis, additional conversions can be calculated within a single equation by inserting the appropriate conversion factors.

LEARNING ACTIVITY 14-9 Refer to each order and supply to calculate the heparin dose in units/h and the heparin infusion rate in mL/h.

1. **Order:** heparin 20 units/kg/h IV infusion (maximum rate 2,000 units/h) for a patient who weighs 90 kg
    Supply: Heparin 25,000 units in 5% dextrose in water 500 mL (50 units/mL)
2. **Order:** heparin 16 units/kg/h IV infusion for a patient who weighs 100 kg
    Supply: Heparin 25,000 units in 5% dextrose in water 250 mL (100 units/mL)

Weight-Based Heparin Protocol

A **weight-based heparin protocol** is an order set of weight-based IV heparin orders (TABLE 14-4). The protocol orders changes in rate or additional IV bolus doses based on the patient's aPTT. The frequency of aPTT blood testing is included in the protocol order set. A **loading dose**, the initial bolus dose, is given to achieve a therapeutic blood level, and the continuous infusion is given to maintain the therapeutic level. As previously mentioned, the therapeutic blood level of heparin is based on the aPTT blood test.

TABLE 14-4   Heparin Protocol for DVT, PE, and High-Intensity Indications* GOAL: aPTT 70=100 Seconds

- Use premixed heparin sodium 25,000 units in 500 mL D$_5$W (50 units/mL) for infusion.
- Use heparin sodium 1,000 units/mL for bolus doses.
- Obtain baseline CBC and aPTT prior to administering heparin.
- Obtain aPTT daily while receiving heparin and while aPTT remains between 70 and 100.
- Initial bolus dose: 80 units/kg (maximum 8,000 units)
- Initial rate: 18 units/kg/h (maximum 1,800 units/h = 36 mL/h)

aPTT Result (in seconds)	IV Bolus Dose	# Minutes to Hold Infusion	Amount to Change Current Infusion Rate
Less than 55: Notify prescriber	80 units/kg (max 8,000 units)	Do not hold.	Increase by 4 units/kg/h. Repeat aPTT in 6 hours.
55–60	40 units/kg (max 4,000 units)	Do not hold.	Increase by 2 units/kg/h. Repeat aPTT in 6 hours.
61–69	40 units/kg (max 4,000 units)	Do not hold.	Increase by 1 unit/kg/h. Repeat aPTT in 6 hours.
70–100 goal	**No bolus dose**	**Do not hold.**	**Do not change current infusion rate. Repeat aPTT in 6 hours. If aPTT result remains between 70-100 seconds, obtain aPTT daily.**
101–114	No bolus dose	Do not hold.	Decrease by 1 unit/kg/h.
115–134	No bolus dose	30	Decrease by 2 unit/kg/h and repeat aPTT 6 hours after infusion resumed.
135–150	No bolus dose	60	Decrease by 3 units/kg/h and repeat aPTT 6 hours after infusion resumed.
151–200: Notify prescriber	No bolus dose	90	Decrease by 4 unit/kg/h and repeat aPTT 6 hours after infusion resumed.

*Sample only: not to be used in clinical practice.

aPTT = activated partial thromboplastin time; CBC = complete blood count; DVT = deep vein thrombosis; PE = pulmonary embolism

Initial Bolus Dose Calculation

The protocol calls for an initial bolus dose of 80 units/kg. The initial bolus dose calculation is a two-step process:

Step 1: Calculate the weight-based bolus dose by multiplying the loading dose, 80 units/kg, by the patient's weight. Note that the maximum loading dose is 8,000 units.

Step 2: Calculate the volume to administer using the heparin supply 1,000 units/mL.

Example 1A: Using the heparin protocol in Table 14-4, calculate the loading dose (initial bolus dose) for a patient weighing 74 kg.

C: *Convert*—Because the order and supply are both in units, there is no conversion.

A: *Approximate*

Step 1: The ordered dose is 80 units/kg and the patient weighs between 50 and 100 kg; therefore the patient will need between 4,000 and 8,000 units.

Step 2: Because there are 1,000 units of heparin per 1 mL, the volume to administer will be between 4 and 8 mL.

S: *Solve*

Ratio-Proportion	Formula Method
Step 1: Calculate the bolus dose in units:	Step 1: Calculate the bolus dose in units:
$\dfrac{80\ units}{1\ kg} = \dfrac{x\ units}{74\ kg}$ or	$\dfrac{80\ units}{1\ \cancel{kg}} \times 74\ \cancel{kg} = x\ (units)$
$80\ units : 1\ kg = x\ unit : 74\ kg$	$80\ units \times 74 = x$
$x = 80 \times 74$	$5,920\ units = x$
$x = 5,920\ units$	The patient's bolus dose is 5,920 units.
The patient's bolus dose is 5,920 units.	Step 2: Calculate the volume to administer:
Step 2: Calculate the volume to administer:	$\dfrac{5,920\ \cancel{units}}{1,000\ \cancel{units}} \times 1\ mL = x\ (mL)$
$\dfrac{1,000\ units}{1\ mL} = \dfrac{5,920\ units}{x\ mL}$ or	$\dfrac{5,920\ mL}{1,000} = x$
$1,000\ units : 1\ mL = 5,920\ units : x\ mL$	$5.92\ mL = x$
$1,000x = 5,920$	The volume to administer is 5.9 mL.
$\dfrac{\cancel{1,000}\,x}{\cancel{1,000}} = \dfrac{5,920}{1,000}$	
$x = 5.92\ mL$	
The volume to administer is 5.9 mL.	

Dimensional Analysis

Step 1 and step 2 are combined:

$$x \, (\text{mL}) = \frac{1 \, \text{mL}}{1{,}000 \, \cancel{\text{units}}} \times \frac{80 \, \cancel{\text{units}}}{1 \, \cancel{\text{kg}}} \times \frac{74 \, \cancel{\text{kg}}}{1}$$

$$x = \frac{5{,}920 \, \text{mL}}{1{,}000}$$

$$x = 5.92 \, \text{mL}$$

The volume to administer is 5.9 mL.

E: *Evaluate*

Ratio-Proportion

Step 1: Calculate the bolus dose in units:

$$\frac{80 \, \text{units}}{1 \, \text{kg}} = \frac{5{,}920 \, \text{units}}{74 \, \text{kg}}$$

$$80 \, \text{units} : 1 \, \text{kg} = 5{,}920 \, \text{units} : 74 \, \text{kg}$$

$$80 \times 74 = 5{,}920$$

$$5{,}920 = 5{,}920$$

Step 2: Calculate the volume to administer:

$$\frac{1{,}000 \, \text{units}}{1 \, \text{mL}} = \frac{5{,}920 \, \text{units}}{5.92 \, \text{mL}} \quad \text{or}$$

$$1{,}000 \, \text{units} : 1 \, \text{mL} = 5{,}920 \, \text{units} : 5.92 \, \text{mL}$$

$$1{,}000 \times 5.92 = 5{,}920$$

$$5{,}920 = 5{,}920$$

Formula Method

Step 1: Calculate the bolus dose in units:

$$\frac{80 \, \text{units}}{1 \, \cancel{\text{kg}}} \times 74 \, \cancel{\text{kg}} = 5{,}920 \, \text{units}$$

$$5{,}920 \, \text{units} = 5{,}920 \, \text{units}$$

Step 2: Calculate the volume to administer:

$$\frac{5{,}920 \, \cancel{\text{units}}}{1{,}000 \, \cancel{\text{units}}} \times 1 \, \text{mL} = 5.92 \, \text{mL}$$

$$\frac{5{,}920 \, \text{mL}}{1{,}000} = 5.92 \, \text{mL}$$

$$5.92 \, \text{mL} = 5.92 \, \text{mL}$$

Dimensional Analysis

Step 1 and step 2 are combined:

$$5.92 \, \text{mL} = \frac{1 \, \text{mL}}{1{,}000 \, \cancel{\text{units}}} \times \frac{80 \, \cancel{\text{units}}}{1 \, \cancel{\text{kg}}} \times \frac{74 \, \cancel{\text{kg}}}{1}$$

$$5.92 \, \text{mL} = \frac{5{,}920 \, \text{mL}}{1{,}000}$$

$$5.92 \, \text{mL} = 5.92 \, \text{mL}$$

The calculated dose is less than the maximum dose, so the calculated dose can be administered. Because the calculated dose, 5,920 units, accurately completes the (Step 1) equation and is consistent with the approximated dose, the answer is confirmed. Because the calculated volume, 5.92 mL, accurately completes the (Step 2) equation and is consistent with the approximated volume, the rounded answer, 5.9 mL, is confirmed. The nurse will administer the 5.9 mL heparin bolus through the IV access port on the primary IV tubing (**Figure 14-49**).

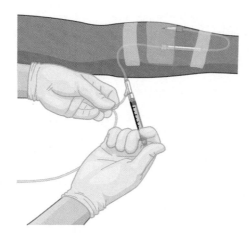

FIGURE 14-49   IV push or bolus medications are administered via the IV access port closest to the patient.

Initial Infusion Rate Calculation

The protocol calls for an initial weight-based hourly infusion dose of 18 units/kg/h with a maximum of 1,800 units/h (36 mL/h). The initial infusion rate calculation is a two-step process:

Step 1: Calculate the weight-based hourly infusion dose by multiplying 18 units/kg/h by the patient's weight.

Step 2: Calculate the IV infusion rate in mL/h using the supply of heparin 25,000 units in 500 mL of D_5W 500 mL (50 units/mL).

Example 1B: Using the heparin protocol in Table 14-4, calculate the initial infusion rate for a patient weighing 74 kg.

C: *Convert*—Because the order and supply are both in units, there is no conversion.

A: *Approximate*

Step 1: The ordered dose is 18 units/kg/h, so the patient will need more than 740 units/h (10 units/h × 74 kg) but less than 1,480 units/h (20 units/h × 74 kg).

Step 2: Because there are 50 units of heparin per 1 mL, the rate to administer 740–1,480 units/h will be between 14 mL/h and 30 mL/h (i.e. 700 units/h divided by 50 units/mL = 14 mL/h; 1500 units/h divided by 50 units/mL = 30 mL/h).

S: *Solve*

Ratio-Proportion	Formula Method
Step 1: Calculate the dose in units/h:	Step 1: Calculate the dose in units/h:
$\dfrac{18 \text{ units/h}}{1 \text{ kg}} = \dfrac{x \text{ units/h}}{74 \text{ kg}}$ or 18 units/h : 1 kg = x units/h : 74 kg $x = 18 \times 74$ $x = 1{,}332$ units/h The patient's dose is 1,332 units/h.	$18 \text{ units/~~kg~~/h} \times 74 \text{ ~~kg~~} = x(\text{units/h})$ $1{,}332 \text{ units/h} = x$ The patient's dose is 1,332 units/h.

Step 2: Calculate the volume to administer 1,332 units:

$$\frac{50 \text{ units}}{1 \text{ mL}} = \frac{1,332 \text{ units}}{x \text{ mL}} \text{ or}$$

$$50 \text{ units} : 1 \text{ mL} = 1,332 \text{ units} : x \text{ mL}$$

$$50x = 1,332$$

$$\frac{50x}{50} = \frac{1,332}{50}$$

$$x = 26.64 \text{ or } 26.6 \text{ mL}$$

To deliver 1,332 units/h, set the rate to 26.6 mL/h.

Step 2: Calculate the rate in mL/h:

$$\frac{1,332 \text{ units}/\text{h}}{50 \text{ units}} \times 1 \text{ mL} = x(\text{mL}/\text{h})$$

$$\frac{1,332 \text{ mL}/\text{h}}{50} = x$$

$$26.64 \text{ mL}/\text{h} = x$$

The rate to deliver 1,332 units/h is 26.6 mL/h

Dimensional Analysis

Step 1 and step 2 are combined:

$$x \text{ (mL/h)} = \frac{1 \text{ mL}}{50 \text{ units}} \times \frac{18 \text{ units}}{1 \text{ kg}} \times \frac{74 \text{ kg}}{1} \times \frac{1}{1 \text{ h}}$$

$$x = \frac{1,332 \text{ mL}}{50 \text{ h}}$$

$$x = 26.64 \text{ mL}/\text{h}$$

The rate to deliver 1,332 units/h is 26.6 mL/h.

E: *Evaluate*

Ratio-Proportion

Step 1: Calculate the rate in units/h:

$$\frac{18 \text{ units}/\text{h}}{1 \text{ kg}} = \frac{1,332 \text{ units}/\text{h}}{74 \text{ kg}} \text{ or}$$

$$18 \text{ units}/\text{h} : 1 \text{ kg} = 1,332 \text{ units}/\text{h} : 74 \text{ kg}$$

$$18 \times 74 = 1,332$$

$$1,332 = 1,332$$

Step 2: Calculate the volume to administer 1,332 units:

$$\frac{50 \text{ units}}{1 \text{ mL}} = \frac{1,332 \text{ units}}{26.64 \text{ mL}} \text{ or}$$

$$50 \text{ units}/\text{h} : 1 \text{ mL} = 1,332 \text{ units} : 26.64 \text{ mL}$$

$$50 \times 26.64 = 1,332$$

$$1,332 = 1,332$$

Formula Method

Step 1: Calculate the rate in units/h:

$$18 \text{ units}/\text{kg}/\text{h} \times 74 \text{ kg} = 1,332 \text{ units}/\text{h}$$

$$1,332 \text{ units}/\text{h} = 1,332 \text{ units}/\text{h}$$

Step 2: Calculate the rate in mL/h:

$$\frac{1,332 \text{ units}/\text{h}}{50 \text{ units}} \times 1 \text{ mL} = 26.64 \text{ mL}/\text{h}$$

$$\frac{1,332 \text{ mL}/\text{h}}{50} = 26.64 \text{ mL}/\text{h}$$

$$26.64 \text{ mL}/\text{h} = 26.64 \text{ mL.h}$$

Dimensional Analysis

Step 1 and step 2 are combined:

$$26.64\,\frac{mL}{h} = \frac{1\,mL}{50\,\cancel{units}} \times \frac{18\,\cancel{units}}{1\,\cancel{kg}} \times \frac{74\,\cancel{kg}}{1} \times \frac{1}{1\,h}$$

$$26.64\,mL/h = \frac{1{,}332\,mL}{50\,h}$$

$$26.64\,mL/h = 26.64\,mL/h$$

Because the calculated dose, 1,332 units/h, accurately completes the (Step 1) equation and is consistent with the approximated amount, the answer is confirmed. Because the calculated rate, 26.64 mL/h (rounded to 26.6 mL or 27 mL/h per pump calibration), accurately completes the (Step 2) equation and is consistent with the approximated rate, the answer is confirmed. The nurse will set the IV rate on the infusion pump to 26.6 mL/h (**Figure 14-50**).

Bolus Dose and Infusion Rate Calculations Based on aPTT

After the heparin protocol is initiated (i.e., after the loading dose is administered and the initial infusion rate is established), additional bolus doses will be administered and IV rate changes will be made according to aPTT results per the heparin protocol in Table 14-4. After an aPTT result is obtained, the nurse will calculate:

- The (next) IV bolus dose in units
- The bolus volume to administer in mL
- The (next) hourly IV dose in units/h
- The (new) IV infusion rate in mL/h

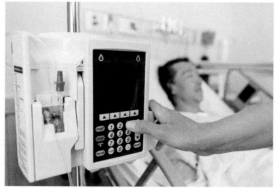

FIGURE 14-50   After administration of the heparin loading dose, the nurse will set the hourly infusion rate on the IV pump.

Example 2:   The aPTT is 65 seconds. The patient weighs 74 kg. The initial weight-based infusion rate, based on 18 units/kg/h is running at 26.6 mL/h. Using the heparin protocol (Table 14-4) determine the following:

- Bolus calculations

    - Bolus dose in units

    - Bolus amount in mL

- Number of minutes to hold the infusion

- Infusion calculations

    - Hourly IV heparin dose in units/h

    - Hourly IV infusion rate in mL/h

Bolus calculations: With an aPTT of 65 seconds, the weight-based bolus dose will be calculated using 40 units/kg. The bolus amount will be calculated using the heparin supply 1,000 units/mL:

C: *Convert*—Because the order and supply are both in units, there is no conversion.

A: *Approximate*

Step 1: The ordered dose is 40 units/kg and the patient weighs between 50 and 100 kg; therefore, the patient will need between 2,000 and 4,000 units.

Step 2: Because there are 1,000 units of heparin per 1 mL, the volume to administer will be between 2 and 4 mL.

S: *Solve*

Ratio-Proportion	Formula Method
Step 1: Calculate the bolus dose in units:	Step 1: Calculate the bolus dose in units:
$$\frac{40 \text{ units}}{1 \text{ kg}} = \frac{x \text{ units}}{74 \text{ kg}} \text{ or}$$ $$40 \text{ units} : 1 \text{ kg} = x \text{ units} : 74 \text{ kg}$$ $$x = 40 \times 74$$ $$x = 2.960$$	$$\frac{40 \text{ units}}{1 \text{ kg}} \times 74 \text{ kg} = x \text{ (units)}$$ $$40 \text{ units} \times 74 = x$$ $$2{,}960 \text{ units} = x$$
The patient's bolus dose is 2,960 units.	The patient's bolus dose is 2,960 units.
Step 2: Calculate the volume to administer:	Step 2: Calculate the volume to administer:
$$\frac{1{,}000 \text{ units}}{1 \text{ mL}} = \frac{2{,}960}{x \text{ mL}} \text{ or}$$ $$1{,}000 \text{ units} : 1 \text{ mL} = 2{,}960 \text{ units} : x \text{ mL}$$ $$1{,}000x = 2{,}960$$ $$\frac{1{,}000x}{1{,}000} = \frac{2{,}960}{1{,}000}$$ $$x = 2.96 \text{ mL}$$	$$\frac{2{,}960 \text{ units}}{1{,}000 \text{ units}} \times 1 \text{ mL} = x \text{ (mL)}$$ $$\frac{2{,}960 \text{ mL}}{1{,}000} = x$$ $$2.96 \text{ mL} = x$$
The volume to administer is 3 mL.	The volume to administer is 3 mL.

Dimensional Analysis

Step 1 and step 2 are combined:

$$x(mL) = \frac{1 \, mL}{1{,}000 \, \text{units}} \times \frac{40 \, \text{units}}{1 \, \text{kg}} \times \frac{74 \, \text{kg}}{1}$$

$$x = \frac{2{,}960 \, mL}{1{,}000}$$

$$x = 2.96 \, mL$$

The volume to administer is 3 mL.

E: *Evaluate*

Ratio-Proportion	Formula Method
Step 1: Calculate the bolus dose in units:	Step 1: Calculate the bolus dose in units:
$\dfrac{40 \, units}{1 \, kg} = \dfrac{2{,}960 \, units}{74 \, kg}$ or $40 \, units : 1 \, kg = 2{,}960 \, units : 74 \, kg$ $40 \times 74 = 2{,}960$ $2{,}960 = 2{,}960$	$\dfrac{40 \, units}{1 \, kg} \times 74 \, kg = 2{,}960 \, units$ $40 \, units \times 74 = 2{,}960 \, units$ $2{,}960 \, units = 2{,}960 \, units$
Step 2: Calculate the volume to administer:	Step 2: Calculate the volume to administer:
$\dfrac{1{,}000 \, units}{1 \, mL} = \dfrac{2{,}960}{2.96 \, mL}$ or $1{,}000 \, units : 1 \, mL = 2{,}960 \, units : 2.96 \, mL$ $1{,}000 \times 2.96 = 2{,}960$ $2{,}960 = 2{,}960$	$\dfrac{2{,}960 \, \text{units}}{1{,}000 \, \text{units}} \times 1 \, mL = 2.96 \, mL$ $\dfrac{2{,}960 \, mL}{1{,}000} = 2.96 \, mL$ $2.96 \, mL = 2.96 \, mL$

Dimensional Analysis

Step 1 and step 2 are combined:

$$2.96 \, mL = \frac{1 \, mL}{1{,}000 \, \text{units}} \times \frac{40 \, \text{units}}{1 \, \text{kg}} \times \frac{74 \, \text{kg}}{1}$$

$$2.96 \, mL = \frac{2{,}960 \, mL}{1{,}000}$$

$$2.96 \, mL = 2.96 \, mL$$

The calculated dose is less than the maximum dose, so the calculated dose can be administered. Because the calculated dose, 2,960 units, accurately completes the (Step 1) equation and is consistent with the approximate volume, the answer is confirmed. Because the calculated volume, 2.96 mL, accurately completes the (Step 2) equation and is consistent with the approximated volume, the rounded answer, 3 mL, is confirmed.

Number of minutes to hold infusion: With an aPTT of 65 seconds, the infusion will not be held.

Infusion calculations: With an aPTT of 65 seconds, the current weight-based infusion rate, 18 units/kg/h will be increased by 1 unit/kg/h. The new infusion rate, 19 units/kg/h, will be calculated using a supply of heparin 25,000 units in 500 mL D_5W 500 (50 units/mL).

C: *Convert*—Because the order and supply are both in units, there is no conversion.

A: *Approximate*

Step 1: The ordered dose is 19 units/kg/h, so the patient will need more than 740 units/h (10 units/h times 74 kg) but less than 1,480 units/h (20 units/h times 74 kg).

Step 2: Because there are 50 units of heparin per 1 mL, the rate to administer 740–1,480 units/h will be between 14 mL/h and 30 mL/h (i.e. 700 units/h divided by 50 units/mL = 14 mL/h; 1500 units/h divided by 50 units/mL = 30 mL/h).

S: *Solve*

Ratio-Proportion	**Formula Method**
Step 1: Calculate the dose in units/h:	Step 1: Calculate the dose in units/h:
$$\frac{19\ \text{units/h}}{1\ \text{kg}} = \frac{x\ \text{units/h}}{74\ \text{kg}}\ \text{or}$$ $$19\ \text{units/h}: 1\ \text{kg} = x\ \text{units/h}: 74\ \text{kg}$$ $$x = 19 \times 74$$ $$x = 1.406$$	$$19\ \text{units/kg/h} \times 74\ \text{kg} = x\ (\text{units/h})$$ $$1,406\ \text{units/h} = x$$
The patient's dose is 1,406 units/h.	The patient's dose is 1,406 units/h.
Step 2: Calculate the volume to administer 1,406 units:	Step 2: Calculate the rate in mL/h:
$$\frac{50\ \text{units}}{1\ \text{mL}} = \frac{1,406\ \text{units}}{x\ \text{mL}}\ \text{or}$$ $$50\ \text{units}: 1\ \text{mL} = 1,406\ \text{units}: x\ \text{mL}$$ $$50x = 1,406$$ $$\frac{50x}{50} = \frac{1,406}{50}$$ $$x = 28.12\ \text{mL}$$	$$\frac{1,406\ \text{units/h}}{50\ \text{units}} \times 1\ \text{mL} = x\ (\text{mL/h})$$ $$\frac{1,406\ \text{mL/h}}{50} = x$$ $$28.12\ \text{mL/h} = x$$
To deliver 1,406 units/h, set the rate to 28.1 mL/h.	The rate to deliver 1,406 units/h is 28.1 mL/h.

Dimensional Analysis

Step 1 and step 2 are combined:

$$x\ (\text{mL/h}) = \frac{1\ \text{mL}}{50\ \text{units}} \times \frac{19\ \text{units}}{1\ \text{kg}} \times \frac{74\ \text{kg}}{1} \times \frac{1}{1\ \text{h}}$$

$$x = \frac{1,406\ \text{mL}}{50\ \text{h}}$$

$$x = 28.12\ \text{mL/h}$$

The rate to deliver 1,406 units/h is 28.1 mL/h.

E: *Evaluate*

Ratio-Proportion	Formula Method
Step 1: Calculate the dose in units/h: $\dfrac{19 \text{ units/h}}{1 \text{ kg}} = \dfrac{1,406 \text{ units/h}}{74 \text{ kg}}$ or $19 \text{ units/h}: 1 \text{ kg} = 1,406 \text{ units/h}: 74 \text{ kg}$ $19 \times 74 = 1,406$ $1,406 = 1,406$ Step 2: Calculate the volume to administer 1,406 units: $\dfrac{50 \text{ units}}{1 \text{ mL}} = \dfrac{1,406 \text{ units}}{28.12 \text{ mL}}$ or $50 \text{ units}: 1 \text{ mL} = 1,406 \text{ units}: 28.12 \text{ mL}$ $50 \times 28.12 = 1,406$ $1,406 = 1,406$	Step 1: Calculate the rate in units/h: $19 \text{ units/\cancel{kg}/h} \times 74 \cancel{\text{ kg}} = 1,406 \text{ units/h}$ $1,406 \text{ units/h} = 1,406 \text{ units/h}$ Step 2: Calculate the rate in mL/h: $\dfrac{1,406 \cancel{\text{ units}}/h}{50 \cancel{\text{ units}}} \times 1 \text{ mL} = 28.12 \text{ mL/h}$ $\dfrac{1,406 \text{ mL/h}}{50} = 28.12 \text{ mL/h}$ $28.12 \text{ mL/h} = 28.12 \text{ mL/h}$

Dimensional Analysis
Step 1 and step 2 are combined: $28.12 \text{ mL/h} = \dfrac{1 \text{ mL}}{50 \cancel{\text{ units}}} \times \dfrac{19 \cancel{\text{ units}}}{1 \cancel{\text{ kg}}} \times \dfrac{74 \cancel{\text{ kg}}}{1} \times \dfrac{1}{1 \text{ h}}$ $28.12 \text{ mL/h} = \dfrac{1,406 \text{ mL}}{50 \text{ h}}$ $28.12 \text{ mL/h} = 28.12 \text{ mL/h}$

Because the calculated dose, 1,406 units/h, accurately completes the (Step 1) equation and is consistent with the approximated rate, the answer is confirmed. Because the calculated rate, 28.12 mL/h (rounded to 28.1 mL/h), accurately completes the (Step 2) equation and is consistent with the approximated rate, the answer is confirmed.

Example 3:   The aPTT is 135. The patient weighs 74 kg. The current weight-based heparin infusion rate, based on 19 units/kg/h, is running at 28.1 mL/h. Using the heparin protocol (Table 14-4) determine the following:

- Bolus dose and volume to administer
- Number of minutes to hold the infusion
- Hourly IV infusion dose and rate

With an aPTT of 135 seconds, there will be no bolus dose. The infusion will be held for 60 minutes, then decreased by 3 units/kg/h to 16 units/kg/h. To calculate the new infusion rate, use the heparin supply of 25,000 units in D_5W 500 mL (50 units/mL).

C: *Convert*—Because the order and supply are both in units, there is no conversion.

A: *Approximate*

Step 1: The ordered dose is 16 units per kg/h, so the patient will need more than 740 units/h (10 units/h times 74 kg) but less than 1,480 units/h (20 units/h times 74 kg).

Step 2: Because there are 50 units of heparin per 1 mL, the rate to administer 740–1,480 units/h will be between 14.8 mL/h and 30 mL/h.

S: *Solve*

Ratio-Proportion

Step 1: Calculate the dose in units/h:

$$\frac{16 \text{ units/h}}{1 \text{ kg}} = \frac{x \text{ units/h}}{74 \text{ kg}} \text{ or}$$

$$16 \text{ units} : 1 \text{ kg} = x \text{ units/h} : 74 \text{ kg}$$

$$x = 16 \times 74$$

$$x = 1.184$$

The patient's dose is 1,184 units/h.

Step 2: Calculate the volume to administer 1,184 units:

$$\frac{50 \text{ units}}{1 \text{ mL}} = \frac{1,184 \text{ units}}{x \text{ mL}} \text{ or}$$

$$50 \text{ units} : 1 \text{ mL} = 1,184 \text{ units} : x \text{ mL}$$

$$50x = 1,184$$

$$\frac{\cancel{50}x}{\cancel{50}} = \frac{1,184}{50}$$

$$x = 23.68 \text{ mL}$$

To administer 1,184 units/h, set the rate to 23.7 mL/h.

Formula Method

Step 1: Calculate the dose in units/h:

$$16 \text{ units/}\cancel{\text{kg}}\text{/h} \times 74 \text{ }\cancel{\text{kg}} = x \text{ (units/h)}$$

$$1,184 \text{ units/h} = x$$

The patient's dose is 1,184 units/h.

Step 2: Calculate the rate in mL/h:

$$\frac{1,184 \text{ }\cancel{\text{units}}\text{/h}}{50 \text{ }\cancel{\text{units}}} \times 1 \text{ mL} = x \text{(mL/h)}$$

$$\frac{1,184 \text{ mL/h}}{50} = x$$

$$23.68 \text{ mL/h} = x$$

To administer 1,184 units/h, set the rate to 23.7 mL/h.

Dimensional Analysis

Step 1 and step 2 are combined:

$$x \text{ (mL/h)} = \frac{1 \text{ mL}}{50 \text{ }\cancel{\text{units}}} \times \frac{16 \text{ }\cancel{\text{units}}}{1 \text{ }\cancel{\text{kg}}} \times \frac{74 \text{ }\cancel{\text{kg}}}{1} \times \frac{1}{1 \text{ h}}$$

$$x = \frac{1,184 \text{ mL}}{50 \text{ h}}$$

$$x = 23.68 \text{ mL/h}$$

To administer 1,184 units/h, set the rate to 23.7 mL/h.

E: *Evaluate*

Ratio-Proportion	Formula Method
Step 1: Calculate the dose in units/h: $\dfrac{16\ units/h}{1\ kg} = \dfrac{1{,}184\ units/h}{74\ kg}$ or 16 units/h : 1 kg = 1,184 units/h : 74 kg 16 × 74 = 1,184 1,184 = 1,184 Step 2: Calculate the volume to administer 1,184 units: $\dfrac{50\ units}{1\ mL} = \dfrac{1{,}184\ units}{23.68\ mL}$ or 50 units : 1 mL = 1,184 units : 23.68 mL 50 × 23.68 = 1,184 1,184 = 1,184	Step 1: Calculate the dose in units/h: 16 units/~~kg~~/h × 74 kg = 1,184 units/h 1,184 units/h = 1,184 units/h Step 2: Calculate the rate in mL/h: $\dfrac{1{,}184\ \text{~~units~~}/h}{50\ \text{~~units~~}} \times 1\ mL = 23.68\ mL/h$ $\dfrac{1{,}184\ mL/h}{50} = 23.68\ mL/h$ 23.68 mL/h = 23.68 mL/h

Dimensional Analysis

Step 1 and step 2 are combined:

$$23.68\ mL/h = \frac{1\ mL}{50\ \text{~~units~~}} \times \frac{16\ \text{~~units~~}}{1\ \text{~~kg~~}} \times \frac{74\ \text{~~kg~~}}{1} \times \frac{1}{1\ h}$$

$$23.68\ mL/h = \frac{1{,}184\ mL}{50\ h}$$

$$23.68\ mL/h = 23.68\ mL/h$$

Because the calculated dose, 1,184 units/h, accurately completes the (Step 1) calculation and is consistent with the approximated volume, the answer is confirmed. Because the calculated rate, 23.68 mL/h (rounded to 23.7 mL/h), accurately completes the (Step 2) equation and is consistent with the approximated rate, the answer is confirmed.

Clinical CLUE

When a calculated dose is higher than the maximum dose listed in the heparin protocol, the maximum dose should be administered, not the calculated dose. Double-check a "smart pump" to be sure the lower rate is infusing. These pumps have increased the rate to that calculated by the pump, administering too much heparin to the patient.

LEARNING ACTIVITY 14-10 Use the heparin protocol (Table 14-4) to calculate bolus dose in units, bolus amount to administer in mL, hourly IV dose in units/h, and hourly IV rate in mL/h.

1. Calculate the loading dose and initial infusion rate for a patient weighing 103 kg.
    Bolus dose: _____ Bolus volume: _____
    Hourly IV dose: _____ IV rate: _____

2. Determine the protocol changes for a patient weighing 56 kg whose aPTT is 58 seconds and current heparin drip is infusing at 17 units/kg/h, including length of time to hold the infusion, if necessary.
    Bolus dose: _____ Bolus volume: _____
    Hourly IV dose: _____ IV rate: _____
    Minutes to hold infusion: _____

Clinical CLUE

Different healthcare agencies may use different heparin protocols. Always follow an agency's protocol. Do not substitute one agency's protocol for another.

What's in a Unit? ... Case Closure

The nurse selected the wrong strength of insulin. The correct insulin was U-100 (100 units/mL) regular insulin (**Figure 14-51**). Because U-100 insulin syringes are designed to be used with U-100 concentration insulin, the dose was not accurately measured when U-500 insulin (500 units/mL) was used.

1. Using a U-100 insulin syringe, the nurse drew up and administered 0.04 mL (at the 4 unit calibration mark) of U-500 regular insulin instead of U-100 regular insulin. A ratio-proportion calculation reveals that 0.04 mL of U-500 insulin is 20 units:

$$\frac{500 \text{ units}}{1 \text{ mL}} = \frac{x \text{ units}}{0.04 \text{ mL}}$$
$$x = 20 \text{ units}$$

    The patient received five times the appropriate dose of insulin.

2. This could be avoided by reading the label three times, understanding that U-500 means 500 units/mL and that insulin syringes are only for U-100 (100 units/mL) insulin. Also, because insulin is a high-alert medication, the nurse should have had another nurse verify the units and the insulin used to prepare the dose to prevent this error. The pharmacy should stock only U-100 insulin on the unit; U-500 insulin should be sent to the floor labeled for the specific patient, if ordered.

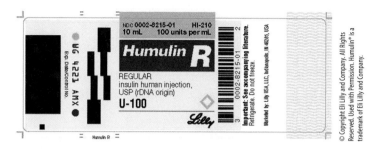

FIGURE 14-51   U-100 regular insulin.

Chapter Summary

Learning Outcomes	Points to Remember

14-1 Determine appropriate insulin, amount, and device.	Types of Insulin
	• Basal covers basic metabolic needs only:
	  o Intermediate-acting
	  o Long-acting
	• Mealtime (bolus dose) insulin is used to *prevent* increased blood glucose.
	• Correction (bolus dose) insulin covers increases in blood glucose levels that have *already occurred* from food or stressors:
	  o Rapid-acting
	  o Short-acting
	• Fixed combination:
	  o Premixed intermediate-acting and mealtime insulin
	Insulin Concentrations
	• U-100 (100 units/mL) is the standard insulin concentration; administer with U-100 insulin syringes calibrated in units.
	• Regular insulin comes in two concentrations:
	  o U-100 (100 units/mL) administered with U-100 insulin syringe, calibrated in units
	  o U-500 (500 units/mL); calculate amount and administer with 1 mL syringe
	Mixing intermediate and mealtime insulin in the same syringe: Withdraw mealtime before basal insulin: "clear before cloudy" or "fast first."

Correctional (Sliding Scale Insulin) Coverage
- PRN insulin orders are based on ranges of blood glucoses.
- The type and route of insulin are ordered.
- The frequency of blood glucose checks and PRN insulin dosages are ordered.

Insulin Pens
- Single patient use
- Prime before use, according to manufacturer's directions.
- Digital readouts can be misinterpreted if read upside down.
- Calculations for number of pens are based on the number of full doses per pen and the expiration date on the pen. Expiration may be earlier once pen is activated.

Insulin Pumps
- Infuse a basal rate of insulin 24 h/day.
- Patient can administer bolus doses to correct blood glucose elevations:
  - Total mealtime bolus dose = carbohydrate insulin dose + high blood glucose correction dose
  - Blood glucose correction factor = amount of insulin required to decrease the blood glucose by 50 mg/dL (determined by prescriber)
  - High blood glucose correction dose: amount of insulin required to lower the blood glucose (BG) to desired range:

$$\frac{\text{current BG (g/dL)} - \text{target BG(g/dL)}}{50 \text{ g/dL}} \times \text{BG correction factor (units)}$$
$$= \text{high BG correction dose (units)}$$

  - Carbohydrate insulin dose = amount of insulin required to dispose of the carbohydrates in the meal
  - Insulin-to-carbohydrate ratio (unit/g): amount of carbohydrates disposed by 1 unit of rapid-acting insulin (value provided by the prescriber)

$$\text{carbohydrate in meal (g)} \times \text{insulin to carb ratio (unit/g)}$$
$$= \text{carbohydrate insulin dose (units)}$$

14-2 Calculate heparin dosages for subcutaneous and intravenous administration.

Heparin—an anticoagulant (inhibits formation of blood clots):
- Unfractionated heparin (UF) has large molecules
- Low molecular weight heparin (LMWH) has small molecules

Calculating weight-based heparin IV boluses and hourly infusion
Step 1: Determine # of units patient requires.
Step 2: Determine # of mL to administer ordered dose.
IV Bolus Dose

Step 1:

$$\frac{\text{ordered units}}{1\,\text{kg}} = \frac{x\ \text{units to administer}}{\text{pt wt in kg}}$$

Step 2:
Ratio-Proportion

$$\frac{\text{units}}{1\,\text{mL}} = \frac{\text{units to administer}}{x\ \text{mL to adm}}$$

Formula Method

$$\frac{\text{units to adm}}{\text{units in supply}} \times \text{mL of supply} = x\ (\text{mL to adm})$$

Dimensional Analysis (combines Steps 1 and 2)

$$x\ (\text{mL to adm}) = \frac{\text{supply mL}}{\text{supply units}} \times \frac{\text{ordered units}}{1\,\text{kg}} \times \frac{\text{pt kg}}{1}$$

IV Infusion Rate
Step 1:

$$\frac{\text{ordered units/h}}{1\,\text{kg}} = \frac{x\ \text{units to administer/h}}{\text{pt wt in kg}}$$

Step 2:
Ratio-Proportion

$$\frac{\text{units/h}}{1\,\text{mL/h}} = \frac{\text{units to administer/h}}{x\ \text{mL/h to adm}}$$

Formula Method

$$\frac{\text{units/h to adm}}{\text{units in supply}} \times \text{mL of supply} = x\ (\text{mL/h to adm})$$

Dimensional Analysis (combines Steps 1 and 2)

$$x\ (\text{mL/h to adm}) = \frac{\text{supply mL}}{\text{supply units}} \times \frac{\text{ordered units}}{1\,\text{kg}} \times \frac{\text{pt's kg}}{1} \times \frac{1}{1\,\text{h}}$$

Weight-Based Heparin Protocol: Order set of weight-based PRN bolus doses and continuous infusion rates in response to activated partial thromboplastin time (aPTT), an anticoagulation blood test.
Rounding Rules:
- Weights are rounded to tenths.
- Infusion rates are rounded to the calibration of the infusion pump (tenths or whole number).

Homework

For exercises 1–6, refer to the following insulin labels and identify the brand and generic names of the insulin that correspond to each statement. (LO 14-1)

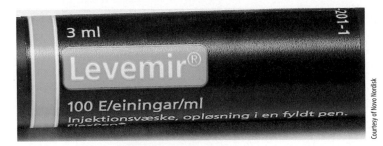

Courtesy of Novo Nordisk

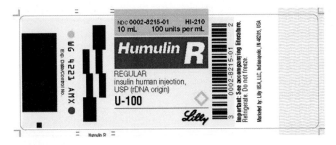

© Copyright Eli Lilly and Company. All Rights Reserved. Used with Permission. Humulin® is a trademark of Eli Lilly and Company.

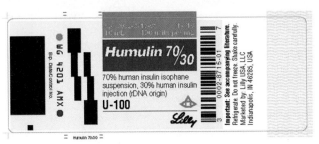

© Copyright Eli Lilly and Company. All Rights Reserved. Used with Permission. Humulin® is a trademark of Eli Lilly and Company.

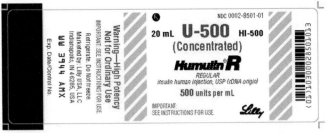

© Copyright Eli Lilly and Company. All Rights Reserved. Used with Permission. Humulin® is a trademark of Eli Lilly and Company.

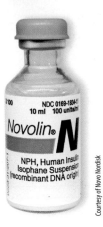

Courtesy of Novo Nordisk

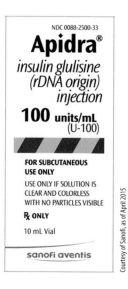

NDC 0088-2500-33

Apidra®

insulin glulisine
(rDNA origin)
injection

100 units/mL
(U-100)

FOR SUBCUTANEOUS
USE ONLY

USE ONLY IF SOLUTION IS
CLEAR AND COLORLESS
WITH NO PARTICLES VISIBLE

℞ ONLY

10 mL Vial

sanofi aventis

Courtesy of Sanofi, as of April 2015

1. Basal insulin that can be mixed with a mealtime insulin in the same syringe
2. Regular insulin that can be administered IV
3. Regular insulin that is administered in a syringe calibrated in milliliters
4. Rapid-acting insulin
5. Basal insulin that cannot be mixed with any other insulin in the same syringe
6. Contains both basal and mealtime insulin

For exercises 7–8, verify that the volume to administer yields the prescribed dose. If it does not, indicate the next action the nurse should take. (LO 14-1)

7. Humulin R U-500 regular insulin 280 units (0.52 mL) subcut before breakfast
8. Humulin R U-500 regular insulin 325 units (0.65 mL) subcut before breakfast

For exercises 9–16, mark the appropriate syringe with the ordered amount. (LO 14-1)

9. **Order:** Novolin N 30 units subcut bid before breakfast and dinner

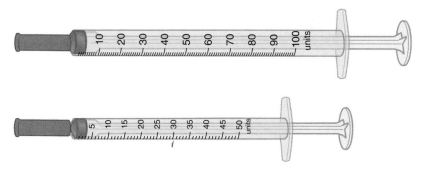

10. Levemir 50 units subcut daily before breakfast

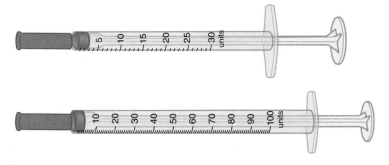

11. Novolin 70/30 insulin 32 units subcut bid before breakfast and dinner

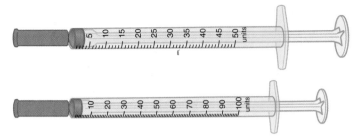

12. Novolin R regular insulin 4 units subcut qid ac and bedtime

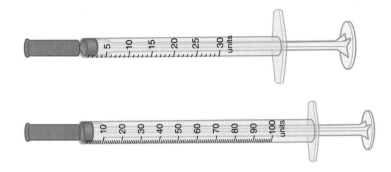

13. Insulin aspart 5 units subcut qid ac and bedtime

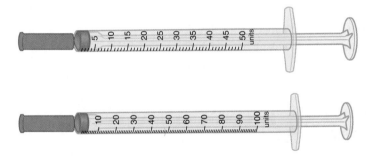

14. NovoLog 50/50 insulin 45 units subcut bid before breakfast and dinner

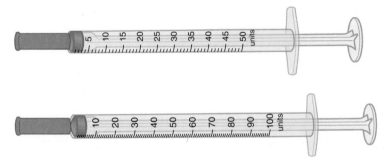

15. Insulin glulisine 10 units subcut tid ac

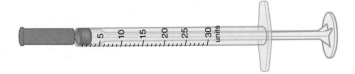

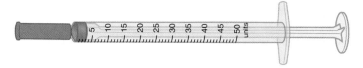

16. Humalog 75/25 37 units subcut bid before breakfast and dinner

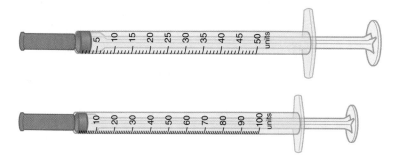

For exercises 17–23, indicate the amount of Humalog insulin using the moderate dose insulin scale. Refer to the following sliding scale insulin coverage order. (LO 14-1)

17. The blood glucose at 1200 is 360 mg/dL.
18. The blood glucose at 2100 is 196 mg/dL.
19. The blood glucose at 1800 is 84 mg/dL.
20. The blood glucose at 0800 is 273 mg/dL.
21. The blood glucose at 1100 is 52 mg/dL.
22. The blood glucose at 1730 is 333 mg/dL.
23. The blood glucose at 2130 is 420 mg/dL.

Humalog® Sliding Scale Subcutaneous Insulin Coverage

Capillary Blood Glucose (mg/dL)	▢ Low Dose	▢ Moderate Dose	▢ High Dose
Less than 70	Institute hypoglycemic protocol	Institute hypoglycemic protocol	Institute hypoglycemic protocol
Less than 145	No coverage	No coverage	No coverage
145–185	1 unit	2 units	3 units
186–225	2 units	3 units	4 units
226–245	3 units	4 units	5 units
246–275	4 units	5 units	6 units
276–315	5 units	6 units	7 units
Greater than 315	6 units	7 units	8 units

For exercises 24–28, mark the calibrations on the U-100 insulin syringe to which the plunger must be pulled to withdraw the basal and mealtime insulins. (LO 14-1)

24. Humulin N NPH insulin 20 units plus Humalog insulin 8 units subcut bid before breakfast and dinner

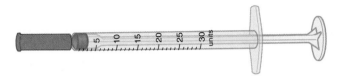

25. Novolin N NPH insulin 27 units plus Novolin R regular insulin 12 units subcut bid before breakfast and dinner

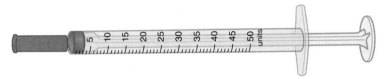

26. Humulin N NPH insulin 17 units plus Humulin R regular insulin 27 units subcut bid before breakfast and dinner

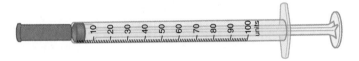

27. Novolin N NPH insulin 32 units plus NovoLog insulin 16 units subcut bid before breakfast and dinner

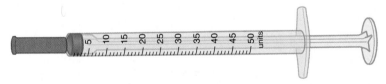

28. Humulin N NPH insulin 28 units plus insulin lispro 6 units subcut bid before breakfast and dinner

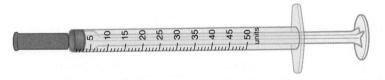

For exercises 29–32, calculate the high blood glucose correction dose, carbohydrate insulin dose, and the total mealtime insulin dose. (LO 14-1)

29. Current blood glucose 320 g/dL; target blood glucose 120 mg/dL; carbohydrate load 50 g; blood glucose correction factor 1 unit; insulin-to-carbohydrate ratio 1 unit/12 g

30. Current blood glucose 185 g/dL; target blood glucose 110 mg/dL; carbohydrate load 70 g; blood glucose correction factor 1 unit; insulin-to-carbohydrate ratio 1 unit/15 g

31. Current blood glucose 100 g/dL; target blood glucose 120 mg/dL; carbohydrate load 60 g; blood glucose correction factor 2 units; insulin-to-carbohydrate ratio 1 unit/14 g

32. Current blood glucose 150 g/dL; target blood glucose 120 mg/dL; carbohydrate load 45 g; blood glucose correction factor 2 units; insulin-to-carbohydrate ratio 1 unit/13 g

For exercises 33–36, determine the number of pens and packs needed for the time frames and orders. (LO 14-1)

33. **Time frame:** 8 weeks

    Order: Humalog cartridge 6 units subcut tid ac

34. **Time frame:** 12 weeks

    Order: Humalog Mix 75/25 53 units subcut bid before breakfast and dinner

35. **Time frame:** 4 weeks

    Order: Humalog KwikPen 8 units subcut tid ac

36. **Time frame:** 6 weeks

    Order: Humalog Mix 50/50 4 units subcut bid before breakfast and dinner

For examples 37–43, calculate the weight-based heparin IV bolus dose. Use heparin 1,000 units/mL. (LO 14-2)

37. **Patient's weight:** 45 kg

    Dose: heparin 35 units/kg

38. **Patient's weight:** 97 kg

    Dose: heparin 40 units/kg

39. **Patient's weight:** 72 kg

    Dose: heparin 80 units/kg

40. **Patient's weight:** 110 kg

    Dose: heparin 65 units/kg

41. **Patient's weight:** 50 kg

    Dose: heparin 78 units/kg

42. **Patient's weight:** 67 kg

    Dose: heparin 80 units/kg

43. **Patient's weight:** 80 kg

    Dose: heparin 40 units/kg

For examples 44–50, calculate the weight-based heparin IV infusion rate in mL/h. The infusion pump is calibrated to the tenth. (LO 14-2)

44. **Patient's weight:** 90 kg

    Hourly dose: heparin 18 units/kg/h

    Supply: heparin 25,000 units in D_5W 500 mL

45. **Patient's weight:** 86 kg

    Hourly dose: heparin 18 units/kg/h

    Supply: heparin 25,000 units in D_5W 250 mL

46. **Patient's weight:** 70 kg

    Hourly dose: heparin 21 units/kg/h

    Supply: heparin 25,000 units in D_5W 500 mL

47. **Patient's weight:** 80 kg

    Hourly dose: heparin 22 units/kg/h

    Supply: heparin 25,000 units in D_5W 500 mL

48. **Patient's weight:** 98 kg

    Hourly dose: heparin 20 units/kg/h

    Supply: heparin 25,000 units in D_5W 250 mL

49. **Patient's weight:** 65 kg

    Hourly dose: heparin 19 units/kg/h

    Supply: heparin 25,000 units in D_5W 500 mL

50. **Patient's weight:** 120 kg

    Hourly dose: heparin 17 units/kg/h

    Supply: heparin 25,000 units in D_5W 250 mL

NCLEX-Style Review Questions

For questions 1–6, select the best response.

1. The doctor orders Humulin R U-500 regular insulin 240 units subcut now. The nurse should: (LO 14-1)

   a. Fill a low-dose insulin syringe to the 5 mark.

   b. Fill a standard insulin syringe to the 50 mark.

   c. Fill a 1 mL syringe to the 0.48 mark.

   d. Fill a 5 mL syringe to the 4.8 mark.

2. The patient's blood glucose is 150 g/dL, the target blood glucose is 120 g/dL, and the blood glucose correction factor is 2 units. The high blood glucose correction dose of Humalog subcut is: (LO 14-1)

   a. 1 unit

   b. 1.2 units

   c. 2 units

   d. 2.1 units

3. The doctor ordered: Humalog Mix 75/25 KwikPen 70 units subcut before breakfast and 56 units subcut before dinner. Each pen lasts 10 days. How many packs of pens (5 pens, 3 mL each/pack) should the nurse order for a 28-day supply? (LO 14-1)

   a. 1 pack

   b. 2 packs

   c. 3 packs

   d. 4 packs

   e. 5 packs

4. The doctor orders an infusion of heparin 21 units/kg/h IV for a patient weighing 85 kg. The pharmacy supplies heparin 25,000 units in D_5W 500 mL. The available infusion pump is calibrated to the tenths.

The nurse sets the rate of the infusion pump for: (LO 12-2)

a. 17 mL/h
b. 17.9 mL/h
c. 21 mL/h
d. 35.7 mL/h
e. 36 mL/h

5. The doctor orders heparin 2,500 units IV subcut. The most appropriate concentration of heparin is: (LO 14-2)

a. 100 units/mL prefilled 10 mL syringe
b. 1,000 units/mL multi-dose vial
c. 5,000 units/mL multi-dose vial
d. 10,000 units/mL single-dose vial
e. 20,000 units/mL single-dose vial

6. The patient, weighing 60 kg, has heparin 25,000 units in D_5W 500 mL infusing at 20 units/kg/h. At 1300 the aPTT is 170 seconds. The protocol orders: aPTT 150–200 seconds, no bolus dose, hold infusion 90 minutes, decrease infusion by 4 units/kg/h, and repeat aPTT 6 hours after infusion resumed. The nurse should turn the infusion off, and at 1430 resume the infusion at: (LO 14-2)

a. 16 mL/h, recheck aPTT at 1930
b. 19 mL/h, recheck aPTT at 2030
c. 20 mL/h, recheck aPTT at 1930
d. 20.7 mL/h, recheck aPTT at 2030

REFERENCES

Becker, R.C., Cannon, C.P., Tracy, R.P., Thompson, B., Bovill, E. G., Desvigne-Nickens, P., … Braunwald, E. (1996). Relation between systemic anticoagulation as determined by activated partial thromboplastin time and heparin measurements and in-hospital clinical events in unstable angina and non-Q wave myocardial infarction. Thrombolysis in myocardial ischemia III B investigators. *American Heart Journal, 131*(3), 421–433.

Davis, E. M., Foral, P. A., Dull, R. B., Smith, A. N. (2013). Review of insulin therapy and pen use in hospitalized patients. *Hospital Pharmacy, 48*(5), 396–405. doi:10.1310/hpj4805-396. Retrieved from http://www.ncbi.nlm.nih.gov/pmc/articles/PMC3839460/

Gebel, E. (2012). 2012 Insulin pens. *Diabetes Forecast.* Retrieved from http://forecast.diabetes.org/magazine/features/2012-insulin-pens

Hammami, M. B. (2013). Partial thromboplastin time, activated. Retrieved from http://emedicine.medscape.com/article/2085837-overview

Institute for Safe Medication Practices. (2011). *ISMP quarterly action agenda.* Retrieved from http://www.ismp.org/Newsletters/acutecare/articles/ActionAgenda1104.doc

Institute for Safe Medication Practices. (2012a). Action needed to prevent dangerous heparin-insulin confusion. *ISMP Medication Safety Alert.* Retrieved from http://www.ismp.org/Newsletters/acutecare/articles/20070503.asp

Institute for Safe Medication Practices. (2012b). *ISMP list of high-alert medications.* Retrieved from http://www.ismp.org/tools/institutionalhighAlert.asp

Institute for Safe Medication Practices. (2015). A clinical reminder about the safe use of insulin vials. *IMSP medication safety alert.* Retrieved from http://www.ismp.org/Newsletter/acutecare/showarticle.aspx?id=42

Jacobi, J., Bircher, N., Krinsley, J., Agus, M., Braithwaite, S. S., Deutschman, C., … Schunemann, H. (2012). Guidelines for the use of an insulin infusion for the management of hyperglycemia in critically ill patients. *Critical Care Medicine, 40*(12), 3251–3276.

Keller, J. E. (2011). Insulin dosing made simple. *Correct Care Journal.* National Commission on Correctional Health. Retrieved from http://www.ncchc.org/puBG/CC/insulin_dosing.html

Lehman, C. M., & Frank, E. L. (2009). Laboratory monitoring of heparin therapy: Partial thromboplastin time or anti-Xa assay? *LabMedicine, 40*, 47–51. doi: 10.1309/LM9NJGW2ZIOLPHY6

Magaji, V., & Johnston, J. M. (2011). Inpatient management of hyperglycemia and diabetes. *Clinical Diabetes, 29*, (1), 3–9.

Neithercott, T. (2012). 2012 consumer guide: Insulin pumps. *Diabetes Forecast.* Retrieved from http://forecast.diabetes.org/magazine/features/2012-insulin-pumps

Spollet, G. R. (2012). Improved disposable insulin pen devices provide an alternative to vials and syringes for insulin administration. *Diabetes Spectrum, 25*(2), 117–122. Retrieved from http://spectrum.diabetesjournals.org/content/25/2/117.full.pdf+html

Chapter 14   ANSWER KEY

Learning Activity 14-1

1.   Novolin N (Figure 14-19)
2.   NovoLog (Figure 14-20)

Learning Activity 14-2

1.   Lantus insulin (Figure 14-26)

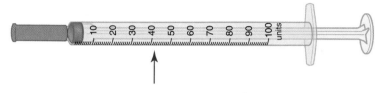

2.   Humulin R U-500 insulin (Figure 14-22)

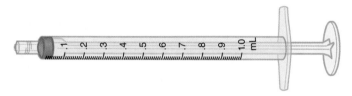

3.   Humalog 50/50 insulin (Figure 14-24)

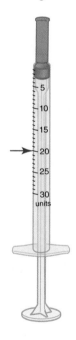

Learning Activity 14-3

1.   7 units
2.   5 units
3.   3 units

Learning Activity 14-4

1.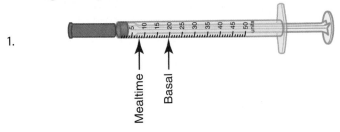

2.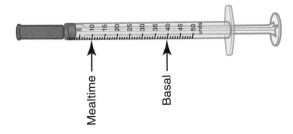

3.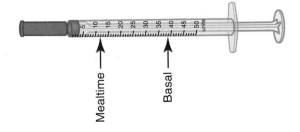

Learning Activity 14-5
1. Two pens required, one pen pack required
2. Two pens required, one pen pack required

Learning Activity 14-6
1. High blood sugar correction dose: 2.4 units
   Carbohydrate insulin dose: 8 units
   Total mealtime bolus dose: 10 units
2. High blood sugar correction dose: 0 units
   Carbohydrate insulin dose: 9 units
   Total mealtime bolus dose: 9 units

Learning Activity 14-7
1. Heparin 5,000 units/mL (Figure 14-48)   1 mL or
   Heparin 10,000 units/mL (Figure 14-46)   0.5 mL
2. Heparin 10,000 units/mL (Figure 14-46)   0.8 mL

Learning Activity 14-8
1. Dose: 2,400 units
   Administer: 2.4 mL
2. Calculated dose: 4,200 units; maximum dose 3,500 units; give 3,500 units
   Administer: 3.5 mL

Learning Activity 14-9

1. Dose: 1,800 units/h
   Rate: 36 mL/h
2. Dose: 1,600 units/h
   Rate: 16 mL/h

Learning Activity 14-10

1. Bolus dose calculation—8,240 units; maximum amount 8,000 units, administer 8 mL
   IV rate calculation—1,854 units/h; maximum rate 1,800 units/h, set rate at 36 mL/h
2. Bolus dose—2,240 units; bolus volume—2.2 mL
   Hourly IV dose: 19 units/kg/h = 1,064 units/h; IV rate—21.3 mL/h or 21 mL/h
   Minutes to hold: none

Homework

1. Novolin N NPH insulin
2. Humulin R regular insulin U-100
3. Humulin R regular insulin U-500
4. Apidra insulin glulisine
5. Levemir insulin detemir
6. Humulin 70/30 insulin
7. 0.52 mL is incorrect, volume should be 0.56 mL; call the prescriber to clarify dose before proceeding.
8. 0.65 mL is correct volume to administer.

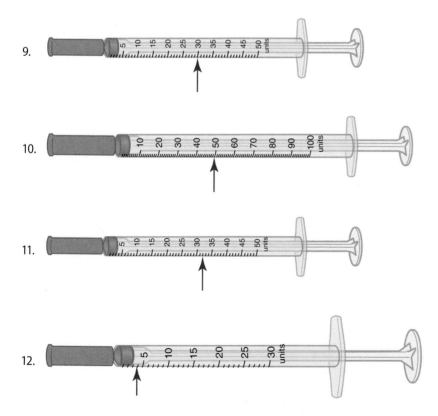

9.

10.

11.

12.

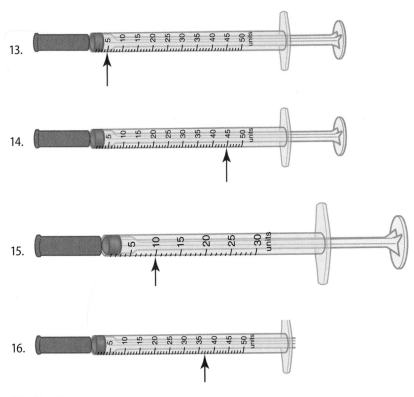

13.
14.
15.
16.

17. 7 units
18. 3 units
19. No coverage
20. 5 units
21. Institute hypoglycemic protocol
22. 7 units
23. 7 units

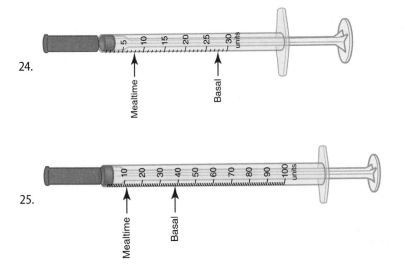

24.
25.

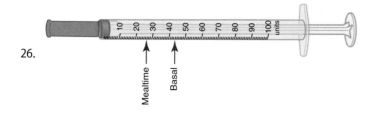

26.

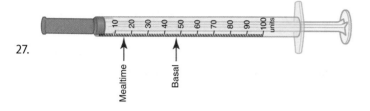

27.

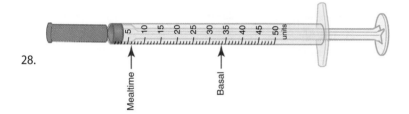

28.

29. High blood sugar correction dose: 4 units
    Carbohydrate insulin dose: 4 units
    Total mealtime insulin dose: 8

30. High blood sugar correction dose: 1.5 units
    Carbohydrate insulin dose: 4.6 units
    Total mealtime insulin dose: 6 units

31. High blood sugar correction dose: 0 units
    Carbohydrate insulin dose: 3 units
    Total mealtime insulin dose: 3 units

32. High blood sugar correction dose: 1.2 units
    Carbohydrate insulin dose: 5.6 units
    Total mealtime insulin dose: 6 units

33. Pens: 4
    Packages: 1

34. Pens: 34
    Packages: 7

35. Pens: 3
    Packages: 1

36. Pens: 5 (20 doses per pen due to 10-day expiration)
    Packages: 1

37. 1,575 units; 1.6 mL
38. 3,880 units; 3.9 mL
39. 5,760 units; 5.8 mL
40. 7,150 units; 7.2 mL
41. 3,900 units; 3.9 mL
42. 5,360 units; 5.4 mL
43. 3,200 units; 3.2 mL

44. 1,620 units/h; 32.4 mL/h
45. 1,548 units/h; 15.5 mL/h
46. 1,470 units/h; 29.4 mL/h
47. 1,760 units/h; 35.2 mL/h
48. 1,960 units/h; 19.6 mL/h
49. 1,235 units/h; 24.7 mL/h
50. 2,040 units/h; 20.4 mL/h

NCLEX-Style Review Questions

1. c
   Rationale: $x \text{ (mL)} = \frac{1 \text{ mL}}{500 \text{ units}} \times \frac{240 \text{ units}}{1}$; $x = 0.48$ mL. To administer 240 units from a supply of 500 units/mL, draw up 0.48 mL in a 1 mL syringe.

2. b
   Rationale:

$$\frac{\text{current BS} (150 \text{ mg/dL}) - \text{target BS}(120 \text{ mg/dL})}{50 \text{ mg/dL}}$$

$$\times \text{ BS correction factor (2 units)}$$

$$= \text{high BS correction dose (1.2 units)}$$

3. c
   Rationale: The daily dose is 126 units, and there are 300 units in each pen, yielding 2 full daily doses. Because each pen is good for 2 days, 14 pens are required for 28 days. Each package contains 5 pens, so there are 15 pens in 3 packages. 3 packages will provide 28 days, with 1 pen remaining.

4. d
   Rationale: 21 units/kg/h multiplied by the patient's weight of 85 kg yields 1,785 units/h. This rate divided by the concentration of heparin, 50 units/mL, is 35.7 mL/h.

5. c
   Rationale: The 5,000 unit/mL concentration provides the ordered dose in 0.5 mL and is in a multi-dose vial. This is the only choice that provides the dose in less than 1 mL, as needed for subcut injections, without wasting the remaining heparin. The other choices that meet the volume requirement are in single-dose vials and would need to be discarded after one use.

6. b
   Rationale: At 1430, after holding the infusion for 1.5 hours, the heparin should infuse at 16 units/kg/h, which is 960 units/h. With a concentration of 50 units/mL, the new rate is 19.2 mL/h, which can round down to 19 mL/h. Adding 6 hours to the start time of 1430 gives a lab time for aPTT of 2030.

© Forfunlife/Shutterstock

Chapter 15

Critical Care Calculations

CHAPTER OUTLINE

LEARNING OUTCOMES

Upon completion of the chapter, the student will be able to:

15-1 Calculate intravenous infusion flow rate based on dosage per time.

15-2 Calculate intravenous infusion flow rate based on dosage per body weight and time.

15-3 Calculate the dose delivered by a specified intravenous rate.

15-4 Calculate titrated intravenous infusion flow rates within prescribed parameters.

KEY TERMS

analgesic

antiarrhythmic

anxiolytic

neuromuscular blocking
   agent

titrate

total volume

vasoactive

Case Consideration ... Multiple Mix-Up

The patient's blood pressure was falling and the provider ordered a continuous IV infusion of dopamine 5 mcg/kg/min for a patient who weighed 188 lb. The nurse was supplied a premixed bag of dopamine with the approved concentration of 1,600 mcg/mL. Based on the following calculations, the nurse started the infusion at 18 mL/h.

Convert: $188 \text{ lb} \times \frac{1 \text{ kg}}{2.2 \text{ lb}} = 85.4545 \text{ kg}$, which rounds to 85.5 kg

Calculate the weight-based dose: 5 mcg × 85.5 kg = 427.5 mcg/min

Calculate the per minute rate:

$$427.5 \text{ mcg/min} \div 1,600 \text{ mcg/mL} = 0.26719 \text{ mL/min, which rounds to } 0.3 \text{ mL/min}$$

Calculate the hourly rate: 0.3 mL/min × 60 min/h = 18 mL/h

1. What went wrong?
2. How could this situation been avoided?

■ INTRODUCTION

Stabilizing critically ill patients can require multiple potent intravenous (IV) medications to regulate heart rate and rhythm, blood pressure, and cardiac output. Continuous infusions of narcotics, sedatives, and **neuromuscular blocking agents** (paralytic medications) may be infused. As with heparin, these high-alert medications are prescribed as a dose over time, or as a weight-based dose over time. Although there have been some instances in the past in which critical care medications have been administered through volume-control tubing with microdrop calibration, critical care medications should be administered via infusion pumps. Most infusion pumps used in these settings are calibrated to tenths of a milliliter, so infusion rates in this chapter will be rounded to tenths.

15-1   Intravenous Infusion Flow Rate Calculations for Dosage per Time

Medication dosages can be written as continuous IV infusions with amount of medication per hour (e.g., 10 mg/h) or per minute (e.g., 5 mcg/min). The nurse then converts this amount into a rate to program the infusion device in mL/h.

Rounding RULES!

- Round weights to tenths, because most digital scales in critical care settings are calibrated to measure weights to tenths (0.1) of a kilogram or tenths of a pound.
- Round infusion rates according to the infusion pump calibration (whole number or tenths). Because most infusion devices in critical care areas are calibrated to tenths, round critical care infusions to tenths (0.1) of a milliliter.
- If a calculation requires multiple steps, rounding should occur once at the end or as the last step of the equation.

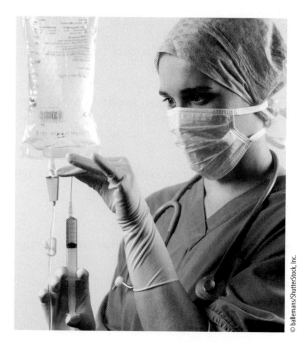

© ballemans/ShutterStock, Inc.

FIGURE 15-1   To prepare a medicated IV, the nurse first withdraws from the solution container the amount of fluid equal to the volume to be added.

Clinical CLUE

Care must be taken to ensure accuracy in dosage calculation and administration. To facilitate calculating the proper dose, the **total volume** of medication and IV solution is used for the supply volume. For simplicity, when preparing a medicated IV solution, the same volume of medication to be added to the IV solution will be removed from the IV bag prior to adding the medication (see **Figure 15-1**). For example, if the amount of medication to be added to the IV solution in a 500 mL bag is 20 mL, then 20 mL of IV solution will be removed from the bag before adding the 20 mL of medication to the bag. By doing this, the total volume in the IV bag will remain 500 mL. For additional examples, see Clinical Applications 1–3 in first section of chapter.

WARNING!

Miscalculation and Infusion Pump Operator Error Can Cause Overdose!

The U.S. Food and Drug Administration (FDA, 2012) issued this nursing-related postmarketing adverse reaction alert for an IV cardiac medication administered in critical care units: "Overdose with … therapy has been reported and is primarily the result of either a *miscalculated … dose* or a mechanical error such as an infusion-pump malfunction or an *infusion-pump programming error* [emphasis added]."

Nurses can and do make errors when working with high-alert medications. Never make assumptions; verify calculations and programming with a second nurse before administering high-alert medications.

Clinical CLUE

To simplify the math, critical care nurses often reduce the supply ratio to lowest terms. When delivering a medication over time, the supply is the IV solution. If the IV solution is 500 mL containing 500 mg, the supply is reduced to 1 mg per 1 mL.

Medications Infused per Hour

When calculating the infusion rate for medication dosages of continuous IV medication per time, use the IV solution as the supply and apply the CASE method.

Example 1:   Use the following order and supply to calculate the infusion rate in mL/h.

Order: morphine sulfate 2.5 mg/h

Supply: morphine sulfate 50 mg in normal saline, total volume 100 mL

Reduced supply: 1 mg/2 mL because $\frac{50 \text{ mg}}{100 \text{ mL}} = \frac{1 \text{ mg}}{2 \text{ mL}}$

C: *Convert*—Not applicable (N/A): The order and supply are both in milligrams.

A: *Approximate*—The ordered dose is 2.5 mg/h. Because there is 1 mg of morphine per 2 mL, the administration rate will be twice as large as the dose (2.5) or 5 mL/h.

S: *Solve*

Ratio-Proportion	Formula Method
$\frac{1 \text{ mg}}{2 \text{ mL}} = \frac{2.5 \text{ mg/h}}{x \text{ mL/h}}$ or 1 mg : 2 mL = 2.5 mg/h : x mL/h $x = 2.5 \times 2$ $x = 5$ mL/h	$\frac{2.5 \text{ mg/h}}{1 \text{ mg}} \times 2 \text{ mL} = x \text{ (mL/h)}$ $\frac{5 \text{ mL / h}}{1} = x$ 5 mL / h = x

Dimensional Analysis	
$x \text{ (mL/h)} = \frac{2 \text{ mL}}{1 \text{ mg}} \times \frac{2.5 \text{ mg}}{1 \text{ h}}$ $x = \frac{5 \text{ mL}}{1 \text{ h}}$ $x = 5$ mL/h	

E: *Evaluate*

Ratio-Proportion	Formula Method
$\frac{1 \text{ mg}}{2 \text{ mL}} = \frac{2.5 \text{ mg/h}}{5 \text{ mL/h}}$ or 1 mg : 2 mL = 2.5 mg/h : 5 mL/h $2 \times 2.5 = 1 \times 5$ 5 = 5	$\frac{2.5 \text{ mg/h}}{1 \text{ mg}} \times 2 \text{ mL} = 5 \text{ mL/h}$ $\frac{5 \text{ mL/h}}{1} = 5$ mL/h 5 mL/h = 5 mL/h

Dimensional Analysis

$$5 \text{ mL/h} = \frac{2 \text{ mL}}{1 \text{ mg}} \times \frac{2.5 \text{ mg}}{1 \text{ h}}$$

$$5 \text{ mL/h} = \frac{5 \text{ mL}}{1 \text{ h}}$$

$$5 \text{ mL/h} = 5 \text{ mL/h}$$

Because the calculated amount, 5 mL/h, accurately completes the equation, and the calculated rate is consistent with the approximated rate of 5 mL/h, the answer is confirmed (see Clinical Application 1 for mixing the supply).

Clinical Application 1 ... Mix the Ordered IV Solution

Morphine 50 mg in normal saline 100 mL is ordered. Prepare the IV solution so that the total volume remains 100 mL.

Supply: morphine 10 mg/mL in a 10 mL multiple dose vial; normal saline 100 mL infusion bag

Step 1: Apply the CASE method and calculate the volume of morphine to remove from the vial, which is 5 mL.

Step 2: Remove 5 mL of normal saline from the IV bag and discard.

Step 3: Withdraw 5 mL of morphine from the multiple-dose vial and inject it into the bag containing normal saline 95 mL. Morphine 5 mL + normal saline 95 mL = 100 mL total volume.

Example 2: Use the following order and supply to calculate the infusion rate in mL/h.

Order: octreotide 25 mcg/h

Supply: octreotide 600 mcg in normal saline, total volume 250 mL

Reduced supply: 2.4 mcg/1 mL because $\frac{600 \text{ mcg}}{250 \text{ mL}} = \frac{2.4 \text{ mcg}}{1 \text{ mL}}$

C: *Convert*—N/A: The order and supply are both in micrograms.

A: *Approximate*—Because the ordered dose of 25 is a little more than 10 times 2.4, the rate to administer will be a little more than 10 mL/h (24 mg/h).

S: *Solve*

Ratio-Proportion	Formula Method
$\dfrac{2.4 \text{ mcg}}{1 \text{ mL}} = \dfrac{25 \text{ mcg/h}}{x \text{ mL/h}}$ or 2.4 mcg: 1mL = 25 mcg/h : x mL/h $2.4x = 25$ $\dfrac{2.4x}{2.4} = \dfrac{25}{2.4}$ $x = 10.41667$	$\dfrac{25 \; \cancel{\text{mcg}}/h}{2.4 \; \cancel{\text{mcg}}} \times 1 \text{ mL} = x \text{ (mL/h)}$ $\dfrac{25 \text{ mL/h}}{2.4} = x$ $10.41667 \text{ mL/h} = x$

Dimensional Analysis

$$x \text{ (mL/h)} = \frac{1 \text{ mL}}{2.4 \; \cancel{\text{mcg}}} \times \frac{25 \; \cancel{\text{mcg}}}{1 \text{ h}}$$

$$x = \frac{25 \text{ mL}}{2.4 \text{ h}}$$

$$x = 10.41667 \text{ mL/h}$$

E: *Evaluate*

Ratio-Proportion	Formula Method
$\dfrac{2.4 \text{ mcg}}{1 \text{ mL}} = \dfrac{25 \text{ mcg/h}}{10.41667 \text{ mL/h}}$ or 2.4 mcg : 1 mL = 25 mcg/h : 10.41667 mL/h $2.4 \times 10.41667 = 1 \times 25$ $25.00001 \cong 25$	$\dfrac{25 \; \cancel{\text{mcg}}/h}{2.4 \; \cancel{\text{mcg}}} \times 1 \text{ mL} = 10.41667$ $\dfrac{25 \text{ mL/h}}{2.4} = 10.41667$ $10.41667 \text{ mL/h} = 10.41667$

Dimensional Analysis

$$10.41667 \text{ mL/h} = \frac{1 \text{ mL}}{2.4 \; \cancel{\text{mcg}}} \times \frac{25 \; \cancel{\text{mcg}}}{1 \text{ h}}$$

$$10.41667 \text{ mL/h} = \frac{25 \text{ mL}}{2.4 \text{ h}}$$

$$10.41667 \text{ mL/h} = 10.41667 \text{ mL/h}$$

Because the calculated amount, 10.4 mL/h, accurately completes the equation, and the calculated rate is consistent with the approximated rate of a little more than 10 mL/h, the answer is confirmed (see Clinical Application 2 to mix the supply).

Clinical Application 2 ... Mix the Ordered IV Solution

Octreotide 600 mcg in normal saline 250 mL is ordered. Prepare the IV solution so that the total volume remains 250 mL.

Supply: octreotide 200 mcg/mL in a 500 mL multi-dose vial

Step 1: Apply the CASE method and calculate the volume of octreotide to remove from the vial, which is 3 mL.

Step 2: Remove 3 mL of normal saline from the IV bag and discard.

Step 3: Withdraw 3 mL of octreotide from the multiple dose vial and inject it into the bag containing normal saline 247 mL. Octreotide 3 mL + normal saline 247 mL = 250 mL total volume.

Example 3: Use the following order and supply to calculate the infusion rate in mL/h.

Order: lorazepam 0.5 mg/h

Supply: lorazepam 4 mg in D_5W 40 mL total volume

Reduced supply: 0.1 mg/1 mL because $\dfrac{4 \text{ mg}}{40 \text{ mL}} = \dfrac{0.1 \text{ mg}}{1 \text{ mL}}$

C: *Convert*—N/A: The order and supply are both in milligrams.

A: *Approximate*—Because the ordered dose of 0.5 is a 5 times 0.1, the rate to administer will be 5 mL/h (0.5mg/h).

S: *Solve*

Ratio-Proportion	Formula Method
$\dfrac{0.1 \text{ mg}}{1 \text{ mL}} = \dfrac{0.5 \text{ mg/h}}{x \text{ mL/h}}$ or $0.1 \text{ mg} : 1 \text{ mL} = 0.5 \text{ mg/h} : x \text{ mL/h}$ $0.1x = 0.5$ $\dfrac{0.1x}{0.1} = \dfrac{0.5}{0.1}$ $x = 5 \text{ mL/h}$	$\dfrac{0.5 \; \cancel{\text{mg}}/h}{0.1 \; \cancel{\text{mg}}} \times 1 \text{ mL} = x \text{ (mL/h)}$ $\dfrac{0.5 \text{ mL/h}}{0.1} = x$ $5 \text{ mL/h} = x$

Dimensional Analysis
$x \text{ (mL/h)} = \dfrac{1 \text{ mL}}{0.1 \; \cancel{\text{mg}}} \times \dfrac{0.5 \; \cancel{\text{mg}}}{1 \text{ h}}$ $x = \dfrac{0.5 \text{ mL}}{0.1 \text{ h}}$ $x = 5 \text{ mL/h}$

Clinical Application 3 ... Mix the Ordered IV Solution

Lorazepam 4 mg in D_5W 40 mL is ordered. Prepare the IV solution so that the total volume remains 40 mL.

Supply: Lorazepam 4 mg/mL ampule; D_5W 50 mL IV bag

Step 1: Apply the CASE method and calculate the volume of lorazepam to remove from the vial, which is 1 mL.

Step 2: Remove 11 mL of normal saline from the IV bag and discard. Because the IV bag contains 10 mL more than the total volume ordered, 10 mL of D_5W must be removed in addition to the 1 mL that would be removed to accommodate the 1 mL of lorazepam, which will be added.

Step 3: Withdraw 1 mL of lorazepam from the ampule and inject it into the bag containing D_5W 39 mL. Lorazepam 1 mL + D_5W 39 mL = 40 mL total volume.

E: *Evaluate*

Ratio-Proportion	Formula Method
$\dfrac{0.1\,mg}{1\,mL} = \dfrac{0.5\,mg/h}{5\,mL/h}$ or 0.1 mg : 1 mL = 0.5 mg/h : 5 mL/h $0.1 \times 5 = 1 \times 0.5$ $0.5 = 0.5$	$\dfrac{0.5\,\cancel{mg}/h}{0.1\,\cancel{mg}} \times 1\,mL = 5\,mL/h$ $\dfrac{0.5\,mL/h}{0.1} = 5\,mL/h$ $5\,mL/h = 5\,mL/h$

Dimensional Analysis
$5\,mL/h = \dfrac{1\,mL}{0.1\,\cancel{mg}} \times \dfrac{0.5\,\cancel{mg}}{1\,h}$ $5\,mL/h = \dfrac{0.5\,mL}{0.1\,h}$ $5\,mL/h = 5\,mL/h$

Because the calculated amount, 5 mL/h, accurately completes the equation, and the calculated rate is consistent with the approximated rate of 5 mL/h, the answer is confirmed (see Clinical Application 3 to mix the supply).

LEARNING ACTIVITY 15-1 Using the following orders and supplies, determine the reduced supply (lowest terms), then calculate the infusion rate in mL/h.

1. **Order:** morphine sulfate 1.5 mg/h
   Supply: morphine sulfate 25 mg in normal saline, total volume 100 mL

2. **Order:** octreotide 30 mcg/h
   Supply: octreotide 0.5 mg in normal saline, total volume 500 mL

3. **Order:** lorazepam 0.1 mg/h IV
   Supply: lorazepam 2 mg in NS 50 mL total volume

Medications Infused per Minute

When using ratio-proportion and the formula method, calculating an infusion rate when the dose is ordered in mcg or mg per minute is a two-step process, because the order first needs to be converted from minutes to 1 hour. The following examples convert the order from "per 1 minute" to "per 1 hour," by multiplying it by 60 min/h. When using dimensional analysis, step 1 and step 2 are combined by including the conversion factor, 60 min/1 h, in the equation.

Example 1:   Use the following order and supply to calculate the infusion rate in mL/h, rounded to tenths.

Order: amiodarone 1 mg/min, to infuse IV over 6 hours

Supply: amiodarone 900 mg in D_5W 500 mL total volume

Reduced supply: 1.8 mg/1 mL

C: *Convert*—N/A: The order and supply are both milligrams.

A: *Approximate*

Step 1: Estimate the hourly dose.

The ordered dose is 1 mg per minute, and there are 60 minutes in 1 hour, so the patient will need 60 mg/h.

Step 2: Estimate the hourly rate.

There are 1.8 mg/mL, which is close to but less than 2 mg/mL. 60 is 30 times larger than 2, so the IV will infuse at more than 30 mL/h.

S: *Solve*

Ratio-Proportion	Formula Method
Step 1: Calculate the hourly dose: $$\frac{1\ mg}{1\ min} = \frac{x\ mg/h}{60\ min/h}\ \ \text{or}$$ 1 mg : 1 min = x mg/h : 60 min/h x = 60 mg/h **Hourly dose is 60 mg/h.**	Step 1: Calculate the hourly dose: $$\frac{1\ mg}{1\ \cancel{min}} \times 60\ \cancel{min}/h = x\ (mg/h)$$ 1 mg × 60 / h = x 60 mg/h = x **Hourly dose is 60 mg/h.**
Step 2: Calculate the hourly rate: $$\frac{1.8\ mg}{1\ mL} = \frac{60\ mg/h}{x\ mL/h}\ \ \text{or}$$ 1.8 mg : 1 mL = 60 mg/h : x mL/h 1.8x = 60 $$\frac{\cancel{1.8}x}{\cancel{1.8}} = \frac{60}{1.8}$$ x = 33.33 mL/h **Hourly rate is 33.3 mL/h** to infuse for 6 h.	Step 2: Calculate the hourly rate: $$\frac{60\ \cancel{mg}/h}{1.8\ \cancel{mg}} \times 1\ mL = x\ (mL/h)$$ $$\frac{60\ mL/h}{1.8} = x$$ 33.33 mL/h = x **Hourly rate is 33.3 mL/h** to infuse for 6 h.

Dimensional Analysis

Step 1 and step 2 are combined:

$$x \text{ (mL/h)} = \frac{1 \text{ mL}}{1.8 \text{ mg}} \times \frac{1 \text{ mg}}{1 \text{ min}} \times \frac{60 \text{ min}}{1 \text{ h}}$$

$$x = \frac{60 \text{ mL}}{1.8 \text{ h}}$$

$$x = 33.33 \text{ mL/h}$$

Hourly rate is 33.3 mL/h to infuse for 6 h.

E: *Evaluate*

Ratio-Proportion

Step 1: Calculate the hourly dose:

$$\frac{1 \text{ mg}}{1 \text{ min}} = \frac{60 \text{ mg/h}}{60 \text{ min/h}} \quad \text{or}$$

1 mg : 1 min = 60 mg/h : 60 min/h

$$\mathbf{60 = 60}$$

Step 2: Calculate the hourly rate:

$$\frac{1.8 \text{ mg}}{1 \text{ mL}} = \frac{60 \text{ mg/h}}{33.33 \text{ mL/h}}$$

1.8 mg : 1 mL = 60 mg/h : 33.33 mL/h

$$1.8 \times 33.33 = 1 \times 60$$

$$\mathbf{59.994 \cong 60}$$

Formula Method

Step 1: Calculate the hourly dose:

$$\frac{1 \text{ mg}}{1 \text{ min}} \times 60 \text{ min/h} = 60 \text{ mg/h}$$

$$1 \text{ mg} \times 60 \text{ /h} = 60 \text{ mg/h}$$

$$\mathbf{60 \text{ mg/h} = 60 \text{ mg/h}}$$

Step 2: Calculate the hourly rate:

$$\frac{60 \text{ mg/h}}{1.8 \text{ mg}} \times 1 \text{ mL} = 33.3 \text{ mL/h}$$

$$\frac{60 \text{ mL/h}}{1.8} = 33.33 \text{ mL/h}$$

$$\mathbf{33.33 \text{ mL/h} = 33.33 \text{ mL/h}}$$

Dimensional Analysis

Step 1 and step 2 are combined:

$$33.33 \text{ mL/h} = \frac{1 \text{ mL}}{1.8 \text{ mg}} \times \frac{1 \text{ mg}}{1 \text{ min}} \times \frac{60 \text{ min}}{1 \text{ h}}$$

$$33.33 \text{ mL/h} = \frac{60 \text{ mL}}{1.8 \text{ h}}$$

$$\mathbf{33.33 \text{ mL/h} = 33.33 \text{ mL/h}}$$

Because the calculated dose, 60 mg/h, accurately completes the (Step 1) equation and is consistent with the approximated dose, the answer to step 1 is confirmed. Because the calculated rate, 33.3 mL/h, accurately completes the (Step 2) equation and is consistent with the approximated rate, the hourly rate is confirmed.

Example 2:   Use the following order and supply to calculate the infusion rate in mL/h.

Order: nitroglycerin 5 mcg/min IV infusion

Supply: nitroglycerin 25 mg in D$_5$W 250 mL total volume

Reduced supply: 1 mg/10 mL

C: *Convert*—Because the order is in micrograms and supply is in milligrams, convert 1 mg/10 mL to 1,000 mcg/10 mL and reduce to 100 mcg/1 mL.

A: *Approximate*

Step 1: Estimate the hourly dose.

The ordered dose is 5 mcg per minute, and there are 60 minutes in 1 hour: $5 \times 60 = 300$, so the patient will need 300 mcg/h.

Step 2: Estimate the hourly rate.

There are 100 mcg/mL. 300 is three times larger than 100, so the IV will infuse at 3 mL/h.

S: *Solve*

Ratio-Proportion	Formula Method
Step 1: Calculate the hourly dose:	Step 1: Calculate the hourly dose:
$\dfrac{5\ \text{mcg}}{1\ \text{min}} = \dfrac{x\ \text{mcg/h}}{60\ \text{min/h}}$ or	$\dfrac{5\ \text{mcg}}{1\ \cancel{\text{min}}} \times 60\ \cancel{\text{min}}/\text{h} = x\ (\text{mcg/h})$
5 mcg: 1 min $= x$ mcg/h: 60 min/h	$5\ \text{mcg} \times 60/\text{h} = x$
$x = 300$ mcg/h	$300\ \text{mcg/h} = x$
Hourly dose is 300 mcg/h.	**Hourly dose is 300 mcg/h.**
Step 2: Calculate hourly rate:	Step 2: Calculate the hourly rate:
$\dfrac{100\ \text{mcg}}{1\ \text{mL}} = \dfrac{300\ \text{mcg/h}}{x\ \text{mL/h}}$	$\dfrac{300\ \cancel{\text{mcg}}/\text{h}}{100\ \cancel{\text{mcg}}} \times 1\ \text{mL} = x\,(\text{mL/h})$
$300x = 100$	$\dfrac{300\ \text{mL/h}}{100} = x$
$\dfrac{\cancel{300}x}{\cancel{300}} = \dfrac{100}{300}$	$3\ \text{mL/h} = x$
$x = 3$ mL/h	**Hourly rate is 3 mL/h.**
Hourly rate is 3 mL/h.	

Dimensional Analysis

Step 1 and step 2 are combined:

$$x \, (mL/h) = \frac{1 \, mL}{100 \, \cancel{mcg}} \times \frac{5 \, \cancel{mcg}}{1 \, \cancel{min}} \times \frac{60 \, \cancel{min}}{1 \, h}$$

$$x = \frac{300 \, mL}{100 \, h}$$

$$x = 3 \, mL/h$$

Hourly rate is 3 mL/h.

E: *Evaluate*

Ratio-Proportion	**Formula Method**
Step 1: Calculate the hourly dose: $\dfrac{5 \, mcg}{1 \, min} = \dfrac{300 \, mcg/h}{60 \, min/h}$ or 5 mcg: 1 min = 3 mcg/h: 60 min/h $300 = 5 \times 60$ **300 = 300** Step 2: Calculate the hourly rate: $\dfrac{100 \, mcg}{1 \, mL} = \dfrac{300 \, mcg/h}{3 \, mL/h}$ $100 \times 3 = 1 \times 300$ **300 = 300**	Step 1: Calculate the hourly dose: $\dfrac{5 \, mcg}{1 \, \cancel{min}} \times 60 \, \cancel{min}/h = 300 \, mcg/h$ $5 \, mcg \times 60/h = 300 \, mcg/h$ **300 mcg/h = 300 mcg/h** Step 2: Calculate the hourly rate: $\dfrac{300 \, \cancel{mcg}/h}{100 \, \cancel{mcg}} \times 1 \, mL = 3 \, mL/h$ $\dfrac{300 \, mL/h}{100} = 3 \, mL/h$ **3 mL/h = 3 mL/h**

Dimensional Analysis

Step 1 and step 2 are combined:

$$3 \, mL/h = \frac{1 \, mL}{100 \, \cancel{mcg}} \times \frac{5 \, \cancel{mcg}}{1 \, \cancel{min}} \times \frac{60 \, \cancel{min}}{1 \, h}$$

$$3 \, mL/h = \frac{300 \, mL}{100 \, h}$$

3 mL/h = 3 mL/h

Because the calculated dose, 300 mcg/h, accurately completes the (Step 1) equation and is consistent with the approximated dose, the hourly dose is confirmed. Because the calculated rate, 3 mL/h, accurately completes the (Step 2) equation and is consistent with the approximated rate, the hourly rate is confirmed.

LEARNING ACTIVITY 15-2 For each of the following orders and supplies, determine the reduced supply (lowest terms), then calculate the infusion rate in mL/h.

1.   **Order:** amiodarone 0.5 mg/min, to infuse IV over 18 hours
       Supply: amiodarone 900 mg in D$_5$W 500 mL total volume

2.   **Order:** nitroglycerin 15 mcg/min IV
        Supply: nitroglycerin 25 mg in D$_5$W 500 mL total volume
3.   **Order:** lidocaine 2 mg/min
        Supply: lidocaine 1g in D$_5$W 250 mL

Clinical CLUE

To determine if advanced dosage calculation is required, identify whether the *dose* is administered as a continuous rather than as an intermittent infusion. Although an antibiotic dose may be based on the patient's weight, the entire dose will be administered over a limited period of time (e.g., 30 minutes or 2 hours). Time limited, intermittent infusion rates are calculated using standard IV calculations that consider only the *volume over time* to be infused (e.g., 50 mL/30 min). However, a continuous infusion of a *dose over time* requires an advanced dosage calculation, in which the amount of medication and the volume are considered. In advanced dosage calculation, the supply is the concentration of the IV bag to be infused (e.g., 1,600 mcg/mL).

15-2   Intravenous Infusion Flow Rate Calculations for Dosage per Body Weight and Time

When IV infusions are weight based per unit of time (e.g., mg/kg/min), the infusion rate calculation might be a three- to five-step process. First, if the weight is measured in pounds, convert it to kilograms. Next, convert the order and supply to the same unit of measurement, if necessary. Then determine the hourly dose, and follow the two steps outlined for per-minute IV rates.

Example 1:   Use the following order and supply to calculate the infusion rate in mL/h.

Order: dopamine 3 mcg/kg/min IV infusion

Supply: dopamine 400 mg in 250 mL D$_5$W

Reduced supply: 1.6 mg/1 mL

Patient's weight: 154 lb

C: *Convert*

Step 1: Convert the patient's weight from lb to kg: $154 \, \cancel{lb} \times \frac{1 \, kg}{2.2 \, \cancel{lb}} = 70 \, kg$

This step is not needed if using dimensional analysis, because the conversion factor, 1 kg/2.2 lb, can be inserted into the equation.

Step 2: Convert the order and supply to the same unit of measurement.

Because the order is in mcg and supply is in mg, convert 1.6 mg/1 mL to 1,600 mcg/1 mL. (Although a weight conversion factor can be inserted into the dimensional analysis equation, this step is needed to perform the "approximate" step of the CASE method.)

Step 3: Convert the per-minute dose to an hourly dose:

$$3 \, mcg/kg/\cancel{min} \times 60 \, \cancel{min}/h = 180 \, mcg/kg/h$$

This step is not needed if using dimensional analysis, because the conversion factor, 60 min/1 h, can be inserted into the equation.

A: *Approximate*

Step 1: Estimate the hourly weight-based dose.

The patient weighs 70 kg. 70 is close to 50 kg and 180 mcg is close to 200 mcg, so the patient will need roughly 10,000 mcg/h.

Step 2: Estimate the hourly rate.

There are 1,600 mcg/mL. 10,000 is more than six times larger than 1,600, therefore the IV rate will be greater than 6 mL/h.

S: *Solve*

Ratio-Proportion	Formula Method
Step 1: Calculate the hourly weight-based dose:	Step 1: Calculate the hourly weight-based dose:
$$\frac{180 \text{ mcg/h}}{1 \text{ kg}} = \frac{x \text{ mcg/h}}{70 \text{ kg}} \text{ or}$$	$$180 \text{ mcg/\cancel{kg}/h} \times 70 \text{ \cancel{kg}} = x \text{ (mcg/h)}$$
$$180 \text{ mcg/h}: 1 \text{ kg} = x \text{ mcg/h}: 70 \text{ kg}$$	$$180 \text{ mcg/h} \times 70 = x$$
$$x = 12,600 \text{ mcg}$$	$$12,600 \text{ mcg/h} = x$$
Weight-based dose is 12,600 mcg/h.	**Weight-based dose is 12,600 mcg/h.**
Step 2: Calculate the hourly rate:	Step 2: Calculate the hourly rate:
$$\frac{1,600 \text{ mcg}}{1 \text{ mL}} = \frac{12,600 \text{ mcg/h}}{x \text{ mL/h}} \text{ or}$$	$$\frac{12,600 \text{ \cancel{mcg}/h}}{1,600 \text{ \cancel{mcg}}} \times 1 \text{ mL} = x \text{ (mL/h)}$$
$$1,600 \text{ mcg}: 1 \text{ mL} = 12,600 \text{ mcg/h}: x \text{ mL/h}$$	$$7.875 \text{ mL/h} = x$$
$$1,600x = 12,600$$	**Hourly rate is 7.9 mL/h.**
$$\frac{\cancel{1,600}x}{\cancel{1,600}} = \frac{12,600}{1,600}$$	
$$x = 7.875 \text{ mL/h}$$	
Hourly rate is 7.9 mL/h.	

Dimensional Analysis

All steps are combined:

$$x \text{ (mL/h)} = \frac{1 \text{ mL}}{1,600 \text{ \cancel{mcg}}} \times \frac{3 \text{ \cancel{mcg}}}{1 \text{ \cancel{kg}}} \times \frac{1 \text{ \cancel{kg}}}{2.2 \text{ \cancel{lb}}} \times \frac{154 \text{ \cancel{lb}}}{1} \times \frac{1}{1 \text{ \cancel{min}}} \times \frac{60 \text{ \cancel{min}}}{1 \text{ h}}$$

$$x = \frac{27,720 \text{ mL}}{3,520 \text{ h}}$$

$$x = 7.875 \text{ mL/h}$$

Hourly rate is 7.9 mL/h.

E: *Evaluate*

Ratio-Proportion	Formula Method
Step 1: Calculate the hourly weight-based dose: $$\frac{180 \text{ mcg/h}}{1 \text{ kg}} = \frac{12,600 \text{ mcg/h}}{70 \text{ kg}} \text{ or}$$ 180 mcg/h: 1 kg = 12,600 mcg/h: 70 kg $$180 \times 70 = 12,600$$ **12,600 = 12,600** Step 2: Calculate the hourly rate: $$\frac{1,600 \text{ mcg}}{1 \text{ mL}} = \frac{12,600 \text{ mcg/h}}{7.875 \text{ mL/h}}$$ $$1,600 \times 7.875 = 1 \times 12,600$$ **12,600 mcg/h = 12,600 mcg/h**	Step 1: Calculate the hourly weight-based dose: 180 mcg/~~kg~~/h × 70 ~~kg~~ = 12,600 mcg/h 180 mcg/h × 70 = 12,600 mcg/h **12,600 mcg / h = 12,600 mcg / h** Step 2: Calculate the hourly rate: $$\frac{12,600 \text{ ~~mcg~~/h}}{1,600 \text{ ~~mcg~~}} \times 1 \text{ mL} = 7.875 \text{mL/h}$$ **7.875 mL / h = 7.875 mL / h**

Dimensional Analysis

All steps are combined:

$$7.875 \text{ mL/h} = \frac{1 \text{ mL}}{1,600 \text{ ~~mcg~~}} \times \frac{3 \text{ ~~mcg~~}}{1 \text{ ~~kg~~}} \times \frac{1 \text{ ~~kg~~}}{2.2 \text{ ~~lb~~}} \times \frac{154 \text{ ~~lb~~}}{1} \times \frac{1}{1 \text{ ~~min~~}} \times \frac{60 \text{ ~~min~~}}{1 \text{ h}}$$

$$7.875 \text{ mL/h} = \frac{27,720 \text{ mL}}{3,520 \text{ h}}$$

7.875 mL / h = 7.875 mL / h

Because the calculated dose, 12,600 mcg/h, accurately completes the (Step 1) equation and is consistent with the roughly approximated dose of 10,000 mcg/h, the answer is confirmed. Because the calculated rate, 7.875 mL/h, accurately completes the (Step 2) equation and is consistent with the approximated rate of greater than 6 mL/h, the answer is confirmed.

Example 2:   Use the following order and supply to calculate the infusion rate in mL/h.

Order: dobutamine 10 mcg/kg/min IV infusion

Supply: dobutamine 500 mg in 250 mL D$_5$W

Reduced supply: 2 mg/1 mL

Patient's weight: 50 kg

C: *Convert*

Step 1: Convert the patient's weight from lb to kg.

N/A: The patient's weight is provided in kg.

Step 2: Convert the order and supply to like units.

Because the order is in mcg and supply is in mg, convert 2 mg/mL to 2,000 mcg/mL.

Step 3: Convert the per-minute dose to an hourly dose:

$$10 \text{ mcg/kg/}\cancel{\text{min}} \times 60 \text{ } \cancel{\text{min}}\text{/h} = 600 \text{ mcg/kg/h}$$

This step is not needed if using dimensional analysis, because the conversion factor, 60 min/1 h, can be inserted into the equation.

A: *Approximate*

Step 1: Estimate the hourly weight-based dose.

The patient weighs 50 kg and the ordered dose is 600 mcg/kg/h: $50 \times 600 = 30,000$, so the patient will need 30,000 mcg/h.

Step 2: Estimate the hourly rate.

There are 2,000 mcg/mL. 30,000 is 15 times larger than 2,000, so the IV will infuse at 15 mL/h.

S: *Solve.*

Ratio-Proportion	Formula Method
Step 1: Calculate the hourly dose:	Step 1: Calculate the hourly dose:
$$\frac{600 \text{ mcg/h}}{1 \text{ kg}} = \frac{x \text{ mcg/h}}{50 \text{ kg}} \text{ or}$$	$$600 \text{ mcg/}\cancel{\text{kg}}\text{/h} \times 50 \text{ } \cancel{\text{kg}} = x \text{ (mcg/h)}$$
$600 \text{ mcg/h} : 1 \text{ kg} = x \text{ mcg/h} : 50 \text{ kg}$	$30,000 \text{ mcg/h} = x$
$x = 30,000 \text{ mcg/h}$	
Hourly dose is 30,000 mcg/h.	**Hourly dose is 30,000 mcg/h.**
Step 2: Calculate the hourly rate:	Step 2: Calculate the hourly rate:
$$\frac{2,000 \text{ mcg}}{1 \text{ mL}} = \frac{30,000 \text{ mcg/h}}{x \text{ mL/h}} \text{ or}$$	$$\frac{30,000 \text{ } \cancel{\text{mcg}}\text{/h}}{2,000 \text{ } \cancel{\text{mcg}}} \times 1 \text{ mL}$$
$2,000 \text{ mcg} : 1 \text{ mL} = 30,000 \text{ mcg/h} : x \text{ mL/h}$	$= x \text{ (mL/h)}$
$$\frac{\cancel{2,000}x}{\cancel{2,000}} = \frac{30,000}{2,000}$$	$15 \text{ mL/h} = x$
$x = 15 \text{ mL/h}$	**Hourly rate is 15 mL/h.**
Hourly rate is 15 mL/h.	

Dimensional Analysis

Steps 1, 2, and 3 are combined:

$$x \, (mL/h) = \frac{1 \, mL}{2,000 \, \cancel{mcg}} \times \frac{10 \, \cancel{mcg}}{1 \, \cancel{kg}} \times \frac{50 \, \cancel{kg}}{1} \times \frac{1}{1 \, \cancel{min}} \times \frac{60 \, \cancel{min}}{1 \, h}$$

$$x = \frac{30,000 \, mL}{2,000 \, h}$$

$$x = 15 \, mL/h$$

Hourly rate is 15 mL/h.

E: *Evaluate*

Ratio-Proportion

Step 1: Calculate the hourly dose:

$$\frac{600 \, mcg/h}{1 \, kg} = \frac{30,000 \, mcg/h}{50 \, kg} \quad \text{or}$$

600 mcg/h : 1 kg = 30,000 mcg/h : 50 kg

30,000 = 30,000

Step 2: Calculate the hourly rate:

$$\frac{2,000 \, mcg}{1 \, mL} = \frac{30,000 \, mcg/h}{15 \, mL/h}$$

$$2,000 \times 15 = 1 \times 30,000$$

30,000 = 30,000

Formula Method

Step 1: Calculate the hourly dose:

600 mcg/$\cancel{kg}$/h × 50 $\cancel{kg}$ = 30,000 mcg/h

30,000 mcg/h = 30,000 mcg/h

Step 2: Calculate the hourly rate:

$$\frac{30,000 \, \cancel{mcg}/h}{2,000 \, \cancel{mcg}} \times 1 \, mL = 15 \, mL/h$$

15 mL / h = 15 mL / h

Dimensional Analysis

Steps 1, 2, and 3 are combined:

$$15 \, mL/h = \frac{1 \, mL}{2,000 \, \cancel{mcg}} \times \frac{10 \, \cancel{mcg}}{1 \, \cancel{kg}} \times \frac{50 \, \cancel{kg}}{1} \times \frac{1}{1 \, \cancel{min}} \times \frac{60 \, \cancel{min}}{1 \, h}$$

$$15 \, mL/h = \frac{30,000 \, mL}{2,000 \, h}$$

15 mL / h = 15 mL / h

Example 3:   Use the following order and supply to calculate the infusion rate in mL/h.

Order: milrinone 0.5 mcg/kg/min IV infusion

Supply: milrinone 10 mg/D$_5$W 50 mL total volume

Reduced supply: 0.2 mg/mL

Patient's weight: 163 lb

C: *Convert*

Step 1: Convert the patient's weight from lb to kg:

$$163 \;\cancel{lb} \times \frac{1 \text{ kg}}{2.2 \;\cancel{lb}} = 74.09091 \text{ kg; round to 74.1 kg}$$

This step is not needed if using dimensional analysis, because the conversion factor, 1 kg/2.2 lb, can be inserted into the equation.

Step 2: Convert the order and supply to like units.

Because the order is in mcg and supply is in mg, convert 0.2 mg/mL to 200 mcg/mL.

Step 3: Convert the per-minute dose to an hourly dose:

$$0.5 \text{ mcg/kg/}\cancel{\text{min}} \times 60 \;\cancel{\text{min}} = 30 \text{ mcg/kg/h}$$

This step is not needed if using dimensional analysis, because the conversion factor, 60 min/1 h, can be inserted into the equation.

A: *Approximate*

Step 1: Estimate the hourly weight-based dose.

The patient weighs about 75 kg and the ordered dose is 30 mcg/kg/h; 75 × 30 is approximately 2,250 mcg/h.

Step 2: Estimate the hourly rate.

There are 200 mcg/mL. 2,225 mcg/h is more than 10 times larger than 200 mcg/mL, so the IV will infuse at a little more than 10 mL/h.

S: *Solve*

Ratio-Proportion	Formula Method
Step 1: Calculate the hourly dose:	Step 1: Calculate the hourly dose:
$$\frac{30 \text{ mcg/h}}{1 \text{ kg}} = \frac{x \text{ mcg/h}}{74.1 \text{ kg}} \text{ or}$$	$$30 \text{ mcg/}\cancel{\text{kg}}\text{/h} \times 74.1 \;\cancel{\text{kg}} = x(\text{mcg/h})$$
30 mcg: 1 kg/h: *x* mcg/h: 74.1 kg	2,223 mcg/h = *x*
x = 2,223 mcg/h	
Hourly dose is 2,223 mcg/h.	**Hourly dose is 2,223 mcg/h.**

Step 2: Calculate the hourly rate:

$$\frac{200 \text{ mcg}}{1 \text{ mL}} = \frac{2,223 \text{ mcg / h}}{x \text{ mL / h}} \quad \text{or}$$

200 mcg : 1 mL = 2,223 mcg/h : x mL/h

$$\frac{\cancel{200}x}{\cancel{200}} = \frac{2,223}{200}$$

$$x = 11.115 \text{ mL/h}$$

Hourly rate is 11.1 mL/h.

Step 2: Calculate the hourly rate:

$$\frac{2,223 \cancel{\text{mcg}}/h}{200 \cancel{\text{mcg}}} \times 1 \text{ mL} = x$$

$$11.115 \text{ mL/h} = x$$

Hourly rate is 11.1 mL/h.

Dimensional Analysis

Steps 1, 2, and 3 are combined:

$$x(\text{mL/h}) = \frac{1 \text{ mL}}{200 \cancel{\text{mcg}}} \times \frac{0.5 \cancel{\text{mcg}}}{1 \cancel{\text{kg}}} \times \frac{1 \cancel{\text{kg}}}{2.2 \cancel{\text{lb}}} \times \frac{163 \cancel{\text{lb}}}{1} \times \frac{1}{1 \cancel{\text{min}}} \times \frac{60 \cancel{\text{min}}}{1 \text{ h}}$$

$$x = \frac{4,890 \text{ mL}}{440 \text{ h}}$$

$$x = 11.11364 \text{ mL/h}$$

Hourly rate is 11.1 mL/h.

E: *Evaluate*

Ratio-Proportion	Formula Method

Ratio-Proportion

Step 1: Calculate the hourly weight-based dose:

$$\frac{30 \text{ mcg/h}}{1 \text{ kg}} = \frac{2,223 \text{ mcg/h}}{74.1 \text{ kg}} \quad \text{or}$$

30 mcg : 1 kg/h = 2,223 mcg/h : 74.1 kg

$$1 \times 2,223 = 1 \times 2,223$$

$$\mathbf{2,223 = 2,223}$$

Step 2: Calculate the hourly rate:

$$\frac{200 \text{ mcg}}{1 \text{ mL}} = \frac{2,223 \text{ mcg/h}}{11.115 \text{ mL/h}}$$

$$200 \times 11.115 = 1 \times 2,223$$

$$\mathbf{2,223 = 2,223}$$

Formula Method

Step 1: Calculate the hourly weight-based dose:

30 mcg/$\cancel{\text{kg}}$/h $\times$ 74.1 $\cancel{\text{kg}}$ = 2,223 mcg/h

$$\mathbf{2,223 \text{ mcg / h} = 2,223 \text{ mcg / h}}$$

Step 2: Calculate the hourly rate:

$$\frac{2,223 \cancel{\text{mcg}}/h}{200 \cancel{\text{mcg}}} \times 1 \text{ mL} = 11.115 \text{ mL/h}$$

$$\mathbf{11.115 \text{ mL / h} = 11.115 \text{ mL / h}}$$

Dimensional Analysis

Steps 1, 2, and 3 are combined:

$$11.11364 \text{ mL/h} = \frac{1 \text{ mL}}{200 \text{ mcg}} \times \frac{0.5 \text{ mcg}}{1 \text{ kg}} \times \frac{1 \text{ kg}}{2.2 \text{ lb}} \times \frac{163 \text{ lb}}{1} \times \frac{1}{1 \text{ min}} \times \frac{60 \text{ min}}{1 \text{ h}}$$

$$11.11364 \text{ mL/h} = \frac{4,890 \text{ mL}}{440 \text{ h}}$$

11.11364 mL / h = 11.11364 mL / h

Clinical CLUE

In an emergency, a nurse may need to rapidly convert the concentration of an IV medication to smaller units. To easily determine how many mcg are in 1 mL of IV fluid when the concentration is in milligrams, mentally enlarge the quantity of fluid to 1 liter (1,000 mL). **The number of mg in 1 L is the same as the number of mcg in 1 mL.** This is because the ratio of mL to L (1,000:1) is the same as the ratio of mcg to mg (1,000:1).

Example: Determine the number of mcg in 1 mL for the following IV solution.

Supply: dopamine 400 mg in 250 mL D₅W

Step 1: Enlarge the quantity 250 mL to 1,000 mL (1 L), keeping the concentration the same.

$$\frac{400 \text{ mg} \times 4}{250 \text{ mL} \times 4} = \frac{1,600 \text{ mg}}{1,000 \text{ mL}}$$

Step 2: Since mg/L is equivalent to mcg/mL: 1,600 mg/L = 1,600 mcg/mL

The calculated rate, prior to rounding, for administering milrinone 0.5 mcg/kg/min to a 163 lb patient was 11.115 mL/h when determined by ratio-proportion and the formula method, but it was 11.11364 mL/h when determined by dimensional analysis. What accounts for the difference?

Converting the patient's weight from lb to kg resulted in a number that needed to be rounded to tenths (i.e., 163 lb $\times \frac{1 \text{ kg}}{2.2 \text{ lb}}$ = 74.09091 kg, which rounds to 74.1 kg). The rounded weight was inserted into the ratio-proportion and formula equations, but the patient's actual weight was inserted into dimensional analysis equation. Not only does dimensional analysis require fewer steps when performing advanced dosage calculation, it is also more accurate. For this reason, many critical care nurses use dimensional analysis when performing these calculations.

LEARNING ACTIVITY 15-3
For the following orders and supplies, determine the supply reduced to mcg/mL by first enlarging the quantity to 1000 mL (1 L), then reducing to 1 mL and calculate the infusion rate in mL/h.

1.   **Order:** norepinephrine 0.5 mcg/kg/min
      Supply: norepinephrine 4 mg/250 mL D$_5$NS
      Patient weight: 45 lb

2.   **Order:** nitroprusside 0.3 mcg/kg/min
      Supply: nitroprusside 50 mg/500 mL D$_5$W
      Patient weight: 185 lb

3.   **Order:** milrinone 0.375 mcg/kg/min
      Supply: milrinone 20 mg/100 mL D$_5$W
      Patient weight: 90 kg

15-3   Intravenous Infusion Dosage Calculations Based on a Specified Volume per Time

Nurses also have to determine the amount of medication that is currently infusing. When one nurse accepts a patient from another caregiver, as in change of shift, the oncoming nurse should determine the amount of medication delivered at the existing rate. To calculate the dose delivered by a specified rate:

1. Calculate the amount of medication delivered in 1 mL.

2. Determine the delivered hourly dose.
    *   Multiply the rate by the amount of medication in 1 mL.

3. Determine the delivered weight-based dose (if order is weight-based).
    *   Divide the hourly dose by the patient's weight in kg.

4. Determine the delivered per-minute dose.
    *   Divide the hourly weight-based dose by 60 minutes (if weight-based dose is ordered per minute).
    *   Divide the hourly dose by 60 minutes if the hourly dose is not weight based.

Example 1:   Verify that the current rate delivers the ordered dose.

Order: dopamine 3 mcg/kg/min IV infusion

Supply: dopamine 400 mg in 250 mL D$_5$W

Patient's weight: 70 kg

Current rate: 7.9 mL/h

1. Calculate the amount of medication delivered in 1 mL.
    *   Divide the amount of medication in the supply by the supply volume:

$$400 \text{ mg} \div 250 \text{ mL} = 400{,}000 \text{ mcg}/250 \text{ mL} = 1{,}600 \text{ mcg/mL}$$

2. Determine the hourly dose.
    *   Multiply the rate by the amount of medication in 1 mL:

$$7.9 \text{ } \cancel{\text{mL}}/\text{h} \times 1{,}600 \text{ mcg}/\cancel{\text{mL}} = 12{,}640 \text{ mcg/h}$$

3. Determine the delivered weight-based dose (if order is weight based).
   - Divide the hourly dose by the patient's weight in kg:

$$12{,}640 \text{ mcg/h} \div 70 \text{ kg} = 180.57143 \text{ mcg/kg/h}$$

4. Determine the delivered per-minute dose.
   - Divide the hourly weight-based dose by 60 minutes (if weight-based dose is ordered per minute):

$$180.57143 \text{ mcg/kg/\cancel{h}} \div 60 \text{ min/\cancel{h}} = 3.00952 \text{ or } 3 \text{ mcg/kg/min}$$

The current rate is delivering the ordered dose.

    Example 2:   Verify that the current rate delivers the ordered dose.

        Order: milrinone 0.5 mcg/kg/min IV infusion

     Supply: milrinone 10 mg/D_5W 50 mL total volume

Patient's weight: 163 lb

   Current rate: 11.1 mL/h

1. Calculate the amount of medication delivered in 1 mL.
   - Convert lb to kg:

$$163 \text{ \cancel{lb}} \times \frac{1 \text{ kg}}{2.2 \text{ \cancel{lb}}} = 74.09, \text{ rounds to } 74.1 \text{ kg}$$

   - Divide the amount of medication in the supply by the supply volume:

$$10 \text{ mg} \div 50 \text{ mL} = 0.2 \text{ mg/mL} = 200 \text{ mcg/mL}$$

2. Determine the hourly dose.
   - Multiply the rate by the amount of medication in 1 mL:

$$11.1 \text{ \cancel{mL}/h} \times 200 \text{ mcg/\cancel{mL}} = 2{,}220 \text{ mcg/h}$$

3. Determine the delivered weight-based dose (if order is weight-based).
   - Divide the hourly dose by the patient's weight in kg:

$$2{,}220 \text{ mcg/h} \div 74.1 \text{ kg} = 29.9595 \text{ mcg/kg/h}$$

4. Determine the delivered per-minute dose.
   - Divide the hourly weight-based dose by 60 minutes (if weight-based dose is ordered per minute):

$$29.9595 \text{ mcg/kg/\cancel{h}} \div 60 \text{ min/\cancel{h}} = 0.49933, \text{ rounds to } 0.5 \text{ mcg/kg/min}$$

The current rate is delivering the ordered dose.

LEARNING ACTIVITY 15-4 Verify whether the following rates deliver the ordered dosages. If the current rate is inaccurate, calculate the correct rate to deliver the ordered dose.

1.   **Order:** nitroglycerin 10 mcg/min IV infusion
   Supply: nitroglycerin 25 mg in D_5W 500 mL total volume
   Current rate: 7 mL/h

2.   **Order:** procainamide 1 mg/min
        Supply: procainamide 1g in NS 250 mL total volume
        Current rate: 15 mL/h

3.   **Order:** dobutamine 7.5 mcg/kg/min IV infusion
        Supply: dobutamine 500 mg in 250 mL D$_5$W
        Patient's weight: 85 kg
        Current rate: 20 mL/h

15-4   Titrated Intravenous Dosage Calculation

Critical care nurses often administer potent medications to obtain a vital effect. These continuous IV infusion dosages are **titrated** (adjusted for desired effect) by the nurse. In addition to the standard requirements for a medication order, the order for a titrated medication must include three criteria: measurable outcome, starting dose, and dosage parameters. The measurable outcome depends on the type of drug. For example, the outcome for:

- An **antiarrhythmic** (medication that normalizes the heart rate or rhythm) would be a heart rate (HR) or rhythm

- A **vasoactive** medication (medication the dilates or constricts blood vessels) would be blood pressure

- An **analgesic** (medication to relieve pain) would be pain level

- An **anxiolytic** (sedative or anti-anxiety medication) would be sedation or anxiety level

The prescriber orders a starting dosage rate to achieve a specific response and end points (parameters) for administering the infusion. Generally, the infusion is ordered to begin at the lowest dose and the nurse will increase the infusion (dosage) rate if the outcome has not been met. The nurse stops increasing the medication dosage if the maximal ordered dose is reached or a negative outcome described in the ordered parameters is reached. If the desired outcome is exceeded, the nurse decreases the rate to deliver less medication. If the desired outcome is not achieved within the parameters, the prescriber should be notified.

Upon receiving a titration order, the nurse calculates the rate for the minimum and maximum prescribed dose. By immediately calculating the rate that delivers the maximum dose, the nurse can make rapid increases without exceeding the prescribed amount.

Example 1:   Using the following order, perform these calculations:

     a.   Minimum hourly weight-based dose and rate

     b.   Maximum hourly weight-based dose and rate

     c.   Titration rate increment

Order: Start dopamine 400 mg in 250 mL D$_5$W continuous IV infusion at 3 mcg/kg/min (the minimum dose). Titrate at 5 mcg/kg/min increments to achieve a mean arterial pressure (MAP) of 65 mm Hg. Maximum dose 20 mcg/kg/min. Keep HR less than 100.

Patient weight: 220 lb

To determine the correct amounts, apply all steps of the CASE method as in previous examples. Only the "Convert" and "Solve" steps are shown here.

Clinical CLUE

In essence, a weight-based heparin protocol is a titrated IV infusion, because the dose is adjusted to achieve a measurable result (activated partial thromboplastin time [aPTT] value). Unlike heparin, the medications that are titrated exclusively in the critical care setting can affect the heart rate and/or respiratory rate and blood pressure. For that reason, the patient's vital signs and response must be continuously monitored.

C: *Convert*—Convert the supply to 400,000 mcg/250 mL and reduce to 1,600 mcg/mL.

S: *Solve*

1. *Minimum* hourly weight-based dose and rate calculation:

Ratio-Proportion	Formula Method
Step 1: Convert the per-minute dose to an hourly dose:	Step 1: Convert the per-minute dose to an hourly dose:
$$\frac{3 \text{ mcg/kg}}{1 \text{ min}} = \frac{x \text{ mcg/kg}}{60 \text{ min}} \text{ or}$$ $$3 \text{ mcg/kg}: 1 \text{ min} = x \text{ mcg/kg}: 60 \text{ min}$$ $$x = 180 \text{ mcg/kg/h}$$	$$3 \text{ mcg/kg/min} \times 60 \text{ min/h} = x \text{ (mcg/kg/h)}$$ $$180 \text{ mcg/kg/h} = x$$
Step 2: Calculate the hourly weight-based dose:	Step 2: Calculate the hourly weight-based dose:
$$\frac{180 \text{ mcg/h}}{1 \text{ kg}} = \frac{x \text{ mcg/h}}{100 \text{ kg}} \text{ or}$$ $$180 \text{ mcg/h} : 1 \text{ kg} : x \text{ mcg/h} : 100 \text{ kg}$$ $$x = 18,000 \text{ mcg/h}$$	$$180 \text{ mcg/kg/h} \times 100 \text{ kg} = x \text{ (mcg/h)}$$ $$18,000 \text{ mcg/h} = x$$
Minimum hourly dose is 18,000 mcg/h.	**Minimum hourly dose is 18,000 mcg/h.**
Step 3: Calculate the hourly rate:	Step 3: Calculate the hourly rate:
$$\frac{1,600 \text{ mcg}}{1 \text{ mL}} = \frac{18,000 \text{ mcg/h}}{x \text{ mL/h}}$$ $$1,600 \text{ mcg} : 1 \text{ mL} = 18,000 \text{ mcg/h} : x \text{ mL/h}$$ $$\frac{1,600x}{1,600} = \frac{18,000}{1,600}$$ $$x = 11.25 \text{ mL/h}$$	$$\frac{18,000 \text{ mcg/h}}{1,600 \text{ mcg}} \times 1 \text{ mL} = x \text{ (mL/h)}$$ $$11.25 \text{ mL} / \text{h} = x$$
Minimum hourly rate is 11.3 mL/h.	**Minimum hourly rate is 11.3 mL/h.**

Dimensional Analysis

Steps 1, 2, and 3 are combined:

$$x(\text{mL/h}) = \frac{1\,\text{mL}}{1{,}600\,\cancel{\text{mcg}}} \times \frac{3\,\cancel{\text{mcg}}}{1\,\cancel{\text{kg}}} \times \frac{1\,\cancel{\text{kg}}}{2.2\,\cancel{\text{lb}}} \times \frac{220\,\cancel{\text{lb}}}{1} \times \frac{1}{1\,\cancel{\text{min}}} \times \frac{60\,\cancel{\text{min}}}{1\,\text{h}}$$

$$x = \frac{39{,}600\,\text{mL}}{3{,}520\,\text{h}}$$

$$x = 11.25\,\text{mL/h}$$

Minimum hourly rate is 11.3 mL/h.

2. *Maximum* hourly weight-based dose and rate calculation:

Ratio-Proportion

Step 1: Convert the per-minute dose to an hourly dose:

$$\frac{20\,\text{mcg/kg}}{1\,\text{min}} = \frac{x\,\text{mcg/kg}}{60\,\text{min}} \quad \text{or}$$

20 mcg/kg : 1 min = x mcg/kg : 60 min

$$x = 1{,}200\,\text{mcg/kg/h}$$

Step 2: Calculate the hourly weight-based dose:

$$\frac{1{,}200\,\text{mcg/h}}{1\,\text{kg}} = \frac{x\,\text{mcg/h}}{100\,\text{kg}} \quad \text{or}$$

1,200 mcg/h : 1 kg = x mcg/h : 100 kg

$$x = 120{,}000\,\text{mcg/h}$$

Maximum hourly dose is 120,000 mcg/h.

Step 3: Calculate the hourly rate:

$$\frac{1{,}600\,\text{mcg}}{1\,\text{mL}} = \frac{120{,}000\,\text{mcg/h}}{x\,\text{mL/h}}$$

1,600 mcg : 1 mL = 120,000 mcg/h : x mL/h

$$\frac{\cancel{1{,}600}\,x}{\cancel{1{,}600}} = \frac{120{,}000}{1{,}600}$$

$$x = 75\,\text{mL/h}$$

Maximum hourly rate is 75 mL/h.

Formula Method

Step 1: Convert the per-minute dose to an hourly dose:

$$20\,\text{mcg/kg/}\cancel{\text{min}} \times 60\,\cancel{\text{min}}\text{/h} = x\,(\text{mcg/kg/h})$$

$$1{,}200\,\text{mcg/kg/h} = x$$

Step 2: Calculate the hourly weight-based dose:

$$1{,}200\,\text{mcg/}\cancel{\text{kg}}\text{/h} \times 100\,\cancel{\text{kg}} = x\,(\text{mcg/h})$$

$$120{,}000\,\text{mcg/h} = x$$

Maximum hourly dose is 120,000 mcg/h.

Step 3: Calculate the hourly rate:

$$\frac{120{,}000\,\cancel{\text{mcg}}\text{/h}}{1{,}600\,\cancel{\text{mcg}}} \times 1\,\text{mL} = x\,(\text{mL/h})$$

$$75\,\text{mL/h} = x$$

Maximum hourly rate is 75 mL/h.

Dimensional Analysis

Steps 1, 2, and 3 are combined:

$$x \,(\text{mL/h}) = \frac{1 \, \text{mL}}{1,600 \, \cancel{\text{mcg}}} \times \frac{20 \, \cancel{\text{mcg}}}{1 \, \cancel{\text{kg}}} \times \frac{1 \, \cancel{\text{kg}}}{2.2 \, \cancel{\text{lb}}} \times \frac{220 \, \cancel{\text{lb}}}{1} \times \frac{1}{1 \, \cancel{\text{min}}} \times \frac{60 \, \cancel{\text{min}}}{1 \, \text{h}}$$

$$x = \frac{264,000 \, \text{mL}}{3,520 \, \text{h}}$$

$$x = 75 \, \text{mL/h}$$

Maximum hourly rate is 75 mL/h.

3. *Titration* dose and rate increment calculation:

Ratio-Proportion	Formula Method
Step 1: Convert the minute dose to an hourly dose: $$\frac{5 \, \text{mcg/kg}}{1 \, \text{min}} = \frac{x \, \text{mcg/kg}}{60 \, \text{min}} \quad \text{or}$$ $$5 \, \text{mcg/kg} : 1 \, \text{min} = x \, \text{mcg/kg} : 60 \, \text{min}$$ $$x = 300 \, \text{mcg/kg/h}$$	Step 1: Convert the minute dose to an hourly dose: $$5 \, \text{mcg/kg/}\cancel{\text{min}} \times 60 \, \cancel{\text{min}}/\text{h} = x \,(\text{mcg/kg/h})$$ $$300 \, \text{mcg/kg/h} = x$$
Step 2: Calculate the hourly weight-based dose: $$\frac{300 \, \text{mcg/h}}{1 \, \text{kg}} = \frac{x \, \text{mcg/h}}{100 \, \text{kg}} \quad \text{or}$$ $$300 \, \text{mcg/h} : 1 \, \text{kg} = x \, \text{mcg/h} : 100 \, \text{kg}$$ $$x = 30,000 \, \text{mcg/h}$$	Step 2: Calculate the hourly weight-based dose: $$300 \, \text{mcg/}\cancel{\text{kg}}/\text{h} \times 100 \, \cancel{\text{kg}} = x \,(\text{mcg/h})$$ $$30,000 \, \text{mcg/h} = x$$
Titration dose increment is 30,000 mcg/h.	**Titration dose increment is 30,000 mcg/h.**
Step 3: Calculate the hourly rate: $$\frac{1,600 \, \text{mcg}}{1 \, \text{mL}} = \frac{30,000 \, \text{mcg/h}}{x \, \text{mL/h}}$$ $$1,600 \, \text{mcg} : 1 \, \text{mL} = 30,000 \, \text{mcg/h} : x \, \text{mL/h}$$ $$\frac{\cancel{1,600}\,x}{\cancel{1,600}} = \frac{30,000}{1,600}$$ $$x = 18.75 \, \text{mL/h}$$	Step 3: Calculate the hourly rate: $$\frac{30,000 \, \cancel{\text{mcg}}/\text{h}}{1,600 \, \cancel{\text{mcg}}} \times 1 \, \text{mL} = x \,(\text{mL/h})$$ $$18.75 \, \text{mL/h} = x$$
Titration rate increment is 18.8 mL/h.	**Titration rate increment is 18.8 mL/h.**

Dimensional Analysis

Steps 1, 2, and 3 are combined:

$$x\,(mL/h) = \frac{1\,mL}{1{,}600\,\cancel{mcg}} \times \frac{5\,\cancel{mcg}}{1\,\cancel{kg}} \times \frac{1\,\cancel{kg}}{2.2\,\cancel{lb}} \times \frac{220\,\cancel{lb}}{1} \times \frac{1}{1\,\cancel{min}} \times \frac{60\,\cancel{min}}{1\,h}$$

$$x = \frac{66{,}000\,mL}{3{,}520\,h}$$

$$x = 18.75\,mL/h$$

Titration rate increment is 18.8 mL/h.

The infusion will be started at 11.3 mL/h and will be increased by 18.8 mL/h until the patient's MAP is 65 mm Hg or the HR is 100, or the maximum dosage rate of 75 mL/h is reached. If the HR of 100 or the maximum hourly rate of 75 mL/h is reached before the desired MAP is achieved, the prescriber would be notified for a change in treatment plan.

Clinical CLUE

MAP is the average blood pressure throughout the cardiac cycle. MAP is useful in determining if the blood pressure is high enough to perfuse the entire body. Cardiac index (CI) is a measurement of blood volume. The CI is helpful in determining if the amount of blood pumped out of the heart each minute generates an adequate circulating volume. Adequate blood volume and pressure are needed to deliver oxygen-rich blood to the cells.

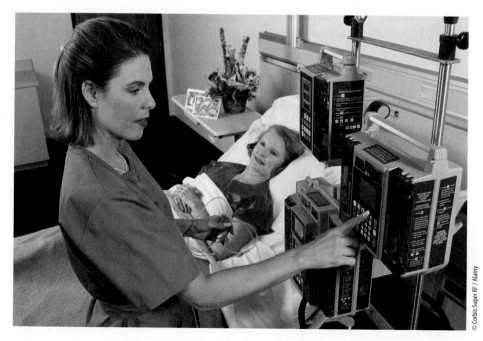

© Corbis Super RF / Alamy

FIGURE 15-2   The nurse checks the titration increment before adjusting the IV flow rate.

Example 2: Use the following order to perform these calculations:

    a. Minimum hourly weight-based dose and rate

    b. Maximum hourly weight-based dose and rate

    c. Titration rate increment

    d. Highest HR

    e. New infusion rate after 4 minutes of infusing at the minimum hourly rate when the MAP is 62 mm Hg

Order: Start dobutamine 250 mg in 500 mL D₅W continuous IV infusion at 5 mcg/kg/min. Titrate at 2.5 mcg/kg/min increments to achieve a cardiac index (CI) of 2.5 mmHg. Maximum dose is 20 mcg/kg/min. Heart rate may not exceed more than 10% of the starting HR.

Patient weight: 100 kg

Starting HR: 90 beats per minute (bpm)

To determine the correct amounts, apply all steps of the CASE method as in previous examples. Only the Convert and Solve steps are shown here.

C: *Convert*—Reduce the supply, 250 mg/500 mL, to 0.5 mg/mL; convert to 500 mcg/mL.

S: *Solve*

1. *Minimum* hourly weight-based dose and rate calculation:

Ratio-Proportion	Formula Method
Step 1: Convert the minute dose to an hourly dose: $$\frac{5 \text{ mcg/kg}}{1 \text{ min}} = \frac{x \text{ mcg/kg}}{60 \text{ min}} \text{ or}$$ $$5 \text{ mcg/kg} : 1 \text{ min} = x \text{ mcg/kg} : 60 \text{ min}$$ $$x = 300 \text{ mcg/kg/h}$$ Step 2: Calculate the hourly weight-based dose: $$\frac{300 \text{ mcg/h}}{1 \text{ kg}} = \frac{x \text{ mcg/h}}{100 \text{ kg}} \text{ or}$$ $$300 \text{ mcg/h}: 1 \text{ kg} = x \text{ mcg/h}: 100 \text{ kg}$$ $$x = 30{,}000 \text{ mcg/h}$$ **Minimum hourly dose is 30,000 mcg/h.**	Step 1: Convert the minute dose to an hourly dose: $$5 \text{ mcg/kg/} \cancel{\text{min}} \times 60 \text{ } \cancel{\text{min}}/\text{h} = x \text{ (mcg/kg/h)}$$ $$300 \text{ mcg/kg/h} = x$$ Step 2: Calculate the hourly weight-based dose: $$300 \text{ mcg/} \cancel{\text{kg}}/\text{h} \times 100 \text{ } \cancel{\text{kg}} = x \text{ (mcg/h)}$$ $$30{,}000 \text{ mcg/h} = x$$ **Minimum hourly dose is 30,000 mcg/h.** Step 3: Calculate the hourly rate: $$\frac{30{,}000 \text{ } \cancel{\text{mcg}}/\text{h}}{500 \text{ } \cancel{\text{mcg}}} \times 1 \text{ mL} = x \text{ (mL/h)}$$ $$60 \text{ mL/h} = x$$ **Minimum hourly rate is 60 mL/h.**

Step 3: Calculate the hourly rate:

$$\frac{500 \text{ mcg}}{1 \text{ mL}} = \frac{30,000 \text{ mcg/h}}{x \text{ mL/h}} \text{ or}$$

$$500 \text{ mcg} : 1 \text{ mL} = 30,000 \text{ mcg/h} : x \text{ mL/h}$$

$$\frac{\cancel{500}x}{\cancel{500}} = \frac{30,000}{500}$$

$$x = 60 \text{ mL/h}$$

Minimum hourly rate is 60 mL/h.

Dimensional Analysis

Steps 1, 2, and 3 are combined:

$$x\,(\text{mL/h}) = \frac{1 \text{ mL}}{500 \,\cancel{\text{mcg}}} \times \frac{5 \,\cancel{\text{mcg}}}{1 \,\cancel{\text{kg}}} \times \frac{100 \,\cancel{\text{kg}}}{1} \times \frac{1}{1 \,\cancel{\text{min}}} \times \frac{60 \,\cancel{\text{min}}}{1 \text{ h}}$$

$$x = \frac{30,000 \text{ mL}}{500 \text{ h}}$$

$$x = 60 \text{ mL/h}$$

Minimum hourly rate is 60 mL/h.

2. *Maximum* hourly weight-based dose and rate calculation:

Ratio-Proportion	Formula Method
Step 1: Convert the minute dose to an hourly dose:	Step 1: Convert the minute dose to an hourly dose:
$$\frac{20 \text{ mcg/kg}}{1 \text{ min}} = \frac{x \text{ mcg/kg}}{60 \text{ min}} \text{ or}$$ $$20 \text{ mcg/kg} : 1 \text{ min} = x \text{ mcg/kg} : 60 \text{ min}$$ $$x = 1,200 \text{ mcg/kg/h}$$	$$20 \text{ mcg/kg/}\cancel{\text{min}} \times 60 \,\cancel{\text{min}}\text{/h} = x \,(\text{mcg/kg/h})$$ $$1,200 \text{ mcg/kg/h} = x$$
Step 2: Calculate the hourly weight-based dose:	Step 2: Calculate the hourly weight-based dose:
$$\frac{1,200 \text{ mcg/h}}{1 \text{ kg}} = \frac{x \text{ mcg/h}}{100 \text{ kg}}$$ $$300 \text{ mcg/h} : 1 \text{ kg} = x \text{ mcg/h} : 100 \text{ kg}$$ $$x = 120,000 \text{ mcg/h}$$	$$1,200 \text{ mcg/}\cancel{\text{kg}}\text{/h} \times 100 \,\cancel{\text{kg}} = x \,(\text{mcg/h})$$ $$120,000 \text{ mcg/h} = x$$
Maximum hourly dose is 120,000 mcg/h.	**Maximum hourly dose is 120,000 mcg/h.**

Step 3: Calculate the hourly rate:

$$\frac{500 \text{ mcg}}{1 \text{ mL}} = \frac{120,000 \text{ mcg/h}}{x \text{ mL/h}}$$

$$500 \text{ mcg}: 1 \text{ mL} = 120,000 \text{ mcg/h}: x \text{ mL/h}$$

$$\frac{\cancel{500}x}{\cancel{500}} = \frac{120,000}{500}$$

$$x = 240 \text{ mL} / \text{h}$$

Maximum hourly rate is 240 mL/h.

Step 3: Calculate the hourly rate:

$$\frac{120,000 \cancel{\text{ mcg}}/\text{h}}{500 \cancel{\text{ mcg}}} \times 1 \text{ mL} = x \text{ (mL/h)}$$

$$240 \text{ mL/h} = x$$

Maximum hourly rate is 240 mL/h.

Dimensional Analysis

Steps 1, 2, and 3 are combined:

$$x \text{ (mL/h)} = \frac{1 \text{ mL}}{500 \cancel{\text{ mcg}}} \times \frac{20 \cancel{\text{ mcg}}}{1 \cancel{\text{ kg}}} \times \frac{100 \cancel{\text{ kg}}}{1} \times \frac{1}{1 \cancel{\text{ min}}} \times \frac{60 \cancel{\text{ min}}}{1 \text{ h}}$$

$$x = \frac{120,000 \text{ mL}}{500 \text{ h}}$$

$$x = 240 \text{ mL/h}$$

Maximum hourly rate is 240 mL/h.

3. *Titration* dose and rate increment calculation:

Ratio-Proportion

Step 1: Convert the minute dose to an hourly dose:

$$\frac{2.5 \text{ mcg/kg}}{1 \text{ min}} = \frac{x \text{ mcg/kg}}{60 \text{ min}} \quad \text{or}$$

$$2.5 \text{ mcg/kg} : 1 \text{ min} = x \text{ mcg/kg} : 60 \text{ min}$$

$$x = 150 \text{ mcg/kg/h}$$

Step 2: Calculate the hourly weight-based dose:

$$\frac{150 \text{ mcg/h}}{1 \text{ kg}} = \frac{x \text{ mcg/h}}{100 \text{ kg}}$$

$$150 \text{ mcg/h} : 1 \text{ kg} : x \text{ mcg/h} : 100 \text{ kg}$$

$$x = 15,000 \text{ mcg/h}$$

Titration dose increment is 15,000 mcg/h.

Formula Method

Step 1: Convert the minute dose to an hourly dose:

$$2.5 \text{ mcg/kg}/\cancel{\text{min}} \times 60 \cancel{\text{ min}}/\text{h} = x \text{ (mcg/kg/h)}$$

$$150 \text{ mcg/kg/h} = x$$

Step 2: Calculate the hourly weight-based dose:

$$150 \text{ mcg}/\cancel{\text{kg}}/\text{h} \times 100 \cancel{\text{ kg}} = (\text{mcg/h})$$

$$15,000 \text{ mcg/h} = x$$

Titration dose increment is 15,000 mcg/h.

Step 3: Calculate the hourly rate:

$$\frac{15,000 \cancel{\text{ mcg}}/\text{h}}{500 \cancel{\text{ mcg}}} \times 1 \text{ mL} = x \text{ (mL/h)}$$

$$30 \text{ mL/h} = x$$

Titration rate increment is 30 mL/h.

Step 3: Calculate the hourly rate:

$$\frac{500 \text{ mcg}}{1 \text{ mL}} = \frac{15,000 \text{ mcg/h}}{x \text{ mL/h}}$$

$$500 \text{ mcg} : 1 \text{ mL} = 120,000 \text{ mcg/h} : x \text{ mL/h}$$

$$\frac{\cancel{500}x}{\cancel{500}} = \frac{15,000}{500}$$

$$x = 30 \text{ mL/h}$$

Titration rate increment is 30 mL/h.

Dimensional Analysis

Steps 1, 2, and 3 are combined:

$$x \,(\text{mL/h}) = \frac{1 \text{ mL}}{500 \text{ mcg}} \times \frac{2.5 \text{ mcg}}{1 \text{ kg}} \times \frac{100 \text{ kg}}{1} \times \frac{1}{1 \text{ min}} \times \frac{60 \text{ min}}{1 \text{ h}}$$

$$x = \frac{15,000 \text{ mL}}{500 \text{ h}}$$

$$x = 30 \text{ mL/h}$$

Titration rate increment is 30 mL/h.

4. HR parameter calculation:

$$10\% \text{ of } 90 \text{ is } 0.1 \times 90 = 9$$

Because the heart rate can increase no more than 10% from the starting rate, add that value to starting heart rate to determine that the maximum HR is 99 bpm:

$$90 + 9 = 99$$

5. New infusion rate calculation: To obtain the new IV rate, add the titration increment (30 mL/h) to the current rate (60 mL/h):

$$30 \text{ mL/h} + 60 \text{ mL/h} = 90 \text{ mL/h}$$

NOTE: The prescriber might consider concentrating the IV supply if high doses are needed, because the volume per hour is so large.

The infusion will start at 60 mL/h and will be increased by 30 mL/h until the patient's MAP is 65 mm Hg or the HR is 99 bpm, or the maximum dosage rate of 240 mL/h is reached. If the HR of 99 or the maximum hourly rate of 240 mL/h is reached before the desired MAP is achieved, the prescriber should be notified for a change in treatment plan.

LEARNING ACTIVITY 15-5 Use the following order and supply to calculate the infusion rate in mL/h.

1.   **Order:** Start norepinephrine 4 mg in 500 mL D$_5$W continuous IV infusion at 2 mcg/min (the minimum dose). Titrate at 1 mcg/min increments every 2 minutes to achieve an MAP of 65 mm Hg. Maximum dose 10 mcg/min.

   a.   Calculate the minimum hourly rate.

   b.   Calculate the maximum hourly rate.

   c.   Calculate the titration rate increment.

   d.   After 2 minutes of infusing at the minimum hourly rate, the MAP is 62 mm Hg; calculate the new rate.

2.   **Order:** nitroprusside 0.1 to 5 mcg/kg/min IV; titrate 0.05 mcg/kg/min every 3 min to achieve an MAP less than 100
      Supply: nitroprusside 50 mg in D$_5$W 250 mL total volume
      Patient weight: 80 kg

   a.   Calculate the minimum hourly rate.

   b.   Calculate the maximum hourly rate.

   c.   Calculate the titration rate increment.

   d.   After 3 minutes of infusing at the minimum hourly rate, the MAP is 120 mm Hg; calculate the new rate.

Multiple Mix-Up ... Case Closure

When a nurse needs to perform calculations under pressure (the patient's blood pressure was not stable, and the infusion needed to be started quickly), it is important that the process is simple and systematic.

1.   What went wrong? The nurse started the infusion at 18 mL/h when it should have been started at 16 mL/h.

2.   How could this situation be avoided?

   a.   Convert the ordered weight-based dose per minute (5 mcg/kg/min) to an hourly dose (300 mcg/kg/hour) prior to performing the calculations using the patient's weight. Because the minute rate was rounded from 0.26719 mL/min to 0.3 mL/min, the inaccurate rate was increased 60 times when converted to an hourly rate. Although the rate would have been correct if the nurse did not round the minute rate before multiplying by 60 minutes, there is less chance for error if the per-minute order is converted to an hourly order before performing calculations with the patient's weight.

$$5 \text{ mcg/kg/} \cancel{\text{min}} \ \times \ 60 \ \cancel{\text{min}} \text{/h} = 300 \text{ mcg/kg/h}$$

$$300 \text{ mcg/} \cancel{\text{kg}} \text{/h} \times 85.5 \ \cancel{\text{kg}} \ = 25,650 \text{ mcg/h}$$

$$25,650 \ \cancel{\text{mcg}} \text{/h} \div \ 1,600 \ \cancel{\text{mcg}} \text{/mL} = 16.03125 \text{ mL/h, rounds to } 16 \text{ mL/h}$$

   b.   Had a second nurse calculated the rate independently, the error might have been caught.

c. If the nurse had performed the calculation using dimensional analysis, in which all of the conversion factors are incorporated into the equation, the answer would have been accurate. This is why many critical care nurses use dimensional analysis when performing calculations for high-alert medications and multiple-factor problems.

$$x \text{ (mL/h)} = \frac{1 \text{ mL}}{1,600 \text{ \cancel{mcg}}} \times \frac{5 \text{ \cancel{mcg}}}{1 \text{ \cancel{kg}}} \times \frac{1 \text{ \cancel{kg}}}{2.2 \text{ \cancel{lb}}} \times \frac{188 \text{ \cancel{lb}}}{1} \times \frac{1}{1 \text{ \cancel{min}}} \times \frac{60 \text{ \cancel{min}}}{1 \text{ h}}$$

$$x = \frac{56,400 \text{ mL}}{3,520 \text{ h}}$$

$$x = 16.02273 \text{ mL/h, rounds to } 16 \text{ mL/h}$$

Chapter Summary

Learning Outcomes	Points to Remember
15-1 Calculate IV infusion flow rate based on dosage per time.	Use the IV solution as the supply and apply the CASE method.
	To simplify the math, reduce the supply to lowest terms, for example, $\frac{1000 \text{ mg}}{500 \text{ mL}} = \frac{2 \text{ mg}}{1 \text{ mL}}$.
15-2 Calculate IV infusion flow rate based on dosage per body weight and time.	Step 1: Convert the patient's weight from lb to kg. This step is not needed if using dimensional analysis, because the conversion factor, 1 kg/2.2 lb, can be inserted into the equation.
	Step 2: Convert the order and supply to like units. Although a weight conversion factor can be inserted into the dimensional analysis equation, this step is needed to perform the "Approximate" step of the CASE method.
	1. Determine the hourly weight-based dose.
	• Multiply the per-minute dose by 60 min/h.
	• Calculate the hourly dose.
	2. Determine the hourly rate.
	• The concentration of the IV solution is the "supply."
	• The hourly dose is the ordered dose.

15-3 Calculate the dose delivered by a specified IV rate.	1. Calculate the amount of medication delivered in 1 mL.
	2. Determine the delivered hourly dose.
	• Divide the rate by the amount of medication in 1 mL.
	3. Determine the delivered weight-based dose (if order is weight based).
	• Multiply the hourly dose by the patient's weight in kg.
	4. Determine the delivered per-minute dose.
	• Divide the hourly weight-based dose by 60 min/h (if weight-based dose is ordered per minute).
	• Divide the hourly dose by 60 min/h if the hourly dose is not weight based.
15-4 Calculate titrated IV infusion flow rates within prescribed parameters.	Continuous IV infusions of potent medications are *titrated* (adjusted for desired effect) by the nurse. In addition to the standard requirements for a medication order, the order for a titrated medication must include three criteria:
	• Measurable outcome
	• Starting dose
	• Dosage parameters

Homework

For exercises 1–2, refer to the following: (LO 15-1)
Order: nitroglycerin 40 mcg/min IV
Supply: nitroglycerin 50 mg in D_5W 250 mL
  1. What is the hourly dose?
  2. What is the hourly rate?

For exercises 3–4, refer to the following: (LO 15-1)
Order: procainamide HCl 3mg/min IV
Supply: procainamide HCl 1 g in D_5W 500 mL
  3. What is the hourly dose?
  4. What is the hourly rate?

For exercises 5–6, refer to the following: (LO 15-1)
Order: epinephrine 10 mcg/min IV
Supply: epinephrine 1 mg in D_5W 500 mL
  5. What is the hourly dose?
  6. What is the hourly rate?

For exercises 7–8, refer to the following: (LO 15-1)
Order: lidocaine 4 mg/min IV
Supply: lidocaine 1 g in D_5W 250 mL
  7. What is the hourly dose?
  8. What is the hourly rate?

For exercises 9–10, refer to the following: (LO 15-1)
Order: vasopressin 0.01 units/min IV
Supply: vasopressin 40 units in NS 40 mL
  9. What is the hourly dose?
 10. What is the hourly rate?

For exercise 11, refer to following: (LO 15-1)
Order: lorazepam 0.5 mg/h IV
Supply: lorazepam 10 mg in D_5W 100 mL
 11. What is the hourly rate?

For exercise 12, refer to the following: (LO 15-1)
Order: morphine 1.5 mg/h IV
Supply: morphine 10 mg in NS 100 mL
 12. What is the hourly rate?

For exercises 13–14, refer to the following: (LO 15-1)
Order: lidocaine 1 mg/min IV
Supply: lidocaine 1 g in D_5W 500 mL
 13. What is the hourly dose?
 14. What is the hourly rate?

For exercises 15–16, refer to the following: (LO 15-1)
Order: norepinephrine 2.5 mcg/min IV
Supply: norepinephrine 4 mg in D_5W 250 mL
Patient weight: 250 lb
 15. What is the hourly dose?
 16. What is the hourly rate?

For exercises 17–18, refer to the following: (LO 15-2)
Order: cisatracurium 3 mcg/kg/min
Supply: cisatracurium besylate 200 mg in D_5W 500 mL
Patient weight: 70 kg
 17. What is the hourly weight-based dose?
 18. What is the hourly rate?

For exercises 19–20, refer to the following: (LO 15-2)
Order: fentanyl 2 mcg/kg/h IV
Supply: fentanyl 1.25 mg in NS 250 mL
Patient weight: 75 kg
 19. What is the hourly weight-based dose?
 20. What is the hourly rate?

For exercises 21–23, refer to the following: (LO 15-2)
Order: esmolol 50 mcg/kg/minIV
Supply: esmolol 2,000 mg in NS 100 mL
Patient weight: 145 lb
 21. What is the patient's weight in kg?
 22. What is the hourly weight-based dose?
 23. What is the hourly rate?

For exercises 24–26, refer to the following: (LO 15-2)
Order: nitroprusside 0.3 mcg/kg/min IV
Supply: nitroprusside 50 mg in D_5W 500 mL
Patient weight: 198 lb
 24. What is the weight in kg?
 25. What is the hourly weight-based dose?
 26. What is the hourly rate?

For exercises 27–29, refer to the following: (LO 15-2)
Order: vecuronium 50 mcg/kg/h IV
Supply: vecuronium 10 mg in NS 100 mL
Patient weight: 135 lb
 27. What is the patient's weight in kg?
 28. What is the hourly dose?
 29. What is the hourly rate?

For exercises 30–32, refer to the following: (LO 15-2)
Order: midazolam 0.02 mg/kg/h IV
Supply midazolam 25 mg in NS 50 mL
Patient weight: 150 lb
 30. What is the patient's weight in kg?
 31. What is the hourly dose?
 32. What is the hourly rate?
 33. The patient's weight is 220 lb. Pancuronium bromide 500 mg in NS 250 mL is infusing at 3 mL/h IV. Determine how many mg/kg/h are infusing. (LO 15-3)

34. Nitroglycerin 100 mg in D_5W 500 mL is infusing at 6 mL/h IV. Determine how many mcg/h are infusing. (LO 15-3)

For exercises 35–42, refer to the following: (LO 15-4)

The patient weighs 140 lb. Dopamine 400 mg/500 mL NS is infusing at 3 mcg/kg/min, which is the lowest ordered dose. There is a titration order to increase the dose by 5 mcg/kg/min every 10–30 minutes as needed to achieve an MAP greater than or equal to 65 mm Hg. Do not exceed a maximum dose of 10 mcg/kg/min or a maximum HR of 100. After 30 minutes, the patient's MAP is 60 mm Hg and the HR is 52.

35. What is the patient's weight in kg?
36. What is the maximum hourly weight-based dose?
37. What is the maximum hourly rate?
38. What is the current hourly weight-based dose?
39. What is the current hourly rate?
40. What is the titration dose?
41. What is the titration rate?
42. Based on the current MAP and HR, to what new rate should the nurse set the IV infusion?

For exercises 43–50, refer to the following: (LO 15-4)

The patient weighs 175 lb. Nitroprusside 50 mg in D_5W 250 mL is infusing at 0.3 mcg/kg/min (the minimum dose). There is a titration order to increase the dose by 0.1 mcg/kg/min every 2 minutes as needed to keep the blood pressure less than or equal to 180/90 mm Hg. The maximum dose is 10 mcg/kg/min. After 2 minutes the patient's blood pressure (BP) is 200/108 mm Hg.

43. What is the patient's weight in kg?
44. What is the maximum hourly weight-based dose?
45. What is the maximum hourly rate?
46. What is the current hourly weight-based dose?
47. What is the current hourly rate?
48. What is the titration dose?
49. What is the titration rate?
50. Based on the current BP, to what new rate should the nurse set the IV infusion?

NCLEX-Style Review Questions

For questions 1–6 select the best response.

1. **Order:** isoproterenol 2 mcg/min IV
   Supply: isoproterenol 1 mg in NS 250 mL total volume

   What is the hourly dose?
   a. 0.12 mg
   b. 0.002 mg
   c. 1 mg
   d. 1.2 mg

2. **Order:** isoproterenol 0.5 mcg/min IV
   Supply: isoproterenol 1 mg in NS 250 mL total volume

   What is the hourly rate?
   a. 5 mL/h
   b. 7.5 mL/h
   c. 10 mL/h
   d. 12.5 mL/h

For questions 3–4, refer to the following: (LO 15-2)
Order: cisatracurium 3 mcg/kg/min
Supply: cisatracurium besylate 200 mg in D_5W 500 mL
Patient weight: 65 kg

3. What is the hourly weight-based dose?
   a. 180 mcg/h
   b. 195 mcg/h
   c. 11,700 mcg/h
   d. 12,600 mcg/h

4. What is the hourly rate?
   a. 9.8 mL/h
   b. 13.2 mL/h
   c. 29.3 mL/h
   d. 31.5 mL/h

5. The patient weighs 95 kg; nesiritide 1.5 mg in $D_5\frac{1}{2}$ NS 250 mL is infusing at 9.5 mL/h IV. Determine how many mcg/kg/min are infusing.
   a. 0.01
   b. 0.1
   c. 1
   d. 10

6. **Ordered:** epinephrine 2–10 mcg/min to attain HR greater than 60, but less than 80 and an MAP 65–100.

   Supply: epinephrine 2 mg/500 mL D_5W. Titrate in 1 mcg/min increments every 5 min as needed. The infusion is delivering 2 mcg/min. After 5 min the HR is 50 and the MAP is 62. At what rate should the nurse should set the infusion pump? (LO 15-4)
   a. 15 mL/h
   b. 30 mL/h
   c. 45 mL/h
   d. 60 mL/h

REFERENCE

U.S. Food and Drug Administration. (2012). Safety: Natrecor (nesiritide) for injection. *MedWatch*. Retrieved from http://www.fda.gov/Safety/ MedWatch/SafetyInformation/ucm169897.htm

Chapter 15   ANSWER KEY

Learning Activity 15-1
1. Reduced supply: 1 mg/4 mL; rate: 6 mL/h
2. Reduced supply: 1 mcg/1 mL; rate: 30 mL/h
3. Reduced supply: 1 mg/25 mL; rate: 2.5 mL/h

Learning Activity 15-2
1. Reduced supply: 1 mg/5 mL; rate: 16.7 mL/h
2. Reduced supply: 50 mcg/1 mL; rate: 18 mL/h
3. Reduced supply: 4 mg/1 mL; rate: 30 mL/h

Learning Activity 15-3
1. Supply in mcg/mL: 16 mcg/mL; rate: 38.4 mL/h
2. Supply in mcg/mL; 100 mcg/mL; rate: 15.1 mL/h
3. Supply in mcg/mL; 200 mcg/mL; rate: 10.1 mL/h

Learning Activity 15-4
1. Rate is *not* accurate; it should be 12 mL/h.
2. Rate is accurate.
3. Rate is *not* accurate; it should be 19.1 mL/h (19.125 rounded).

Learning Activity 15-5
1. a. 15 mL/h
   b. 75 mL/h
   c. 7.5 mL/h
   d. 22.5 mL/h

2. a. 2.4 mL/h
   b. 120 mL/h
   c. 1.2 mL/h
   d. 3.6 mL/h

Homework

1. 2,400 mcg/h
2. 12 mL/h
3. 180 mg/h
4. 90 mL/h
5. 600 mcg/h
6. 300 mL/h
7. 240 mg/h
8. 60 mL/h
9. 0.6 units/h
10. 0.6 mL/h
11. 5 mL/h
12. 15 mL/h
13. 60 mg/h
14. 30 mL/h
15. 150 mcg/h
16. 9.4 mL/h
17. 12,600 mcg/h
18. 31.5 mL/h
19. 150 mcg/h
20. 30 mL/h
21. 65.9 kg
22. 197,700 mcg/h
23. 9.9 mL/h (rounded from 9.885 mL/h)
24. 90 kg
25. 1,620 mcg/h
26. 16.2 mL/h
27. 61.4 kg (rounded from 61.3636)
28. 3,070 mcg/h
29. 30.7 mL/h
30. 68.2 kg
31. 1.364 mg/h
32. 2.7 mL/h
33. 0.06 mg/kg/h
34. 1,200 mcg/h
35. 63.6 kg
36. 38,160 mcg/h
37. 47.7 mL/h
38. 11,448 mcg/h
39. 14.3 mL/h (rounded from 14.31 mL/h)
40. 19,080 mcg/h
41. 23.9 mL/h (rounded from 23.85 mL/h)
42. 38.2 mL/h (current rate 14.3 mL/h + titration increment 23.9 mL/h)
43. 79.5 kg
44. 47,700 mcg/h
45. 238.5 mL/h
46. 1,431 mcg/h
47. 7.2 mL/h (rounded from 7.155 mL/h)
48. 477 mcg/h
49. 2.4 mL/h
50. 9.6 mL/h (current rate 7.2 mL/h + titration increment 2.4 mL/h)

NCLEX-Style Review Questions

1. a. 0.12 mg (120 mcg)

$$\frac{2 \text{ mcg}}{1 \text{ min}} \times \frac{60 \text{ min}}{1 \text{ h}} = \frac{120 \text{ mcg}}{1 \text{ h}}$$

$$\frac{120 \text{ mcg}}{1 \text{ h}} \times \frac{1 \text{ mg}}{1,000 \text{ mcg}} = 0.12 \text{ mg/h}$$

Note: The supply is not considered when solving this problem, because the question was about the dose, not the rate.

2. b. 7.5 mL/h

Rationale:

$$x(\text{mL/h}) = \frac{250 \text{ mL}}{1 \text{ mg}} \times \frac{1 \text{ mg}}{1,000 \text{ mcg}} \times \frac{0.5 \text{ mcg}}{1 \text{ min}} \times \frac{60 \text{ min}}{1 \text{ h}} = \frac{7,500 \text{ mL}}{1,000 \text{ h}} = 7.5 \text{ mL/h}$$

3. c. 11,700 mcg/h

$$x(\text{mcg/kg/h}) = \frac{3 \text{ mcg}}{1 \text{ kg}} \times \frac{65 \text{ kg}}{1} \times \frac{1}{1 \text{ min}} \times \frac{60 \text{ min}}{1 \text{ h}} = 11,700 \text{ mcg/h}$$

4. c. 29.3 mL/h (29.25 rounded)

$$x(\text{mL/h}) = \frac{500 \text{ mL}}{200 \text{ mg}} \times \frac{1 \text{ mg}}{1,000 \text{ mcg}} \times \frac{3 \text{ mcg}}{1 \text{ kg}} \times \frac{65 \text{ kg}}{1} \times \frac{1}{1 \text{ min}} \times \frac{60 \text{ min}}{1 \text{ h}} = \frac{5,850,000 \text{ mL}}{200,000 \text{ h}}$$

$$\frac{5,850,000 \text{ mL}}{200,000 \text{ h}} = \frac{29.25 \text{ mL}}{1 \text{ h}} \text{ which rounds to 29.3 mL/h}$$

5. a. 0.01

$$x \text{ (mcg/kg/min)} = \frac{1,000 \text{ mcg}}{1 \text{ mg}} \times \frac{1.5 \text{ mg}}{250 \text{ mL}} \times \frac{9.5 \text{ mL}}{1 \text{ h}} \times \frac{1 \text{ h}}{60 \text{ min}} \times \frac{1}{95 \text{ kg}} = \frac{14,250 \text{ mcg}}{1,425,000 \text{ kg/min}}$$

$$= 0.01 \text{ mcg/kg/min}$$

6. c. 45 mL/h

Because the HR is below 80 and the MAP is below 65, increase the current dose (2 mcg/min) by the titration increment of 1 mcg/min. Calculate the hourly rate using the new dose of 3 mcg/min:

$$x(\text{mL/h}) = \frac{500 \text{ mL}}{2 \text{ mg}} \times \frac{1 \text{ mg}}{1,000 \text{ mcg}} \times \frac{3 \text{ mcg}}{1 \text{ min}} \times \frac{60 \text{ min}}{1 \text{ h}} = \frac{90,000 \text{ mL}}{2,000 \text{ h}} = 45 \text{ mL/h}$$

© Forfunlife/Shutterstock

Appendix A

Calculating with Complex Fractions

A complex fraction is a fraction in which the numerator and/or the denominator is a fraction (e.g., $\dfrac{\frac{1}{2}}{1\frac{1}{4}}$, $\dfrac{\frac{3}{5}}{2}$, or $\dfrac{1}{\frac{2}{3}}$). To perform calculations with complex fractions, first reduce the complex fraction to a simple fraction or whole number. This is done by multiplying the numerator of the complex fraction by the reciprocal of the denominator. Follow the steps in Chapter 1 for dividing fractions. The numerator becomes the dividend (first number in a linear division equation) and the denominator is the divisor (second number in a linear division equation).

Example: $\dfrac{\frac{1}{2}}{1\frac{1}{4}} + \dfrac{\frac{3}{5}}{2}$

Step 1: Simplify the first complex fraction.

$$\frac{\frac{1}{2}}{1\frac{1}{4}} = \frac{1}{2} \div 1\frac{1}{4} = \frac{1}{2} \div \frac{5}{4} = \frac{1}{2} \times \frac{4}{5} = \frac{4}{10}$$

Step 2: Simplify the divisor.

$$\frac{\frac{3}{5}}{2} = \frac{3}{5} \div 2 = \frac{3}{5} \times \frac{1}{2} = \frac{3}{10}$$

Step 3: Add the simplified fractions.

$$\frac{4}{10} + \frac{3}{10} = \frac{7}{10}$$

© Forfunlife/Shutterstock

Appendix B

Apothecary System

As noted in Chapter 2, the apothecary system is an antiquated system of measurement based on the weight of one grain of wheat; therefore, the base unit of weight is one grain. The smallest measure of volume is one minim, which is a drop of water that weighs the same amount as one grain of wheat. Unlike the Metric System, there are no length measurements/equivalencies in the Apothecary System. Apothecary symbols, used for abbreviations, are on The Joint Commission's "Do Not Use" list, and will not be displayed here. Amounts are indicated by Roman numerals placed after the apothecary unit. For example, two grains (gr) is written as gr ii.

Volume Equivalencies	
Within Apothecary System	**Apothecary to Metric**
60 minims (m) = 1 fluidram 8 fluidrams = 1 fluid ounce 1 fluid ounce = 480 minims 16 fluid ounces = 1 pint (pt)	15–16 minims = 1 mL

Weight Equivalencies	
With Apothecary System	**Apothecary to Metric**
60 grains (gr) = 1 dram (dr) 8 drams (dr) = 1 ounce (oz) 1 ounce (oz) = 480 grains (gr) 16 ounce (oz) = 1 pound (lb)	1 grain (gr) = 60 mg or 65 mg 15 grain (gr) = 1 g 2.2 pound (lb) = 1 kg

© Forfunlife/Shutterstock

Appendix C

The Joint Commission's Do Not Use List

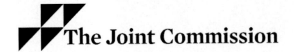

The Joint Commission

Official "Do Not Use" List[1]

Do Not Use	Potential Problem	Use Instead
U (unit)	Mistaken for "0" (zero), the number "4" (four) or "cc"	Write "unit"
IU (International Unit)	Mistaken for IV (intravenous) or the number 10 (ten)	Write "International Unit"
Q.D., QD, q.d., qd (daily)	Mistaken for each other	Write "daily"
Q.O.D., QOD, q.o.d, qod (every other day)	Period after the Q mistaken for "I" and the "O" mistaken for "I"	Write "every other day"
Trailing zero (X.0 mg)* Lack of leading zero (.X mg)	Decimal point is missed	Write X mg Write 0.X mg
MS	Can mean morphine sulfate or magnesium sulfate	Write "morphine sulfate" Write "magnesium sulfate"
MSO_4 and $MgSO_4$	Confused for one another	

[1] Applies to all orders and all medication-related documentation that is handwritten (including free-text computer entry) or on pre-printed forms.

*Exception: A "trailing zero" may be used only where required to demonstrate the level of precision of the value being reported, such as for laboratory results, imaging studies that report size of lesions, or catheter/tube sizes. It may not be used in medication orders or other medication-related documentation.

Additional Abbreviations, Acronyms and Symbols
(For possible future inclusion in the Official "Do Not Use" List)

Do Not Use	Potential Problem	Use Instead
> (greater than) < (less than)	Misinterpreted as the number "7" (seven) or the letter "L" Confused for one another	Write "greater than" Write "less than"
Abbreviations for drug names	Misinterpreted due to similar abbreviations for multiple drugs	Write drug names in full
Apothecary units	Unfamiliar to many practitioners Confused with metric units	Use metric units
@	Mistaken for the number "2" (two)	Write "at"
cc	Mistaken for U (units) when poorly written	Write "mL" or "ml" or "milliliters" ("mL" is preferred)
µg	Mistaken for mg (milligrams) resulting in one-thousand-fold overdose	Write "mcg" or "micrograms"

Updated 3/5/09

© Joint Commission Resources: The Joint Commission official: "Do Not Use List". Oakbrook Terrace, IL: Joint Commission on Accreditation of Healthcare Organizations, (2009). Reprinted with permission.

© Forfunlife/Shutterstock

Appendix D

ISMP's List of Error-Prone Abbreviations, Symbols, and Dose Designations

Institute for Safe Medication Practices

ISMP's List of *Error-Prone Abbreviations, Symbols,* and *Dose Designations*

The abbreviations, symbols, and dose designations found in this table have been reported to ISMP through the ISMP National Medication Errors Reporting Program (ISMP MERP) as being frequently misinterpreted and involved in harmful medication errors. They should **NEVER** be used when communicating medical information. This includes internal communications, telephone/verbal prescriptions, computer-generated labels, labels for drug storage bins, medication administration records, as well as pharmacy and prescriber computer order entry screens.

Abbreviations	Intended Meaning	Misinterpretation	Correction
μg	Microgram	Mistaken as "mg"	Use "mcg"
AD, AS, AU	Right ear, left ear, each ear	Mistaken as OD, OS, OU (right eye, left eye, each eye)	Use "right ear," "left ear," or "each ear"
OD, OS, OU	Right eye, left eye, each eye	Mistaken as AD, AS, AU (right ear, left ear, each ear)	Use "right eye," "left eye," or "each eye"
BT	Bedtime	Mistaken as "BID" (twice daily)	Use "bedtime"
cc	Cubic centimeters	Mistaken as "u" (units)	Use "mL"
D/C	Discharge or discontinue	Premature discontinuation of medications if D/C (intended to mean "discharge") has been misinterpreted as "discontinued" when followed by a list of discharge medications	Use "discharge" and "discontinue"
IJ	Injection	Mistaken as "IV" or "intrajugular"	Use "injection"
IN	Intranasal	Mistaken as "IM" or "IV"	Use "intranasal" or "NAS"
HS	Half-strength	Mistaken as bedtime	Use "half-strength" or "bedtime"
hs	At bedtime, hours of sleep	Mistaken as half-strength	
IU**	International unit	Mistaken as IV (intravenous) or 10 (ten)	Use "units"
o.d. or OD	Once daily	Mistaken as "right eye" (OD–oculus dexter), leading to oral liquid medications administered in the eye	Use "daily"
OJ	Orange juice	Mistaken as OD or OS (right or left eye); drugs meant to be diluted in orange juice may be given in the eye	Use "orange juice"
Per os	By mouth, orally	The "os" can be mistaken as "left eye" (OS–oculus sinister)	Use "PO," "by mouth," or "orally"
q.d. or QD**	Every day	Mistaken as q.i.d., especially if the period after the "q" or the tail of the "q" is misunderstood as an "i"	Use "daily"
qhs	Nightly at bedtime	Mistaken as "qhr" or every hour	Use "nightly"
qn	Nightly or at bedtime	Mistaken as "qh" (every hour)	Use "nightly" or "at bedtime"
q.o.d. or QOD**	Every other day	Mistaken as "q.d." (daily) or "q.i.d." (four times daily) if the "o" is poorly written	Use "every other day"
q1d	Daily	Mistaken as q.i.d. (four times daily)	Use "daily"
q6PM, etc.	Every evening at 6 PM	Mistaken as every 6 hours	Use "daily at 6 PM" or "6 PM daily"
SC, SQ, sub q	Subcutaneous	SC mistaken as SL (sublingual); SQ mistaken as "5 every;" the "q" in "sub q" has been mistaken as "every" (e.g., a heparin dose ordered "sub q 2 hours before surgery" misunderstood as every 2 hours before surgery)	Use "subcut" or "subcutaneously"
ss	Sliding scale (insulin) or ½ (apothecary)	Mistaken as "55"	Spell out "sliding scale;" use "one-half" or "½"
SSRI	Sliding scale regular insulin	Mistaken as selective-serotonin reuptake inhibitor	Spell out "sliding scale (insulin)"
SSI	Sliding scale insulin	Mistaken as Strong Solution of Iodine (Lugol's)	
i/d	One daily	Mistaken as "tid"	Use "1 daily"
TIW or tiw	3 times a week	Mistaken as "3 times a day" or "twice in a week"	Use "3 times weekly"
U or u**	Unit	Mistaken as the number 0 or 4, causing a 10-fold overdose or greater (e.g., 4U seen as "40" or 4u seen as "44"); mistaken as "cc" so dose given in volume instead of units (e.g., 4u seen as 4cc)	Use "unit"
UD	As directed ("ut dictum")	Mistaken as unit dose (e.g., diltiazem 125 mg IV infusion "UD" misinterpreted as meaning to give the entire infusion as a unit [bolus] dose)	Use "as directed"

Dose Designations and Other Information	Intended Meaning	Misinterpretation	Correction
Trailing zero after decimal point (e.g., 1.0 mg)**	1 mg	Mistaken as 10 mg if the decimal point is not seen	Do not use trailing zeros for doses expressed in whole numbers
"Naked" decimal point (e.g., .5 mg)**	0.5 mg	Mistaken as 5 mg if the decimal point is not seen	Use zero before a decimal point when the dose is less than a whole unit
Abbreviations such as mg. or mL. with a period following the abbreviation	mg mL	The period is unnecessary and could be mistaken as the number 1 if written poorly	Use mg, mL, etc., without a terminal period

Courtesy of the Institute for Safe Medication Practices.

Institute for Safe Medication Practices

ISMP's List of *Error-Prone Abbreviations, Symbols,* and *Dose Designations* (continued)

Dose Designations and Other Information	Intended Meaning	Misinterpretation	Correction
Drug name and dose run together (especially problematic for drug names that end in "l" such as Inderal40 mg; Tegretol300 mg)	Inderal 40 mg Tegretol 300 mg	Mistaken as Inderal 140 mg Mistaken as Tegretol 1300 mg	Place adequate space between the drug name, dose, and unit of measure
Numerical dose and unit of measure run together (e.g., 10mg, 100mL)	10 mg 100 mL	The "m" is sometimes mistaken as a zero or two zeros, risking a 10- to 100-fold overdose	Place adequate space between the dose and unit of measure
Large doses without properly placed commas (e.g., 100000 units; 1000000 units)	100,000 units 1,000,000 units	100000 has been mistaken as 10,000 or 1,000,000; 1000000 has been mistaken as 100,000	Use commas for dosing units at or above 1,000, or use words such as 100 "thousand" or 1 "million" to improve readability

Drug Name Abbreviations	Intended Meaning	Misinterpretation	Correction
To avoid confusion, do not abbreviate drug names when communicating medical information. Examples of drug name abbreviations involved in medication errors include:			
APAP	acetaminophen	Not recognized as acetaminophen	Use complete drug name
ARA A	vidarabine	Mistaken as cytarabine (ARA C)	Use complete drug name
AZT	zidovudine (Retrovir)	Mistaken as azathioprine or aztreonam	Use complete drug name
CPZ	Compazine (prochlorperazine)	Mistaken as chlorpromazine	Use complete drug name
DPT	Demerol-Phenergan-Thorazine	Mistaken as diphtheria-pertussis-tetanus (vaccine)	Use complete drug name
DTO	Diluted tincture of opium, or deodorized tincture of opium (Paregoric)	Mistaken as tincture of opium	Use complete drug name
HCl	hydrochloric acid or hydrochloride	Mistaken as potassium chloride (The "H" is misinterpreted as "K")	Use complete drug name unless expressed as a salt of a drug
HCT	hydrocortisone	Mistaken as hydrochlorothiazide	Use complete drug name
HCTZ	hydrochlorothiazide	Mistaken as hydrocortisone (seen as HCT250 mg)	Use complete drug name
MgSO4**	magnesium sulfate	Mistaken as morphine sulfate	Use complete drug name
MS, MSO4**	morphine sulfate	Mistaken as magnesium sulfate	Use complete drug name
MTX	methotrexate	Mistaken as mitoxantrone	Use complete drug name
PCA	procainamide	Mistaken as patient-controlled analgesia	Use complete drug name
PTU	propylthiouracil	Mistaken as mercaptopurine	Use complete drug name
T3	Tylenol with codeine No. 3	Mistaken as liothyronine	Use complete drug name
TAC	triamcinolone	Mistaken as tetracaine, Adrenalin, cocaine	Use complete drug name
TNK	TNKase	Mistaken as "TPA"	Use complete drug name
ZnSO4	zinc sulfate	Mistaken as morphine sulfate	Use complete drug name

Stemmed Drug Names	Intended Meaning	Misinterpretation	Correction
"Nitro" drip	nitroglycerin infusion	Mistaken as sodium nitroprusside infusion	Use complete drug name
"Norflox"	norfloxacin	Mistaken as Norflex	Use complete drug name
"IV Vanc"	intravenous vancomycin	Mistaken as Invanz	Use complete drug name

Symbols	Intended Meaning	Misinterpretation	Correction
℥ ♏	Dram Minim	Symbol for dram mistaken as "3" Symbol for minim mistaken as "mL"	Use the metric system
x3d	For three days	Mistaken as "3 doses"	Use "for three days"
> and <	Greater than and less than	Mistaken as opposite of intended; mistakenly use incorrect symbol; "< 10" mistaken as "40"	Use "greater than" or "less than"
/ (slash mark)	Separates two doses or indicates "per"	Mistaken as the number 1 (e.g., "25 units/10 units" misread as "25 units and 110" units)	Use "per" rather than a slash mark to separate doses
@	At	Mistaken as "2"	Use "at"
&	And	Mistaken as "2"	Use "and"
+	Plus or and	Mistaken as "4"	Use "and"
°	Hour	Mistaken as a zero (e.g., q2° seen as q 20)	Use "hr," "h," or "hour"
Φ or ⦰	zero, null sign	Mistaken as numerals 4, 6, 8, and 9	Use 0 or zero, or describe intent using whole words

**These abbreviations are included on The Joint Commission's "minimum list" of dangerous abbreviations, acronyms, and symbols that must be included on an organization's "Do Not Use" list, effective January 1, 2004. Visit www.jointcommission.org for more information about this Joint Commission requirement.

© ISMP 2013. Permission is granted to reproduce material with proper attribution for internal use within healthcare organizations. Other reproduction is prohibited without written permission from ISMP. Report actual and potential medication errors to the ISMP National Medication Errors Reporting Program (ISMP MERP) via the Web at www.ismp.org or by calling 1-800-FAIL-SAF(E).

www.ismp.org

Courtesy of the Institute for Safe Medication Practices.

© Forfunlife/Shutterstock

Appendix E

ISMP's List of Confused Drug Names

Institute for Safe Medication Practices

ISMP's List of *Confused Drug Names*

This list of confused drug names, which includes look-alike and sound-alike name pairs, consists of those name pairs that have been published in the *ISMP Medication Safety Alert!* and the *ISMP Medication Safety Alert!* Community/Ambulatory Care Edition. Events involving these medications were reported to ISMP through either the ISMP National Medication Errors Reporting Program (ISMP MERP) or ISMP National Vaccine Errors Reporting Program (ISMP VERP). We hope you will use this list to determine which medications require special safeguards to reduce the risk of errors. This may include strategies such as: using both the brand and generic names on prescriptions and labels; including the purpose of the medication on prescriptions; configuring computer selection screens to prevent look-alike names from appearing consecutively; and changing the appearance of look-alike product names to draw attention to their dissimilarities. Both the FDA-approved and the ISMP-recommended tall man (mixed case) letters have been included in the list below.

Updated February 2015

Drug Name	Confused Drug Name
Abelcet	amphotericin B
Accupril	Aciphex
acetaZOLAMIDE	acetoHEXAMIDE
acetic acid for irrigation	glacial acetic acid
acetoHEXAMIDE	acetaZOLAMIDE
Aciphex	Accupril
Aciphex	Aricept
Activase	Cathflo Activase
Activase	TNKase
Actonel	Actos
Actos	Actonel
Adacel (Tdap)	Daptacel (DTaP)
Adderall	Inderal
Adderall	Adderall XR
Adderall XR	Adderall
ado-trastuzumab emtansine	trastuzumab
Advair	Advicor
Advicor	Advair
Advicor	Altocor
Afrin (oxymetazoline)	Afrin (saline)
Afrin (saline)	Afrin (oxymetazoline)
Aggrastat	argatroban
Aldara	Alora
Alkeran	Leukeran
Alkeran	Myleran
Allegra (fexofenadine)	Allegra Anti-Itch Cream (diphenhydrAMINE/allantoin)
Allegra	Viagra
Allegra Anti-Itch Cream (diphenhydrAMINE/allantoin)	Allegra (fexofenadine)
Alora	Aldara
ALPRAZolam	LORazepam
Altocor	Advicor
amantadine	amiodarone
Amaryl	Reminyl
Ambisome	amphotericin B
Amicar	Omacor

Drug Name	Confused Drug Name
Amikin	Kineret
aMILoride	amLODIPine
amiodarone	amantadine
amLODIPine	aMILoride
amphotericin B	Abelcet
amphotericin B	Ambisome
Anacin	Anacin-3
Anacin-3	Anacin
antacid	Atacand
Anticoagulant Citrate Dextrose Solution Formula A	Anticoagulant Sodium Citrate Solution
Anticoagulant Sodium Citrate Solution	Anticoagulant Citrate Dextrose Solution Formula A
Antivert	Axert
Anzemet	Avandamet
Apidra	Spiriva
Apresoline	Priscoline
argatroban	Aggrastat
argatroban	Orgaran
Aricept	Aciphex
Aricept	Azilect
ARIPiprazole	proton pump inhibitors
ARIPiprazole	RABEprazole
Arista AH (absorbable hemostatic agent)	Arixtra
Arixtra	Arista AH (absorbable hemostatic agent)
Asacol	Os-Cal
Atacand	antacid
atomoxetine	atorvastatin
atorvastatin	atomoxetine
Atrovent	Natru-Vent
Avandamet	Anzemet
Avandia	Prandin
Avandia	Coumadin
AVINza	INVanz
AVINza	Evista
Axert	Antivert
azaCITIDine	azaTHIOprine

* Brand names always start with an uppercase letter. Some brand names incorporate tall man letters in initial characters and may not be readily recognized as brand names. Brand name products appear in black; generic/other products appear in red.

www.ismp.org

Courtesy of the Institute for Safe Medication Practices.

Institute for Safe Medication Practices

ISMP's List of *Confused Drug Names*

Drug Name	Confused Drug Name	Drug Name	Confused Drug Name
azaTHIOprine	azaCITIDine	CeleXA	ZyPREXA
Azilect	Aricept	CeleXA	CeleBREX
B & O (belladonna and opium)	Beano	CeleXA	Cerebyx
BabyBIG	HBIG (hepatitis B immune globulin)	Cerebyx	CeleBREX
Bayhep-B	Bayrab	Cerebyx	CeleXA
Bayhep-B	Bayrho-D	cetirizine	sertraline
Bayrab	Bayhep-B	cetirizine	stavudine
Bayrab	Bayrho-D	chlordiazePOXIDE	chlorproMAZINE
Bayrho-D	Bayhep-B	chlorproMAZINE	chlordiazePOXIDE
Bayrho-D	Bayrab	chlorproMAZINE	chlorproPAMIDE
Beano	B & O (belladonna and opium)	chlorproPAMIDE	chlorproMAZINE
Benadryl	benazepril	Cidex	Cedax
benazepril	Benadryl	CISplatin	CARBOplatin
Benicar	Mevacor	Claritin (loratadine)	Claritin Eye (ketotifen fumarate)
Betadine (with providone-iodine)	Betadine (without providone-iodine)	Claritin-D	Claritin-D 24
Betadine (without providone-iodine)	Betadine (with providone-iodine)	Claritin-D 24	Claritin-D
Bextra	Zetia	Claritin Eye (ketotifen fumarate)	Claritin (loratadine)
Bicillin C-R	Bicillin L-A	Clindesse	Clindets
Bicillin L-A	Bicillin C-R	Clindets	Clindesse
Bicitra	Polycitra	clobazam	clonazePAM
Bidex	Videx	clomiPHENE	clomiPRAMINE
Brethine	Methergine	clomiPRAMINE	clomiPHENE
Bio-T-Gel	T-Gel	clonazePAM	clobazam
Brevibloc	Brevital	clonazePAM	cloNIDine
Brevital	Brevibloc	clonazePAM	LORazepam
Brilinta	Brintellix	cloNIDine	clonazePAM
Brintellix	Brilinta	cloNIDine	KlonoPIN
buPROPion	busPIRone	Clozaril	Colazal
busPIRone	buPROPion	coagulation factor IX (recombinant)	factor IX complex, vapor heated
Capadex [non-US product]	Kapidex	codeine	Lodine
Capex	Kapidex	Colace	Cozaar
Carac	Kuric	Colazal	Clozaril
captopril	carvedilol	colchicine	Cortrosyn
carBAMazepine	OXcarbazepine	Comvax	Recombivax HB
CARBOplatin	CISplatin	Cortrosyn	colchicine
Cardene	Cardizem	Coumadin	Avandia
Cardizem	Cardene	Coumadin	Cardura
Cardura	Coumadin	Covaryx HS	Covera HS
carvedilol	captopril	Covera HS	Covaryx HS
Casodex	Kapidex	Cozaar	Colace
Cathflo Activase	Activase	Cozaar	Zocor
Cedax	Cidex	cyclophosphamide	cycloSPORINE
ceFAZolin	cefTRIAXone	cycloSERINE	cycloSPORINE
cefTRIAXone	ceFAZolin	cycloSPORINE	cyclophosphamide
CeleBREX	CeleXA	cycloSPORINE	cycloSERINE
CeleBREX	Cerebyx	Cymbalta	Symbyax

* Brand names always start with an uppercase letter. Some brand names incorporate tall man letters in initial characters and may not be readily recognized as brand names. Brand name products appear in black; generic/other products appear in red.

www.ismp.org

Institute for Safe Medication Practices

ISMP's List of *Confused Drug Names*

Drug Name	Confused Drug Name	Drug Name	Confused Drug Name
DACTINomycin	**DAPTO**mycin	Durasal	Durezol
Daptacel (DTaP)	Adacel (Tdap)	Durezol	Durasal
DAPTOmycin	**DACTIN**omycin	Duricef	Ultracet
Darvocet	Percocet	Dynacin	Dynacirc
Darvon	Diovan	Dynacirc	Dynacin
DAUNOrubicin	**DAUNO**rubicin citrate liposomal	edetate calcium disodium	edetate disodium
DAUNOrubicin	**DOXO**rubicin	edetate disodium	edetate calcium disodium
DAUNOrubicin	**IDA**rubicin	Effexor	Effexor XR
DAUNOrubicin citrate liposomal	**DAUNO**rubicin	Effexor XR	Enablex
Denavir	indinavir	Effexor XR	Effexor
Depakote	Depakote ER	Enablex	Effexor XR
Depakote ER	Depakote	Enbrel	Levbid
Depo-Medrol	Solu-**MEDROL**	Engerix-B adult	Engerix-B pediatric/adolescent
Depo-Provera	Depo-subQ provera 104	Engerix-B pediatric/adolescent	Engerix-B adult
Depo-subQ provera 104	Depo-Provera	Enjuvia	Januvia
desipramine	disopyramide	e**PHED**rine	**EPINEPH**rine
Desyrel	**SERO**quel	**EPINEPH**rine	e**PHED**rine
dexmethylphenidate	methadone	epirubicin	eribulin
Diabenese	Diamox	eribulin	epirubicin
Diabeta	Zebeta	Estratest	Estratest HS
Diamox	Diabenese	Estratest HS	Estratest
Diflucan	Diprivan	ethambutol	Ethmozine
Dilacor XR	Pilocar	ethaverine [non-US name]	etravirine
Dilaudid	Dilaudid-5	Ethmozine	ethambutol
Dilaudid-5	Dilaudid	etravirine	ethaverine [non-US name]
dimenhy**DRINATE**	diphenhydr**AMINE**	Evista	**AVIN**za
diphenhydr**AMINE**	dimenhy**DRINATE**	factor IX complex, vapor heated	coagulation factor IX (recombinant)
Dioval	Diovan	Fanapt	Xanax
Diovan	Dioval	Farxiga	Fetzima
Diovan	Zyban	Fastin (phentermine)	Fastin (dietary supplement)
Diovan	Darvon	Fastin (dietary supplement)	Fastin (phentermine)
Diprivan	Diflucan	Femara	Femhrt
Diprivan	Ditropan	Femhrt	Femara
disopyramide	desipramine	fenta**NYL**	**SUF**entanil
Ditropan	Diprivan	Fetzima	Farxiga
DOBUTamine	**DOP**amine	Fioricet	Fiorinal
DOPamine	**DOBUT**amine	Fiorinal	Fioricet
Doribax	Zovirax	flavox**ATE**	fluvoxa**MINE**
Doxil	Paxil	Flonase	Flovent
DOXOrubicin	**DAUNO**rubicin	Floranex	Florinef
DOXOrubicin	**DOXO**rubicin liposomal	Florastor	Florinef
DOXOrubicin	**IDA**rubicin	Florinef	Floranex
DOXOrubicin liposomal	**DOXO**rubicin	Florinef	Florastor
Dulcolax (bisacodyl)	Dulcolax (docusate sodium)	Flovent	Flonase
Dulcolax (docusate sodium)	Dulcolax (bisacodyl)	flumazenil	influenza virus vaccine
DULoxetine	**FLU**oxetine	**FLU**oxetine	**PAR**oxetine

* Brand names always start with an uppercase letter. Some brand names incorporate tall man letters in initial characters and may not be readily recognized as brand names. Brand name products appear in black; generic/other products appear in red.

INSTITUTE FOR SAFE MEDICATION PRACTICES

www.ismp.org

Institute for Safe Medication Practices

ISMP's List of *Confused Drug Names*

Drug Name	Confused Drug Name	Drug Name	Confused Drug Name
FLUoxetine	DULoxetine	IDArubicin	DAUNOrubicin
FLUoxetine	Loxitane	IDArubicin	DOXOrubicin
fluvoxaMINE	flavoxATE	Inderal	Adderall
Focalgin B	Focalin	indinavir	Denavir
Focalin	Focalgin B	inFLIXimab	riTUXimab
Folex	Foltx	influenza virus vaccine	flumazenil
folic acid	folinic acid (leucovorin calcium)	influenza virus vaccine	perflutren lipid microspheres
folinic acid (leucovorin calcium)	folic acid	influenza virus vaccine	tuberculin purified protein derivative (PPD)
Foltx	Folex	Inspra	Spiriva
fomepizole	omeprazole	Intuniv	Invega
Foradil	Fortical	INVanz	AVINza
Foradil	Toradol	Invega	Intuniv
Fortical	Foradil	iodine	Lodine
gentamicin	gentian violet	Isordil	Plendil
gentian violet	gentamicin	ISOtretinoin	tretinoin
glacial acetic acid	acetic acid for irrigation	Jantoven	Janumet
glipiZIDE	glyBURIDE	Jantoven	Januvia
Glucotrol	Glycotrol	Janumet	Jantoven
glyBURIDE	glipiZIDE	Janumet	Januvia
Glycotrol	Glucotrol	Janumet	Sinemet
Granulex	Regranex	Januvia	Enjuvia
guaiFENesin	guanFACINE	Januvia	Jantoven
guanFACINE	guaiFENesin	Januvia	Janumet
HBIG (hepatitis B immune globulin)	BabyBIG	K-Phos Neutral	Neutra-Phos-K
Healon	Hyalgan	Kaopectate (bismuth subsalcylate)	Kaopectate (docusate calcium)
heparin	Hespan	Kaopectate (docusate calcium)	Kaopectate (bismuth subsalcylate)
Hespan	heparin	Kadian	Kapidex
HMG-CoA reductase inhibitors ("statins")	nystatin	Kaletra	Keppra
HumaLOG	HumuLIN	Kapidex	Capadex [non-US product]
HumaLOG	NovoLOG	Kapidex	Capex
HumaLOG Mix 75/25	HumuLIN 70/30	Kapidex	Casodex
Humapen Memoir (for use with HumaLOG)	Humira Pen	Kapidex	Kadian
Humira Pen	Humapen Memoir (for use with HumaLOG)	Keflex	Keppra
HumuLIN	NovoLIN	Keppra	Kaletra
HumuLIN	HumaLOG	Keppra	Keflex
HumuLIN 70/30	HumaLOG Mix 75/25	Ketalar	ketorolac
HumuLIN R U-100	HumuLIN R U-500	ketorolac	Ketalar
HumuLIN R U-500	HumuLIN R U-100	ketorolac	methadone
Hyalgan	Healon	Kineret	Amikin
hydrALAZINE	hydrOXYzine	KlonoPIN	cloNIDine
Hydrea	Lyrica	Kuric	Carac
HYDROcodone	oxyCODONE	Kwell	Qwell
Hydrogesic	hydrOXYzine	LaMICtal	LamISIL
HYDROmorphone	morphine	LamISIL	LaMICtal
hydrOXYzine	Hydrogesic	lamiVUDine	lamoTRIgine
hydrOXYzine	hydrALAZINE	lamoTRIgine	lamiVUDine

* Brand names always start with an uppercase letter. Some brand names incorporate tall man letters in initial characters and may not be readily recognized as brand names. Brand name products appear in black; generic/other products appear in red.

Institute for Safe Medication Practices

ISMP's List of *Confused Drug Names*

Drug Name	Confused Drug Name	Drug Name	Confused Drug Name
lamoTRIgine	levETIRAcetam	Lovenox	Levemir
lamoTRIgine	levothyroxine	Loxitane	Lexapro
Lanoxin	levothyroxine	Loxitane	FLUoxetine
Lanoxin	naloxone	Loxitane	Soriatane
lanthanum carbonate	lithium carbonate	Lunesta	Neulasta
Lantus	Latuda	Lupron Depot-3 Month	Lupron Depot-Ped
Lantus	Lente	Lupron Depot-Ped	Lupron Depot-3 Month
Lariam	Levaquin	Luvox	Lasix
Lasix	Luvox	Lyrica	Hydrea
Latuda	Lantus	Lyrica	Lopressor
Lente	Lantus	Maalox	Maalox Total Stomach Relief
Letairis	Letaris [non-US product]	Maalox Total Stomach Relief	Maalox
Letaris [non-US product]	Letairis	Matulane	Materna
leucovorin calcium	Leukeran	Materna	Matulane
leucovorin calcium	levoleucovorin	Maxzide	Microzide
Leukeran	Alkeran	Menactra	Menomune
Leukeran	Myleran	Menomune	Menactra
Leukeran	leucovorin calcium	Mephyton	methadone
Levaquin	Lariam	Metadate	methadone
Levbid	Enbrel	Metadate CD	Metadate ER
levETIRAcetam	lamoTRIgine	Metadate ER	Metadate CD
Levemir	Lovenox	Metadate ER	methadone
levETIRAcetam	levOCARNitine	metFORMIN	metroNIDAZOLE
levETIRAcetam	levofloxacin	methadone	dexmethylphenidate
levOCARNitine	levETIRAcetam	methadone	ketorolac
levofloxacin	levETIRAcetam	methadone	Mephyton
levoleucovorin	leucovorin calcium	methadone	Metadate
levothyroxine	lamoTRIgine	methadone	Metadate ER
levothyroxine	Lanoxin	methadone	methylphenidate
levothyroxine	liothyronine	methadone	metolazone
Lexapro	Loxitane	Methergine	Brethine
Lexiva	Pexeva	methimazole	metolazone
liothyronine	levothyroxine	methylene blue	VisionBlue
Lipitor	Loniten	methylphenidate	methadone
Lipitor	ZyrTEC	metolazone	methadone
lithium	Ultram	metolazone	methimazole
lithium carbonate	lanthanum carbonate	metoprolol succinate	metoprolol tartrate
Lodine	codeine	metoprolol tartrate	metoprolol succinate
Lodine	iodine	metroNIDAZOLE	metFORMIN
Loniten	Lipitor	Mevacor	Benicar
Lopressor	Lyrica	Micronase	Microzide
LORazepam	ALPRAZolam	Microzide	Maxzide
LORazepam	clonazePAM	Microzide	Micronase
LORazepam	Lovaza	midodrine	Midrin
Lotronex	Protonix	Midrin	midodrine
Lovaza	LORazepam	mifepristone	misoprostol

* Brand names always start with an uppercase letter. Some brand names incorporate tall man letters in initial characters and may not be readily recognized as brand names. Brand name products appear in black; generic/other products appear in red.

www.ismp.org

Institute for Safe Medication Practices

ISMP's List of *Confused Drug Names*

Drug Name	Confused Drug Name	Drug Name	Confused Drug Name
Miralax	Mirapex	NovoLIN	HumuLIN
Mirapex	Miralax	NovoLIN	NovoLOG
misoprostol	mifepristone	NovoLIN 70/30	NovoLOG Mix 70/30
mitoMYcin	mitoXANtrone	NovoLOG	HumaLOG
mitoXANtrone	mitoMYcin	NovoLOG	NovoLIN
morphine	HYDROmorphone	NovoLOG Flexpen	NovoLOG Mix 70/30 Flexpen
morphine - non-concentrated oral liquid	morphine - oral liquid concentrate	NovoLOG Mix 70/30 Flexpen	NovoLOG Flexpen
morphine - oral liquid concentrate	morphine - non-concentrated oral liquid	NovoLOG Mix 70/30	NovoLIN 70/30
Motrin	Neurontin	Nuedexta	Neulasta
MS Contin	OxyCONTIN	nystatin	HMG-CoA reductase inhibitors ("statins")
Mucinex	Mucinex Allergy	Occlusal-HP	Ocuflox
Mucinex	Mucomyst	Ocuflox	Occlusal-HP
Mucinex Allergy	Mucinex	OLANZapine	QUEtiapine
Mucinex D	Mucinex DM	Omacor	Amicar
Mucinex DM	Mucinex D	omeprazole	fomepizole
Mucomyst	Mucinex	opium tincture	paregoric (camphorated tincture of opium)
Myleran	Alkeran	Oracea	Orencia
Myleran	Leukeran	Orencia	Oracea
nalbuphine	naloxone	Organan	argatroban
naloxone	Lanoxin	Ortho Tri-Cyclen	Ortho Tri-Cyclen LO
naloxone	nalbuphine	Ortho Tri-Cyclen LO	Ortho Tri-Cyclen
Narcan	Norcuron	Os-Cal	Asacol
Natru-Vent	Atrovent	oxaprozin	OXcarbazepine
Navane	Norvasc	OXcarbazepine	oxaprozin
Neo-Synephrine (oxymetazoline)	Neo-Synephrine (phenylephrine)	OXcarbazepine	carBAMazepine
Neo-Synephrine (phenylephrine)	Neo-Synephrine (oxymetazoline)	oxyCODONE	HYDROcodone
Neulasta	Lunesta	oxyCODONE	OxyCONTIN
Neulasta	Neumega	OxyCONTIN	MS Contin
Neulasta	Nuedexta	OxyCONTIN	oxyCODONE
Neumega	Neupogen	PACLitaxel	PACLitaxel protein-bound particles
Neumega	Neulasta	PACLitaxel protein-bound particles	PACLitaxel
Neupogen	Neumega	Pamelor	Panlor DC
Neurontin	Motrin	Pamelor	Tambocor
Neurontin	Noroxin	Panlor DC	Pamelor
Neutra-Phos-K	K-Phos Neutral	paregoric (camphorated tincture of opium)	opium tincture
NexAVAR	NexIUM	PARoxetine	FLUoxetine
NexIUM	NexAVAR	PARoxetine	piroxicam
niCARdipine	NIFEdipine	Patanol	Platinol
NIFEdipine	niCARdipine	Pavulon	Peptavlon
NIFEdipine	niMODipine	Paxil	Doxil
niMODipine	NIFEdipine	Paxil	Taxol
Norcuron	Narcan	Paxil	Plavix
Normodyne	Norpramin	PAZOPanib	PONATinib
Noroxin	Neurontin	PEMEtrexed	PRALAtrexate
Norpramin	Normodyne	penicillin	penicillAMINE
Norvasc	Navane	penicillAMINE	penicillin

* Brand names always start with an uppercase letter. Some brand names incorporate tall man letters in initial characters and may not be readily recognized as brand names. Brand name products appear in black; generic/other products appear in red.

INSTITUTE FOR SAFE MEDICATION PRACTICES

www.ismp.org

Institute for Safe Medication Practices

ISMP's List of *Confused Drug Names*

Drug Name	Confused Drug Name	Drug Name	Confused Drug Name
Peptavlon	Pavulon	Provera	Proscar
Percocet	Darvocet	Provera	**PRO**zac
Percocet	Procet	**PRO**zac	Prograf
perflutren lipid microspheres	influenza virus vaccine	**PRO**zac	Pri**LOSEC**
Pexeva	Lexiva	**PRO**zac	Provera
PENTobarbital	**PHEN**obarbital	Purinethol	propylthiouracil
PHENobarbital	**PENT**obarbital	Pyridium	pyridoxine
Pilocar	Dilacor XR	pyridoxine	Pyridium
piroxicam	**PAR**oxetine	**QUE**tiapine	**OLANZ**apine
Platinol	Patanol	qui**NID**ine	qui**NINE**
Plavix	Paxil	qui**NINE**	qui**NID**ine
Plavix	Pradax [Non-US Product]	Qwell	Kwell
Plavix	Pradaxa	**RABE**prazole	**ARIP**iprazole
Plendil	Isordil	Ranexa	Prenexa
pneumococcal 7-valent vaccine	pneumococcal polyvalent vaccine	Rapaflo	Rapamune
pneumococcal polyvalent vaccine	pneumococcal 7-valent vaccine	Rapamune	Rapaflo
Polycitra	Bicitra	Razadyne	Rozerem
PONATinib	**PAZOP**anib	Recombivax HB	Comvax
potassium acetate	sodium acetate	Regranex	Granulex
PRALAtrexate	**PEME**trexed	Reminyl	Robinul
Pradax [Non-US Product]	Plavix	Reminyl	Amaryl
Pradaxa	Plavix	Renagel	Renvela
Prandin	Avandia	Renvela	Renagel
Precare	Precose	Reprexain	Zy**PREXA**
Precose	Precare	Restoril	Risper**DAL**
predniso**LONE**	predni**SONE**	Retrovir	ritonavir
predni**SONE**	predniso**LONE**	Rifadin	Rifater
Prenexa	Ranexa	Rifamate	rifampin
Pri**LOSEC**	Pristiq	rifampin	Rifamate
Pri**LOSEC**	**PRO**zac	rifampin	rifaximin
Priscoline	Apresoline	Rifater	Rifadin
Pristiq	Pri**LOSEC**	rifaximin	rifampin
probenecid	Procanbid	Risper**DAL**	Restoril
Procan SR	Procanbid	risperi**DONE**	r**OPINIR**ole
Procanbid	probenecid	Ritalin	ritodrine
Procanbid	Procan SR	Ritalin LA	Ritalin SR
Procardia XL	Protain XL	Ritalin SR	Ritalin LA
Procet	Percocet	ritodrine	Ritalin
Prograf	**PRO**zac	ritonavir	Retrovir
propylthiouracil	Purinethol	ri**TUX**imab	in**FLIX**imab
Proscar	Provera	Robinul	Reminyl
Protain XL	Procardia XL	r**OPINIR**ole	risperi**DONE**
protamine	Protonix	Roxanol	Roxicodone Intensol
proton pump inhibitors	**ARIP**iprazole	Roxanol	Roxicet
Protonix	Lotronex	Roxicet	Roxanol
Protonix	protamine	Roxicodone Intensol	Roxanol

* Brand names always start with an uppercase letter. Some brand names incorporate tall man letters in initial characters and may not be readily recognized as brand names. Brand name products appear in black; generic/other products appear in red.

www.ismp.org

Institute for Safe Medication Practices

ISMP's List of *Confused Drug Names*

Drug Name	Confused Drug Name	Drug Name	Confused Drug Name
Rozerem	Razadyne	sulfADIAZINE	sulfiSOXAZOLE
Salagen	selegiline	sulfaSALAzine	sulfADIAZINE
SandIMMUNE	SandoSTATIN	sulfiSOXAZOLE	sulfADIAZINE
SandoSTATIN	SandIMMUNE	SUMAtriptan	sitaGLIPtin
saquinavir	SINEquan	SUMAtriptan	ZOLMitriptan
saquinavir (free base)	saquinavir mesylate	Symbyax	Cymbalta
saquinavir mesylate	saquinavir (free base)	T-Gel	Bio-T-Gel
Sarafem	Serophene	Tambocor	Pamelor
selegiline	Salagen	Taxol	Taxotere
Serophene	Sarafem	Taxol	Paxil
SEROquel	Desyrel	Taxotere	Taxol
SEROquel	SEROquel XR	TEGretol	TEGretol XR
SEROquel	Serzone	TEGretol	Tequin
SEROquel	SINEquan	TEGretol	TRENtal
SEROquel XR	SEROquel	TEGretol XR	TEGretol
sertraline	cetirizine	Tenex	Xanax
sertraline	Soriatane	Tequin	TEGretol
Serzone	SEROquel	Tequin	Ticlid
silodosin	sirolimus	Testoderm	Testoderm with Adhesive
Sinemet	Janumet	Testoderm	Testoderm TTS
SINEquan	saquinavir	Testoderm with Adhesive	Testoderm
SINEquan	SEROquel	Testoderm with Adhesive	Testoderm TTS
SINEquan	Singulair	Testoderm TTS	Testoderm
SINEquan	Zonegran	Testoderm TTS	Testoderm with Adhesive
Singulair	SINEquan	tetanus diptheria toxoid (Td)	tuberculin purified protein derivative (PPD)
sirolimus	silodosin	Thalomid	Thiamine
sitaGLIPtin	SUMAtriptan	Thiamine	Thalomid
sodium acetate	potassium acetate	tiaGABine	tiZANidine
Solu-CORTEF	Solu-MEDROL	Tiazac	Ziac
Solu-MEDROL	Depo-Medrol	Ticlid	Tequin
Solu-MEDROL	Solu-CORTEF	tiZANidine	tiaGABine
Sonata	Soriatane	TNKase	Activase
Soriatane	Loxitane	TNKase	t-PA
Soriatane	sertraline	Tobradex	Tobrex
Soriatane	Sonata	Tobrex	Tobradex
sotalol	Sudafed	TOLAZamide	TOLBUTamide
Spiriva	Apidra	TOLBUTamide	TOLAZamide
Spiriva	Inspra	Topamax	Toprol-XL
stavudine	cetirizine	Toprol-XL	Topamax
Sudafed	sotalol	Toradol	Foradil
Sudafed	Sudafed PE	t-PA	TNKase
Sudafed 12 Hour	Sudafed 12 Hour Preassure + Pain	Tracleer	Tricor
Sudafed 12 Hour Preassure + Pain	Sudafed 12 Hour	traMADol	traZODone
Sudafed PE	Sudafed	trastuzumab	ado-trastuzumab emtansine
SUFentanil	fentaNYL	traZODone	traMADol
sulfADIAZINE	sulfaSALAzine	TRENtal	TEGretol

* *Brand names always start with an uppercase letter. Some brand names incorporate tall man letters in initial characters and may not be readily recognized as brand names. Brand name products appear in black; generic/other products appear in* red.

INSTITUTE FOR SAFE MEDICATION PRACTICES

www.ismp.org

Institute for Safe Medication Practices

ISMP's List of *Confused **Drug** Names*

Drug Name	Confused Drug Name	Drug Name	Confused Drug Name
tretinoin	ISOtretinoin	Zantac	ZyrTEC
Tricor	Tracleer	Zavesca (escitalopram) [non-US product]	Zavesca (miglustat)
tromethamine	Trophamine	Zavesca (miglustat)	Zavesca (escitalopram) [non-US product]
Trophamine	tromethamine	Zebeta	Diabeta
tuberculin purified protein derivative (PPD)	influenza virus vaccine	Zebeta	Zetia
tuberculin purified protein derivative (PPD)	tetanus diptheria toxoid (Td)	Zegerid	Zestril
Tylenol	Tylenol PM	Zelapar (Zydis formulation)	ZyPREXA Zydis
Tylenol PM	Tylenol	Zerit	ZyrTEC
Ultracet	Duricef	Zestril	Zegerid
Ultram	lithium	Zestril	Zetia
valACYclovir	valGANciclovir	Zestril	ZyPREXA
Valcyte	Valtrex	Zetia	Bextra
valGANciclovir	valACYclovir	Zetia	Zebeta
Valtrex	Valcyte	Zetia	Zestril
Varivax	VZIG (varicella-zoster immune globulin)	Ziac	Tiazac
Vesanoid	Vesicare	Zocor	Cozaar
Vesicare	Vesanoid	Zocor	ZyrTEC
Vexol	Vosol	ZOLMitriptan	SUMAtriptan
Viagra	Allegra	zolpidem	Zyloprim
Videx	Bidex	Zonegran	SINEquan
vinBLAStine	vinCRIStine	Zostrix	Zovirax
vinCRIStine	vinBLAStine	Zovirax	Doribax
Viokase	Viokase 8	Zovirax	Zyvox
Viokase 8	Viokase	Zovirax	Zostrix
Vioxx	Zyvox	Zyban	Diovan
Viracept	Viramune	Zyloprim	zolpidem
Viramune	Viracept	ZyPREXA	CeleXA
Viramune (nevairapine)	Viramune (herbal product)	ZyPREXA	Reprexain
Viramune (herbal product)	Viramune (nevairapine)	ZyPREXA	Zestril
VisionBlue	methylene blue	ZyPREXA	ZyrTEC
Vosol	Vexol	ZyPREXA Zydis	Zelapar (Zydis formulation)
VZIG (varicella-zoster immune globulin)	Varivax	ZyrTEC	Lipitor
Wellbutrin SR	Wellbutrin XL	ZyrTEC	Zantac
Wellbutrin XL	Wellbutrin SR	ZyrTEC	Zerit
Xanax	Fanapt	ZyrTEC	Zocor
Xanax	Tenex	ZyrTEC	ZyPREXA
Xanax	Zantac	ZyrTEC	ZyrTEC-D
Xeloda	Xenical	ZyrTEC (cetirizine)	ZyrTEC Itchy Eye Drops (ketotifen fumarate)
Xenical	Xeloda	ZyrTEC-D	ZyrTEC
Yasmin	Yaz	ZyrTEC Itchy Eye Drops (ketotifen fumarate)	ZyrTEC (cetirizine)
Yaz	Yasmin	Zyvox	Vioxx
Zantac	Xanax	Zyvox	Zovirax

* Brand names always start with an uppercase letter. Some brand names incorporate tall man letters in initial characters and may not be readily recognized as brand names. Brand name products appear in black; generic/other products appear in red.

© ISMP 2015. Permission is granted to reproduce material with proper attribution for internal use within healthcare organizations. Other reproduction is prohibited without written permission from the Institute for Safe Medication Practices (ISMP). Report actual and potential medication or vaccine errors to the ISMP National Medication Errors Reporting Program (ISMP MERP) or ISMP National Vaccine Errors Reporting Program (ISMP VERP) via the Web at www.ismp.org/merp or by calling 1-800-FAIL-SAF(E).

www.ismp.org

Courtesy of the Institute for Safe Medication Practices.

© Forfunlife/Shutterstock

Appendix F

Adult Nomogram

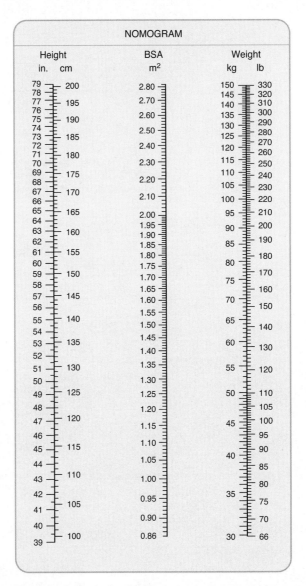

The Adult Nomogram

© Forfunlife/Shutterstock

Glossary

A

absorption In pharmacokinetics, the movement of a drug into the bloodstream.

activated partial thromboplastin time (aPTT) A blood test, measured in seconds, that indicates how long it takes for blood to clot.

addend Numbers that are added together.

ampule A small glass container that contains a single dose of medication.

analgesic Pain-relieving medication.

antiarrhythmic Medication that normalizes heart rate or rhythm.

anticoagulant A medication that decreases blood clot formation.

anxiolytic Sedative or anti-anxiety medication.

apothecary system An antiquated system of measurement based on the weight of one grain of wheat; therefore, the base unit of weight is one grain. Use of the apothecary system has resulted in numerous medication errors, so it is currently out of favor.

B

back-prime To prime from the bottom to the top of the tubing using backflow from the primary IV solution.

bar code A code, required by the U.S. Department of Health and Human Services, on the labels of all human medications and biological agents. It provides the ability to double-check a medication by both reading and scanning the code, an approach that has been demonstrated to reduce medication errors.

Bar Code Medication Administration (BCMA) A system that requires scanning the bar codes of each medication prior to administration. Scanning the label bar code serves as an additional label check.

basal insulin Synthetic human insulin that provides long-term coverage.

basal rate A slow, continuous supply. Related to insulin, it is the rate at which insulin is slowly and continuously released into the bloodstream from the pancreas or by an insulin pump.

blood glucose correction factor Also called the insulin sensitivity factor, this is the dose of insulin required to decrease the blood glucose by 50 mg/dL and is determined by the prescriber.

body surface area (BSA) The total surface area of the body. It is a more sensitive indicator of body size than body weight as it takes into account both height and weight.

BSA-based dosing Medication dosing that varies according to body surface area; assumes that drug dose parameters increase in proportion with increasing body size.

buccal Pertaining to the cheek or mouth; buccal tablets are medications that are placed between the gum and cheek as they are designed to dissolve through the mucous membranes of the mouth to rapidly enter the bloodstream.

C

calibration Lines on equipment that represent a specific unit of measurement.

calibrated spoon A device calibrated in 2.5 mL increments and fractional teaspoons that has a capacity of 10 mL; designed for pediatric medication administration.

caloric requirement The number of calories needed to meet energy needs and sustain growth.

calorie (cal or kcal) A unit of energy used to fuel the body.

cannula A tube inserted into the body used to administer or remove fluids.

caplet (cap) An oval-shaped tablet with a smooth coating to make it tamper resistant.

capsule (cap) An oval or round gelatinous container filled with powder or liquid medication.

carbohydrate One of the three main nutrients that supply energy for the body; manufactured by plants, they are a major source of fuel for the body.

carbohydrate insulin dose The amount of insulin required to dispose of the total number of carbohydrates (in grams) in the meal.

cartridge A device that is prefilled with a typical single dose of medication.

CASE approach An acronym for the four steps of safe dosage calculation: (1) Convert to like units of measurement, (2) Approximate the amount to administer, (3) Solve the equation for the dosage calculation, and (4) Evaluate your work by checking the dosage calculation against the approximated amount.

Celsius scale A temperature scale in which 0 degrees is freezing and 100 degrees is boiling. Also known as centigrade scale.

centigrade Refers to the Celsius scale.

central line An IV catheter that terminates in the great vessels (inferior or superior vena cava, or right atrium). Central lines allow for greater dilution of the IV solution as it enters the body. Certain central lines, such as PICC lines or porta-caths, are used for long–term IV infusions, and can be managed in out patient or homecare settings.

combination medication A combination of two or more medications in one dosage form.

complex carbohydrate A type of carbohydrate that includes starches and is found in grains, cereals, pastas, vegetables, and fruits.

complex fraction A fraction in which the numerator and/or the denominator is a fraction. For example:

$$\frac{\frac{1}{2}}{1\frac{1}{4}}, \frac{\frac{3}{5}}{2}, \frac{1}{\frac{2}{3}}$$

concentration The amount of medication per dosage unit; also known as dosage strength, strength, or supply.

control number A number that is a universal product identifier for human drugs; also known as a National Drug Code (NDC).

controlled substance A drug whose manufacturing or possession is regulated by the federal government because of its potential for abuse.

controlled substance schedule Differentiates controlled substances into five categories according to their potential for abuse or addiction, from Schedule I (substances with the most potential for abuse or addiction with no medicinal benefit, such as heroin) to Schedule V (substances with the lowest potential for abuse or addiction, typically a combination medication in which the addictive substance has low dosage strength, such as some cold medications that contain a small amount of codeine).

controllers Regulators. As it relates to IVs, a manually set, metered device that regulates the rate of intravenous infusions. For example, a dial-a-flow.

conversion factor method A method of converting known quantities to an unknown value by multiplying the known amount by known conversions factors (equivalencies); also known as dimensional analysis.

correction insulin Insulin administered to correct existing high blood glucose from food or other causes such as some medications or illnesses.

creatinine clearance The rate at which creatinine, a byproduct of muscle metabolism, is cleared or filtered by the kidneys and is thereby decreased as a normal part of the aging process.

cross-multiplication Multiplying the numerator of one fraction by the denominator of the other fraction. The product of the numerator of the first fraction and the denominator of the second fraction is equal to the product of the numerator of the second fraction and the denominator of the first fraction when the fractions are equivalent.

D

daily fluid requirement (DFR) The amount of fluid a patient needs to maintain normal hydration; also called maintenance fluids.

decimal Fractions with a denominator that is a multiple of ten (e.g., 0.1 = one-tenth). The decimal point separates a whole number from the fraction. The whole number is placed to the left of the decimal point, and the fraction (quantity ending in *th*) is placed to the right of the decimal point. Also known as decimal fractions.

denominator The part of a fraction that represents that number of equal parts that make up a whole; the number below the division sign in a fraction.

diluent A diluting agent; a liquid mixed with a medication in order to reduce the amount (strength) of the medication in the solution.

dimensional analysis (DA) A way to convert amounts by multiplying the given (known) by the appropriate conversion factor/s (equivalencies); also known as the conversion factor method. For example, to determine the number of seconds in 1 week:

$$x \text{ sec/week} = \frac{60 \text{ sec}}{1 \text{ min}} \times \frac{60 \text{ min}}{1 \text{ h}} \times \frac{24 \text{ h}}{1 \text{ day}} \times \frac{7 \text{ days}}{1 \text{ week}} = 604{,}800 \text{ sec/week}$$

distal port The port farthest from the insertion site (point at which the device enters the patient); this is commonly the connection point for the secondary line used for the infusion of intravenous piggyback medication.

distribution The movement of a medication into body tissues and fluids.

dividend The fraction or number being divided. In a linear equation, the first number (the dividend) is divided by the second number (divisor).

divisor The number the dividend is being divided by. In a linear equation, the first number (dividend) is divided by the second number (the divisor).

dosage strength The amount of medication *per* dosage unit; also referred to as the strength, concentration, or supply. The dosage strength is a ratio or fraction. It is the supply dose/dosage unit or supply dose:dosage unit.

dosage unit Refers to the quantity of solid or liquid in which the supplied dose is contained.

drop factor A number based on the size or calibration of the drop that falls in the drip chamber; also known as the drip factor.

dropper A device used to deliver small quantities of liquid medication.

duration A length of time. Related to medication, it is the length of time the effect of a medication lasts, such as the effect from a dose of insulin.

E

eccentric Off center. An eccentric tip; describes an off-center tip for an oral syringe that distinguishes it from a syringe to be used for injections.

electronic medication administration record (eMAR) Legal records found in a patient's electronic medical record that give information about medication orders and their times for administration.

elimination Removal. As it pertains to medication, the movement of a medication out of the body.

elixir A liquid that contains water, alcohol, and a sweetener.

enteral Gastrointestinal. Refers to medication given through the gastrointestinal tract, including drugs given both orally and through a tube into the stomach or intestines.

enteric-coated Enteric-coated tablets have an outer coating designed to withstand gastric juice, causing the tablet to pass through the stomach and dissolve in the small intestine.

extravasation Leakage of IV fluid from a blood vessel into the surrounding tissue.

F

factor-label method Also known as the dimensional analysis, this calculation determines the amount of medication to administer by multiplying the order and supply by a series of conversion factors.

Fahrenheit scale A measurement of temperature that is calibrated with 212 degrees. Water has a freezing point of 32°F and a boiling point of 212°F.

fat As energy nutrients, fats (also called lipids) provide energy to fuel the body when carbohydrates are not available. They also play an important role in nutrient absorption, insulation, and maintaining body temperature. Fat has a high caloric content, with 9 calories per gram, and should make up no more than 30% of the calories in a healthy diet.

filter needle A needle used to withdraw medication from an ampule that contains a filter inside to separate from the medication any glass fragments that occur as a result of breaking open the ampule.

fixed combination insulin A combination of basal and mealtime insulin premixed by the manufacturer, in one vial or cartridge.

fixed dosing Medication dosing applied to homogenous populations, such as average-sized adults.

fluid resuscitation The administration of a large volume of intravenous fluid over a relatively short period of time; one of the most important aspects in managing care of patients experiencing hypovolemic shock.

form The form of a drug refers to its composition, which may be solid, semisolid (such as creams or ointments), or liquid.

formula method (FM) A simple way of calculating the amount of medication to administer; the supplied dose, ordered dose, and supplied dosage unit are placed into the formula to determine the amount to administer:

$$\frac{\text{ordered dose } (D)}{\text{supplied dose } (H)} \times \text{dosage unit } (Q) = \text{amount to administer } (x)$$

fraction Represents a portion of the whole, written as two quantities: the numerator divided by the denominator.

fractional ratio-proportion Compares two equivalent fractions.

frequency Time interval. As it relates to medication, the spacing or how often a medication is to be administered.

full strength Undiluted. As it relates to liquid enteral formulas, the typical concentration used to meet normal needs.

G

gastrostomy tube (GT, G-tube) A tube inserted directly through the abdomen into the stomach.

gauge Measure of the diameter of a needle. The larger the gauge, the narrower the needle (and lumen).

gelcap Gelatin shells that usually contain liquid medication.

generic name The nonproprietary name assigned to the active substance of a medication.

geriatric Refers to persons ages 65 years or older.

gram (g) The base unit of weight in the metric system.

H

hang time The time an enteral nutrition formula is considered safe for delivery to the patient at room temperature, beginning from the time when the formula was reconstituted, or decanted, or from the time when the original package seal was broken.

heparin lock A venous access device that is periodically flushed with heparin (a blood-thinning substance).

high-alert medications Medication that, if given erroneously, can result in serious harm and possibly death.

hospitalist Doctor who practices in a hospital.

household system The system of measurement currently used in the United States, originally derived from the apothecary system. It requires the measuring tools used for cooking (measuring cups and measuring spoons). The household system is the least accurate system of measurement and is not recommended for medication administration.

hypertonic A solution that has more particles than plasma, therefore it produces a pressure gradient that causes fluid to move from the cells and interstitial spaces back into the vascular bed (circulatory system).

hypodermoclysis Subcutaneous infusion of fluids.

hypotonic A solution that has fewer particles than plasma, producing a pressure gradient that causes fluid to move from the vascular bed (circulatory system) into interstitial space and the cells.

hypovolemic shock A life-threatening condition in which 20% or more of the body's blood or fluid supply is lost.

I

implantable subcutaneous infusion port Internal central venous ports surgically placed below the clavicle with a catheter threaded through the subclavian vein, e.g., a Port-a-cath®.

improper fraction A fraction in which the numerator is greater than the denominator, so the value is greater than 1 (e.g., $\frac{6}{5}$), or the numerator is the same as the denominator, so the value is equivalent to 1 (e.g., $\frac{5}{5}$).

in-line filter A filter usually attached to a primary line of IV tubing meant to remove particulate matter, such as crystals, from the IV solution.

infiltration Swelling at the insertion site that occurs when the IV cannula slips out of or pierces the vein, causing fluid to infuse into the surrounding tissue.

Institute for Safe Medication Practices (ISMP) An organization whose sole mission is to prevent medication errors and promote safe medication administration.

Institute of Medicine (IOM) An independent organization that provides unbiased and authoritative advice to decision makers and the public in order to facilitate good health decisions.

insulin-to-carbohydrate ratio The amount of carbohydrate disposed of by 1 unit of insulin.

insulin pen A prefilled syringe used to administer insulin.

insulin pumps Small, portable continuous subcutaneous infusion devices that are attached to the patient, under the skin, and are designed to infuse insulin 24 hours a day.

insulin sensitivity factor The dose of insulin required to decrease the blood glucose by 50 mg/dL, determined by the prescriber.

International System of Units (SI, *systeme international d'unites*) Official name of the metric system.

international time Based on 24 hours, not 12 hours, so each hour has a unique numerical representation. The day begins after 0000 and ends at 2400 (both of which represent midnight). Also known as military time.

international unit A measure of medication potency for the same medication between nations and manufacturers.

intradermal (ID) Into the dermis. An intradermal injection is inserted into the dermis (connective tissue within the skin) at a 10- to 15-degree angle; abbreviated ID.

intramuscular (IM) Into the muscle. An intramuscular injection is injected directly into a muscle at a 90-degree angle; abbreviated IM.

intravenous (IV) Into the vein. An intravenous injection is administered directly into a vein; abbreviated IV.

intravenous piggyback (IVPB) Medications in mini-bags that are connected (piggybacked) to the primary IV line through secondary (short) tubing.

isotonic Used to expand intravascular volume, these solutions have the same osmolarity as plasma. Therefore, they do not promote the shift of fluid into or out of cells, and the IV solution remains in the blood vessels longer than maintenance fluids.

IV flush A small volume of IV fluid, 10–15 mL, needed to clear the medication from the IV tubing and deliver it completely into the patient's vein.

IV push (bolus medication) Medications that can be directly injected with a syringe into a vein through an IV port; does not require further dilution in an IV bag.

jejunal tube (J-tube) A tube inserted directly though the abdomen into the jejunum.

The Joint Commission (TJC) An organization whose mission is to improve health care by evaluating healthcare organizations for their compliance with federal regulations.

K

KVO An acronym meaning "keep vein open," it refers to a very slow rate used to maintain an IV; also called a TKO ("to keep open") rate. Generally 20 mL/h or 30 mL/h for adult patients, 5–10 mL/h for pediatric patients.

L

leading ring The side of the black rubber tip on a plunger for a syringe that is closest to the needle.

leading zero The zero before the decimal point in a value less than one (0.4). To prevent dosage errors, always use a leading zero.

licensed independent practitioner (LIP) Licensed healthcare professionals that have prescriptive authority, the legal right to prescribe medication, granted by the state in which they are licensed; also called prescribers.

linear ratio-proportion Compares two equivalent ratios.

lipid As energy nutrients, lipids (also known as fats) provide energy to fuel the body when carbohydrates are not available. They also play an important role in nutrient absorption, insulation, and maintaining body temperature.

liter (L) The base unit of volume in the metric system.

loading dose An initial bolus dose given to achieve a therapeutic blood level.

lot number A number on a medication identifying the batch and manufacturing plant. It helps to track medication made in the same lot, enabling them to be recalled if there is a problem with the medication.

low molecular weight heparin (LMWH) A type of heparin (an anticoagulant that decreases blood clot formation) that has small molecules.

lumen A channel through which fluids infuse, e.g., the lumen of a needle. The higher the gauge, the smaller the lumen.

M

maintenance fluids Fluids that are given to maintain normal levels of fluid and electrolytes.

maximum concentration Uses the least amount of diluent; also called minimum dilution. Usually indicated for administration routes requiring smaller volumes, such as IM.

maximum dilution Uses the greatest amount of diluent; also called minimum concentration. Usually indicated for administration routes that could accommodate larger volumes, such as the IV route.

mealtime insulin Faster-acting insulin that provides short-term coverage for the anticipated insulin requirement associated with food intake. Also includes correctional insulin dose (faster-acting insulin used to correct an existing high blood glucose level).

medication administration record (MAR) Legal records that contain the same information as the medication order with the addition of the specified times for medication administration.

medicine cup An open, plastic container used to administer liquid oral medications, usually marked with household and metric calibrations.

meniscus A concave curve in the upper surface of a liquid poured into an open container (due to the surface tension between the liquid and the container).

metabolism Chemical transformation within cells. The transformation of a drug or food into chemicals used by the body.

meter (m) The base unit of length in the metric system.

metric system The preferred system of measurement used in health care. It includes three base units of measurement: liter (volume), gram (weight), and meter (length). The metric system uses powers of 10 and amounts are written as whole numbers or decimals.

microemboli Small blood clots.

military time Based on 24 hours, not 12 hours, so each hour has a unique numerical representation. The day begins after 0000 and ends at 2400 (both of which represent midnight). Also known as international time.

milliequivalent (mEq) A measurement of chemical activity, not molecular weight. It is used to measure the combining power of ions. Electrolytes such as potassium are measured using milliequivalents.

minimum concentration Uses the greatest amount of diluent; also called maximum dilution. Usually indicated for administration routes that can accommodate larger volumes, such as IV

minimum dilution Uses the least amount of diluent; also called maximum concentration. Usually indicated for administration routes that require smaller volumes, such as the IM route.

mixed number A whole number and a fraction (e.g., $1\frac{3}{5}$).

multiple dose A multiple-dose package contains enough medication for more than one dose; also called a multiple-use package. Medications in these containers have preservatives, if necessary, to ensure that each dose is safe to administer.

N

nasogastric tube (NGT) A tube inserted through the nose into the gastric (stomach) region.

nasojejunal (NJT) A tube inserted through the nose into the jejunum (the middle section of the small intestine).

National Drug Code (NDC) A number that is a universal product identifier for human drugs, also known as a control number. All medications and compounds manufactured for public distribution are registered with the FDA and given a three-part numeric code that is unique to the medication.

net weight Refers to the total amount of the medication form within the dosage container (not the dosage strength).

neuromuscular blocking agent Paralytic medications.

numerator The part of a fraction that indicates the portion (number of parts) of a whole quantity; the number above the division sign in a fraction.

nutrient dense Foods that are rich in nutrients but low in calories.

O

onset Starting point. After administering a medication, the length of time before the medication begins to take effect. In terms of insulin, the length of time it takes for the insulin to start lowering blood glucose.

oral syringe A syringe used to administer liquid medication, it is available in two sizes: 5 mL and 10 mL. It is calibrated in tenths of a milliliter and fractional teaspoon measurements. Oral syringes are designed with features that differentiate them from syringes used for injections, such as labeling and off-center tips.

osmolality The number of particles (osmoles) in a kilogram of fluid; used to refer to body fluids because they are often measured by weight.

osmolarity The number of particles (osmoles) in a liter of fluid; used to refer to infusion fluids because they are measured by volume.

P

parenteral Outside the digestive tract; parenteral medication enter the bloodstream without first entering the intestines. Generally understood to mean injection routes.

patient-controlled analgesia (PCA) pump A device that allows the patient to self-administer intravenous pain medication with the press of a button.

peak Highest point. After administering a medication, the point in time at which the medication is most effective. In terms of insulin, the time at which the insulin has its maximum effect.

pediatric Refers to children from birth to the age of 18 years.

percent daily value (%DV) A percentage in one serving of a particular product that contributes to the recommended daily intake of a nutrient.

peripheral venous catheter A small, flexible tube that is inserted over a needle into the vein, after which the needle is withdrawn.

peripherally inserted central catheter (PICC) line Long central venous lines inserted into an arm vein and threaded into a central vein.

pharmacokinetics The study of how drugs move through the body or the study of absorption, distribution, metabolism, and elimination.

polypharmacy Referring to multiple medications taken by one patient, polypharmacy increases the chances of drugs interacting or interfering with one another, which may minimize the intended effect of a drug while increasing its side effects.

port An entry to the intravenous catheter through which an IV infusion or syringe is attached.

prehydration To prevent dehydration, fluids may be infused in advance of an event that causes dehydration, such as chemotherapy.

prescriptive authority The legal right to prescribe medication.

primary line The main IV tubing for an IV infusion.

prime Clearing the air from IV tubing by running a solution of IV fluid through it, according to manufacturer instructions found on the tubing packaging.

proper fraction A fraction where the numerator is less that the denominator, so the value is less than 1 (e.g., $\frac{3}{5}$).

protein Nutrient made up of amino acids, found in foods such as meat, poultry, seafood, dairy, eggs, and many plant-based foods. Proteins perform many functions in the body, including building and repairing tissue.

proximal port An injection port closest to the insertion site used for the administration of medications that can be directly injected (i.e., IV bolus medications).

Q

quotient The result of division, when the dividend is divided by the divisor.

R

reconstitution The process of reforming/transforming (changing the form of) a medication (e.g., liquefying a powdered medication).

replacement fluids Fluids infused into a patient to replenish fluid volume and rehydrate the patient after an event such as surgery or an episode of sweating, vomiting, diarrhea, or hemorrhage.

route The path by which medication enters the body, named by the entry point.

S

safe dose range (SDR) The quantity between a calculated minimum safe dose and a maximum safe dose.

saline lock IV device that is periodically flushed with normal saline to maintain patency, provides access for intermittent infusion therapy.

scored Linear indentations on tablets or caplets that facilitate dividing the dose in halves or quarters as marked.

secondary line IV tubing used for the infusion of intravenous piggyback medications.

simple carbohydrate Nutrient that elevates blood sugar quickly; sugars which are found in foods such as fruits, milk, sugar, honey, and corn syrup.

single dose A single-dose container is made for just one use, with the capacity to hold enough medication for a typical single dose.

single use Also called a single-dose container, a single-use container is made for just one use, with the capacity to hold enough medication for a typical single dose.

smart pump A computerized infusion pump equipped with medication error–prevention software that alarms when infusion settings exceed best practice guidelines.

solute The substance that is dissolved in a solution.

solvent A product that dilutes or dissolves a solute; also call diluent.

souffle cup A small paper or plastic cup used to administer solid oral medication.

spansule Timed-release capsules containing tiny beads of medicine that dissolve at spaced intervals designed for long-acting medications.

strength Dosage strength; the concentration of a medication, which is the amount of medication per dosage unit.

subcutaneous (subcut) Injection route located below all of the layers of the skin (fat, adipose tissue).

sublingual (SL) Route of medication administration requiring placement of medication under the tongue for rapid absorption into the bloodstream.

subtrahend Numbers involved in subtraction.

supply (supply dosage, supply dose) Dosage strength, the amount of medication in each dosage unit (e.g., 325 mg per tablet, 80 mg per mL, 200 mcg per metered spray).

suppository A solid, bullet-shaped medication, usually composed of glycerin, that is design for easy insertion into the rectum or vagina.

suspension A liquid that contains fine particles of a drug that cannot be dissolved and must be stirred or shaken prior to administration to evenly disperse the particles.

sustained-release capsules Timed-release capsules that contain tiny beads of medicine that dissolve at spaced intervals designed for long-acting medications.

syringe pump A small-volume infusion device that delivers fluids and medications directly from a syringe; often used in pediatric and critical care settings.

syrup A liquid that contains water, concentrated sugar, and dissolved medication (e.g., cough syrup).

T

tablet (tab) Compressed powdered medications available in a variety of types, shapes, and sizes.

time-critical medications Medications for which early or late administration may result in harm for patients; determined by each healthcare institution. Examples include hormones, antibiotics, and cardiac medications.

time tape A strip of tape attached to an IV container on which the nurse marks start time, fluid intervals, and end time.

titrate To adjust a continuous IV infusion dosage to achieve the desired effect.

TKO An acronym meaning "to keep open," it refers to a very slow rate used to maintain an IV; also called a KVO ("keep vein open") rate.

tonicity Also known as osmolality, which is the number of particles (osmoles) in a kilogram of fluid.

total mealtime bolus dose The total number of insulin units to administer as the bolus dose.

total number Refers to the total amount of the medication form within the container (not the dosage strength).

total parenteral nutrition (TPN) A means of nourishing a patient intravenously, bypassing the gastrointestinal tract. Due to its high concentration, TPN must be infused through large, central veins.

total volume Refers to the total amount of the medication form within the container (not the dosage strength).

trade name Also called a brand name, it is the name that the manufacturer gives a medication to identify it as made by the manufacturer. The name is registered with the U.S. Department of Commerce so that no other pharmaceutical company can use the same name. Common practice is to capitalize a trade name, while the generic name is usually in lowercase letters.

traditional time Measuring time using a 12-hour clock that repeats, at the meridian, to account for 24 hours of the day. The day begins at midnight (12:00 a.m.) and the second 12 hours begin at noon (12:00 p.m.).

trailing ring The side of the black rubber tip on a plunger for a syringe that is farthest from the needle.

trailing zero The zero at the end of a decimal value. To prevent dosage errors, never use a trailing zero.

transcription The process of copying or entering orders onto the MAR or eMAR, includes the assignments of times for administration.

U

U-100 Signifies an insulin concentration of 100 units per 1 mL.

U-500 Signifies a regular insulin concentration of 500 units per 1 mL.

unfractionated heparin (UH) A type of heparin (an anticoagulant that decreases blood clot formation) that has large molecules.

unit dose Unit dose packages of medications contain enough medication for one dose.

United States Pharmacopeia (USP) A U.S. government agency that sets standards for medicines.

United States Pharmacopeia—National Formulary (USP-NF) A book that contains standards for medicines, dosage forms, drug substances, excipients (inactive substances), medical devices, and dietary supplements.

United States Pharmacopeia units (USP units) A measure of medication potency for the same medication, standardized between manufacturers and determined by the United States Pharmacopeia.

universal solvent Water is called the universal solvent because it is the most commonly used solvent to dilute solutions.

V

vasoactive A medication that dilates or constricts blood vessels.

verbal order (telephone order) A prescription order given orally instead of via documentation.

vesicant A chemical that causes blistering or tissue necrosis with extravasation (leakage from IV cannula into the surrounding tissue).

vial A multiple- or single-dose container of powdered or liquid medication with a rubber stopper on top.

viscosity The thickness of a solution.

volume-control sets A safety device with a maximum capacity of 150 mL that is inserted between the IV bag and the infusion pump to prevent accidental fluid overload due to programming error or pump malfunction; also called burette, Buretrol, or VOLU-trol.

W

warning A label put on medication to protect the patient from medication administration errors.

weight-based dosing Drug dosing based on body weight.

weight-based heparin protocol A set of weight-based IV heparin orders that call for changes in rate or additional IV bolus doses based on the patient's aPTT (how long it takes for a patient's blood to clot).

workarounds Omitted or unauthorized steps in the bar code medication administration process, which can put patients at risk for medication errors.

World Health Organization A United Nations institute that is concerned with public health.

Y

Y-tubing Special tubing that has two spikes that are y-connected to pierce two solution containers.

Z

zero calibration The measurement point at the beginning of a syringe barrel.

Index

© Forfunlife/Shutterstock

Note: Page numbers followed by *f* or *t* indicate material in figures or tables respectively.